W9-AUY-187

This authoritative international text on fetal therapy is the first to cover all three classes of fetal therapy in one book: transplancental drug treatment, invasive procedures and fetal surgery. It emphasizes treatments that have become established in clinical practice in this rapidly developing field, as well as reviewing those that have failed to live up to initial expectation, and discusses the likely impact of new therapies on the horizon. The editors head a team of American, European and Australian authors, all of whom are leading experts in their respective fields. The text is authoritative, evidence based and balanced, finding the common ground between the opposing camps of 'enthusiasts' and 'therapeutic nihilists'. It will be an essential source of reference for all those involved in the care of the unborn child, and particularly for obstetricians training in fetal medicine.

Fetal therapy
Invasive and transplacental

Fetal therapy

Invasive and transplacental

Edited by

Nicholas M. Fisk
Professor of Obstetrics and Gynaecology
Queen Charlotte's and Chelsea Hospital, London

Kenneth J. Moise Jr
Associate Professor of Obstetrics and Gynecology
Baylor College of Medicine, Houston, USA

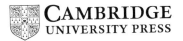
CAMBRIDGE
UNIVERSITY PRESS

PUBLISHED BY THE PRESS SYNDICATE OF THE UNIVERSITY OF CAMBRIDGE
The Pitt Building, Trumpington Street, Cambridge CB2 1RP United Kingdom

CAMBRIDGE UNIVERSITY PRESS
The Edinburgh Building, Cambridge CB2 2RU, United Kingdom
40 West 20th Street, New York, NY 10011–4211, USA
10 Stamford Road, Oakleigh, Melbourne 3166, Australia

© Cambridge University Press 1997

This book is in copyright. Subject to statutory exception
and to the provisions of relevant collective licensing agreements,
no reproduction of any part may take place without
the written permission of Cambridge University Press.

First published 1997

Printed in the United Kingdom at the University Press, Cambridge

Typeset in Ehrhardt 9/12pt

A catalogue record for this book is available from the British Library

Library of Congress cataloguing in publication data available

ISBN 0 521 46133 2 hardback

Every effort has been made in preparing this book to provide accurate and
up-to-date information which is in accord with accepted standards and
practice at the time of publication. Nevertheless, the authors, editors and
publisher can make no warranties that the information herein is totally
free from error, not least because clinical standards are constantly changing
through research and regulation. The authors, editors and publisher
therefore disclaim all liability for direct or consequential damages
resulting from the use of the material contained in this book. The reader is
strongly advised to pay careful attention to information provided by the
manufacturer of any drugs or equipment that they plan to use.

To our wives Ann and Karen, and our children
Catriona and Angus, and Rachael, Kaitlyn and Erin
for their unconditional love and support during the
gestation and delivery of this work.

Also to our mentors, Rodney Shearman and
Frank Boehm. Through their example and guidance
we chose to pursue the field of fetal medicine.

Contents

Contributors

N. Scott Adzick
Center for Fetal Diagnosis and Treatment, Children's
Hospital of Philadelphia, Philadelphia, PA 19104, USA

Phillip Bennett
Royal Postgraduate Medical School, Institute of
Obstetrics and Gynaecology, Queen Charlotte's and
Chelsea Hospital, London W6 0XG, UK

Carol Bower
Western Australian Research Institute for Child
Health, GPO Box D 184, Perth, Western Australia
6001

Frank A. Chervenak
The New York Hospital – Cornell Medical Centre,
Department of Obstetrics and Gynecology, New York
NYS 10021, USA

Joshua A. Copel
Department of Obstetrics and Gynecology, Yale
University School of Medicine, New Haven, CT
06520, USA

Caroline A. Crowther
The University of Adelaide, Department of Obstetrics
and Gynaecology, Queen Victoria Hospital, Rose
Park, South Australia 5067

Mark I. Evans
Division of Reproductive Genetics, Hutzel Hospital
Detroit, MI 48201, USA

Nicholas M. Fisk
Royal Postgraduate Medical School, Institute of
Obstetrics and Gynaecology, Queen Charlotte's and
Chelsea Hospital, London W6 0XG, UK

W. D. Andrew Ford
Department of Paediatric Surgery, Adelaide
Children's Hospital, South Australia 5005

James D. Goldberg
Department of Obstetrics, Gynecology, and
Reproductive Sciences, University of California, San
Francisco, CA 94143, USA

Michael R. Harrison
Fetal Treatment Center, University of California, San
Francisco, CA 94143–0570, USA

Marc H. Hedrick
Division of Plastic Surgery, University of California,
Los Angeles, CA 90096–1665, USA

Roderick F. Hume, Jr
Department of Obstetrics and Gynecology, Madigan
Army Medical Center, Dacoma, Washington 98431,
USA

Mark P. Johnson
Division of Reproductive Genetics, Hutzel Hospital,
Detroit, MI 48210, USA

Helen Kelsey
Watford General Hospital, Watford WD1 8HB, UK

Charles S. Kleinman
Fetal Cardiovascular Center, Yale University School
of Medicine, New Haven, CT 06520, USA

Phillipa M. Kyle
Centre for Fetal Care, Queen Charlotte's and Chelsea
Hospital, London W6 0XG, UK

Abraham Ludomirsky
Department of Obstetrics, Gynecology and
Reproductive Sciences, School of Medicine, Temple
University, Philadelphia, PA 19140, USA

Lauren Lynch
Department of Obstetrics, Gynecology and
Reproductive Sciences, Mount Sinai Medical Centre,
New York, 10029, USA

David C. Merrill
Department of Obstetrics and Gynecology, University
of Iowa Hospitals and Clinics, Iowa City, IA 52242–
1080, USA

Laura S. Martin
Department of Pathology, Pediatrics, and Obstetrics/
Gynecology, Wayne State University, Detroit, MI
48201, USA

Laurence McCullough
Baylor College of Medicine, Center for Ethics,
Medicine, and Public Issues, Houston, TX 77030,
USA

Kenneth J. Moise, Jr
Department of Obstetrics and Gynecology, Baylor
College of Medicine, Houston, TX 77030, USA

Rodolfo Montemagno
Department of Obstetrics and Gynaecology,
University College London Medical School, London
WC1P 9LN, UK

Kypros H. Nicolaides
Harris Birthright Research Centre for Fetal Medicine,
King's College Hospital School of Medicine, London
SE5 8RX, UK

Umberto Nicolini
Istituto Ostetrico Ginecologico, Universita di Milano,
Milano 20122, Italy

Heverton N. Pettersen
Harris Birthright Research Centre for Fetal Medicine,
King's College Hospital School of Medicine, London
SE5 8RX, UK

William F. Rayburn
Department of Obstetrics and Gynecology, University
of Oklahoma College of Medicine, Oklahoma City, OK
73190, USA

Henry E. Rice
Fetal Treatment Center,
University of California,
San Francisco CA 94143, USA

Charles Rodeck
Department of Obstetrics and Gynaecology,
University College London Medical School, London
WC1P 9LN, UK

Shelley Rowlands
Department of Obstetrics, Gynaecology and
Neonatology, The University of Sydney at Westmead
Hospital, Westmead NSW 2145, Australia

George R. Saade
Department of Obstetrics and Gynecology, University
of Texas Medical Branch at Galveston, Galveston, TX
77555, USA

Bernd Schumacher
Department of Obstetrics and Gynecology, Baylor
College of Medicine, Houston, TX 77030, USA

Peter Soothill
Maternal and Fetal Medicine Unit, Department of
Obstetrics and Gynaecology, Bristol University, St
Michael's Hospital, Bristol BS2 8BJ, UK

J. Guy Thorpe-Beeston
Department of Obstetrics and Gynaecology, St Mary's
Hospital, London W2 1NY, UK

Jean-Louis Touraine
Transplantation and Clinical Immunology Unit,
INSERM U 80, Hôpital Edouard Herriot, 69437
Lyon Cedex 03, France

Brian J. Trudinger
Department of Obstetrics, Gynaecology and
Neonatology, University of Sydney at Westmead
Hospital, Westmead, NSW 2145, Australia

Nicholas J. Wald
Deapartment of Environmental and Preventive
Medicine, Wolfson Institute of Preventive Medicine,
The Medical College of St Bartholomew's Hospital,
London EC1M 6BQ, UK

Carl P. Weiner
Department of Obstetrics and Gynecology, and
Reproductive Sciences, University of Maryland,
Baltimore, MD 21201, USA

Preface

Maternal-fetal medicine or perinatology has emerged over the last 10 years as the major clinical discipline in modern obstetric practice, with the establishment in most developed countries of specific training programmes and career structures in this field. *Fetal Therapy: Invasive and Transplacental* arose out of several concerns we had with the source material available to our fellows and subspecialty trainees.

First, perinatologists had no standard reference work available to them on fetal therapy. This is because the field has traditionally been divided into transplacental drug therapy employed by general obstetricians, and invasive therapies employed by fetal physicians and surgeons. Books on drug treatment in pregnancy have concentrated on teratology or the treatment of maternal disease while those on invasive procedures have dealt mainly with diagnosis. Their marriage in textbooks of perinatal medicine was necessarily superficial because of the breadth of cover.

Second, attempts at fetal therapy have long been regarded as experimental. This reflected the priorities of the 1980s when attention focused on the intrauterine treatment of fetal abnormalities made possible by technical advances in ultrasound and invasive procedures. Despite sound theoretical bases for the surgical treatments, not all lived up to expectations, and indeed many remain the subject of controversy. Several fetal medical treatments, however found an accepted role in perinatal practice. During the same time, there were significant advances in drug therapy. Most recent examples include folate to prevent neural tube defects, and thyrotrophin-releasing hormone (TRH) to promote lung maturity, which are now set to have a major impact on fetal disease in the late 1990s. These changing emphases had the effect of blurring the distinction between different types of fetal therapy, all areas of which are now relevant to the modern perinatologist.

Finally those seeking to consult authoritative reviews on fetal therapy were often confused by apparent conflicts between, on the one hand, articles by enthusiastic but uncritical promoters of new interventions and, on the other, negative overviews denigrating such procedures as experimental. In most cases, there is a sensible middle ground. Clearly scientific evaluation by randomized controlled trials is not always achievable with infrequent fetal interventions, yet this should be no excuse for avoiding critical evaluation. Given the emotionally and ethically charged nature of fetal therapies, a collection of balanced overviews addressing the risk benefit ratio of each treatment seemed desirable.

Here we combine the three classes of fetal therapy, transplacental drug treatment, invasive procedures and fetal surgery, within the one book. The aim is to emphasize those treatments which have become established in clinical practice, while reviewing the reasons others have failed to live up to initial expectation. The format is disease based, as this is how problems are encountered in clinical practice. Defining the boundaries of fetal therapy will always prove problematic, especially when anything which promotes or maintains maternal health can be considered indirectly as fetal therapy. We chose boundaries which exclude primarily maternal therapies, such as insulin for diabetes, or primarily postnatal therapies, such as prophylaxis against periventricular haemorrhage. Finding the common ground between the opposing camps of 'enthusiasts' and 'therapeutic nihilists' proved challenging, and meta-analysis is employed wherever relevant. Finally, novel treatments on the horizon, together with speculation on their likely impact, are examined.

We intend this book to appeal to those primarily interested in fetal medicine, be they novices or seasoned practitioners. Nevertheless, we have strived to avoid an overly restrictive remit and trust that others with secondary interest, such as neonatologists, radiologists and paediatric surgeons, will also find it of value.

Nicholas M. Fisk
Kenneth J. Moise Jr

Foreword

Compared with the revolution in molecular biology, the fetal therapy revolution is a minor one but they have in common a similar life history beginning from humble origins in the 1960s and having an exponential rise in the rate of acquisition of knowledge. The impetus to the progress in both disciplines stems from technological advances that provide the tools for discovery. Fetal physiology, the foundation on which rational therapy is based, received a great boost from the development in the 1960s of chronic experimental preparations in animals, particularly vascular catheterization. And it is salutary to ponder on where our present understanding of human fetal anatomy and physiology would be in the absence of ultrasound imaging and the techniques such as blood sampling that have stemmed from it.

The foundation of fetal therapy can be fairly attributed to the pioneering effects of D. C. A. Bevis and A. W. Liley, who developed amniocentesis for the diagnosis of Rh haemolytic disease. As so often happens, the ability to diagnose accurately provided the spur to finding effective treatment. Liley, frustrated by helplessness in altering the course of the disease in fetuses predicted by amniocentesis to become hydropic before rescue by preterm delivery was feasible, turned to fetal peritoneal transfusion. His success in 1963 was not only a major contribution to the management of haemolytic disease but equally importantly was the unambiguous signal that the fetus should be regarded as a patient accessible for diagnosis and therapy as in extra-uterine life. Medical (non-invasive) therapy had to await progress in fetal physiology but made a good start in 1972 with the first report of the effectiveness of transplacental corticosteroid administration in preventing neonatal respiratory distress syndrome.

In theory, the fetus is a candidate for any therapy used in adults. Indeed, the sterile life support system supplied by the placenta could extend the range of potential therapies. In practice, however, the reader of this book will meet the many problems that limit the scope of the more extensive invasive procedures and the application of molecular genetics. None of these seems insurmountable and continuing exciting progress can be expected. Meantime, this text written by authors who are working at the cutting edge of their respective fields makes it abundantly clear that the range and complexity of fetal therapies already available justifies the creation of centres employing specialists devoted to the care of the fetus and to the research that will maintain the momentum of recent progress.

As the 20th century moves towards the 21st, one wonders what lies ahead for fetal therapy. It is hard to believe that the pace can be kept up, and yet one only has to look at what is happening in other disciplines to realise that the next generation of fetal therapists will look back on present practices with wonder that they could be so primitive and unimaginative. They may wonder why robotic, computer-controlled surgery was so slow in being adapted to the intrauterine environment. Completion of the Human Genome Project will have identified a multitude of genetic disorders amenable to correction *in utero*. Will the present ethical limitation of genetic transplantation to somatic cells be still in force or will germ-cell transplantation with its potential benefits to future generations become acceptable? Surely, growth of the fetus and placenta will become amenable to effective manipulation, thereby reducing the risk of cardiovascular disease in adult life as a long-term consequence of fetal growth retardation. Hopefully, the early promise of neuroprotection will come to fruition in preventing the disastrous consequences of asphyxial brain damage. Perhaps the threat of vertical transmission of HIV will have disappeared with the conquering of AIDS.

Had this book been prepared 10 years ago, it would have been a very slim volume indeed and I expect this present edition to have a similar lifespan before a new edition is needed to reflect progress. Meantime, this text, which contains everything worth saying about fetal therapy at the present time, will occupy a place on the bookshelf of everyone, be they jurist, ethicist or fetalist, who has pecuniary, moral or medical interest in the welfare of the fetus.

> *G. C. Liggins*
> *University of Auckland, New Zealand*

Part one

Approaches

1 Transplacental drug therapy

WILLIAM F. RAYBURN

Introduction

Drug therapy appears promising for a broad spectrum of fetal conditions and may become the pillar of fetal therapy. Drugs intended for the fetus are those used for the primary or sole purpose of treating a fetal disorder or of improving the capacity of the fetus for later intra-uterine or postnatal adaptation (Rayburn & Payne, 1993). The 1990s may revolutionize the care of the fetus and create new options in drug therapy, gene control and immunotherapy which will serve to identify susceptible populations and treat them selectively without increasing the risk to the mother.

This chapter will discuss transplacental passage of drugs and principles of fetal pharmacology. Select fetal and neonatal conditions will be cited to illustrate how drugs delivered transplacentally have aroused interest because of their individual beneficial effects and their contribution to our understanding of fetal physiology and developmental pharmacology. Advantages of trans-placental therapy and problems with direct fetal therapy will be discussed.

Principles of perinatal pharmacology

Maternal pharmacokinetics

Drug pathways in the maternal, placental, and fetal units are illustrated in Fig. 1.1. The pharmacokinetics of drugs during pregnancy have been reviewed by Noschel et al. (1982). The concentration of any drug is diminished in the maternal circulation during late gestation as a result of an increase in extracellular fluid. The volume of distribution is enlarged because of inclusion of the fetoplacental unit. The decrease in maternal serum drug concentration and increase in the volume of distribution also depend on the chemical properties of the drug. Water-soluble com-pounds may be diluted in the larger volume of distribu-tion, while lipid-soluble compounds may concentrate in the added membrane layers of the fetoplacental unit. Total clearance is expected to rise in late gestation, which further accentuates a reduction in serum and tissue concentrations of water-soluble drugs and metabolites.

Most drugs are expected to have a shorter half-life during late pregnancy than in the nonpregnant state. This is especially true for antibiotics and barbiturates. Drugs are eliminated more rapidly during pregnancy because of transplacental passage and increased renal perfusion and glomerular filtration. Renal blood flow increases 25% to 50% during pregnancy because of the increased cardiac output, while glomerular filtration is increased by 50% (Bynum, 1977).

Placenta transfer

The placental transfer of drugs and other substances is complex, and no method of study is ideal. Several models have been used to increase our understanding of placental transfer. However, drugs move across the placenta primarily by simple diffusion, and the process is dependent on the chemical properties and concentration gradients of the free drug (Juchau & Dyer, 1972). Most drugs have a molecular weight of 250 to 500. An un-bound and unionized drug of molecular weight less than 1000 usually is lipid soluble and rapidly penetrates the trophoblast, connective and endothelial tissues that separate the fetal and maternal circulations.

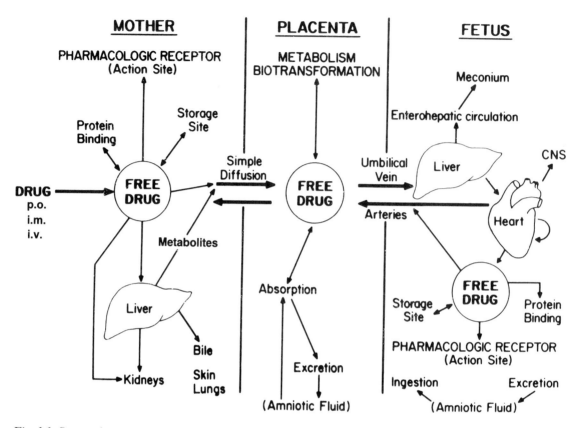

Fig. 1.1 *Drug pathways within the maternal, placental, and fetal units. (From Livezey, G. and Rayburn, W.: Principles of perinatal phamacology. In Rayburn W., Zuspan, F. (eds.) (1992).* Drug Therapy in Obstetrics and Gynecology. *St. Louis: CV Mosby, p. 5. Used with permission.)*

Drug transfer is greater during late gestation (Juchau & Dyer, 1972), and explanations for this increased transfer are listed in Table 1.1. Any drug in sufficient concentrations will eventually cross the placenta, especially when maternal therapeutic blood levels of the drug have been maintained for an extended period. Pathological processes causing inflammation, hypoxia, vascular degeneration, or partial separation of the placental implantation can affect uteroplacental blood flow and thus drug transfer.

Placental metabolism of drugs is not well understood, but in vivo studies have shown the placenta to be capable of significant drug biotransformation (Rayburn *et al.*,

1984). Further, the metabolites formed are often similar to those formed within the adult human liver (Bynum, 1977) and may be similar to those of the fetal liver. Differences in the formation of principal metabolites between adult liver and the placenta may relate to differing concentrations of microsomal enzymes in the tissues and to each tissue's specific regulation of enzymatic activity. Enzymatic reactions at both the placenta and fetal liver may be necessary to explain any effects within the fetus.

Certain substances may cross the placenta only after biotransformation. The synthetic capabilities of the placenta have not been well demonstrated. Drugs can induce or inhibit placental enzymes necessary for the metabolic conversion of endogenous substances. Drugs may act on the fetus and placenta to reduce placental blood flow or to interfere with active transport or other nutritive functions of the placenta (Juchau, 1976).

Table 1.1 *Reasons for increased drug transfer across the placenta in late pregnancy*

Increased unbound drug available for transport
Increased uteroplacental blood flow (500 ml/min)
Increased placental surface area
Decreased thickness of the semipermeable lipid membranes (2 µg at term) between the placental capillaries
Greater physical disruption of placental membranes
More acidic fetal circulation to 'trap' basic drugs

Fetal pharmacokinetics

For most drugs that cross the placenta, fetal levels reach 50% to 100% of maternal serum concentrations (Mirkin & Singh, 1976). Once the levels reach steady state, fetal serum levels can be higher than those in the mother. The total exposure to a drug and its metabolites in the fetus is more important than the rate of transplacental transport. Long-term drug exposure, rather than single-dose therapy, may influence fetal cell growth during early hyperplasia or later hypertrophy stages of development (Juchau, 1976; Enesco & Leblond, 1962).

Drugs transported in the umbilical vein travel to the fetal liver via the portal vein or are shunted through the liver to the right side of the heart via the ductus venosus. Factors determining the flow direction through the ductus venosus or portal vein are not well understood. Cardiac output is proportionally greater in the fetus than in the adult, and blood is circulated preferentially to the essential organs such as the brain, heart and placenta through less resistant pathways. Blood–brain permeability is greater in the fetus than in the adult. Therefore, the developing brain is more vulnerable to circulating drug levels. Mitochondria, the main intracellular sites for metabolism, increase in number and enzyme content with age in the fetal brain and heart (Winick & Noble, 1965). More than half of the cardiac output is directly returned to the placenta through the umbilical arteries. The proportion returned is greater when fetal acidosis is present. The maternal-fetal concentration gradient is, therefore, decreased, and further transfer of drug or metabolite is retarded (Smith, 1964).

Despite preferential circulation to the heart and brain, drug distribution in the fetus eventually becomes diffuse. Total body water increases with fetal maturity but decreases proportionally with total body mass from 95% at mid-gestation to 75% at term. Plasma protein concentrations and protein-binding capacities are lower in the fetus than in the mother. More free drug is, therefore, available for tissue penetration or competitive protein binding with other drugs or endogenous compounds. Consequently, conclusions about drug disposition in the fetus based on maternal or fetal serum levels may not accurately reflect fetal pharmacokinetics or drug distribution patterns.

Concentrations of drugs in the fetus vary but are progressively lower in samples from the umbilical vein, umbilical artery and fetal tissue such as the fetal scalp. The rate of tissue permeability of a drug is unknown but probably increases with gestation (Waddell & Marlowe, 1976). Studies of fetal animals have shown that autonomic receptors are present in the ileum, carotid artery and aortic arch sinuses in the early second trimester. Those receptors are responsive to catecholamine stimulation (Waddell & Marlowe, 1976; Boreus, 1967; McMurphy & Boreus, 1968). Binding affinities remain relatively constant throughout gestation (Massotti *et al.*, 1980). However, the strength of the receptor response increases remarkably with fetal development, probably because of a combination of increased receptor complement and the ontogeny of effector molecules coupled to the receptors (Boreus, 1967). Some drugs may also have a higher affinity for specific target tissues owing to receptor distribution or chemical conditions.

Many fetal organs are capable of substantial metabolic activity, but drug metabolism occurs primarily in the liver. Human fetal liver microsomes have significant P-450 levels and nicotinamide-adenine dinucleotide phosphate (NADPH)–cytochrome *c* reductase, which can be measured as early as the 14th week of gestation (Waddell & Marlowe, 1976). Oxidation and reduction reactions have been observed as early as the 16th week (McMurphy & Boreus, 1968). The activity and concentrations of certain hepatic microsomal enzymes and the rate of oxidative and conjugative reactions are probably less than in the adult (McMurphy & Boreus, 1968). Therefore, direct effects from drugs may be more pronounced and more prolonged in the fetus than in the mother. Certain drugs, such as phenobarbital or ethanol, which readily cross the placenta, may induce specific fetal liver enzymes (Mirkin & Singh, 1976). With chronic exposure, enzyme induction increases the amount of smooth endoplasmic reticulum, and the hepatic drug-metabolizing capabilities of the fetus are activated. Prolonged phenobarbital, narcotic or ethanol exposure has been shown to stimulate glucuronyl transferase to conjugate circulating bilirubin over several days and thereby diminish the amount of conjugated bilirubin in the neonate (Mirkin, 1974). This also may result in the reduction of endogenous substrates for further conjugation of drugs and metabolites. However, by stimulating hepatic enzymes, phenobarbital may enhance the metabolism of other exogenous drugs, such as phenytoin (Pippenger & Rosen, 1975). The absence or excess of one or more enzymes may go unrecognized if the embryo or fetus does not survive; thus potentially toxic drug effects may go undiagnosed.

The excretion of most drugs is slower in the fetus than in the adult, since many systems are not fully developed. The primary routes of elimination involve the placenta and fetal urine. The placental transfer of drugs from the fetus to the mother is the primary route of drug elimination in early pregnancy and is dependent on simple diffusion, free-drug chemical properties and concentration gradients. In the latter part of pregnancy, drug elimination is determined by the immature fetal kidneys contributing to the amniotic fluid. In the absence of an upper gastrointestinal atresia, great amounts of amniotic fluid can be swallowed by the fetus and recirculated in the enterohepatic circulation. Although clinical application is very limited, some drugs and metabolites may be measured by amniotic fluid sampling and by meconium analysis.

Modes of administration

The transplacental route is the standard means of administering drugs to the fetus. Exceptions to this are circumstances in which (i) the drug crosses the placenta poorly, such as thyroxine; (ii) transplacental passage is adversely affected by the fetal disease state such as hydrops; (iii) the fetus is moribund such that rapid drug effects are desirable; and (iv) maternal administration is associated with undesirable side-effects in the mother.

Direct fetal routes are limited by the invasive nature of the procedure especially given the need for repeated drug administration. There is little available information regarding the pharmacokinetics of drugs administered directly to the fetal compartment. It is, therefore, understandable that this approach has been pursued with great caution.

The intraamniotic route would appear to be associated with the lowest loss rate. It may in addition act as a reservoir for drugs by recirculation via the fetal gastrointestinal and urinary tracts. Absorption is presumably by swallowing and possibly by the intramembranous route. An example of this application is the intraamniotic injection of thyroid hormones to treat hypothyroid fetal goitre (see Chapter 15).

The direct fetal intravascular route, although the most invasive, has the advantages of immediacy and allows the concomitant measurement of drug levels and disease parameters. Clinical experience has shown that the half-life of drugs administered intravascularly to the fetus are substantially shorter than when the same drugs are used neonatally. This is felt to reflect placenta binding, placental metabolism, increased volume of distribution owing to placental circulation, and transplacental transfer back into the maternal circulation. Consequently, most investigators would administer larger doses per kilogram estimated fetal weight than would be given to preterm neonates. The usual indication is antiarrythmic therapy, as discussed in Chapter 12.

In an attempt to reduce the risk of repeated fetal blood samplings, the direct fetal intramuscular and intraperitoneal routes have been proposed. The intramuscular route may carry a risk of fetal nerve damage. However, it has been shown to lead to more prolonged drug levels of digitoxin, thereby reducing the cumulative number of procedures (Weiner & Thompson, 1988). The intraperitoneal route has also been proposed as vehicle for even slower absorption and the need for fewer procedures. Many fetal physicians have experience with this technique secondary to the use of intraperitoneal transfusion. However, there are no published pharmacokinetic data and there is some concern regarding absorption in the presence of the ascites.

Specific fetal conditions

These are discussed in detail in the respective chapters. The indications for fetal drug therapy can be classified into the three distinct groups.

The first category is prophylactic use to prevent fetal malformations. Examples include folic acid to prevent neural tube defects (Chapter 4) and steroids to prevent virilization in cases of congenital adrenal hyperplasia (Chapter 5). Antibiotics are widely used to prevent fetal damage from toxoplasmosis and syphilis (Chapter 8).

The second category comprises prophylactic use during late pregnancy to prevent specific neonatal conditions. Examples include glucocorticoids and thyrotrophin-releasing hormone to prevent respiratory distress syndrome (Chapter 7). In addition, a variety of antimicrobial agents can be used to minimize vertical transmission of infection, such as zidovudine against human immunodeficiency virus and antibiotics in pre-term prelabour rupture of the membranes or maternal Group B streptococcal carriage (Chapter 8).

Finally, drugs can be used to treat specific fetal conditions in utero. Examples include aspirin in intra-uterine growth retardation (Chapter 9), immuno-globulins in alloimmune thrombocytopenia (Chapter 11), anti-arrhythmics in supraventricular tachycardia (Chapter 12), prostaglandin synthetase inhibitors in polyhydramnios (Chapter 13) and thyroid hormones for fetal goitre (Chapter 15).

Conclusion

The mother and fetus undergo many unique and progressive changes in pharmacokinetics and pharmacodynamics during pregnancy. The result can be a greater total drug burden for the fetus than for the mother. In addition, the intermediate state of many immature fetal tissues permits special tissue specific accumulations. This often results in the need for different dosage regimens to treat the fetus via the mother than would be used in the non-pregnant woman.

Drugs can be administered by intraamniotic instillation or direct intraperitoneal, intramuscular or intra-umbilical injection if transplacental passage is ineffective. The direct route has clear invasive risks but would quickly aid the fetus if transplacental drug transfer is slow. Our limited understanding of fetal pharmacokinetics forces us to proceed cautiously in this direction.

Drug therapy directed toward the fetus is intended for either the treatment of a fetal disorder or improvement of capacity for later intrauterine or postnatal adaptation. Many reported studies involve single cases or small numbers of fetuses after the first trimester. However, there are increasing numbers of large randomized controlled trials of drug therapy in late pregnancy. Clearly drug administration has proven beneficial to the fetus in many circumstances.

References

Boreus, L. O. (1967). Pharmacology of the human fetus: Dose-effect relationship for acetylcholine during ontogenesis. *Biologia Neonatorum*, 11, 328–37.

Bynum, T. E. (1977). Hepatic and gastrointestinal disorders in pregnancy. *Medical Clinics of North America*, 61, 129–38.

Davidson, K. M., Richards, D. S., Schatz, D. A. & Fischer, D. A. (1991). Successful in utero treatment of fetal goiter and hypothyroidism. *New England Journal of Medicine*, 324, 543–6.

Enesco, M. & Leblond, C. P. (1962). Increase in cell number as a factor in the growth of the organs and tissues of the young male rat. *Journal of Embryology and Experimental Morphology*, 10, 530–62.

Juchau, M. R. (1976). Drug biotransformation reactions in the placenta. In *Perinatal Pharmacology and Therapeutics*, ed. B. L. Mirkin, p. 71. New York: Academic Press.

Juchau, M. R. & Dyer, D. C. (1972). Pharmacology of the placenta. *Pediatric Clinics of North America*, 19, 65–9.

Massotti, M., Alleva, F. R., Balazs, T. & Guidotti, A. (1980). GABA and benzodiazepine receptors in the offspring of dams receiving diazepam: ontogenetic studies. *Neuropharmacology*, 19, 951–6.

McMurphy, D. M. & Boreus, L. O. (1968). Pharmacology of the human fetus: adrenergic receptor function in small intestine. *Biologia Neonatorum*, 13, 325–39.

Mirkin, B. L. (1974). Biological maturation and drug disposition. In *Perinatal Pharmacology: Mead Johnson Symposium on Perinatal and Developmental Medicine*, No 5, pp. 31–8. Oradell, NJ: Medical Economic Books.

Mirkin, B. L. & Singh, S. (1976). Placental transfer of pharmacologically active molecules., In *Perinatal Pharmacology and Therapeutics*, ed. B. L. Mirkin, pp. 1–70. New York: Academic Press.

Noschel, H., Peiker, G., Muller, B., Schroder, S., Bonow, A., Meinhold, P., Voigt, R. & Tittel, R. (1982). Pharmacokinetics during pregnancy and delivery. *International Journal of Biological Research*, 3, 66–73.

Pippenger, C. E. & Rasen, T. S. (1975). Phenobarbital plasma levels in neonates. *Clinics in Peritatology*, 2, 111–15.

Rayburn, W. F., Holsztynska, E. F. & Dommino, E. F. (1984). Phencyclidine: biotransformation by the human placenta. *American Journal of Obstetrics and Gynecology*, 148, 111–12.

Rayburn, W. F. & Payne, G. F. (1993). *In utero* drug therapy. *Pharmacology and Therapeutics*, 58, 237–47.

Smith, R. J. (1964). Mitochondria in fetal tissue. *Journal of Embryology and Experimental Morphology*, 11, 424.

Waddell, W. J. & Marlowe, G. C. (1976). Disposition of drugs in the fetus. In *Perinatal Pharmacology and Therapeutics*, ed. B. L. Mirkin, pp. 119–268. New York: Academic Press.

Weiner, C. P. & Thompson, M. I. (1988). Direct treatment of fetal supraventricular tachycardia after failed transplacental therapy. *American Journal of Obstetrics and Gynecology*, 158, 570–3.

Winick, M. & Noble, A. (1965). Quantitative changes in DNA and RNA and protein during prenatal and postnatal growth in the rat. *Developmental Biology*, 12, 451–66.

2 Invasive procedures

RODOLFO MONTEMAGNO
AND PETER SOOTHILL

Introduction

The development of ultrasound allows inspection and examination of the unborn. The wide range of invasive procedures available allows the principles of medicine to be applied to the fetus. Tissues can be sampled in order to confirm or refute a suspected diagnosis, but increasingly these techniques can also be used to treat the unborn. Prenatal diagnosis of a fetal abnormality is not always a preliminary step to termination of pregnancy, and improved perinatal management or treatment *in utero* in the fetal interest are equally important. The implications of prenatal events for postnatal and even adult disease (Barker *et al.*, 1989) are becoming more clearly defined and may be more far reaching than previously realized. Since birth is often too late, understanding and preventing future pathology requires access to the fetus.

In this chapter, we review the invasive procedures that are part of the process of treating the unborn. We will not consider the pathologies leading to the indications since these are the subject of other chapters.

General aspects

Many aspects of undertaking invasive procedures apply to all the different techniques and so these are dealt with together.

Detailed ultrasound scanning

Before counselling a patient about the need for an invasive procedure, the operator should undertake a detailed ultrasound scan. This will provide important information such as gestational age, the number of fetuses, viability and the presence of any structural abnormalities. This information may influence the patient's decision to have a test or technical aspects of the procedure. For example, it is bad practice to undertake an amniocentesis for maternal age without looking for structural abnormalities of sufficient severity that the patient would not wish to wait for the karyotype result. The finding of a multiple pregnancy before an invasive procedure causes counselling and technical problems. Zygosity will affect the chance of having an abnormal baby and chorionicity the post-procedure pregnancy risk. Therefore, it is useful information if twins can be shown to be dizygotic by being different sex on ultrasound and to assess chorionicity by separation of placental masses and thickness of the inter-fetal septum. If the fetuses are the same sex, one cannot exclude monozygosity and so the risk of chromosomal abnormality is about 1.7 times the maternal age-specific risk (Chudleigh & Pearce, 1992). If the twins are dizygotic, the risk of one twin being chromosomally abnormal is double the maternal age-related risk.

Counselling

Counselling is a vital part of any invasive procedure in pregnancy. It is the only time in medicine in which access to one patient requires permission to cause discomfort and some risk to another. Counselling involves helping the individual and, if she wishes, her family to comprehend as fully as possible the indication for the procedure, the consequences of the results and alternative management options as well as the advantages, limitations and risks of any proposed test. The practical aspects should be carefully explained both before and during the procedure in order to obtain informed consent and to reassure her while the procedure is done that it is going as planned. Counselling should be done in an environment where privacy and confidentiality are guaranteed. The counsellor must have the time, patience and skills to convey information and concepts in understandable language considering the patient's education and ethical beliefs. In particular, the attitude of the patient to termination of pregnancy should be understood by the counsellor. When the patient decides to have an invasive test, written consent should be obtained.

Clinical setting and operator training

The environment and staff behaviour should be organized to achieve both an efficient and rapid invasive procedure but also to reduce the psychological stress for the patient. The general atmosphere should be calm and confident and the personal approach relaxed and informal. It is essential that the operator and the support staff are trained to work together in a co-ordinated manner. Careful arrangements for sample labelling, processing and transport are an important part of the procedure, as is rapid and accurate communication of results from the laboratories to the fetal medicine unit and then to the patient and referring doctors.

Invasive techniques should be undertaken only by operators with considerable experience in other aspects of obstetric ultrasound. Since almost all procedures use a very similar technique, trainees can be taught how to do an easier procedure properly (e.g. amniocentesis) and then move with experience to more difficult targets. Units offering this service should have sufficient throughput to maintain expertise, usually a considerable number of referrals from other hospitals for anomaly scanning and fetal medicine opinions.

Preparation

Maternal supine hypotension, hyperventilation and sedation should be avoided. Anything that gives the patient an image of an 'operation' (surgical masks, hats, drapes' etc.) should be limited to the minimum required unless the procedure involves a significant risk of intra-

uterine infection, e.g. insertion of a foreign body as in shunting. The length of the needle or trochar required depends on obesity, liquor volume and the positions of the fetus and placenta. Maternal obesity affects both the distance to the target and the quality of the ultrasound image. If there is any doubt, it is important to measure the depth from the skin surface to the target by ultrasound before the procedure so a needle of sufficient length can be used.

The skin insertion site is scrupulously cleaned with an antiseptic solution such as chlorhexidine. If local anaesthetic is used, it should be injected into the skin and the abdominal and uterine peritoneum. When using a free-hand technique, the anaesthetic injection can help to confirm the needle angle required to follow the intended path and so reduce the need to change the sampling needle direction during the procedure. However, patients who have had invasive tests repeatedly, e.g. for Rh disease, say the local anaesthetic may be more painful than the procedure done quickly without anaesthetic. Furthermore, by the time the anaesthetic has been given time to work it can produce a uterine contraction sufficient to interfere with the intended needle path and move the position of the target tissue. A small scalpel blade can be used to incise the skin after anaesthetic if a large cannula or needle is to be used or if the patient's skin is unusually tough.

One or two operators?

Some operators prefer to have a different person controlling the scanning transducer from the needle. We strongly disagree with this approach since the operator may lose sight of the intended needle path. The 'single operator' technique means that one hand holds the needle and the other the ultrasound transducer; a skilled assistant is required to withdraw the needle stylet, fix a syringe, aspirate at the right time or do other actions such as transfusing blood or inserting a catheter.

Fetal paralysis/analgesia

Occasionally fetal activity is a concern when it threatens to dislodge the needle. Some centres use temporary immobilization of the fetus by intramuscular or intravascular injection of a neuromuscular blocker such as pancuronium (0.1 to 0.3 mg/kg) (de Crespigny *et al.*, 1985b; Moise *et al.*, 1989) but in our experience this procedure is rarely necessary. Fetal paralysis is complete, lasts 60 to 120 minutes and seems quite safe as the problems which can result from reduced fetal movements, such as lung development and joint problems, should not occur in such a short time. Recently 1.0 mg/kg atracurium has been used as an alternative to pancuronium because of quicker induction of fetal paralysis and then faster return to normal fetal movements (Bernstein *et al.*, 1988). This is discussed in more detail in Chapter 10.

Recent data have shown that the fetus can mount a hormonal stress response to invasive procedures with excretion of cortisol and β-endorphin (Giannakoulopoulos *et al.*, 1994). They raise the possibility that human fetuses may feel pain *in utero* and so might benefit from anaesthesia and analgesia. However, further study is needed to answer such questions before any practice guidelines are advised.

After the procedure

The fetal heart beat should be checked and demonstrated to the woman. Both uterine and fetal puncture sites should be observed ultrasonically for bleeding. If bleeding is seen, the fetal heart rate should be checked again and monitored until the bleeding has stopped. If local anaesthetic has been used, she should be warned to expect a bruised sensation in a few hours and reassured that paracetamol can be used safely. If the fetus is previable, the patient should allowed to wait in the hospital until she feels well but can return home with no special precautions or restrictions in her activity. When the fetus is viable, heart rate monitoring by cardiotocography for about half an hour may be sensible, although if pancuronium has been used a non-reactive trace may be expected. In the rare event that fetal bleeding is prolonged and sufficient to compromise the fetal circulation, emergency fetal blood transfusion of O negative blood should be considered.

Anti-D is given to Rh-negative women unless they are known to be D alloimmunized. Doses used range from 250 to 1500 IU, equivalent to 50 to 300 mg, depending on national guidelines in individual countries. The risk of causing or worsening alloimmunization can be mini-

mized by avoiding transplacental approaches and using small-gauge needles. If an unusual amount of placental trauma occurs in a Rh-negative woman, Kleihauer testing should be considered to assess if further doses of anti-D are required.

Complications

Assessing the risk of an invasive procedure is highly complex. The use of the term 'procedure-related loss' to mean a fetal death within two weeks should be discouraged since some of these deaths will be the result of the indication for sampling, e.g. hydrops or growth retardation, rather than the procedure. It is also possible, although less likely, that some complications caused by the procedure might be first detected after 14 days. Observed post-procedure loss rates are determined by the procedure risk, both intrinsic and operator-dependent, added to the pre-procedure risk, which is in turn dependent on gestational age, maternal age and the indication for sampling (Ghidini *et al.*, 1993).

Gestational age at the procedure is an important determinant of observed fetal loss rates because the earlier the pregnancy, the greater the pre-procedure risk of miscarriage. For example, at 9–11 weeks, approximately 2% of women will miscarry after a viable fetus has been seen on ultrasound without any invasive procedure, while later in pregnancy the background loss rate is less. Therefore, the spontaneous pregnancy loss rate should be subtracted from the observed total post-procedure loss rate to estimate the procedure-related rate. Furthermore, when procedures are done in the late second or third trimesters, serious complications may be under-estimated because of emergency delivery of viable fetuses. If a problem occurs, emergency caesarean section may salvage the fetus, but by the time the complication has failed to resolve spontaneously and delivery has been organized, the fetus may survive permanently damaged or die in the neonatal rather than fetal period.

A second determinant of observed fetal loss rate is the indication for the procedure. For fetal blood sampling, the best estimate of pre-procedure risk comes after classification by indication (Maxwell *et al.*, 1991): (i) prenatal diagnosis; (ii) structural abnormalities; (iii) fetal assessment; and (iv) hydrops fetalis. In 202 pregnancies not electively terminated, the number of fetal losses within 14 days of the procedure were 1 of 76 (1.5%) of fetuses in group 1, 5 of 76 (7%) in group 2, 4 in 29 (14%) in group 3 and 9 in 35 (25%) in group 4. It would be useful if other investigators reported loss rates in such a way.

The difficulties in evaluating the post-procedure loss rates have been clearly shown by the controversial results of several multicentre trials done in order to compare safety and accuracy of different invasive techniques (Rhoads *et al.*, 1989; Canadian Collaborative CVS-Amniocentesis Clinical Trial Group, 1989; Medical Research Council, 1991; Smidt-Jensen & Philip, 1991; Jackson *et al.*, 1992). Whereas the Canadian, American and the Danish studies did not reveal a significant difference in fetal loss rates comparing first trimester chorion villus sampling (CVS) and mid-trimester amniocentesis, the randomized MRC European trial showed a significantly lower rate of surviving infants in the CVS group. Equally controversial results have been reported when comparing the risks of transcervical and transabdominal CVS. With such complicated multifactorial problems, we recommend giving most weight to trials and series from single groups rather than pooled data from different centres.

The main risk to the mother is red cell alloimmunization. However, chorioamnionitis or emergency caesarean section as a result of the procedure can result in secondary maternal problems. When an invasive procedure is undertaken and the fetus is considered viable, maternal aspects of emergency delivery should be considered. Significant morbidity from needle injury to maternal intra-abdominal organs such as intestines or vessels has not been reported.

Research

Fetal medicine is a new and rapidly changing area of medicine. Some of the indications for invasive procedures are being replaced by non-invasive techniques. It is, therefore, important that when these techniques are indicated, we should have ethically approved means of obtaining a small surplus sample for research with no additional risk to the pregnancy. Such samples should be stored and made available for research.

Access to the fetus

Three techniques are used: 'blind' needling, endoscopic guidance and ultrasound guidance.

Blind needling

Amniocentesis is still done in some centres without ultrasound imaging at all or as a separate procedure after identification of a pool of fluid and marking the overlying skin. A pioneering group of Chinese investigators reported experience with blind, transcervical CVS (Tietung Hospital, 1975). Simultaneous ultrasound monitoring during amniocentesis has been shown to reduce the number of dry and bloody taps (Romero *et al.*, 1985; de Crespigny and Robinson, 1986) and has thus replaced the older technique of 'semi-blind' insertion following ultrasonic identification of a pool.

Most authorities consider that ultrasound has an essential place in the performance of any invasive procedure and is important in avoiding damage to developing tissues.

Endoscopy

Endoscopic techniques allow visualization inside the uterus and guidance for tissue sampling (Hobbins & Mahoney, 1974; Rodeck & Campbell, 1978; Rodeck *et al.*, 1980) or therapy (Rodeck *et al.*, 1985; Ville *et al.*, 1995). Advances in ultrasound techniques have limited application, but laser photocoagulation either in twin-to-twin transfusion syndrome or in fetal structural abnormalities may be new indications. Direct inspection of fetal anatomy beyond the resolution of ultrasound may be useful occasionally in some inherited conditions such as Door syndrome, in which nail hypoplasia is associated with mental retardation (Fig. 2.1). The size of endoscopes used varies from about 0.7 mm to 6.8 mm depending on gestational age, the indication and operator experience. Embryoscopy differs from fetoscopy in that it uses a transcervical approach, is done at an earlier gestational age and the amnion is not punctured but the fetus viewed through the amniotic membrane (Dumez, Oury & Duchetel, 1988).

Transabdominal fetoscopy is easiest between 15–20 weeks' gestation because after 20 weeks the amniotic fluid is cloudy, but fetoscopy is possible until late in the third trimester. It is really an ultrasound-guided technique as well because scanning is used to allow entry without damage to the placenta, umbilical cord or fetus and give access to the fetal part being examined or biopsied. Under local anaesthesia and full aseptic technique, a trochar and cannula are inserted into the amniotic cavity and a fetoscope replaces the trochar. If required, a blood sampling needle or biopsy forceps can be passed through the side channel of the cannula. Recently a thin-gauge embryo-fetoscope (TGEF) technique has been developed (Quintero et al., 1993a). An 18- or 19-gauge needle is placed under ultrasound guidance into the amniotic or extra-coelomic cavity. A flexible fibre optic endoscope (≤0.7 mm in diameter) is then passed through the lumen to the distal end of the needle and the eyepiece connected to a video camera. This technique has recently been extended to allow fetal cystoscopy, for direct inspection of the trigone and ureteric orifices and access to the upper urethra for therapeutic procedures (Quintero et al., 1995).

No major maternal complications have been reported in over 6000 fetoscopies. The risks to the pregnancy depend on operator experience and the size of endoscope used; in centres that have performed more than 100 fetoscopies, the fetal mortality is less than 5% and in the largest series it is about 2%. Morbidity includes preterm labour in 8–10%, amniotic fluid leakage in 10% and amnionitis in 0.5%. Because of its recent introduction, complete data on the safety of the TGEF technique do not exist but may be similar to that reported for amniocentesis (Quintero, Karoline & Puder, 1993b). However, because of the potential teratogenic or harmful effect of light and heat on the developing conceptus, primarily on the central nervous and visual systems, embryoscopy is not recommended before 9–10 weeks' gestation.

Ultrasound guided techniques

Ultrasound guidance means that the needle is made to follow a pre-determined path and its position is continuously observed throughout the procedure. After identifying the target ultrasonically, the transducer is rotated

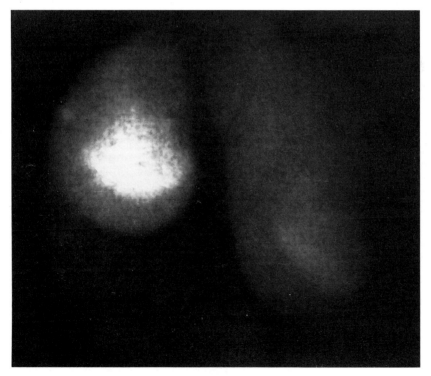

Fig. 2.1 *Fetoscopic picture of the fingernails of an 18 week fetus. These appear normally formed, providing reassurance in a pregnancy at risk of Door syndrome (severe mental retardation and nail hypoplasia).*

through 90° and the path selected to avoid fetal parts, maternal vessels and, where possible, the placenta. There are two variations in the technique, needle-guide and free-hand.

A needle-guide technique uses a sector-type ultrasound transducer with a needle guide channel attached. Lines on the ultrasound screen indicate the path the needle will follow when inserted down the guide. The transducer is moved until these lines cross the intended target. This approach has the advantage of allowing thinner 22–26 gauge needles to be used than those needed for a free-hand technique. However, it limits the

operator's ability to adjust to difficulties or changes that may occur during the procedure by altering the position of the needle tip. It is also not possible to use this approach in some of the larger procedures such as shunting.

With a free-hand technique, a curvilinear or linear ultrasound transducer is moved until the intended sampling site and skin insertion point appear on opposite sides of the ultrasound screen. The needle path will then be nearly perpendicular to the ultrasound beam to facilitate imaging of the whole needle length (Fig. 2.2). The stiffness of a 20–22 gauge needle is needed to allow the needle direction to be changed. The advantages of this technique are the flexibility it gives to make adjustments during the procedure and that once learned the same technique can be used for all ultrasound-guided invasive procedures.

Colour Doppler

Colour Doppler imaging is sometimes of value in invasive procedures. It is especially suitable for identifying the umbilical cord insertion in difficult cases and to avoid accidental injury to fetal vessels. The problem with colour Doppler is that it reduces the quality of the conventional image. This is because for ideal imaging the object should be at right angles to the sound, whereas the Doppler shift is greater if the sound is parallel with the vessel. We use it before a procedure to help plan the path but not during a procedure. It is also not required to confirm good flow during a transfusion since this can be clearly seen by conventional imaging anyway, although it can be used to monitor arterial pulsation at the sampling site and thus fetal heart rate. Others have used it as an alternative technique to determine whether the artery or vein is sampled within the umbilical cord.

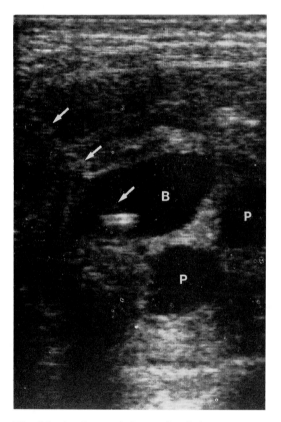

Fig. 2.2 *An ultrasound picture taken during an ultrasound-guided needling procedure. The needle is designated by the arrows. The needle tip is seen within the bladder (B) adjacent to dilated renal pelves (P) in a case of urinary tract obstruction (from Fisk & Rodeck, 1990, reproduced with permission).*

Specific techniques

This chapter concentrates on therapeutic techniques, although several diagnostic techniques are relevant for fetal therapy being used either to diagnose diseases amenable to treatment or to monitor medical treatment of the fetus.

Amniocentesis

Amniocentesis means aspiration of amniotic fluid. Although therapeutic amniocentesis was introduced more than 100 years ago for the symptomatic relief of polyhydramnios, it was not until the 1950s that the diagnostic capabilities began to be addressed when Bevis (1952) demonstrated that spectrophotometric analysis of amniotic fluid could be used to predict the severity of Rh alloimmunization. The timing of amniocentesis depends on the indication but can be between eight weeks and term. For karyotyping, amniocentesis is usually performed at 14–16 weeks' gestation. Recently it has been shown that cytogenetic culture is successful after 10 weeks but the miscarriage rate may be higher than with CVS so this technique is unlikely to become widely used (Nicolaides *et al.*, 1994). Amniocentesis in the late second and third trimester is usually undertaken for the investigation of Rh alloimmunization or assessment of fetal lung maturity.

Amniocentesis should be done under continuous ultrasound guidance. A pool of amniotic fluid is identified, as described earlier. An anterior placenta rarely covers the entire anterior uterine wall so there is usually a 'window' available for a lateral approach. If not, then the needle may be passed through the anterior placenta, avoiding the placental edge and the cord insertion, and bleeding only occasionally results. The fine needle used (22 gauge) makes local anaesthesia more painful than the procedure. The needle is passed through the abdominal wall and along the required path. When the needle tip is identified in the middle of the target pool, the stylet is removed and amniotic fluid aspirated. To prevent maternal contamination, the first 1–2 ml are discarded and the syringe removed from the needle before it is withdrawn.

Sampling problems

If the needle appears properly placed in the target pool but no amniotic fluid can be aspirated, the needle should be rotated through 180 and then aspiration retried. If this fails, the needle may be blocked or the membranes 'tented' around the needle. Reinserting the stylet, advancing the needle under ultrasound guidance or injection of a small volume of normal saline may help.

When blood is aspirated, careful inspection should indicate if the fluid is pure blood or blood-stained amniotic fluid. If pure fresh blood, the position of the needle tip should be re-checked, the fetal heart beat observed and the needle usually withdrawn. If fresh blood staining is found, there is likely to be bleeding from the uterine puncture site so after checking the tip of the needle it can be moved into a different pool of amniotic fluid and clear fluid obtained.

If two attempts fail, the procedure should be abandoned. The patient should be re-scanned and the procedure postponed for several days or a week to give time for any blood staining to clear. Other techniques such as CVS or fetal blood sampling may need to be considered

Many regard amniocentesis as the procedure of choice for fetal karyotyping in multiple pregnancies, since sampling the same twin twice appears less likely than with CVS. Either two separate abdominal punctures can be made or the needle passed through the septum internally. Recently, septal disruption has been associated with a higher perinatal mortality consistent with that of true monoamniotic gestations (Gilbert *et al.*, 1991). However, only in one case was the amniotic rupture related to amniocentesis and others have reported that traversing the septum in a single abdominal puncture technique may be quicker and safer (Jeanty, Shah & Roussis, 1990). In case of results discordant for abnormality, it is important to be able to identify which specimen came from which fetus. This is achieved at the time of the procedure by detailed mapping of septal and placental anatomy in three dimensions in relation to each twin, and labelling the specimens accordingly. Some operators inject indigo carmine into the first sac after aspiration to ensure that the same sac is not tapped twice. Methylene blue injection was more widely used but is now contraindicated because of the risk of causing intestinal atresia in the fetus (Nicolini & Monni, 1990). We have not found dye injection necessary.

Complications

Some studies have reported a small but significant association with neonatal respiratory distress and it has been suggested that this could be the result of oligohydramnios following chronic leakage of fluid (Medical Research Council, 1978; Tabor *et al.*, 1986).

The British collaborative study also found an increase in postural deformities such as talipes and congenital dislocation of the hip following amniocentesis (Medical Research Council, 1978). Both these observations have not been found in the other trials (National Institute of Child Health and Human Development, 1976; Hunter, 1987). There are no large studies defining the risk of amniocentesis after 20 weeks' gestation. Between 15–20 weeks, the only randomized controlled trial reported a 1% increase in the miscarriage rate (Tabor *et al.*, 1986).

Therapy

Therapeutic indications for amniocentesis include the injection of drugs to correct fetal disorders (e.g. thyroxine in fetal hypothyroidism, or anti-arrhythmics in the treatment of some fetal cardiovascular disorders). However, the main therapeutic use is to drain large volumes of amniotic fluid in severe polyhydramnios. Effective treatment of polyhydramnios should consider the possible cause of the abnormal amniotic fluid production and so maternal diabetes, severe fetal anaemia or structural fetal anomalies should be excluded or treated and fetal karyotyping offered (Chapter 13). The placement of the needle is the same as for amniocentesis but the time taken to remove the fluid should be kept to a minimum because the patients often become uncomfortable. Therefore, at least an 18 gauge needle should be used and after obtaining fluid a 50 ml syringe can be attached to the needle via a three-way tap and plastic tubing. An alternative is to use a plastic catheter, which is then taped into position and left on free drainage to a collector bag. The amount of fluid removed depends on gestational age and the severity of the polyhydramnios but 3–4 litres may be required to achieve an amniotic fluid index within the normal range. Some have used amniotic pressure monitoring to guide the amount of fluid to be withdrawn, aiming to reduce the increased intrauterine pressure back to normal. The frequency with which the procedure should be repeated depends on maternal discomfort and the rate of reaccumulation.

Potential complications of amnioreduction include placental abruption, chorioamnionitis, premature rupture of membranes and premature labour (Meagher & Fisk, 1994). However it is impossible to determine when these occur whether they resulted from the procedure or the polyhydramnios. The risks of labour soon after the procedure are high and counselling about this risk (whether treatment is given or not) is important. The value of this technique is difficult to assess because the fluid often reaccumulates and the procedure may need to be repeated frequently. However, there is evidence that this technique can reduce intra-amniotic pressure in both singleton and twin gestations, prolong gestation and, therefore, improve perinatal survival rates (Queenan & Gadow, 1970; Mahoney *et al.*, 1990; Saunders, Snijders & Nicolaides, 1992). Certainly amnioreduction improves maternal discomfort.

Fetal blood sampling

Fetal blood sampling (FBS) was initially used for prenatal diagnosis of severe inherited disease with a view to termination of affected fetuses. More recently, a medical approach to diseases of the unborn has developed and the role of phlebotomy in fetal medicine is becoming more comparable to its place in postnatal medicine. Not only has direct access to the fetal circulation allowed effective therapies such as fetal transfusion, it has also become important for the assessment of placental drug transfer and monitoring the success of transplacental therapy. Examples include anti-arrhythmic agents to correct fetal tachyarrhythmias, gammaglobulin and steroids to improve low fetal platelet counts and hyperoxygenation to increase low pO_2 levels (Nicolini *et al.*, 1990; Rayburn, 1991; Hansmann *et al.*, 1991, Nicolaides *et al.*, 1987).

The operator must first choose the intended sampling target and guide technique. At times, these decisions are affected by the indication but generally they depend on the operators' personal experience. The most commonly used FBS site is the umbilical cord. A variety of terms have been used to describe this technique, such as 'cordocentesis', 'funipuncture' or 'PUBS'.

Umbilical cord

A transplacental approach is the easiest route to the placental cord insertion unless the placenta is entirely posterior. The best sampling site is usually the umbilical cord about 1 cm from the placental umbilical cord insertion as it seems to have a low risk of haemorrhage, perhaps as a result of the relatively thick Wharton's jelly. Attempts to puncture free loops often result in the cord being pushed away by the needle and if the fetal umbilicus is needled without paralysis, fetal movements may be dangerous. To enter the umbilical cord, the needle is brought close in line with the umbilical vein and then advanced sharply the remaining distance. A slow advance can push the tissues away even at this relatively fixed sampling site. On confirmation that the needle tip is in the umbilical cord, the assistant withdraws the stylet and, if the needle is ideally sited, blood will be seen filling the needle hub. A syringe is applied tightly and the desired volume of blood withdrawn. At 18 weeks, 2–4 ml can be taken safely and larger volumes can be taken at later gestations.

Often no blood is obtained initially; then the needle is briskly advanced or gently withdrawn and rotated between the operator's finger and thumb while suction is maintained with the syringe. If amniotic fluid is obtained, the needle will be either completely through the cord or alongside it. The needle should be carefully imaged again to assess the position of the tip and using the free-hand technique the needle can be moved from side to side looking for resulting movements of the cord. Should the needle be through the cord it should be withdrawn until no more amniotic fluid is aspirated, then the syringe changed, since even a small amount of amniotic fluid is a powerful coagulant, and the procedure described above repeated. If the needle has passed to the side of the cord, the needle is withdrawn a little and the needle path adjusted. A slow careful advance can be used to touch the cord with the needle before the sharp movement to puncture the vessels is repeated.

Zoom magnification and colour Doppler can be used to determine which vessel is sampled. However, changing the ultrasound settings during the procedure can be distracting and can reduce the quality of the image as discussed earlier. After aspiration of the required volume of blood, if blood gases studies are needed the umbilical vessel should be confirmed as artery or vein by a 'flush' technique in which 1 ml normal saline is rapidly injected and the resulting turbulence seen ultrasonically in the vessel (Nicolaides *et al.*, 1986a).

Other sites

These include the intrahepatic umbilical vein and fetal heart, although fetal paralysis/analgesia may need to be

considered. Blood can be successfully sampled from vessels within the substance of the liver (Bang, Bock & Trolle, 1982; de Crespigny *et al.*, 1985a; Nicolini *et al.*, 1990). The techniques for needle path selection and guidance are as described for the umbilical cord, but the fetal chest or abdomen is entered first, the direction checked and then the needle advanced into the sampling site as a separate movement. Some have used a double needle technique, the first to enter the fetal body cavity and a second finer needle passed within the first to puncture the target, but this is not necessary. Although good results have been reported, most suggest hepatic vein sampling is technically more difficult than FBS at the cord insertion, and this is usually used when the latter is difficult.

The heart is larger than the cord vessels, making ultrasound-guided needling relatively easy. Fears of damaging this organ have not been substantiated in the available series (Bang, 1983; Westgren, Selbing & Stangenberg, 1988). The heart should be entered through the anterior chest and so through the thick muscle of the ventricles, thereby avoiding damage to the valves or electrical conducting system. The heart is an alternative sampling site in the unusual event that the placental cord insertion or intrahepatic vein cannot be used safely or when access to the fetal circulation must be obtained at a gestational age less than 17–18 weeks' gestation. It can also be useful if an emergency blood transfusion is required; for instance to treat procedure-related bleeding, or for fetocide when potassium is injected for advanced or selective termination of pregnancy.

Laboratory testing

Various laboratory techniques for rapid confirmation that the blood obtained is fetal and pure have been reported. The most common is comparison of mean red cell volumes, which are bigger in the fetus. These become unnecessary if the technique described above is used, especially if a saline 'flush' confirms the vessel sampled, and may be impossible if fetal blood is replaced with adult blood following transfusions.

Complications

The complications of FBS that can threaten the fetus are bleeding or haematoma, and thus obstruction to flow at the site of needling (Jauniaux *et al.*, 1989), and fetal bradycardia (Benacerraf *et al.*, 1987), often associated with vasospasm after puncture of the umbilical artery (Weiner, 1987). As the hepatic vein is surrounded by neither cord nor arteries, its complication rate may theoretically be lower (Nicolini *et al.*, 1990). There is also a theoretical risk of transmitting microorganisms from the mother's blood, e.g. hepatitis or human immunodeficiency virus, to the fetus. Although this does not appear to have been documented, invasive procedures should be avoided when a mother is known to be infective. A further complication is intrauterine infection. Amniotic fluid leakage appears rare but should occur at the same frequency as after amniocentesis.

Several groups using different techniques and of varying experience have reported post-fetal blood sampling pregnancy loss rates excluding elective termination of pregnancy of about 1% with a range 0–2.5% (Soothill, 1994) but this is strongly influenced by the indication for sampling, as discussed earlier. A review of the published large series in 1993 (Ghidini *et al.*, 1993) showed a total loss rate, including perinatal deaths, of 2.7%.

Liver biopsy

Fetal liver biopsy has been used to diagnose inborn errors of metabolism when this tissue is the only site of expression of the enzymes, such as ornithine transcarbamylase deficiency, glucose 6-phosphatase deficiency, carbamyl phosphatase synthetase deficiency and alanine glycoxalate deficiency (Rodeck *et al.*, 1982; Golbus *et al.*, 1988; Piceni-Sereni *et al.*, 1988), although the indications have declined in frequency with advances in molecular diagnosis. In addition, fetal liver is of interest because it can be used for stem-cell harvesting and so possibly bone marrow transplantation (Chapter 20). Fetal liver biopsy is usually done between 17 and 20 weeks' gestation when the liver enzyme activities are adequately expressed. A needle is introduced into the fetal trunk, under the right costal margin, and is advanced into the liver substance. Although a single-needle technique has been shown to be successful, usually a double-needle system is preferred. The stylet of the needle is removed within the liver parenchyma and the longer sampling needle introduced with a 10–20 ml

syringe attached. A strong negative pressure is exerted while the needle is moved back and forth within the liver. The needle is then withdrawn and flushed in order to check the adequacy of the sample microscopically. Several attempts may be necessary in order to obtain the 10–25 mg tissue that are usually required. Reference ranges for enzyme activities have been established in mid-trimester fetuses (Rodeck *et al.*, 1982; Dampure *et al.*, 1989) and technical failures can be checked against other liver enzymes as controls.

Too few fetal liver biopsies have been performed to assess the safety of the procedure, but serious hepatic bleeding seems to be rare. To date, no failed procedures have been reported.

Urine sampling

In fetal urinary tract obstruction, fetal urine sampling and biochemical analysis may help to indicate the prognosis, be used for karyotyping and help to select patients for vesico-amniotic shunting (Golbus *et al.*, 1985). Under ultrasound guidance, a needle is introduced into the fetal bladder and the urine removed by aspiration. Subsequent serial imaging of the bladder will allow evaluation of the refilling rate and thus urine production. Risks and complications are as for all ultrasound-guided procedures. As injury to the umbilicus or umbilical arteries passing around the bladder could occur, colour Doppler can be helpful to identify and avoid these vessels.

Amnioinfusion

Amnioinfusion involves the introduction of fluid into the amniotic cavity because of severe oligohydramnios, but we will not consider amnioinfusion during labour in this chapter. Before labour, it is currently used as a diagnostic procedure that can help to establish the cause of severe oligohydramnios. Amnioinfusion helps ultrasound imaging; it may provide a sample for further investigation (Gembruch & Hansmann, 1988; Fisk *et al.*, 1991), while dye injection can help diagnose ruptured membranes.

Even with severe oligohydramnios, careful ultrasound and colour Doppler imaging will usually identify a pool of amniotic fluid around loops of cord. Ultrasound-guided needling of this area may obtain blood from the cord that can be used for diagnostic tests, but if amniotic fluid is aspirated the operator is sure the tip is placed correctly. If nothing is obtained, great care must be taken to avoid injection of fluid into the cord and thus tamponade; delicate movement of the needle, however, should allow it to be drawn into the amniotic cavity. If no amniotic fluid is present at all, an injection of 1–2 ml of normal saline while visualising the needle tip may help. The needle is attached to plastic tubing, a three-way tap and a 50 ml syringe, and a warm sterile physiological solution such as normal saline or Hartmann's is infused. Care should be taken to avoid the injection of air bubbles which makes subsequent imaging difficult. The volume infused is the minimum required to make the diagnosis and depends on gestational age but is usually about 200–400 ml (Sepulveda et al., 1994). Indigocarmine (0.5 ml 0.8% diluted 1:20) can be added to the fluid in order to reveal ruptured membranes by pad checks. If the patient continues with the pregnancy, oligohydramnios will usually return in 0.5–2 weeks and a single procedure is unlikely to have any significant therapeutic effect on lung development (Chapter 13).

Intraperitoneal or thoracic infusion

Following the observation that intra-abdominal organs are clearly visualized when a fetus has ascites, intra-peritoneal saline injection has been used occasionally to facilitate ultrasonic visualization. For example, un-equivocal demonstration of renal agenesis might in-fluence management (Nicolini et al., 1989b). The needle is inserted into the fetal intraperitoneal cavity by ultrasound-guided needling. After checking that the saline infusion is entering the peritoneal cavity and not distending the fetal gut, enough is given to create signifi-cant ascites. Scanning 30 minutes after the procedure provides good quality imaging as the fluid tracks around and separates the different tissue layers. Occasionally this technique is also useful to distinguish cystic adenomatoid malformation of the lung from diaphragmatic hernia.

Fetal transfusion

Fetal anaemia or thrombocytopenia can be treated by transfusion with blood or platelets. These procedures

are dealt with more fully in Chapters 10 and 11, although their technical aspects are summarized below.

Intravascular transfusion

The procedure of intravascular transfusion (IVT) is the same for blood, platelet or drug infusion (Rodeck et al., 1985; Bang et al., 1982; Nicolaides et al., 1986b). Intra-vascular access is achieved as described for FBS. Having aspirated blood, the tip of the needle is kept still and observed continuously within the sampling site. If blood or platelets are to be used fresh antigen-negative, packed, irradiated, cytomegalovirus- and HIV-negative products compatible with the mother are infused with a 5–10 ml syringe using a three-way tap to avoid injecting air bubbles. Blood products are packed to reduce the volume transfused, typically blood to a haematocrit of 70–80%.

Transfusion results in turbulence, which can be seen in the vessel and is monitored during the procedure. The fetal heart rate is monitored intermittently either by arterial pulsation on colour Doppler, or by visualization of the fetal heart. The transfusion must be stopped immediately should flow not be seen or the heart rate changes significantly, because if the needle is displaced and fluid transfused into Wharton's jelly a 'haematoma' will develop. This can occlude blood flow and lead to fetal death. For the same reason, if the pressure on the syringe required to maintain the transfusion suddenly becomes greater, it is wise to stop, disconnect the trans-fusion tubing and check that blood can be aspirated through the needle with a syringe. If not, the needle should be rotated or slightly repositioned until this is achieved. The rate the transfusion is given is usually as fast as can be passed through the needle without causing disturbance to the heart rate. If tachy- or bradycardia develops, the transfusion should be stopped until this corrects and the transfusion then restarted at a slower rate.

The teamwork, clinical setting and counselling aspects described earlier are especially important for the safety of this procedure. The operator must stay very still and vigilant and the assistant must be capable of under-taking all other aspects of the transfusion. A third skilled person is required to receive and process the samples, calculate the volume of transfusion required and be available to support the patient. It is vital to have the patient's co-operation and she should be as comfortable as possible to help her stay very still.

The volume of blood or platelets required to correct the deficit is derived from nomograms constructed from gestational age and thus feto-placental blood volume, the initial fetal measurement and past experience (Chapters 10 and 11). After giving the predicted volume a post-transfusion measurement should be made and the transfusion continued if necessary.

Intraperitoneal transfusion

Although intraperitoneal transfusion (IPT) was the first example of successful fetal therapy, it has been replaced as the route of choice for transfusion by intravascular procedures, as these are safer, more quickly effective, more easily monitored and give more accurate information on the need for transfusion. Nevertheless, IPT is considerably easier and may still be used when access to the fetal circulation is difficult, for example at early gestational ages. IPT also has a role in combination with IVT to increase the total volume administered, as discussed in Chapter 10.

The techniques involves ultrasound-guided insertion of a needle into the fetal peritoneal cavity between the umbilicus and the bladder, as for intraperitoneal saline infusion, and slow injection of blood as previously described for IVT. At the beginning of the transfusion, the tip of the needle and the fetal abdomen should be carefully inspected to ensure ascites is produced and the transfusion is not distending the fetal gut or bladder. The fetal heart rate should be observed repeatedly during the transfusion and if a sustained abnormality occurs this may be caused by venous obstruction from increased intra-abdominal pressure (Nicolini *et al.*, 1989c); reaspiration in this event is sometimes associated with recovery.

Complications and risks

Alloimmunized patients can be expected to have an increase in the amount of antibody and thus disease severity if the placenta is transgressed. However, with repeated transfusion, the blood in the fetal circulation becomes antigen negative so this rise is not so important immediately but may have significant adverse effects on future pregnancies. The survival rates for severely affected fetuses requiring transfusion have increased to

78–95% (Nicolaides *et al.*, 1986b; Poissonier *et al.*, 1989; Nicolini *et al.*, 1989a). However, many of the fetuses who do not survive die as a result of the procedure-related complications already described.

Drainage procedures

Needle aspiration

Fluid collections can cause dilatation and damage to both the primary organ and the adjacent structures. Decompression may prevent secondary damage until spontaneous resolution or delivery and definitive surgery can occur. Aspiration of fluid-filled cysts using ultrasound-guided needling provides temporary relief while awaiting a karyotype result. However, almost always the fluid reaccumulates and either the procedures have to be repeated regularly or a shunting procedure used.

Shunting

The placement of a plastic tube to provide a shunt from the fetus to the amniotic fluid is also an outpatient ultrasound-guided procedure, but maternal sedation is often needed. There is a case for prophylactic antibiotics because a foreign body is being left in the uterus. The Rodeck catheter of London (Rodeck *et al.*, 1988) (Fig. 2.3) or the Harrison catheter of San Francisco are most commonly used, the latter having an external curl at a right angle to sit flat on the fetal exterior.

A cannula with a trochar is introduced transabdominally into the amniotic cavity and then through the antero-lateral aspect of the fetus. The tip of the cannula should reach the centre of the fluid collection or cyst to be drained. The trochar is then removed and a double 'pigtail' plastic catheter with radio-opaque ends inserted into the cannula. Care must be taken to avoid kinking the metal wire within the catheter or it may not pass through the cannula. When the catheter has been fully inserted, the wire within the catheter is withdrawn and fluid should start to flow out. It is important to loose as little fluid from within the obstructed system as possible since this provides the space into which the catheter can be passed. If too much fluid is lost it is possible to distend the cyst again by instillation of saline. The short introducer is then used to push the catheter down the cannula so the first part passes into the fetal chest and the end

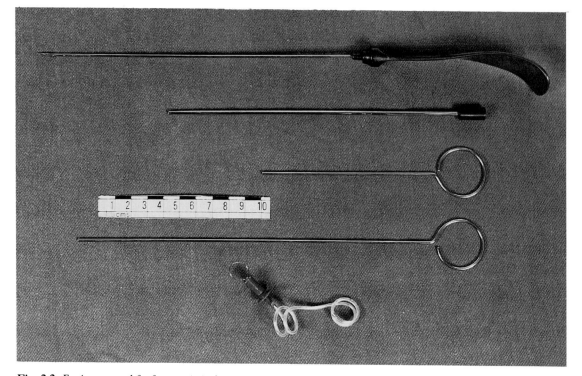

Fig. 2.3 *Equipment used for feto-amniotic shunting. The sharp introducer is shown at the top which is placed inside the trochar below for insertion into the uterus. The plastic catheter is pushed out of the trochar as shown in Fig. 2.4 by the pusher rods, the long one for the intra-amniotic portion.*

curls up inside. The introducer must be placed onto the end of the catheter with care because if it is pushed into the side of the catheter and distorts its shape the catheter may block in the cannula. Having achieved good placement of the distal end in the chest, the cannula is pulled back into the amniotic fluid. In the presence of severe oligohydramnios, amnioinfusion may be required first to give space for the catheter outside the fetus. The long introducer is then used to push the rest of the catheter out of the cannula so the proximal end will then curl in the amniotic fluid (Fig. 2.4). Monitoring by serial scans will reveal if the obstruction remains decompressed, whether the normal tissue expands and if secondary effects such as hydrops resolve.

Drainage procedures have been used for pathology in the chest and renal tract, as detailed in Chapters 16 and 17. Shunt placement in the bladder is more difficult than in the chest because of the absence of ribs. Also the severe oligohydramnios often present makes scanning and intra-amniotic deposition of the catheter difficult, so that preliminary amnioinfusion is usually required. Unless the bladder is extremely distended, the lack of rigidity may make insertion of the shunt impossible so it is important to loose as little urine from the bladder as possible during the procedure. Once the shunt is sited, ultrasound monitoring is important to detect problems of displacement or blockage.

Ventriculo-amniotic shunts have also been done using ultrasound-guided needling through the parietal bone into the lateral ventricle. A specially designed shunt with a one-way valve allowing cerebro-spinal fluid out of the brain but preventing back-flow of amniotic fluid has been developed. However, experience with this device was followed by the delivery of such severely handicapped children that its use has been abandoned (Chapter 19).

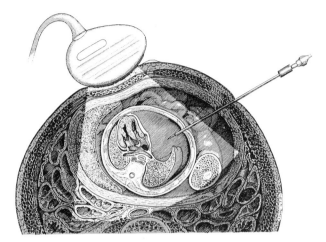
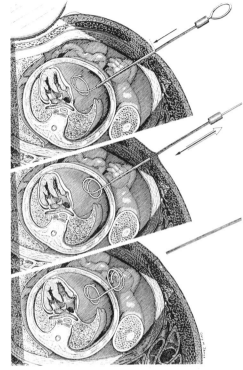

Fig. 2.4 *A drawing illustrating how feto-amniotic shunting is undertaken. The trochar is inserted into the fetal space to be drained (in this case the chest) (a) and one end of the of the plastic catheter is pushed out with the shorter probe to curl up within the fetal thorax (b). The trochar is then withdrawn into the amniotic cavity (c) while the catheter is kept still by downward pressure with the longer probe, the latter then being used to pass the catheter completely out of the trochar (d) so that the other end curls up within the amniotic fluid.*

Concluson

A wide range of invasive procedures have been described which provide access for many diagnostic and therapeutic possibilities, as described in more detail in the other sections of this book. They must not be performed in isolation from the concepts and practice of fetal medicine but, instead, are only effective when combined with good non-invasive investigation. Even apparently simple invasive procedures should be undertaken in tertiary centres with experience. Sometimes the greatest skill is to recognize when not to undertake the procedures described in this chapter.

References

Bang, J. (1983). Intrauterine needle diagnosis. In: *Interventional Ultrasound*, ed. J. Bang, pp. 122–8. Copenhagen: Munksgaard.

Bang, J., Bock, J. E. & Trolle, D. (1982). Ultrasound-guided fetal intravascular transfusion for severe rhesus haemolytic disease. *British Medical Journal*, 284, 373–4.

Barker, D., Osmond, C., Golding, J., Kuh, D. & Wadsworth, M. (1989). Growth *in utero*, blood pressure in childhood and adult life, and mortality from cardiovascular disease. *British Medical Journal*, 298, 564–7.

Benacerraf, B., Baras, V. A., Saltzman, D. H., Grene, M. F., Penso, C. A. & Frigoletto, F. D. (1987). Acute fetal distress associated with percutaneous umbilical blood sampling. *American Journal of Obstetrics and Gynecology*, 156, 1218–20.

Bernstein, H. H., Chitkara, U., Plosker, H., Gettes, M. & Berkowitz, R. L. (1988). Use of atracium besylate to arrest fetal activity during intrauterine intravascular transfusions. *Obstetrics and Gynecology*, 72, 813–16.

Bevis, D. C. A. (1952). The antenatal prediction of haemolytic disease of the newborn. *Lancet*, 1, 395.

Canadian Collaborative CVS-Amniocentesis Clinical Trial Group (1989). Multicentre randomized clinical trial of chorionic villus sampling and amniocentesis. *Lancet*, i, 1–6.

Chudleigh, P. & Pearce, J. M. (1992). Invasive procedures performed under ultrasound guidance: twin amniocentesis. In: *Obstetric Ultrasound*, 2nd edn, ed. S. Campbell, pp. 174–5. London: Churchill Livingstone.

Dampure, C. J., Jennnings, P. J., Penketh, R. J., Wise, P. J. & Rodeck, C. H. (1989). Fetal liver alanine: glycoxalate aminotransferase and the prenatal diagnosis of primary hyperoxaluria type 1. *Prenatal Diagnosis*, 9, 271–81.

de Crespigny, L. C. H. & Robinson, H. P. (1986). Amniocentesis: a comparison of 'monitored' versus 'blind' needle insertion techniques. *Australian and New Zealand Journal of Obstetrics and Gynaecology*, 26, 124–8.

de Crespigny, L. C. H., Robinson, H. P., Ross, A. W. & Quinn, M. (1985b) Curarisation of fetus for intrauterine procedures. *Lancet*, i, 1164.

de Crespigny, L. C. H., Robinson, H. P., Quinn, M., Doyle, L., Ross, A. & Cauchi, M. (1985a). Ultrasound guided fetal blood transfusions for severe red cell isoimmunisation. *Obstetrics and Gynecology*, 66, 529–32.

Dumez, Y., Oury, J. & Duchetel, F. (1988). Embryoscopy and congenital malformations. In *Proceedings of the International Conference on Chorionic Villus Sampling and Early Prenatal Diagnosis*, Athens, Greece.

Fisk, N. M. & Rodeck, C. H. (1990). Detection of congenital anomalies of the renal and urinary tract by ultrasound. In *Modern Antenatal Care of the Fetus*, ed. G. V. Chamberlain, pp. 359–88, Oxford: Blackwell Scientific.

Fisk, N. M., Ronderos-Dumit, D., Soliani, A., Nicolini, U., Vaughan, J. & Rodeck, C. H. (1991). Diagnostic and therapeutic transabdominal amnioinfusion in oligohydramnios. *Obstetrics and Gynecology*, 78, 270–8.

Gembruch, U. & Hansmann, M. (1988). Artificial instillation of amniotic fluid as a new technique for the diagnostic evaluation of cases of oligohydramnios. *Prenatal Diagnosis*, 8, 33–45.

Ghidini, A., Sepulveda, W., Lockwood, C. J. & Romero, R. (1993). Complications of fetal blood sampling. *American Journal of Obstetrics and Gynecology*, 168, 1339–43.

Giannakoulopoulos, H., Sepulveda, W., Kourtis, P., Glover, V. & Fisk, N. M. (1994). Fetal plasma cortisol and fl-endorphin response to intrauterine needling. *Lancet*, 344, 77–81.

Gilbert, W. M., Stanley, E. D., Kaplan, C., Pretorius, D., Merritt, A. & Benirschke, K. (1991). Morbidity associated with prenatal disruption of the dividing membrane in twin gestations. *Obstetrics and Gynecology*, 78, 623–30.

Golbus, M. S., Filly, R. A., Callen, P. W., Glick, P. L., Harrison, M. R. & Anderson, R. L. (1985). Fetal urinary tract obstruction: management and selection for treatment. *Seminars in Perinatology*, 9, 91.

Golbus, M. S., Simpson, T. J., Koresawa, M., Appelman, Z. & Alpers, C. E. (1988). The prenatal determination of glucose-6-phosphatase activity by fetal liver biopsy. *Prenatal Diagnosis*, 8, 401–4.

Hansmann, M., Gembruch, U., Bald, R., Manz, M., & Redel, A. (1991). Fetal tachy-arrhythmias: transplacental and direct treatment of the fetus – a report of 60 cases. *Ultrasound in Obstetrics and Gynecology*, 1, 162–70.

Hobbins, J. C. & Mahoney, M. J. (1974). *In utero* diagnosis of hemoglobinopathies. *New England Journal of Medicine*, 290, 1065–7.

Hunter, A. G. W. (1987). Neonatal lung function following mid-trimester amniocentesis. *Prenatal Diagnosis*, 7, 431–41.

Jackson, L. G., Zachary, M., Fowler, S. E., Desnick, R. J., Golbus, R. S., Ledbetter, D. H., Mahoney, M. J., Pergament, E., Simpson, J. L., Black, S., Wapner, R. J. & the US National Institute of Child Health and Human Development Chorion Villus Sampling and Amniocentesis Study Group (1992). A randomized comparison of transcervical and transabdominal chorionic villus sampling. *New England Journal of Medicine*, 327, 594–8.

Jauniaux , E., Donner, C., Simon, P., Vanesse, M., Hustin, J. & Rodesch, F. (1989). Pathological aspects of the umbilical cord after percutaneous umbilical blood sampling. *Obstetrics and Gynecology*, 73, 215–18.

Jeanty, P., Shah, D. & Roussis, P. (1990). Single-needle insertion in twin amniocentesis. *Journal of Ultrasound in Medicine*, 9, 511–17.

Mahoney, B. S., Petty, C. N., Nyberg, D. A., Luthy, D. A., Hickok, D. E. & Hirsch, J. H. (1990). The 'stuck twin' phenomenon: ultrasonographic findings, pregnancy outcome, and management with serial amniocenteses. *American Journal of Obstetrics and Gynecology*, 163, 1513–22.

Maxwell, D., Johnson, P., Hurley, P., Neales, K., Allan, L. & Knott, P. (1991). Fetal blood sampling and pregnancy loss in relation to indication. *British Journal of Obstetrics and Gynaecology*, 98, 892–7.

Meagher, S. E. & Fisk, N. M. (1994). Hydramnios, Oligohydramnios. In *High Risk Pregnancy, Management Options*, ed. D. K. James, P. J. Steer, C. P. Weiner & B. Gonik, pp. 827–40. London: W.B. Saunders.

Medical Research Council (1978). An assessment of the hazards of amniocentesis. *British Journal of Obstetrics and Gynaecology*, 85 (suppl), 1–41.

Medical Research Council European Trial of chorion villus sampling (1991). MRC working party on the evaluation of chorion villus sampling. *Lancet*, 337, 1491–9.

Moise, K. J., Deter, R. L., Kishorn, B., Adam., K., Patton, D. E. & Carpenter, R. J. (1989). Intravenous pancuronium bromide for fetal neuromuscular blockade during intrauterine transfusion for red cell alloimmunization. *Obstetrics and Gynecology*, 74, 905–8.

NICHD: National Institute of Child Health and Human Development National Registry for Amniocentesis Study Group (1976). Amniocentesis for prenatal diagnosis: safety and accuracy. *Journal of American Medical Association*, 236, 1471–76.

Nicolaides, K., Brizot, M. L., Patel, F. & Snijders, R. (1994). Comparison of chorionic villus sampling and amniocentesis for fetal karyotyping at 10–13 weeks' gestation. *Lancet*, 8, 435–9.

Nicolaides, K. H., Campbell, S., Bradley, R. J., Bilardo, C. M., Soothill, P. W. & Gibb, D. (1987). Maternal oxygen therapy for intrauterine growth retardation. *Lancet*, i, 942–5.

Nicolaides, K. H., Soothill, P. W., Rodeck, C. H. & Campbell, S. (1986a). Ultrasound-guided sampling of umbilical cord and placental blood to assess fetal wellbeing. *Lancet*, i, 1065–7.

Nicolaides, K. H., Soothill, P. W., Rodeck, C. H. & Clewell, W. (1986b). Rh disease: intravascular fetal blood transfusion by cordocentesis. *Fetal Therapy*, 1, 185–92.

Nicolini, U., Kochenouer, N. K., Greco, P., Letsky, E. & Rodeck, C. H. (1989a). When to perform the next intrauterine transfusion in patients with Rh alloimmunisation: combined intravascular and intraperitoneal transfusion allows longer intervals. *Fetal Therapy*, 4, 14–20.

Nicolini, U. & Monni, G. (1990). Intestinal obstruction in babies exposed *in utero* to methylene blue. *Lancet*, 336, 1258–9.

Nicolini, U., Nicolaidis, P., Fisk, N. M., Tannirandorn, Y. & Rodeck, C. H. (1990). Fetal blood sampling from the intrahepatic vein: analysis of safety and clinical experience with 214 procedures. *Obstetrics and Gynecology*, 76, 47–53.

Nicolini, U., Santolaya, J., Hubinont, C., Fisk, N. M., Maxwell, D. & Rodeck, C. H. (1989b). Visualisation of fetal intra-abdominal organs in second trimester severe oligohydramnios by intraperitoneal infusion. *Prenatal Diagnosis*, 9, 191–4.

Nicolini, U., Talbert, D. G., Fisk, N. M. & Rodeck, C. H. (1989c). Pathophysiology of pressure changes during intrauterine transfusion. *American Journal of Obstetrics and Gynecology*, 160, 1139–45.

Piceni Sereni, L., Bachmann, C., Pfister, U., Buscaglia, M. & Nicolini, U. (1988). Prenatal diagnosis of carbamoyl-phosphate synthetase deficiency by fetal liver biopsy. *Prenatal Diagnosis*, 8, 307.

Poissonnier, M. H., Brossard, Y., Demedeiros, N., Vassileva, J., Parnet, F., Larsen, M., Gosset, M., Chavinie, J. & Hechet, J. (1989). Two hundred intrauterine exchange transfusions in severe blood incompatibilities. *American Journal of Obstetrics and Gynecology*, 161, 709–13.

Queenan, J. T. & Gadow, E. C. (1970). Polyhydramnios: chronic versus acute. *American Journal of Obstetrics and Gynecology*, 108, 349–55.

Quintero, R., Abuhamad, A., Hobbins, J. C. & Mahoney, M. J. (1993a). Transabdominal thin-gauge embryo-fetoscopy: a technique for early prenatal diagnosis and its use in the diagnosis of case of Meckel–Gruber syndrome. *American Journal of Obstetrics and Gynecology*, 168, 1552–7.

Quintero, R.A., Puder, K. S., Cottom, D. B. (1993b). Embryoscopy and fetoscopy. In *Prenatal Diagnosis: Present and Future Perspectives. Obstetrics and Gynecology Clinics of North America*, vol. 20, pp. 563–81.

Quintero, R. A., Romero, R., Johnson, M. P., Smith, C., Arias, F., Guevara-Zuloaga, F., Cotton, D. B. & Evans, M. I. (1995). In-utero percutaneous cystoscopy in the management of fetal lower obstructive uropathy. *Lancet*, 346, 537–40.

Rayburn, W. F. (1991). Fetal drug therapy: an overview of selected conditions. *Obstetrics and Gynecology Survey*, 47, 1–9.

Rhoads, G. G., Jackson, L. G., Schlesselman, S. E., de la Cruz, F. F., Desnick, R. J., Golbus, M. S.,

Ledbetter, D. H., Lubs, H. A., Mahoney, M. J., Pergament, J. L., Simpson, J. L., Carpenter, R. J., Elias, S., Ginsberg, N. A., Goldberg, J. D., Hobbins, J. C., Lynch, L., Shiongo, P. H., Wapner, R. J. & Zachary, J. M. (1989). The safety and efficacy of chorionic villus sampling for early prenatal diagnosis of cytogenetic abnormality. *New England Journal of Medicine*, 320, 609–14.

Robertson, E. G., Brown, A., Ellis, M. I. & Walker, W. (1976). Intrauterine transfusion in the management of severe rhesus isoimmunisation. *British Journal of Obstetrics and Gynaecology*, 83, 694–7.

Rodeck, C. H. (1980). Fetoscopy guided by real time ultrasound for pure fetal blood samples, fetal skin sample and examination of the fetus *in utero*. *British Journal of Obstetrics and Gynaecology*, 87, 449–56.

Rodeck, C. H. & Campbell, S. (1978). Sampling pure fetal blood by fetoscopy in second trimester of pregnancy. *British Medical Journal*, ii, 728–30.

Rodeck, C. H., Fisk, N. M., Fraser, D. E. & Nicolini, U. (1988). Long-term *in utero* drainage of fetal hydrothorax. *New England Journal of Medicine*, 319, 1135–8.

Rodeck, C.H., Holman, C.A., Karnicki, J., Kemp, J., Whitmore, D.N. & Austin, M.A. (1985). Direct intravascular fetal blood transfusion by fetoscopy in severe rhesus isoimmunisation. *Lancet*, i, 625–7.

Rodeck, C. H., Patrick, A. D., Pembrey, M. E., Tzannatos, C. & Whitfield, A. E. (1982). Fetal liver biopsy for prenatal diagnosis of ornithine carbamyl transferase deficiency. *Lancet*, ii, 297–9.

Romero, R., Jeanty, P., Reece, E. A., Grannum, P., Bracken, M., Berkowitz, R. & Hobbins, J. C. (1985) Sonographically monitored amniocentesis to decrease intraperitoneal complications. *Obstetrics and Gynecology*, 65, 426–30.

Saunders, N. J., Snijders, R. M. & Nicolaides, K. H. (1992). Therapeutic amniocentesis in twin-twin transfusion syndrome appearing in the second trimester of pregnancy. *American Journal of Obstetrics and Gynecology*, 166, 820–4.

Sepulveda, W., Flack, N. J. & Fisk, N. M. (1994). Direct volume measurement at midtrimester amnioinfusion in relation to ultrasonographic indexes of amniotic fluid volume. *American Journal of Obstetrics and Gynecology*, 170, 1160–3.

Smidt-Jensen, S. & Philip, J. (1991). Comparison of transabdominal and transcervical CVS and amnio-centesis: sampling success and risk. *Prenatal Diagnosis*, 11, 529–37.

Soothill, P. W. (1994). Fetal blood sampling before labor. In *High Risk Pregnancy, Management Options*, ed. D. K. James, P. J. Steer, C. P. Weiner & B. Gonik, pp. 745–55, London: W. B. Saunders.

Tabor, A., Philip, J., Madsen, M., Obel, E. B. & Norgaard-Pedersen, B. (1986). Randomized controlled trial of genetic amniocentesis in 4606 low risk women. *Lancet*, i, 1287–93.

Tietung Hospital. Department of Obstetrics and Gynecology of Anshan Iron and Steel Co. Anshan China. (1975). Fetal sex prediction by sex chromatin of chorionic villi cells during early pregnancy. *Journal of Chinese Medicine*, 1, 117.

Ville Y., Hyett J., Hecher K. & Nicolaides K. H. (1995) Preliminary experience with endoscopic lazer surgery for severe twin-to-twin transfusion syndrome. *New England Journal of Medicine*, 332, 224–7.

Weiner, C. P. (1987). Cordocentesis for diagnostic indications: two years' experience. *Obstetrics and Gynecology*, 70, 664–8.

Westgren, M., Selbing, A. & Stangenberg, M. (1988). Fetal intracardiac transfusions in patients with severe rhesus isoimmunisation. *British Medical Journal*, 296, 885–6.

3 Open fetal surgery

HENRY E. RICE AND MICHAEL R. HARRISON

Introduction

Although most malformations diagnosed prenatally are best managed after birth, a few severe anomalies may be better treated by correction before birth. Extensive experimental work in animals and new innovative technologies have supported the recent growth of human fetal surgery. At present, only a few life-threatening malformations have been successfully corrected. Several major obstacles exist, including control of preterm labour and lack of chronic intravascular access to the fetus. Further research on the pathophysiology of fetal anomalies and development of less invasive methods of intervention should lead to the successful treatment of more fetal disorders.

Continued major advancements in prenatal diagnosis have led to new approaches to prenatal therapy. Routine obstetrical sonography has enabled us to 'see' the fetus in the womb and diagnose fetal anatomic malformations before irreversible organ damage can occur. With the use of this knowledge, we have gained insight into the natural history of severe fetal disorders and have begun to consider whether some diseases are better treated before birth.

In the late 1970s, we began an extensive research program at the Fetal Treatment Center, University of California, San Francisco (UCSF) to examine prenatal anomalies induced experimentally in animal models. The natural history of these anomalies in humans was determined by longitudinal surveys of human fetuses, and selection criteria for potential prenatal intervention were developed (Harrison, Golbus & Filly, 1981). Later research began to define the anesthetic, tocolytic, and surgical techniques for hysterotomy and fetal surgery

(Harrison & Adzick, 1991; Longaker *et al.*, 1991). Recently, more fundamental research has been devoted to understanding the developmental pathophysiology of several fetal anomalies and the maternal and fetal responses to fetal surgery.

Although only a few defects are amenable to surgical correction at present, the enterprise of fetal surgery has produced some unexpected spin-offs that have widespread interest. For paediatricians and neonatologists, the developmental pathology and abnormal function of many newborn conditions have been clarified by following the natural history of the disease *in utero*. For example, diseases such as diaphragmatic hernia, cystic adenomatoid malformation and cystic hygroma have a worse outcome if the defect is detected in a fetus than if the disease is diagnosed after birth, a phenomenon termed 'hidden mortality'. For obstetricians and perinatologists, many formidable technical problems in obtaining access to a fetus have been solved. Techniques for opening and closing a gravid uterus without disrupting the pregnancy or jeopardizing a mother's health or reproductive potential have been developed (Longaker *et al.*, 1991). More recently, the development of endoscopic techniques allows fetal manipulation without hysterotomy, potentially expanding the indications for fetal intervention (Estes *et al.*, 1992a). For the physiologist and obstetrician, an intense effort to solve the problem of labour after hysterotomy for fetal surgery has yielded new insights into the molecular mediators of myometrial relaxation and new approaches to the treatment of preterm labour using nitric oxide donors (Jennings, MacGillivray & Harrison, 1993b).

Many innovative techniques have been developed especially for fetal surgery, each of which has a wide-ranging impact. An absorbable stapling device for control of bleeding during the hysterotomy has been applied to routine caesarean sections. Sophisticated radiotelemetric monitoring of the fetal electrocardiogram and uterine contractions may prove useful in managing other high-risk pregnancies. New approaches to long-term access to the fetal vasculature may lead to improved care for fetuses with many different disorders.

Experimental research on fetal surgery has yielded advances in understanding fetal biology with implications beyond fetal therapy. An example of this was the observation that the fetus heals without scar formation. This has provided new insight into the natural history of wound healing and stimulated efforts to mimic the fetal process to inhibit scar formation (Adzick & Longaker, 1992).

Maternal–fetal management

Fetal surgery requires caring for two patients, the mother and the fetus; the focus on this 'maternal–fetal unit' is an essential approach to safe and effective care. Maternal safety is paramount with the optimal management of both the mother and fetus requiring perioperative maternal support in an intensive care setting (Fig. 3.1). Maternal arterial blood pressure, central venous pressure, urine output, and transcutaneous oxygen saturation are continuously monitored. More invasive measurement of maternal cardiac output is performed as necessary to ensure optimal maternal haemodynamic function.

Monitoring of the fetus is performed by tocodynomometry, ultrasonography and echocardiography. Fetal cardiac monitoring has been greatly improved by the development of an implanted radiotelemeter that continuously transmits the fetal electrocardiogram to a radio antenna and converts it to a real-time signal which is displayed at a bedside computer (Jennings et al., 1992; 1993a). Recently this telemeter has been modified to measure continuously and transmit the intrauterine pressure, and it has proved to be a very sensitive method to detect preterm contractions.

Managing preterm labour has proven to be the Achilles' heel of fetal surgery. Our tocolytic regimens have included preoperative indomethacin, halogenated inhalational agents for intraoperative anaesthesia and tocolysis, and postoperative betamimetics and magnesium sulphate; all of these have proved less than satisfactory. The depth of anaesthesia required to achieve intraoperative uterine relaxation can produce fetal and maternal myocardial depression and affect placental perfusion (Sabik, Assad & Hanley, 1993). Indomethacin can constrict the fetal ductus arteriosus, producing right-sided heart failure (Besinger & Niebyl, 1990). All tocolytics can contribute to maternal pulmonary oedema, while fluid restriction to avoid pulmonary oedema often compromises placental blood flow thereby worsening preterm labour (Besinger et al., 1990). The search for less toxic tocolytics has led to the experimental finding that exogenous nitric oxide can ablate preterm labour induced by hysterotomy in monkeys (Jennings et al., 1993b). Ongoing research in rats, sheep and monkeys is consistent with the hypothesis that nitric oxide is a fundamental mediator of preterm labour and myometrial relaxation. This work has suggested that the pharmacologic manipulation of nitric oxide may provide an effective treatment of preterm labour. We are pursuing the use of the nitric oxide donor nitroglycerine for perioperative tocolysis and are hopeful that this approach will reduce the major obstacle to successful fetal surgery, preterm labour.

The technical aspects of the hysterotomy procedure have evolved over 15 years of experimental and clinical work (Harrison & Longaker, 1990; Harrison & Adzick, 1993). The uterus is exposed though a low transverse abdominal incision. Intraoperative sonography is used to delineate the fetal position and placental location. The uterus is opened with a specially developed stapler that is fast, haemostatic and seals the amnion and chorion to the myometrium, limiting the risk of dissection of the fetal membranes (Adzick et al., 1985). Specially designed compression clamps are placed around the incision, and the fetus and uterus are continually bathed in warm Ringer's lactate solution. A miniaturized pulse oximeter is wrapped around the fetal palm. The radiotelemetric monitor is implanted subcutaneously on the fetal flank or back and transmits the fetal heart rate and intrauterine pressure both intraoperatively and postoperatively (Jennings et al., 1993a). The appropriate fetal part is exposed and the defect repaired. After repair, the fetus is returned to the uterus, the staples are incised from the

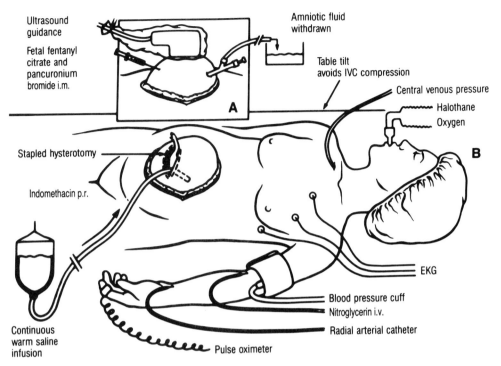

Ultrasound
guidance

Fetal fentanyl
citrate and
pancuronium
bromide i.m.

Amniotic fluid
withdrawn

Table tilt
avoids IVC compression

Central venous pressure

Halothane

Oxygen

A

B

Stapled hysterotomy

Indomethacin p.r.

EKG

Blood pressure cuff

Nitroglycerin i.v.

Radial arterial catheter

Continuous
warm saline
infusion

Pulse oximeter

Fig. 3.1 *Technical aspects of fetal surgery. With the maternal abdomen open, ultrasonography is used to localize the placenta and draw a fetal blood specimen before some amniotic fluid is withdrawn. The uterus is opened away from the placenta, and only the pertinent fetal anatomy exposed. Maternal monitoring is shown; the fetus is monitored by radiotelemetry. (Reprinted with permission from Adzick & Harrison, 1994.)*

uterine edge, and the hysterotomy is closed in layers with fibrin glue to seal the membranes (Fig. 3.2). Warm Ringer's lactate solution with broad-spectrum antibiotics is used to replenish the amniotic fluid volume. The maternal skin is closed with subcuticular sutures and a transparent dressing is placed so that sonography can be performed through the maternal abdomen postoperatively.

After the patient emerges from anaesthesia, the monitoring of maternal haemodynamics, fetal condition, and uterine contractions continues in the intensive care unit. Parenteral narcotics are used, usually in the form of patient-controlled analgesia, to assist with postoperative pain control. Tocolytics are administered and their effect on uterine irritability and contractions closely monitored. When labour is controlled and both the mother and fetus are stabilized, usually after two to three days, the mother is transferred to the obstetrical ward where monitoring continues until discharge, usually after a week. Fetal sonograms are performed frequently in the immediate postoperative period then weekly after discharge. Outpatient tocolysis is provided with subcutaneous terbutaline via a portable pump. Caesarean section is undertaken when there is rupture of membranes or when preterm labour is unresponsive to tocolysis. In our experience, one of these two events is likely to occur prior to 36 completed weeks of gestation.

The learning curve in fetal surgery remains steep. Our group and others continue to develop and test techniques in maternal and fetal anaesthesia, surgical procedures, fetal and uterine monitoring, and fetal resuscitation. Many challenges remain, including the need for reliable long-term fetal intravascular access for blood sampling and medication infusion, methods for maternal and fetal haemodynamic assessment, less invasive methods of intervention and better control of preterm labour.

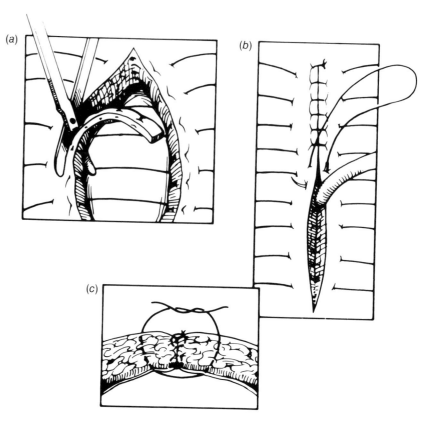

Fig. 3.2 *Uterine closure. (a) Full-thickness stay sutures are placed first, then the staple line is excised to allow muscle-to-muscle apposition. An assistant applies upward traction to the stay sutures in order to minimize bleeding during and after the staple removal. (b) Uterus is closed in two layers of running sutures, and a soft rubber catheter is inserted before completing the first layer to place warm saline solution and antibiotics in the amniotic cavity. (c) The stay sutures are tied last. (Reprinted with permission from Adzick and Harrison, 1994.)*

Risks and benefits

Fetal therapy raises complex issues regarding the risks and benefits for both the fetus and mother. For the fetus, the risk of the procedure is weighed against the benefit of correcting a fatal or debilitating defect. For the mother, the risks and benefits are more difficult to assess. Most fetal malformations do not directly threaten the mother's health, yet she must bear the risks and discomfort from the procedure. She may choose to aid her unborn fetus and thereby alleviate her own burden in raising a child with a severe malformation. The risk of hysterotomy and open fetal surgery is unknown but potentially formidable. In the 1960s, initial experience with surgical exposure of the fetus to catheterize fetal vessels for exchange transfusion was discouraging, and the procedure was quickly abandoned. In the 1980s, after extensive experimental work, newer surgical techniques and improved anaesthetic and tocolytic therapy were developed. For example, at the UCSF Fetal Treatment Center, we have performed more than 1600 procedures in fetal lambs and 400 procedures in fetal monkeys in the course of developing and refining techniques for maternal–fetal management (Harrison & Adzick, 1991). This experimental work has made possible the surgical exposure of more than 49 human fetuses for attempted correction of a variety of anatomical defects, as detailed in Table 3.1.

Because open fetal surgery has been attempted only rarely elsewhere, once each in Boston, Melbourne and Seoul, twice in Denver, and three times in Paris, the cases at UCSF provide the best data on maternal outcome. No maternal deaths have occurred, but our patients have experienced considerable morbidity, primarily related to preterm labour. Three patients developed pulmonary oedema as a result of tocolysis. Five required blood transfusions. The only infectious complications included one case of mild pseudo-

Table 3.1 *Experience with open fetal surgery in 49 patients managed at UCSF before 1993*

Variable	Median	Range
Maternal age (years)	26	18–43
Gestational age of fetus (weeks)	24	17–28
Operative time, total (min)	127	69–182
Blood loss (ml)	455	150–1400
Interval to delivery (weeks)	4	1–15
Gestational age of delivery (weeks)	28	22–36

Adapted from Harrison, 1993.

membranous colitis resulting from antibiotic therapy and one superficial wound infection. Leakage of amniotic fluid through the hysterotomy site in two patients required reoperation and secondary closure. Passage of amniotic fluid from the vagina occurred in three patients, presumably secondary to the dissection of fluid from the hysterotomy site to the cervix. Although not a complication of the operation, two patients have presented with the 'maternal mirror syndrome', a condition in which the mother has severe hypertension, proteinuria and pulmonary failure as a response to the presence of a hydropic fetus (Adzick, Harrison & Flake, 1993).

An important aspect of maternal safety is the effect of hysterotomy on a patient's ability to carry subsequent pregnancies. Because the midgestation hysterotomy is usually located in the upper uterine segment, there is a potential for disruption of the uterine eschar during labour. For this reason, the pregnancy in which fetal surgery is undertaken as well as all subsequent pregnancies should be delivered by caesarean section. In our series, two uterine dehiscences occurred in subsequent pregnancies (Table 3.1) (Longaker *et al.*, 1991). Uterine closure and neonatal outcome were excellent in both patients. The ability to carry and deliver subsequent pregnancies does not appear to be greatly jeopardized by fetal surgery. Although the majority of the fetal operations at our centre have taken place in the past three years, long-term follow-up from earlier patients reveals that 20 women have had normal children in subsequent pregnancies. Two of these women have experienced two subsequent uneventful pregnancies each. Seven patients with a previous history of infertility have either not conceived or had early miscarriages.

Anatomical malformations amenable to surgical correction

The only malformations that warrant consideration for surgical correction are those that interfere with fetal organ growth and development and that, if alleviated, would allow normal growth to proceed (Table 3.2). Open fetal surgery has been performed in human fetuses for diaphragmatic hernia, urinary obstruction, cystic adenomatoid malformation, sacrococcygeal teratoma, twin–twin transfusion syndrome and congenital heart block, as discussed in Chapters 18 and 19. The majority of the experience with open fetal surgery at UCSF has involved the fetus with diaphragmatic hernia (Adzick & Harrison, 1994).

Minimally invasive surgical techniques have changed the practice of surgery and are ideally suited for use in fetal surgery. Fetoscopic surgery may minimize the environmental exposure of the fetus and obviate the need for a full hysterotomy. We have developed fetoscopic techniques in fetal lambs and monkeys for *in utero* bladder decompression, pleural fluid decompression and cleft lip repair (Estes *et al.*, 1992a,b). The Detroit group has treated fetal hydrops from an acardiac twin by fetoscopic ligation of the umbilical cord (Quintero, Reich & Puder, 1994). *In utero* tracheal occlusion with fetoscopic guidance accelerates lung growth in fetal lambs and may be a safe method of limiting the pulmonary hypoplasia associated with congenital diaphragmatic hernia (Hedrick *et al.*, 1993). It is our hope that minimally invasive fetoscopic procedures will result in less uterine irritability and preterm labour, although this remains unproved at present. Several technical problems require experimental resolution before clinical application. The advantages and disadvantages of a gas environment with better visualization yet a greater risk for air embolism must be compared with a liquid environment. In a liquid media, better fetal haemostasis would be likely; however, visualization may be suboptimal. The possibility of fetal eye damage from bright

Table 3.2 *Fetal malformations that may be surgically corrected before birth: rationale for treatment*

Fetal defect	Effect on fetus	Likely result	Treatment
Life threatening			
Urinary obstruction	Hydronephrosis, lung hypoplasia	Renal, pulmonary failure	Percutaneous catheter placement, fetoscopic or open vesicostomy
Cystic adenomatoid malformation	Hydros, lung hypoplasia	Hydrops, fetal demise	Open lung lobectomy
Sacrococcygeal teratoma	Heart failure	Hydrops, fetal demise	Tumour resection, vascular occlusion[a]
Twin–twin transfusion	Vascular steal	Hydrops, fetal demise	Fetectomy, vascular isolation
Tracheal atresia or stenosis	Lung over-distension	Hydrops, fetal demise	Open or fetoscopic tracheostomy[a]
Not life threatening			
Myelomeningocele	Spinal cord damage	Paralysis, neurogenic bladder	Open or fetoscopic repair[a]
Cleft lip and palate	Facial defect	Persistent deformity	Open or fetoscopic repair
Metabolic or cellular			
Stem cell or enzyme defects	Haemoglobinopathy, immunodeficiency, storage disease	Anaemia, hydrops, infection, retardation	Fetal stem cell transplant, gene therapy[a]
Predictable neonatal organ failure	Organ failure	Organ failure	Tolerance induction by fetal stem cell transplantation

[a] Not yet attempted in human fetuses.
Adapted from Harrison 1993.

lights or lasers must be studied. Instruments must be miniaturized. If these techniques are successful, the list of anatomical conditions amenable to fetal surgery may be extended to encompass ventriculomegaly and meningomyelocele (Chapter 19).

Fetal intensive care will probably require chronic access to the fetal circulation to sample blood and allow for the infusion of fluids and medications. We have addressed this problem in the laboratory in both the sheep and primate model (Hedrick *et al.*, 1992; Rice *et al.*, 1993). Fetoscopic extra-amniotic catheterization of placental vessels has been successful and can be used to measure fetal blood pressure, sample fetal blood and infuse medications. These techniques may soon be applicable to human fetuses and may be useful for the chronic delivery of medications or specific cell lines to treat a variety of disorders.

Establishment of a fetal surgery centre

The steep learning curve derived from our experimental and clinical experience with fetal surgery has provided invaluable lessons regarding optimal maternal anaesthesia and uterine relaxation, hysterotomy and fetal exposure techniques, intraoperative fetal monitoring, and reliable methods for closure of amniotic membranes and the uterus. However, many challenges remain. Current issues include the need for better postoperative maternal–fetal monitoring, reliable long-term fetal intravascular access for fetal blood sampling and infusions, non-invasive maternal–fetal haemodynamic assessment, less invasive methods of intervention, including fetoscopy, and effective detection and treatment of preterm labour.

Because fetal surgery jeopardizes the pregnancy and entails potential risk to the mother and the fetus, fetal surgery should be pursued at centres committed to ongoing research concomitant with cautious clinical application. A fetal treatment centre requires the close collaboration of dedicated paediatric surgeons, perinatal obstetricians, ultrasonographers, echocardiographers, neonatologists, intensivists, geneticists, anaesthetists, neonatal and obstetric nurses, and a compassionate

coordinator (Fig. 3.3). The fetal treatment team should make a commitment to have this innovative therapy reviewed by uninvolved professional colleagues, including the local institutional review board, to publish all results, bad as well as good, and to avoid media reports until cases are peer reviewed.

Conclusion

The great promise of fetal therapy is that for some diseases the earliest possible intervention will produce the best possible result. After vigorous development in animals models, open fetal surgical techniques have been successfully applied in human pregnancies. Maternal morbidity remains low although the need for hysterotomy dictates delivery by caesarean section in the index and subsequent pregnancies. Preterm labour frequently

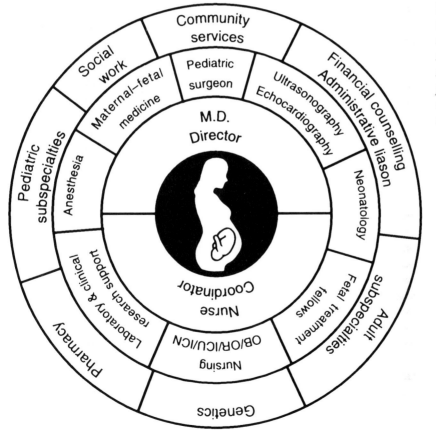

Fig. 3.3 *The fetal treatment centre requires the expertise of many different specialists in an institutional setting that fosters high-level perinatal care, clinical investigation and experimental work.*

complicates fetal surgery and is, therefore, the major determinant of fetal morbidity and mortality. The development of more effective tocolytic agents and the application of minimally invasive techniques may improve the results of fetal surgery and extend application.

References

Adzick, N. S. & Harrison, M. R. (1992). Fetal Surgery Experience. In *Fetal Wound Healing*, 1st edn, ed. N. S. Adzick & M. T. Longaker, pp. 1–23. New York: Elsevier Scientific Press.

Adzick, N. S., Harrison, M. R., Flake, A. W., Glick, P.L. & Bottles, K. (1985). Automatic uterine stapling device in fetal surgery. *Surgical Forum*, 36, 479–81.

Adzick, N. S., Harrison, M. R. & Flake, A. W. (1993). Fetal surgery for cystic adenomatoid malformation of the lung. *Journal of Pediatric Surgery*, 28, 1–6.

Adzick, N. S. & Harrison, M. R. (1994). The unborn surgical patient. *Current Problems in Surgery*, 31, 1–68.

Besinger, R. E. & Niebyl, J. R. (1990). The safety and efficacy of tocolytic agents for the treatment of preterm labour. *Obstetrical and Gynecological Survey*, 45, 415–40.

Estes, J. M., MacGillivray, T. E., Hedrick, M. H., Adzick, N. S. & Harrison, M. R. (1992a). Fetoscopic surgery for the treatment of congenital anomalies. *Journal of Pediatric Surgery*, 27, 950–4.

Estes, J. M., Whitby, D. J., Lorenz, H. P., Longaker, M. T., Szabo, Z., Adzick, N. S. & Harrison, M. R. (1992b). Endoscopic creation and repair of fetal cleft lip. *Plastic and Reconstructive Surgery*, 90, 743–6.

Harrison, M. R. (1993). Fetal surgery. *Western Journal of Medicine*, 159, 341–9.

Harrison, M. R. & Adzick, N. S. (1991). The fetus as a patient: surgical considerations. *Annals of Surgery*, 213, 279–91.

Harrison, M. R. & Adzick, N. S. (1993). Fetal surgical techniques. *Seminars in Pediatric Surgery*, 2, 136–42.

Harrison, M. R., Golbus, M. S. & Filly, R. A. (1981). Management of the fetus with a correctable congenital defect. *Journal of the American Medical Association*, 246, 774–7.

Harrison, M. R. & Longaker M. T. (1990). Maternal risk and development of fetal surgery. In *The Unborn Patient: Prenatal Diagnosis and Treatment*, 2nd edn, ed. M. R. Harrison, M. S. Golbus & R. A. Filly, pp. 189–204. Philadelphia, PA: W. B. Saunders.

Hedrick, M. H., Jennings, R. W., MacGillivray, T. E., Flake, A. W., Lorenz, H. P., Estes, J. M., Roberts, L., Adzick, N. S. & Harrison, M. R. (1992). Endoscopic catheterization of placental vessels for chronic fetal vascular access. *Surgical Forum*, 43, 504–5.

Hedrick, M. H., Estes, J. M., Sullivan, K. M., Bealer, J. F., Kitterman, J. A., Flake, A. W., Adzick, N. S. & Harrison, M. R. (1993). Plug the lung until it grows (PLUG): a new method to treat congenital diaphragmatic hernia *in utero*. *Journal of Pediatric Surgery*, 29, 612–17.

Jennings, R. W., Adzick, N. S., Longaker, M. T., Lorenz, H. P., Estes, J. M. & Harrison, M. R. (1992). New techniques in fetal surgery. *Journal of Pediatric Surgery*, 27, 1329–33.

Jennings, R. W., Adzick, N. S., Longaker, M. T., Lorenz, H. P. & Harrison, M. R. (1993a). Radiotelemetric fetal monitoring during and after open fetal surgery. *Surgery, Gynecology, & Obstetrics*, 176, 59–64

Jennings, R. W., MacGillivray, T. E., & Harrison, M. R. (1993b). Nitric oxide inhibits preterm labour in the rhesus monkey. *Journal of Maternal–Fetal Medicine*, 2, 170–5.

Longaker, M. T., Golbus, M. A., Filly, R. A., Rosen, M. A., Chang, S. W. & Harrison, M. R. (1991). Maternal outcome after open fetal surgery. *Journal of the American Medical Association*, 265, 737–41.

Quintero, R. A., Reich, H., Puder, K. S., Bardicef, M., Evans, M. I., Cotton, D. B. & Romero, R. (1994). Umbilical-cord ligation of an acardic twin by fetoscopy at 19 weeks of gestation. *New England Journal of Medicine*, 330, 469–71.

Rice, H. E., Hedrick, M. H., Bealer, J. F., Zanjani, E. D., Harrison, M. R. & Flake, A. W. (1993). Placental vessel catheterization: a new technique of chronic intravenous access in fetal sheep. *Surgical Forum*, 44, 524–6.

Sabik, J. F., Assad, R. S. & Hanley, F. L. (1993). Halothane as an anesthetic for fetal surgery. *Journal of Pediatric Surgery*, 28, 542–6.

Part two

Preventative therapy

4 Neural tube defects

CAROL BOWER AND NICHOLAS J. WALD

Background

Neural tube defects (anencephaly, spina bifida, encephalocele) result from a failure of closure of the neural tube early in pregnancy. Normally, the neural tube is closed by the end of the sixth week after the last menstrual period. Complete failure of closure at the rostral end of the neural tube results in anencephaly, localized defects in this location result in encephalocele, and failure of closure of the neural tube anywhere along the spine results in spina bifida. All infants with anencephaly are either stillborn or die soon after birth, but most infants with other neural tube defects survive, usually with major lifelong physical disabilities and sometimes intellectual impairment as well.

The birth prevalence of neural tube defects (NTDs) varies geographically around the world, from less than 1 per 1000 to over 4 per 1000 (Little & Elwood, 1992). Some of this variation reflects background differences in the occurrence of NTDs in different populations, and some is the result of the differing availability and uptake of secondary prevention (Fig. 4.1). In England and Wales, the birth prevalence is currently only about one in 10 000 births, because most cases are detected antenatally and the pregnancies terminated.

Women who have had one infant with a NTD have a risk of recurrence some 10-fold greater than women in general, about 3 to 4%. There is a similar risk to the offspring of a parent with spina bifida. The second- or third-degree relatives of an affected individual have a risk of having an affected pregnancy that is similar to the general population risk (Little, 1992). Less than 5% of infants with NTDs are born to families with a family history of the condition.

It has been shown conclusively that the majority of NTDs can be prevented by an increase in maternal folic acid intake around the time of conception and in early pregnancy. The primary prevention of these devastating defects is now a reality.

Primary prevention with folic acid

Maternal diet has long been suspected as a risk factor for NTDs (Elwood, Elwood & Little, 1992). An intervention study showed that women who had already had at least one infant with a NTD and who took a periconceptional multivitamin supplement (Smithells *et al.*, 1980; 1981; 1983; 1989) had a low risk of recurrence of NTDs. There were criticisms of this trial, summarized in Wald and Polani (1985), mainly that there was the opportunity for bias since it was not randomized. It was likely that the women who took part in the study were, in any case, at lower risk of NTDs than the women used as a reference group, and the extent of this self-selection could not be estimated.

At about the same time, two studies from Wales were published. One showed a non-significant reduction in recurrence of NTDs in the offspring of women who were counselled to improve their diet before pregnancy (Laurence *et al.*, 1980). The other was a randomized controlled trial of periconceptional supplementation with either 4 mg folic acid or a placebo (Laurence *et al.*, 1981). There were two recurrences of NTDs amongst the 60 infants born to women allocated to the supplement group, and four recurrences among the 51 births to women in the placebo group. This represented a 60% reduction in recurrence, but because of the small sample

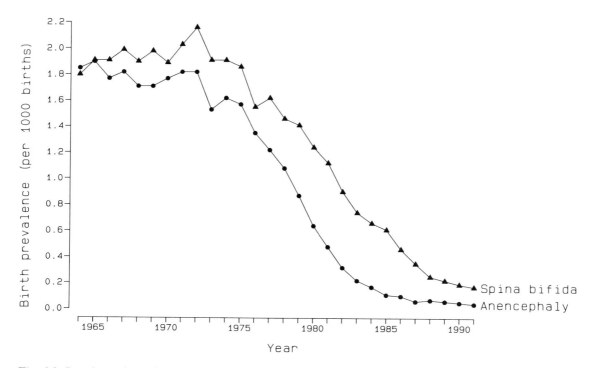

Fig. 4.1 *Prevalence of neural tube defects at birth in England and Wales, 1964–91. Source of data: Office of Population Censuses and Surveys (1991), adjusted for under-reporting as follows:*

anencephaly adjusted = anencephaly observed /0.81
spina bifida adjusted = spina bifida observed /0.87.

size, the difference was not statistically significant.

The results of these studies generated much discussion and prompted further research. Several observational studies, a non-randomized trial and three further randomized controlled trials were undertaken. The results of all these studies are summarized in Figs. 4.2 and 4.3.

The strongest evidence that folic acid prevents NTDs comes from the results of the randomized prevention trials. In order to reduce the sample size required for the study, the MRC Vitamin Study Research Group (1991) recruited women who had already had a pregnancy affected by a NTD and hence were at higher risk of having an affected infant in a subsequent pregnancy. A factorial design was used to investigate both 4.0 mg/day folic acid and a mixture of other vitamins. This trial

showed that folic acid was protective (relative risk 0.29, 95% confidence interval 0.10–0.74). No evidence that the vitamins other than folic acid had any effect in the prevention of NTDs was found; these vitamins with their daily dose were 4000 U vitamin A, 1.5 mg B_1, 1.5 mg B_2, 1.0 mg B_6, 40 mg C, 400 U D and 15 mg nicotinamide. The rate of NTD pregnancies in the women receiving this mixture of vitamins was similar to that in the controls (relative risk 0.8, 95% confidence interval 0.38–1.70).

The second trial was that of Kirke, Daly & Elwood (1992), who used a three-way randomization in women with a previous affected pregnancy of 0.36 mg/day folic acid alone, or folic acid with multivitamins, or multivitamins without folic acid. The multivitamins were the same as those used in the MRC Vitamin Study. The trial was stopped before the required sample size had been reached because of a marked fall in the rate of recruitment. There was one affected pregnancy among the 89 pregnancies in the multivitamin-only arm, and none in either of the folic acid arms (a total of 172 pregnancies).

The third trial was conducted in Hungary. Czeizel & Dudas (1992) reported on 2104 women randomly allocated to receive folic acid (0.8 mg/day) with other vitamins, and 2052 women randomly allocated to receive a trace element supplement daily, for at least one month before a planned pregnancy and for the first three months of pregnancy. These were women embarking on their first pregnancy. There were six incidents of NTDs in children born to the women in the trace element group, and none in children born to the women allocated to the vitamin supplementation group, a significant difference.

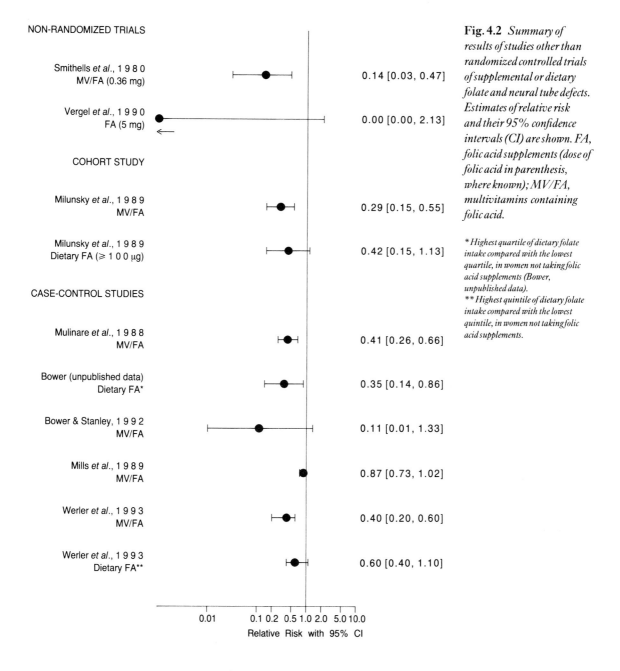

Fig. 4.2 *Summary of results of studies other than randomized controlled trials of supplemental or dietary folate and neural tube defects. Estimates of relative risk and their 95% confidence intervals (CI) are shown. FA, folic acid supplements (dose of folic acid in parenthesis, where known); MV/FA, multivitamins containing folic acid.*

* Highest quartile of dietary folate intake compared with the lowest quartile, in women not taking folic acid supplements (Bower, unpublished data).
** Highest quintile of dietary folate intake compared with the lowest quintile, in women not taking folic acid supplements.

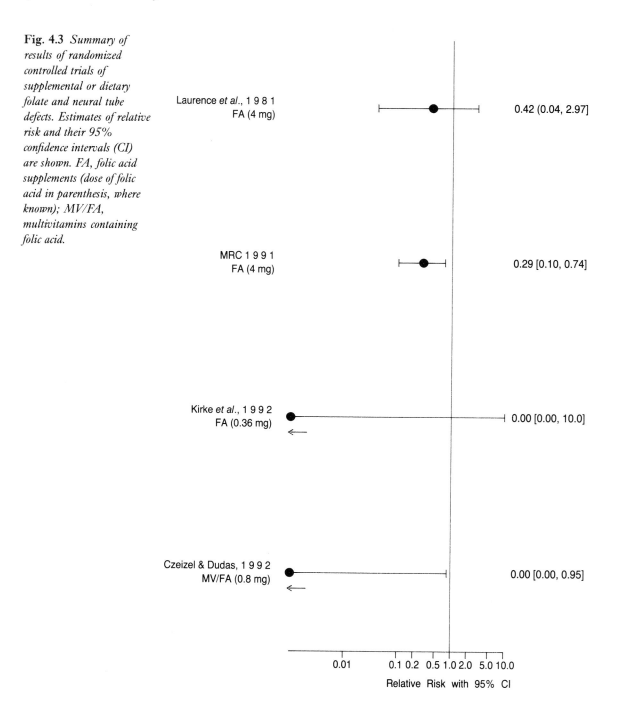

Fig. 4.3 *Summary of results of randomized controlled trials of supplemental or dietary folate and neural tube defects. Estimates of relative risk and their 95% confidence intervals (CI) are shown. FA, folic acid supplements (dose of folic acid in parenthesis, where known); MV/FA, multivitamins containing folic acid.*

Observational studies have also investigated the effect of dietary folate, supplemental folic acid or supplemental multivitamins containing folic acid on occurrent NTDs and all showed a relative risk of less than one (protective), four of which were individually statistically significant (Mulinare *et al.*, 1988; Bower & Stanley, 1989; Milunsky *et al.*, 1989; Mills *et al.*, 1989; Bower & Stanley, 1992; Werler, Shapiro & Mitchell, 1993). A further non-randomized controlled trial similarly suggested a protective effect, albeit non-significant, of a 5 mg folic acid supplement in preventing recurrent NTDs (Vergel *et al.*, 1990).

The results of the randomized trials along with the evidence from the observational and the non-randomized studies all show that folic acid in the periconceptional period prevents the majority of NTDs.

Mechanism of preventing NTDs

Folic acid is pteroylglutamic acid, which consists of a pteridine ring, P-aminobenzoic acid and L-glutamic acid. This parent compound with methyl, hydroxyl and formyl substituents, and up to 10 additional glutamic acid side chains attached are the forms found naturally in foods. Folate is the collective term generally used to refer to folic acid compounds in foods, while the specific term folic acid refers to pteroylglutamic acid, the form used in supplements and food fortification.

Folate is a B group vitamin that is found in leafy green vegetables, many fruits and other vegetables, and in wholegrain cereals and pulses such as beans and peas. With the exception of organ meats such as liver, it is present in only small quantities in meat and dairy products. Folates are easily destroyed by exposure to heat and light, and a considerable amount of the folate in food is lost during cooking. Pure folic acid, however is not degraded by heat or light.

Recent research has suggested a genetic defect of folate metabolism in mothers of affected infants, although the underlying mechanism of action of folic acid in preventing NTDs is still not known precisely (Yates *et al.*, 1987; Steegers-Theunissen *et al.*, 1991; Kirke *et al.*, 1993). Recent evidence suggests that this may be a defect in homocysteine metabolism via the enzyme methionine synthase (Mills *et al.*, 1995). There were

similar rates of miscarriage in women in the folic acid and control groups of the MRC Vitamin Study (1991), and so it is unlikely that folic acid induces the early loss of fetuses with NTDs. There were 92 miscarriages, intrauterine deaths and ectopic pregnancies among the 910 women in the folic acid groups and 84 among the 907 women in the control groups, giving a relative risk of 1.09 and 95% confidence intervals of 0.82–1.44. Folic acid is unlikely to prevent those multiple NTDs that occur as part of a syndrome, such as the autosomal recessive Meckel syndrome, or in association with a chromosomal anomaly such as trisomy 13. Folic acid does not prevent all isolated NTDs. The serum folic acid levels were high in those women in the MRC Vitamin Study (1991) who had been assigned to receive folic acid and who had affected pregnancies, so the lack of a protective effect was not a result of failure to take the folic acid supplement or to absorb it. Although there are likely to be several causes of NTDs, the important fact is that most NTDs can be prevented by consuming sufficient folic acid in the period between planning a pregnancy and about 12 weeks of pregnancy, and there should be no further delay in implementing preventive programmes.

Amount of folic acid

Effectiveness

It may never be possible to determine the minimum effective dose of folic acid needed to prevent NTDs, given the scale and costs of conducting the appropriate studies and concerns about the ethics of using a dose of folic acid less than that which has been shown to be effective in the studies already reported. What is known from these studies is that supplements of between 0.36 mg and 0.8 mg of folic acid daily confer substantial protection and that increasing amounts of dietary folate are also associated with decreasing risk of NTDs within the range of usual intakes of dietary folate (Bower & Stanley, 1989; Werler *et al.*, 1993). Therefore, the increase in folate intake achievable by normal dietary means confers some protection, while the larger intake achievable by supplementation confers even greater protection.

Based on the evidence from the MRC Vitamin Study

(1991), it is reasonable to recommend that women at high risk, defined as a previous pregnancy or NTDs in themselves or their partner, take a 4 mg folic acid supplement daily when planning a pregnancy.

For the majority of women at low risk, the current evidence supports a recommendation of an extra 0.4 mg folic acid daily, in addition to the average dietary intake of folate of about 0.2 mg daily. This target will need to be reviewed as further information becomes available.

The MRC Vitamin Study showed no evidence of a protective effect of other vitamins, and given the association of birth defects with high doses of vitamin A (Teratology Society, 1987), it has been recommended that folic acid be obtained from supplements containing only folic acid and not as part of a multivitamin preparation.

Safety

Folic acid is generally regarded as non-toxic. It is water soluble, very little is stored in the body and excess is excreted in the urine. There has been no evidence of harm to either the fetus or the mother reported from any of the trials, although the power to detect a small effect is limited. Millions of women have taken folic acid supplements in pregnancy with no record of ill-effect.

Concern has been expressed for two particular groups: those with untreated vitamin B_{12} deficiency and those with anticonvulsant-treated epilepsy.

Before the isolation of vitamin B_{12} in 1947, cases of pernicious anaemia, the commonest cause of vitamin B_{12} deficiency, were treated with folic acid in large doses of $\geqslant 5$ mg a day, often administered parenterally (Chanarin, 1979). Many of these patients had a haematological remission, usually only temporarily, and they occasionally had a remission of the neurological features. More commonly, however, the neurological symptoms and signs did not improve, and in many patients progressed. Once vitamin B_{12} was isolated as the specific deficiency in pernicious anaemia, treatment with folic acid fell from favour. The concern now is that in the presence of additional folic acid, the diagnosis of vitamin B_{12} deficiency may be delayed because of the absence of anaemia and, as a result, the neurological abnormalities may become irreversible, even when the correct diagnosis is made and vitamin B_{12} treatment is

instituted. Vitamin B_{12} deficiency is very rare in women of childbearing age, although if food were fortified with folic acid, then some of the high-risk elderly group in the population may have a high intake of folate as a consequence. This theoretical possibility is a good reason for ensuring that B_{12} status is assessed when investigating a patient who presents with a neuropathy – the diagnosis of B_{12} deficiency is made on the presence of a low B_{12} status, not on the presence of macrocytic anaemia. It is not a good reason to limit the fortification of food with folic acid for the prevention of NTDs (Wald & Bower, 1994).

With respect to epilepsy, high doses of folic acid have been reported as reducing anticonvulsant control in some subjects and it has been suggested that very high doses of folic acid may have a convulsant effect in their own right (Reynolds, 1978). However, in a randomized controlled trial of epileptic patients stabilized on phenytoin, there was a significant reduction in seizure frequency in those randomized to receive 5 mg folic acid three times daily, compared with those randomized to receive placebo (Gibberd, Nicholls & Wright, 1981). Moreover, in studies of epileptic women in pregnancy on anticonvulsant therapy, women taking folic acid supplements had normal or supranormal blood folate levels, with no apparent loss of anticonvulsant control (Dansky et al., 1987; Dansky, Rosenblatt & Andermann, 1992). Serum and red cell folic acid levels are reduced in epileptic patients taking anticonvulsant drugs, the rate of birth defects in general is increased amongst the offspring of women taking anticonvulsants (Delgado-Escueta & Janz, 1992), and sodium valproate has been specifically associated with an increased risk of spina bifida (Centers for Disease Control, 1983). For these, and for a number of other reasons, pregnancy in women with epilepsy constitutes a particular problem in management. On balance, an increase in folate is likely to benefit epileptic women and their offspring and should be offered to such women planning a pregnancy, in conjunction with counselling about the risk of birth defects and under medical supervision and monitoring (Delgado-Escueta & Janz, 1992). The actual dose should be decided by the physician. Although 0.4 mg per day may be appropriate, some may wish to give the 4 mg dose in view of the higher risk of NTDs in women with epilepsy.

The amounts of extra folic acid that would be obtained from foods fortified with folic acid are most unlikely to have any effect on the control of epilepsy in the general population.

Strategies for folate supplementation

Individual women at risk of having an affected infant cannot be identified by virtue of their dietary intake of folate, or serum or red cell measures of their folate status (Wald, 1994). Other than those women who have already had an affected infant (or if the women or her partner has spina bifida), there is no way of identifying women at high risk of having an affected pregnancy. This, combined with the fact that the neural tube closes so early in pregnancy, means that public health strategies must aim to increase the folate intake of all women of childbearing age capable of becoming pregnant, so that in the event that they do become pregnant, there will be sufficient folate available for the developing embryo.

Increased intakes of folic acid can be achieved in three complementary ways: by taking a folic acid supplement; by eating more folate-rich foods; and by eating food fortified with folic acid.

Folic acid supplements

While it is reasonable to expect that most women planning a pregnancy would be willing to take a folic acid supplement periconceptionally, it is unrealistic that all women of childbearing age would take a folic acid supplement for their entire fertile life. As many pregnancies are unplanned, this strategy, while effective for the individual women taking a supplement, would have limited impact on the overall prevention of NTDs in the population. Nonetheless, it is sound medical advice to recommend that all women planning a pregnancy should take a 0.4 mg folic acid supplement.

Dietary folic acid

A diet rich in folate can be achieved by increased consumption of vegetables, fruit and wholegrain cereals. As well as being rich in folate, such a diet is also rich in several other vitamins, high in fibre, and usually low in fats, and has health advantages for everyone, not just women of childbearing age. However, it would require a major dietary change on a population basis and is, therefore, unlikely to be achieved in the short term.

Fortification of food with folic acid

The most effective public health strategy is likely to be the fortification of some staple foods with folic acid. Several types of breakfast cereal and bread are fortified already in the UK, and breakfast cereals have been fortified for many years in the USA. However, there is a need for more widespread fortification if average intakes of folate, currently about 0.2 mg/day, are to be raised.

Education and recommendations

All three strategies require education of both health professionals and the public. A survey of women presenting for their first antenatal visit in Leeds, UK, found that only 2.4% of women had been informed about the preventive effects of folate and had either increased their dietary consumption of folate or taken a folic acid supplement before becoming pregnant (Sutcliffe et al., 1993). A study of women attending the antenatal clinic at Queen Charlotte's Hospital, London in 1993 showed that 67% were unaware of the Department of Health recommendations (Clark & Fisk, 1994). These data were collected six months or more after recommendations about folic acid and the prevention of NTDs had been circulated to all doctors with recommendations about folic acid and the prevention of NTDs by the Department of Health in the UK (Expert Advisory Group, 1992).

National bodies in several other countries have also issued recommendations (Centers for Disease Control, 1992; Health and Welfare Canada, 1993; National Health and Medical Research Council Australia, 1993). They have recommended that women of childbearing age increase their dietary folate intake and, if planning a pregnancy, take a folic acid supplement during the periconceptional period, and all but one of the bodies recommend fortification of food with folic acid, although how this is to be accomplished and the level of fortification recommended are not detailed.

Other benefits of folate supplementation

An increased intake of folate may have benefits beyond the prevention of NTDs. An obvious additional benefit would be a reduction in folic acid deficiency, a particular risk in the elderly and in pregnant women (Runcie, 1979; Chanarin, 1979). There is evidence that a metabolic marker of deficient folate intake, plasma homocysteine, is raised in about a quarter of US adults (Selhub et al., 1993). Folic acid deficiency may be more widespread than was previously recognized.

There are a number of other suggested benefits of increased folic acid intake, although the evidence is at present uncertain. The conditions in which folic acid may play a protective or therapeutic role include precancerous lesions of the cervix (Butterworth et al., 1992) and the bronchus (Heimburger et al., 1988), primitive neuroectodermal tumours in children (Bunin et al., 1993), cardiovascular disease (Clarke et al., 1991) and cleft lip (Tolorova, 1982). Indeed, a recent case control study suggests that periconceptual folate supplementation may also reduce the risk of cleft lip/palate (Shaw et al., 1995). High plasma homocysteine levels have been found to be associated with subsequent risk of myocardial infarction (Stampfer et al., 1992) and folic acid can lower homocysteine levels; folic acid may, therefore, help protect against myocardial infarction.

Future developments

It is important to develop effective ways of educating people about the prevention of NTDs, including the need for folate intake to increase before pregnancy. It should become part of undergraduate and postgraduate medical teaching. In addition to prepregnancy counselling, information can be given to women when renewing prescriptions for oral contraceptives, at postnatal checks and following miscarriages (Cuckle, 1994) or, as has recently been suggested (Clark & Fisk, 1994), by leaflets in packets of sanitary wear. Use of the mass media may be an effective means of raising public awareness (News, 1994). It is important to provide the information in a way that can be acted upon with ease. Details of fortified foods should be given, women will need to be informed about where they can obtain supplements and be given

an indication of cost. Dietary sources of folate need to be presented in a simple manner, taking into consideration the usual diet of the target group, and the availability and cost of foods.

The level of fortification should be determined and reviewed by a central authority (Wald, 1994). The most appropriate foods for fortification will vary from population to population, and in some countries, legislative changes may be necessary before folic acid can be added to foods in the amounts likely to provide most women with sufficient to prevent NTDs in their offspring.

This central authority should monitor the extent of supplementation, dietary change and fortification, as well as the incidence of NTDs among births and terminations, and other information on effectiveness and safety (Hall, 1994). This may include a means of monitoring the incidence of neuropathy resulting from vitamin B_{12} deficiency, and the effect on seizure frequency and severity in epileptic patients.

Continued research to find the underlying mechanism of action of folic acid may lead to ways of identifying high-risk groups to whom preventive strategies can be directed. Recent work from Dublin suggests that vitamin B_{12} and folic acid may be independent risk factors for NTDs (Kirke et al., 1993; Mills et al., 1995) and that B_{12} and folate may be required for the most effective NTD prophylaxis. This finding needs to be investigated further.

Conclusion

The majority of NTDs can be prevented by an increase in maternal folic acid intake around the time of conception and in early pregnancy. It would require a major dietary change on a population basis to achieve the required intake of folic acid. While the minimum fully effective dose of folic acid is unknown, current evidence suggests that in addition to the average dietary intake of about 0.2 mg folate per day, supplements of 0.4 mg folic acid per day would be required to confer a benefit for the majority of women. Public health policy is now to recommend that all women planning a pregnancy take a folic acid supplement, but studies have shown that this recommendation has not effectively reached its target population, and many pregnancies are unplanned. The most effective strategy is the fortification of a staple food with folic acid. What is now needed is appropriate public health action to educate the public about the importance of folic acid, make folic acid supplements readily available for women planning to become pregnant and provide practical guidelines on the fortification of food with folic acid.

Not all NTDs are prevented by folic acid. The search for other causes should continue, but not at the expense of implementing effective means of preventing the three quarters of cases amenable right now to prevention by folic acid.

References

Bower, C. & Stanley, F. J. (1989). Dietary folate as a risk factor for neural tube defects: evidence from a case-control study in Western Australia. *Medical Journal of Australia*, 150, 613–19.

Bower, C. & Stanley, F. (1992). Periconceptional vitamin supplementation and neural tube defects: evidence from a case-control study in Western Australia and a review of recent publications. *Journal of Epidemiology and Community Health*, 46, 157–61.

Bunin, G. R., Kuijten, R. R., Buckley, J. D., Rorke, L. B. & Meadows, A. T. (1993). Relation between maternal diet and subsequent primitive neuroectodermal brain tumours in young children. *New England Journal of Medicine*, 329, 536–41.

Butterworth, C. E., Hatch, K. D., Macaluso, M., Cole, P., Sauberlich, H. E., Soong, S. J., Borst, M. & Baker, V. V. (1992). Folate deficiency and cervical dysplasia. *Journal of the American Medical Association*, 267, 528–33.

Centers for Disease Control (1983). Valproate: a new cause of birth defects – report from Italy and follow-up from France. *Morbidity and Mortality Weekly Report*, 32, 438–9.

Centers for Disease Control (1992). Recommendations for the use of folic acid to reduce the number of cases of spina bifida and other neural tube defects. *Morbidity and Mortality Weekly Report*, 41, 1–7.

Chanarin, I. (1979). *The Megaloblastic Anaemias*, 2nd edn. Oxford: Blackwell Scientific.

Clark, N. A. C. & Fisk, N. M. (1994). Minimal compliance with Department of Health recommendation for routine folate prophylaxis to prevent fetal neural tube defects. *British Journal of Obstetrics and Gynaecology*, 101, 709–10.

Clarke, R., Daly, L., Robinson, K., Naughten, E., Cahalane, S., Fowler, B. & Graham, I. (1991). Hyperhomocysteinemia: an independent risk factor for vascular disease. *New England Journal of Medicine*, 324, 1149–55.

Cuckle, H.S. (1994). Discussion. In *Neural Tube Defects*. Ciba Foundation Symposium 181, p. 230. Chichester, UK: John Wiley.

Czeizel, A. & Dudas, I. (1992). Prevention of first occurrence of neural tube defects by periconceptional vitamin supplementation. *New England Journal of Medicine*, 327, 1832–5.

Dansky, L. V., Andermann, E., Rosenblatt, D., Sherwin, A. L. & Andermann, F. (1987). Anticonvulsants, folate levels, and pregnancy outcome: a prospective study. *Annals of Neurology*, 21, 176–82.

Dansky, L. V., Rosenblatt, D. & Andermann, E. (1992). Mechanisms of teratogenesis: folic acid and antiepileptic therapy. *Neurology*, (Suppl. 5), 32–42.

Delgado-Escueta, A. V. & Janz, D. (1992). Consensus guidelines: preconception counselling, management and care of the pregnant woman with epilepsy. Neurology, 42 (Suppl. 5), 149–60.

Elwood, M., Elwood, H. & Little, J. (1992). Diet. In *Epidemiology and Control of Neural Tube Defects*, ed. J. M. Elwood, J. Little & J. H. Elwood, pp. 521–603. Oxford: Oxford University Press.

Expert Advisory Group (1992). *Folic acid and the prevention of neural tube defects*. London: Department of Health.

Gibberd, F. B., Nicholls, A. & Wright, M. G. (1981). The influence of folic acid on the frequency of epileptic attacks. *European Journal of Clinical Pharmacology*, 19, 57–60.

Hall, J. (1994). Final discussion. In *Neural Tube Defects*, Ciba Foundation Symposium 181, p. 287. Chichester, UK: John Wiley.

Health and Welfare Canada (1993). *Issues: Folic Acid, the Vitamin that helps Protect against Neural Tube (birth) Defects*. Ottawa: Health Protection Branch.

Heimburger, D. C., Alexander, B., Birch, R., Butterworth, C. E., Bailey, W. C. & Krumdeick, C. L. (1988). Improvement in bronchial squamous metaplasia in smokers treated with folate and vitamin B_{12}. *Journal of the American Medical Association*, 259, 1525–30.

Kirke, P. N., Daly, L. E. & Elwood, J. H. for the Irish Vitamin Study Group (1992). A randomized trial of low dose folic acid to prevent neural tube defects. *Archives of Disease in Childhood*, 67, 1442–6.

Kirke, P. N., Molloy, A. M., Daly, L. E., Burke, H., Weir, D. G. & Scott, J. M. (1993). Maternal plasma folate and vitamin B_{12} are independent risk factors for neural tube defects. *Quarterly Journal of Medicine*, 86, 703–8.

Laurence, K. M., James, N., Miller, M. & Campbell, H. (1980). Increased risk of recurrence of pregnancies complicated by fetal neural tube defects in mothers receiving poor diets, and possible benefit of dietary counselling. *British Medical Journal*, 281, 1592–4.

Laurence, K. M., James, N., Miller, M. H., Tennant, G. B. & Campbell, H. (1981). Double-blind randomized controlled trial of folate treatment before conception to prevent recurrence of neural-tube defects. *British Medical Journal*, 282, 1509–11.

Little, J. (1992). Risks in siblings and other relatives. In *The Epidemiology and Control of Neural Tube Defects*, ed. J. M. Elwood, J. Little & J. H. Elwood, pp. 604–76. Oxford: Oxford University Press.

Little, J. & Elwood, M. (1992). Geographic variation. In *The Epidemiology and Control of Neural Tube Defects*, ed J. M. Elwood, J. Little & J. H. Elwood, pp. 96–145. Oxford: Oxford University Press.

Medical Research Council Vitamin Study Research Group (1991). Prevention of neural tube defects: results of the Medical Research Council Vitamin Study Research Group. *Lancet*, 338, 131–7.

Mills, J. L., McPartlin, J. M., Kirke, P. N., Lee, Y. J., Conley, M. R., Weir, D. G. & Scott, J. M. (1995). Homocysteine metabolism in pregnancies complicated by neural tube defects. *Lancet*, 345, 149–51.

Mills, J. L., Rhoads, G. G., Simpson, J. L., Cunningham, G. C., Conley, M. R., Lassman, M. R., Walden, M. E., Depp, R. O., Hoffman, H. J. & the National Institute of Child Health and Human Development Neural Tube Defect Study Group (1989). The absence of a relation between the periconceptional use of vitamins and neural-tube defects. *New England Journal of Medicine*, 321, 430–5.

Milunsky, A., Jick, H., Jick, S., Bruell, C., MacLaughlin, D. S., Rothman, K. J. & Willett, W. (1989). Multivitamin/folic acid supplementation in early pregnancy reduces the prevalence of neural tube defects. *Journal of the American Medical Association*, 262, 2847–52.

Mulinare, J., Cordero, J. F., Erickson, J. D. & Berry, R. J. (1988). Periconceptional use of multivitamins and the occurrence of neural tube defects. *Journal of the American Medical Association*, 260, 3141–5.

National Health & Medical Research Council (1993). *Revised Statement on the Relationship between Dietary Folic Acid and Neural Tube Defects such as Spina Bifida*. 115th Session. Australia: The National Health and Medical Research Council.

News (1994). US campaign for women to take folic acid to prevent birth defects. *British Medical Journal*, 308, 223.

Office of Population Censuses and Surveys (1991). *Congenital Malformation Statistics*, Series MB3, No. 7. London: HMSO.

Reynolds, E. H. (1978). How do anticonvulsants work? *British Journal of Hospital Medicine*, 19, 505–12.

Runcie, J. (1979). Folate deficiency in the elderly. In *Folic Acid in Neurology, Psychiatry, and Internal Medicine*, ed. M. I. Botez & E. H. Reynolds, pp. 493–99. New York: Raven Press.

Selhub, J., Jacques, P. F., Wilson, P. W. F., Rush, D. & Rosenberg, I. H. (1993). Vitamin status and intake as primary determinants of homocysteinemia in an elderly population. *Journal of the American Medical Association*, 270, 2693–8.

Shaw, G. M., Lammer, E. J., Wasserman, C. R., O'Malley, C. & Tolarova, M. M. (1995). Risks of orofacial clefts in children born to women using multivitamins containing folic acid periconceptionally. *Lancet*, 346, 393–6.

Smithells, R. W., Seller, M. J., Harris, R., Fielding, D. W., Schorah, C. J., Nevin, N. C., Sheppard, S., Read, A. P., Walker, S. & Wild, J. (1983). Further experience of vitamin supplementation for prevention of neural tube defect recurrences. *Lancet*, i, 1027–31.

Smithells, R. W., Sheppard, S., Schorah, C. J., Seller, M. J., Nevin, N. C., Harris, R., Read, A. P. & Fielding, D. W. (1980). Possible prevention of neural-tube defects by periconceptional vitamin supplementation. *Lancet*, i, 339–40.

Smithells, R. W., Sheppard, S., Schorah, C. J., Seller, M. J., Nevin, N. C., Harris, R., Read, A.P. & Fielding, D.W. (1981). Apparent prevention of neural tube defects by periconceptional vitamin supplementation. *Archives of Disease in Childhood*, 56, 911–18.

Smithells, R. W., Sheppard, S., Wild, J. & Schorah, C. J. (1989). Prevention of neural tube defect recurrences in Yorkshire: final report. *Lancet*, ii, 498–9.

Stampfer, M. J., Malinow, R., Willett, W. C., Newcomer, L. M., Upson, B., Ullmann, D., Tishler P. V. & Hennekens, C. H. (1992). A prospective study of plasma homocyst(e)ine and risk of myocardial infarction in US physicians. *Journal of the American Medical Association*, 268, 877–81.

Steegers-Theunissen, R. P. M., Boers, G. H. J., Trijbels, F. J. M. & Eskes, T. K. A. B. (1991). Neural-tube defects and derangement of homocysteine metabolism. *New England Journal of Medicine*, 324, 199–200.

Sutcliffe, M., Schorah, C. J., Perry, A. & Wild, J. (1993). Prevention of neural tube defects. *Lancet*, 342, 1174.

Teratology Society (1987). Position paper: use of vitamin A during pregnancy. *Teratology*, 35, 267–77.

Tolorova, M. (1982). Periconceptional supplement with vitamins and folic acid to prevent recurrence of cleft lip. *Lancet*, ii, 217.

Vergel, R. G., Sanchez, L. R., Heredero, B. L., Rodriguez, P. L. & Martinez, A. J. (1990). Primary prevention of neural tube defects with folic acid supplementation: Cuban experience. *Prenatal Diagnosis*, 10, 149–52.

Wald, N. J. (1994). Folic acid and neural tube defects: the current evidence and implications for prevention. In *Neural Tube Defects*. Ciba Foundation Symposium 181. Chichester, UK: John Wiley.

Wald, N. J. & Bower, C. (1994). Folic acid, pernicious anaemia, and prevention of neural tube defects. *Lancet*, 343, 307.

Wald, N. & Polani, P. E. (1985). Neural-tube defects and vitamins: the need for a randomized clinical trial. *British Journal of Obstetrics and Gynaecology*, 92, 187–8.

Werler, M., Shapiro, S. & Mitchell, A. (1993). Periconceptional folic acid exposure and risk of occurrent neural tube defects. *Journal of the American Medical Association*, 269, 1257–61.

Yates, J. R. W., Ferguson-Smith, M. A., Shenkin, A., Guzman-Rodriguez, R., White, M. & Clark, B. J. (1987). Is disordered folate metabolism the basis for the genetic predisposition to neural tube defects? *Clinical Genetics*, 31, 279–87.

5 Inborn errors of metabolism

RODERICK F. HUME, JR, LAURA S. MARTIN,
MARK P. JOHNSON AND MARK I. EVANS

Introduction

Fetal therapy of inborn errors of metabolism can be
considered in a number of ways. The maternal metabolic
disorder may be the primary disease, and an adverse fetal
effect secondary (Schulman & Simpson, 1981). Optimal
maternal care is then required for the well-being of both
the mother and her fetus. This is the case in phe-
nyketonuria (PKU) and Wilson's disease, where the
fetus is the passive victim of the maternal metabolic
derangement. The primary goal of maternal therapy is to
optimize the fetal environment to minimize the risk for
fetal damage of an otherwise unaffected fetus. Rarely,
the maternal adaptation to pregnancy may precipitate a
disease state in a previously asymptomatic individual,
such as in the ornithine transcarboxylase heterozygote
(Arn et al., 1990; Horwich & Fenton, 1990), or in acute
intermittent porphyria (Kanaan, Veille & Lakin, 1989).
Even more rarely, the fetus may share the inherited
defect with its mother, e.g. PKU (Levy et al., 1992).
Alternatively, the fetus may have the primary metabolic
disorder. Examples include congenital adrenal hyperplasia (Evans et al., 1985), methylmalonic acidaemia and
multiple carboxylase deficiency. In utero therapy is given
for its beneficial fetal effects and may cause unwanted
maternal effects as a secondary problem.

Maternal metabolic disorders

Background

The most common exposure of the obstetrician to a
metabolic disease in pregnancy pertains to the adverse
fetal effects of a maternal inborn error of metabolism.
Advances in molecular biology have provided new insights into the pathophysiology of many of these
metabolic disorders.

Phenylketonuria

Classic PKU is a molecularly heterogeneous autosomal
recessive metabolic disorder caused by deficient activity
of the enzyme phenylalanine hydroxylase (PAH). The
PAH gene has been localized to chromosome 12q22-
q24. Detailed molecular analysis suggests that genotype
can predict phenotype (Okano et al., 1991; Scriver,
1991). PAH is a hepatic enzyme that catalyses hydrox-
ylation of phenylalanine to tyrosine (Scriver & Clow,
1980a,b). In patients with PKU, a block in phenylalanine
metabolism results in the accumulation of this amino
acid and its metabolites. This in turn leads to progressive, severe, irreversible mental retardation.

Despite screening programmes since the early 1960s,
undiagnosed maternal PKU represents an ongoing public health challenge (Dorland et al., 1993; Hanley,
Clarke & Schoonheyt, 1990). There are more than 1600
known women with PKU in the USA of childbearing
age.

Fetuses of untreated pregnant women with high levels
of phenylalanine may spontaneously abort or exhibit
intrauterine growth retardation (Shaw, Macleod &
Applegarth, 1991). Elevated phenylalanine levels found
in untreated maternal PKU are teratogenic. Children of
PKU women may have mental retardation, dysmorphic
facies, microcephaly and congenital heart disease.
There appears to be a dose–response relationship
between the severity of these manifestations and the

mother's plasma level of phenylalanine during pregnancy (Lenke & Levy, 1980; American Academy of Pediatrics Committee on Genetics, 1991; Matalon et al., 1991; Rouse et al., 1990).

In the preliminary report of an ongoing prospective, longitudinal study involving 213 pregnant women with PKU, treatment initiated in the third trimester showed little benefit. Infants with congenital heart disease were born to mothers with phenylalanine levels greater than 10 mg/dl (Koch et al., 1990; Platt et al., 1992). Levy and coworkers (1992) reported the outcome of two children, one with PKU and one without PKU, who were born after untreated pregnancies in a mother with PKU. Both infants were mentally retarded with an IQ of less than 50. Congenital anomalies exhibited by both children included microcephaly, hypoplasia of the corpus callosum and enlarged cerebral ventricles. However, only the infant affected with PKU exhibited intrauterine growth retardation. This case highlights the need for maternal biochemical control independent of the fetal phenotype (Koch et al., 1990; Platt et al., 1992).

Preconceptional counselling should stress the importance of adherence to diet to prevent deleterious effects in the fetus. The primary goal of nutritional therapy in the pregnant patient with PKU is to maintain the phenylalanine levels below 600 μmol/l or 10 mg/dl. This is achieved through a diet restricted in total protein and phenylalanine, which should be initiated under the guidance of a skilled nutritionist. Optimal fetal outcomes occurred in 134 pregnancies when the phenylalanine level was maintained below these levels during the first trimester (Koch et al., 1990; Platt et al., 1992). Severe protein restriction in pregnancy requires individualization and careful monitoring of fetal growth with serial ultrasounds. Excessive levels of phenylalanine are more dangerous to the fetus than any theoretical protein starvation. A metabolic nutritionist and clinical geneticist working in concert with the obstetrician greatly facilitates the maintenance of dietary therapy.

Wilson's disease

Wilson's disease is an autosomal recessive, multisystem disorder characterized by abnormal tissue accumulations of copper. The putative gene for Wilson's disease

has been mapped to 13q14. Before the introduction of chelation therapy, Wilson's disease was a progressively debilitating and fatal disease. Since the introduction of D-penicillamine, a cupriuretic-chelating agent, several pregnancies have been described (Scheinburg & Sternlief, 1975; Walshe, 1977; 1986; Dupont, Irion & Beguin, 1990; Chin, 1991). Recurrent abortion is not uncommon in untreated Wilson's disease, perhaps on the basis of direct embryotoxicity from elevated tissue copper. Two successful pregnancies have been reported in a woman with Wilson's disease and a history of recurrent abortion subsequently treated with zinc therapy (Schagen-van-Leeuwen, Christiaens & Hoogenraad, 1991).

However, agents which chelate copper may be teratogenic. Lysyl oxidase is a copper-dependent enzyme involved in cross-linking collagen and elastin. A dose-related teratogenesis of penicillamine has been described in rats. Several infants exposed to this drug, including one with Wilson's disease, were found to have transient cutis laxa (Linares et al., 1979; Rosa, 1986). One had inguinal hernias, low-set ears and joint mobility. However, discontinuing therapy may be catastrophic for the mother or have significant neonatal sequelae. One patient, a gravida with two prior successful pregnancies and known Wilson's disease, deliberately stopped penicillamine therapy, developed CNS findings, fulminant hepatic failure, haemolytic crisis and died postpartum (Oga et al., 1993). In a second patient, copper deposition was found on the maternal side of the placenta, but not on the fetal side. Copper levels in umbilical serum and amniotic fluid were remarkably elevated. The neonate showed hepatomegaly (Shimono et al., 1991).

Untreated Wilson's disease may have adverse fetal and neonatal effects; however concerns remain regarding the teratogenic effects of maternal chelating therapy.

Fetal metabolic disorders

Background

The advent of prenatal diagnosis has afforded the opportunity to identify the fetus with an inborn error of metabolism, often in a presymptomatic condition.

Secondary prevention may be the only current available therapeutic option for many untreatable diseases such as Duchenne muscular dystrophy (Evans et al., 1991; 1993), osteogenesis imperfecta (McKusick, 1992), Lesch–Nyan disease (Scriver et al., 1989) and Tay-Sachs disease (Scriver et al., 1989). However, with the parallel advances in molecular genetics (Isada & Blakemore, 1993) and human transplantation (Johnson et al., 1989), human stem cell transplantation has been utilized to create a chimaeric state with enough normal function to offer a genetic solution to a select few of these lethal disorders (Schulman, 1990).

Most inborn errors of metabolism currently treated in utero evolved from successful ex utero therapies for which some irreversible sequelae or fetal maldevelopment remained after the institution of neonatal therapy. The success of neonatal screening programmes for PKU and congenital hypothyroidism have been monumental. The prevention of mental retardation through early recognition and the application of rather simple nutritional therapy or hormonal replacement has proved that inherited errors of metabolism could be corrected. However, irreversible fetal damage could not be addressed by neonatal therapy for some individuals (Fisher & Klein, 1981).

Fetal goitre and congenital hypothyroidism

Advanced sonographic evaluation and biochemical analysis of the amniotic fluid allows in utero diagnosis and therapy of congenital hypothyroidism (Carswell, Kerr & Hutchison, 1970; Davidson et al., 1991; Sagot et al., 1991; Hatjis, 1993). Approximately 20% of congenital hypothyroidism is caused by inborn errors of metabolism or single gene defects (New England Congenital Hypothyroidism Collaborative, 1984). Examples include autosomal recessive familial congenital non-goitrous hypothyroidism (White, Wiedermann & Kirkland, 1981), autosomal dominant peripheral insensitivity to thyroxine (Hamon, Bovier-La & Robert, 1988), and X-linked pseudohypoparathyroidism (Levine, Jap & Hung, 1985). Fetal therapy may be required in these conditions to avoid irreversible damage present at birth, as detailed in Chapter 15.

Congenital adrenal hyperplasia

Congenital adrenal hyperplasia (CAH) offers the first example of an inborn error of metabolism inherited by the fetus that can be treated in utero with prevention of malformation as the primary goal. This disorder has been linked to chromosome 6 using HLA haplotypes as the informative marker. Subsequent gene mapping identified the 21-hydroxylase gene locus to be within the HLA gene cluster. Molecular heterogeneity is the rule, and most CAH individuals are compound heterozygotes at the molecular level. The clinical phenotype does show a correlation with the molecular genotypic abnormality (Miller, 1994). The clinical spectrum of disease associated with CAH ranges from a critically ill salt-wasting variety, to mild virilization precociously in males or ambiguous genitalia in females. Prominent clitoromegaly with labial fusion can resemble the male genitalia so much as to misclassify newborn sex identity. CAH can be life- threatening if the salt-wasting variety of adrenal insufficiency is present. When recognized at birth, steroid-replacement therapy is initiated which decreases the androgen excess.

Since CAH is inherited in an autosomal recessive manner, and only the females will be affected by the anomaly, the birth defect risk is 1 in 8. However, virilization of the female fetus may already have occurred during weeks 10 to 16 of gestation. Therefore, in utero therapy aimed at the prevention of virilization must be begun prior to the determination of gender or disease status (Evans et al., 1985; David & Forest, 1984; Pang et al., 1990; Forest & David, 1992). The fetal adrenal gland can be pharmacologically suppressed by maternal replacement doses of dexamethasone (Evans et al., 1985). The 21-hydroxylase enzyme defect impairs the metabolism of cholesterol to cortisol, creating excessive 17-hydroxyprogesterone (see Fig. 5.1). Alternate pathway metabolism shifts this precursor to androstenedione and other androgens. Consequently, genetic females are exposed to high levels of androgens and can become masculinized. The abnormal differentiation can vary from mild clitoral hypertrophy to complete formation of a phallus and apparent scrotum. In the first attempt to prevent this birth defect, Evans et al. (1985) administered dexamethasone to an at-risk mother beginning in the 10th week of gestation. Maternal oestriol and cortisol

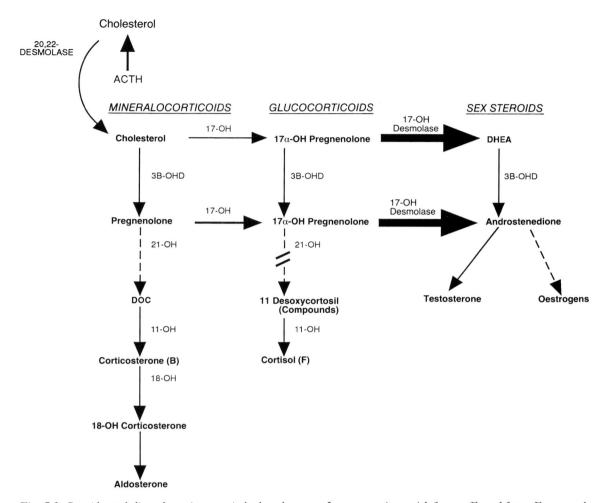

Fig. 5.1 *Steroid metabolic pathway in congenital adrenal hyperplasia: 17-OH, 17a-hydroxylase; 3B-OHD, 3β-hydroxysteroid dehydrogenase; 21-OH, 21a-hydroxylase; 11-OH, 11a-hydroxylase; 18-OH, 18-hydroxylase corticosterone methyl oxidase.*

values indicated rapid and sustained fetal and maternal adrenal gland suppression. Forest and David (David & Forest, 1984; Forest & David, 1992) using the same protocol of 0.25 mg dexamethasone q.i.d. beginning at nine weeks of gestation reported the successful prevention of external genitalia masculinization in several pregnancies at risk for the severe form of 21-hydroxylase deficiency.

In pregnancies at risk for an affected fetus, Forest and coworkers (1989) have recommended that maternal dexamethasone therapy be initiated as early as five weeks' gestation. These investigators suggested a dosage based on maternal first-trimester body weight instead of an empirical daily dose of 1.0 or 1.5 mg and recommended a dosage of 20 μg/kg per day rounded off to the nearest half tablet. At 9–12 weeks of gestation, chorion villus biopsy should be undertaken for DNA analysis to determine if the fetus is affected. Alternatively, the DNA diagnosis can also be made by first- or second-trimester amniocentesis with culture of amniocytes. The older prenatal diagnostic technique of amniotic fluid biochemistry for elevated 17-hydroxyprogesterone levels is not only less reliable but also is uninterpretable in the presence of maternal steroid therapy. The finding of an unaffected fetus of either sex or an affected male fetus warrants discontinuation of maternal dexamethasone therapy. In the case of an affected female fetus, maternal therapy should be continued until delivery. Clinical experience with maternal steroid therapy has been somewhat disappointing, with one third of neonates still exhibiting complete virilization and a further one third exhibiting some degree of virilization (Pang *et al.*, 1990). This may in part be attributed to inadequate dosing or late entry into therapy.

Maternal oestriol levels reflect the conversion of placental pregnenolone to dehydroepiandrosterone sulphate by the fetal adrenals. For this reason, a low maternal oestriol level would indicate adequate fetal adrenal suppression. A second- and third-trimester value should be obtained and compared with normal values for gestational age (Wald *et al.*, 1988; Taylor *et al.*, 1970). If a normal value is noted, consideration should be given to increasing the maternal dose of dexamethasone. Forest *et al.* (1989) have suggested that the maximum dose be limited to 25 µg/kg per day. The obstetrician should be alert to the glucose intolerance that may occur secondary to exogenous steroids. In addition, stress doses of steroids should be administered in labour (hydrocortisone 100 mg intravenously every 8 hours for three doses). Finally, when maternal dexamethasone therapy is to be discontinued, either in the case of an unaffected fetus or in the postpartum period, the dose should be weaned by 0.5 mg/day every 4–5 days.

Methylmalonic acidaemia

Methylmalonic acidaemia (MMA) is related to a functional vitamin B_{12} deficiency. Coenzymatically active B_{12} is required for the conversion of methylmalonyl-coenzyme A to succinyl-coenzyme A. Genetically determined aetiologies for MMA include defects in methylmalonyl-coenzyme A mutase or in the metabolism of vitamin B_{12} to its active coenzyme form, adenosylcobalamin, by the converting enzyme (see Fig. 5.2). Children with MMA present with metabolic acidaemia and mental retardation. Some patients respond to high-dose B_{12} therapy, which can enhance the amount of the

active holoenzyme mutase apoenzyme plus adenosylcobalamin.

Nyhan (1975) has suggested that an increased frequency of minor congenital anomalies may be associated with untreated fetal MMA. Therefore, very early or perhaps even prophylactic treatment with vitamin B_{12} prior to prenatal diagnosis for the at-risk fetus may be indicated for the optimal therapy of B_{12}-responsive MMA. It seems likely that reduction of the fetal burden of MMA should have developmental benefit and could reduce the neonatal risk. However, this remains speculative. Ampola *et al.* (1975) were the first to attempt prenatal diagnosis and treatment of a B_{12}-responsive variant of MMA. The diagnosis of MMA was made posthumously by chemical analysis of blood and urine of the proband who died of severe acidosis and dehydration at three months of age. At 19 weeks' gestation, an amniocentesis revealed elevated levels of methylmalonic acid in amniotic fluid and undetectable adenosylcobalamin levels in cultured amniocytes, indicating an affected fetus. *In vitro* methylmalonyl-coenzyme A mutase activity returned to normal when the active coenzyme of vitamin B_{12} was added. Methylmalonic acid was detected in the maternal urine at 23 weeks' gestation. Since maternal heterozygotes carrying an unaffected fetus do not exhibit elevated level of methylmalonic acid in their urine, this confirmed the diagnosis of fetal MMA. Maternal urine values, therefore, can be utilized as an excellent monitoring tool to assess fetal therapy. Cyanocobalamin at a dose of 10 mg per day was administered orally to the mother in divided doses, producing a slight reduction in maternal urinary methylmalonic acid excretion and only a marginal increase in maternal serum B_{12} levels. Therefore, at 34 weeks' gestation, 5 mg cyanocobalamin per day as an intramuscular injection was initiated. The maternal serum B_{12} level rose sixfold above normal, and the maternal urinary excretion of methylmalonic acid progressively decreased to slightly above normal by delivery. Postnatally, the fetal diagnosis of MMA was confirmed. The neonate suffered no acute neonatal complications, and had an extremely high serum level of B_{12}. In this case, the prenatal therapy certainly improved the fetal and secondarily the maternal biochemistry. Whether there was any significant clinical benefit to this fetus cannot be sufficiently addressed.

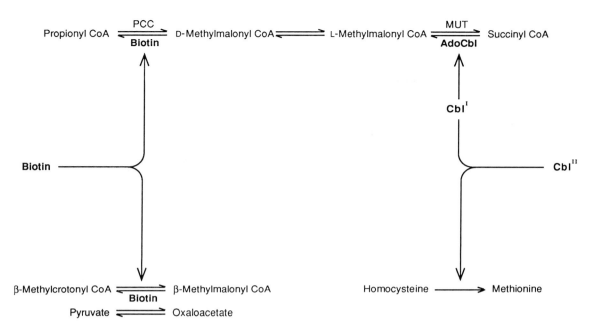

Fig. 5.2 *Summary scheme of inherited defects of propionate and methylmalonate metabolism, which may be biotin or cyanocobalamin (vitamin B_{12}) responsive. PCC, propionyl CoA carboxylase; MUT, methylmalonyl CoA mutase; Cbl, cobalanin with Co(III) or Co(I); AdoCbl, adenosylcobalamin; MeCbl, methylcobalamin.*

Multiple carboxylase deficiency

Biotin-responsive multiple carboxylase deficiency (MCA) is an inborn error of metabolism in which the mitochondrial biotin-dependent enzymes pyruvate carboxylase, propionyl-coenzyme A carboxylase and beta-methylcrotonyl-coenzyme A carboxylase have diminished activity. Metabolism in patients and in *in vitro* cultured cells can be restored toward normal levels by biotin supplementation. Such therapy has been utilized for fetuses affected with this severe disorder of metabolism. Roth *et al.* (Roth, Yang & Allen, 1982) treated a fetus without the benefit of prenatal diagnosis in a case in which two siblings had died of MCA. The first sibling died at three days of age, and in the second sibling the diagnosis was made posthumously in the neonatal period. Because of the severe neonatal manifestations and the relative harmlessness of biotin, oral administration of this compound was given to the mother at a dose

of 10 mg each day. No untoward effects were noted, and the maternal urinary biotin excretion increased 100-fold. Dizygotic twins were subsequently delivered at term. Cord blood and urinary organic acid profiles were normal. Cord blood biotin concentrations were four- and sevenfold greater than normal. Both neonatal courses were unremarkable. Cultured fibroblasts of twin B had virtually complete deficiency of all three carboxylase activities, while the enzyme activity of twin A was normal.

Packman *et al.* (1982) have also reported successful prenatal therapy for a fetus at risk for MCD. These reports provide compelling evidence that biotin administration effectively prevents neonatal complications in certain patients with biotin-responsive multiple carboxylase deficiency. No toxicity has been observed.

Future developments

Vitamin therapy has been utilized in two vitamin-responsive inborn errors of metabolism: methylmalonic acidaemia and multiple carboxylase deficiency. A significant number of other vitamin-responsive defects are known and vitamin supplementation *in utero* may possibly prove to have a role in those conditions associated with neonatal manifestations.

We also speculate that, in addition to these disorders, there may be genetic defects for which prenatal vitamin E administration may be justifiable. Postnatally, vitamin E administration prevents abnormalities of leukocyte function and improves shortened red cell survival in glutathione synthetase deficiency. Most patients with glutathione synthetase deficiency have neurological impairment, which can be progressive. Because grossly lowered intracellular glutathione levels in this mutant state seem to predispose to oxidant-mediated cellular damage, it might be desirable to consider prenatal antioxidant therapy with vitamin E. In abetalipoproteinaemia, which is associated with very low serum vitamin E levels, progressive and fatal neurological impairment develops. It is now known that high-dose vitamin E supplementation can retard or prevent these neurological changes. Prenatal treatment might be justifiable on an experimental basis if fetal damage is possible.

In a third disorder, Menke's kinky hair syndrome, a derangement in copper metabolism produces rapidly progressive neurological injury in neonatal life. Although the disease has proved resistant to postnatal copper therapy, studies in mutant mice support a role for maternal supplementation with copper nitrilotracetate in increasing postnatal survival (Hurley & Bell, 1974).

Prenatal therapy may, therefore, be justifiable in these conditions on an experimental basis in cases where fetal damage is possible.

Conclusion

The fetal metabolic milieu can be manipulated to prevent adverse consequences of maternal or fetal inborn errors of metabolism. Maternal dietary restriction in PKU is recommended to prevent neurodevelopmental impairment but must be rigorously maintained throughout pregnancy. Maternal steroid therapy prevents virilization of some but not all female fetuses with CAH, although treatment needs to be initiated by five weeks of gestation. Although maternal vitamin treatment may have a role in minimizing adverse neonatal effects of vitamin-responsive inborn errors of metabolism, the paucity of data means that such use remains speculative at this time.

References

American Academy of Pediatrics Committee on Genetics (1991). Maternal phenylketonuria. *Pediatrics*, 88, 1284–5.

Ampola, M. G., Mahoney, M. J. & Nakamura, E. (1975). Prenatal therapy of a patient with vitamin B responsive methylmalonic acidemia. *New England Journal of Medicine*, 293, 313–7.

Arn, P. H., Hauser, E. R., Thomas, G. H., Herman, G., Hess, D. & Brusilow, S. W. (1990). Hyperammonemia in women with a mutation at the ornithine carbamoyltransferase locus. A cause of postpartum coma. *New England Journal of Medicine*, 322, 1652–5.

Carswell, F., Kerr, M. M. & Hutchison, J. H. (1970). Congenital goitre and hypothyroidism produced by maternal ingestion of iodides. *Lancet*, i, 1241–3.

Chin, R. K. H. (1991) Pregnancy and Wilson's disease [letter & comment]. *American Journal of Obstetrics and Gynecology*, 165, 488–9.

David, M. & Forrest, M. G. (1984). Prenatal treatment of congenital adrenal hyperplasia resulting from 21-hydroxylase deficiency. *Journal of Pediatrics*, 105, 799–803.

Davidson, K. M., Richards, D. S., Schatz, D. A. & Fisher, D. A. (1991). Successful *in utero* treatment of fetal goiter and hypothyroidism. *New England Journal of Medicine*, 324, 543–6.

Dorland, L., Poll-The, B. T., Duran, M., Smeitink, J. A. & Berger, R. (1993). Phenylpyruvate, fetal damage, and maternal phenylketonuria syndrome. *Lancet*, 341, 1351–2.

Dupont, P., Irion, O. & Beguin, F. (1990). Pregnancy in a patient with treated Wilson's disease: a case report. *American Journal of Obstetrics and Gynecology*, 163, 1527–8.

Evans, M. I., Chrousos, G. P., Mann, D. W., Larsen, J. W., Green, I., McCluskey, J., Loriaux, D. L., Fletcher, J. C., Koons, G., Overpeck, J. & Schulman, J. D. (1985). Pharmacologic suppression of the fetal adrenal gland *in utero*: attempted prevention of abnormal external genital masculinization in suspected congenital adrenal hyperplasia. *Journal of American Medical Association*, 253, 1015.

Evans, M. I., Greb, A., Kunkel, L. M., Sacks, A. J., Johnson, M. P., Boehm, C., Kazazian, H. H. Jr & Hoffman, E. P. (1991). *In utero* fetal muscle biopsy for the diagnosis of Duchenne muscle dystrophy. *American Journal of Obstetrics and Gynecology*, 165, 728–32.

Evans, M. I., Farrell, S. A., Greb, A., Ray, P., Johnson, M. P. & Hoffman, E. P. (1993). *In utero* fetal muscle biopsy for the diagnosis of Duchenne muscular dystrophy in a female fetus suddenly at risk. *American Journal of Medical Genetics*, 46, 309–12.

Fisher, D. A. & Klein, A. H. (1981). Thyroid development and disorders of thyroid function in the newborn. *New England Journal of Medicine*, 304, 702–12.

Forest, M. G., Bétuel, H. & Davis, M. (1989). Prenatal treatment in congenital adrenal hyperplasia due to 21–hydroxylase deficiency: up-date 88 of the French multicentric study. *Endocrine Research*, 15, 277–301.

Forest, M. G. & David, M. (1992). Prevention of sexual ambiguity in children with 21–hydroxylase deficiency by treatment in utero. *Pediatrie*, 47,3 51–7.

Hamon, P., Bovier-La, P. M. & Robert, M. (1988). Hyperthyroidism due to selective pituitary resistance th thyroid hormone in a 15-month old boy: efficacy of D-thyroxine therapy. *Journal of Clinical Endocrinology and Metabolism*, 67, 1089–93.

Hanley, W. B., Clarke, J. T. & Schoonheyt, W. E. (1990). Undiagnosed phenylketonuria in adult women: a hidden public health problem. *Canadian Medical Association Journal*, 143, 513–16.

Hatjis, C. G. (1993). Diagnosis and successful treatment of fetal goitrous hyperthyroidism caused by maternal Grave's disease. *Obstetrics and Gynecology*, 81, 837–9.

Horwich, A. L. & Fenton, W. A. (1990). Precarious balance of nitrogen metabolism in women with a urea-cycle defect. *New England Journal of Medicine*, 322, 1668–70.

Hurley, L. S. & Bell, L. T. (1974). Genetic influence on response to dietary manganese deficiency in mice. *Journal of Nutrition*, 104, 133–7.

Isada, N. B. & Blakemore, K. J. (1993). Basic concept in molecular diagnosis. *Obstetrics and Gynecology Clinics of North America*, 20, 413–20.

Johnson, M. P., Drugan, A., Miller, O. J. & Evans, M. I. (1989). Genetic correction of hereditary disease. *Fetal Therapy*, 4, 28–39.

Johnson, M. P., Compton, A., Drugan, A. & Evans, M. I. (1990). Metabolic control of von Gierke disease (glycogen storage disease type Ia) in pregnancy: maintenance of euglycemia with cornstarch. *Obstetrics and Gynecology*, 75, 507–10.

Kanaan, C., Veille, J. C. & Lakin, M. (1989). Pregnancy and acute intermittent porphyria. *Obstetrical and Gynecological Survey*, 44, 244–9.

Koch, R., Hanley, W., Levy, H., Matalon, R., Rouse, B., de la Cruz, F., Azen, C. & Friedman, E. G. (1990). A preliminary report of the collaborative study of maternal phenylketonuria in the United States and Canada. *Journal of Inherited Metabolic Disease*, 13, 641–50.

Lenke, R. R. & Levy, H. L. (1980). Maternal phenylketonuria and hyperphenylalaninemia: an international survey of the outcome of untreated andtreated pregnancies. *New England Journal of Medicine*, 303, 1202–8.

Levine, M. A., Jap, T. S. & Hung, W. (1985). Infantile hypothyroidism in two sibs: an unusual presentation of pseudohypoparathyroidism type Ia. *Journal of Pediatrics*, 107, 919–22.

Levy, H. L., Lobbregt, D., Sansaricq, C. & Snyderman, S. E. (1992). Comparison of phenylketonuric and non-phenylketonuric sibs from untreated pregnancies in a mother with phenylketonuria. *American Journal of Medical Genetics*, 44, 439–42.

Linares, A., Zarranz, J., Rodriguez-Alarcon, J. & Diaz-Perez, J. (1979). Reversible cutis laxa due to maternal D–penicillamine treatment [letter]. *Lancets*, 2, 43.

Matalon, R., Michals, K., Azen, C., Friedman, E. G., Koch, R., Wenz, E., Levy, H., Rohr, F., Rouse, B., Castiglioni, L., Hanley, W., Austin, V. & de la Cruz, F. (1991). Maternal PKU collaborative study: the effect of nutrient intake on pregnancy outcome. *Journal of Inherited Metabolic Disease*, 14, 371–4.

McKusick, V. A. (1992). *Mendelian Inheritance in Man: Catalogs of Autosomal Dominant, Autosomal Recessive, and X-linked Phenotypes*, 10th edn. Baltimore, MD: Johns Hopkins University Press.

Miller, W. L. (1994). Clinical Review 54: genetics, diagnosis, and management of 21-hydroxylase deficiency. *Journal of Clinical Endocrinology and Metabolism*, 78, 241–6.

New England Congenital Hypothryoidism Collaborative (1984). Characteristics of infantile hypothyroidism discovered on neonatal screening. *Journal of Pediatrics*, 104, 539–44.

Nyhan, W. L. (1975). Prenatal treatment of methylmalonic aciduria. *New England Journal of Medicine*, 293, 353–4.

Oga, M., Matsui, N., Anai, T., Yoshimatsu, J., Inoue, I. & Miyakawa, I. (1993). Copper disposition of the fetus and placenta in a patient with untreated Wilson's disease. *American Journal of Obstetrics and Gynecology*, 169, 196–8.

Okano, Y., Eisensmith, R. C., Guttler, F., Lichter-Konecki, U., Konecki, D. S., Trefz, F. K., Dasovich, M., Wang, T., Henriksen, K., Lou, H. & Woo, S. L. C. (1991). Molecular basis of phenotypic heterogeneity in phenylketonuria. *New England Journal of Medicine*, 324, 1232–8.

Packman, S., Cowan, M. J. & Golbus, M. S. (1982). Prenatal treatment of biotin responsive multiple carboxylase deficiency. *Lancet*, i, 1435–8.

Pang, S. Y., Pollack, M. S., Marshall, R. N. & Immken, L. D. (1990). Prenatal treatment of congenital adrenal hyperplasia due to 21–hydroxylase deficiency. *New England Journal of Medicine*, 322, 111–15.

Platt, L. D., Koch, R., Azen, C., Hanley, W. B., Levy, H. L., Matalon, R., Rouse, B., de la Cruz, F. & Walla, C. A. (1992). Maternal phenylketonuria collaborative study, obstetric aspects and outcome: the first 6 years. *American Journal of Obstetrics and Gynecology*, 166, 1150–62.

Rosa, F. W. (1986). Teratogen update: penicillamine. Teratology, 33, 127–31.

Roth, K. S., Yang, W. & Allen, L. (1982). Prenatal administration of biotin: biotin responsive multiple carboxylase deficiency. *Pediatric Research*, 16, 126–9.

Rouse, B., Lockhart, L., Matalon, R., Azen, C., Koch, R., Hanley, W., Levy, H., de la Cruz, F. & Friedman, E. (1990). Maternal phenylketonuria pregnancy outcome: a preliminary report of facial dysmorphology and major malformations. *Journal of Inherited Metabolic Disease*, 13, 289–91.

Sagot, P., David, A., Yvinec, M., Pousset, P., Papon, V., Mouzard, A. & Boog, G. (1991). Intrauterine treatment of thyroid goiters. *Fetal Diagnosis and Therapy*, 6, 28–33.

Schagen-van-Leeuwen, J. H., Christiaens, G. C. & Hoogenraad, T. U. (1991). Recurrent abortion and the diagnosis of Wilson's disease. *Obstetrics and Gynecology*, 78, 547–9.

Scheinburg, I. H. & Sternlief, I. (1975). Pregnancy in penicillamine-treated patients with Wilson's disease. *New England Journal of Medicine*, 293, 1300–2.

Schulman, J. D. (1990). Treatment of the embryo and the fetus in the first trimester: current status and future possibilities. *American Journal of Medical Genetics*, 35, 197–200.

Schulman, J. D. & Simpson, J. L. (ed.) (1981). In Genetic Diseases in Pregnancy: *Maternal Effects and Fetal Outcome*, pp. 169–96. New York: Academic Press.

Scriver, C.R. (1991). Phenylketonuria – genotypes and phenotypes. *New England Journal of Medicine*, 324, 1280–1.

Scriver, C. R., Beaudet, A. L., Sly, W. S. & Valle, D. (ed.) (1989). *The Metabolic Basis of Inherited Disease*, 6th edn, Vol. 1. New York: McGraw-Hill.

Scriver, C. R. & Clow, C. L. (1980a). Phenylketonuria: epitome of human biochemical genetics. Part I. *New England Journal of Medicine*, 303, 1336–42.

Scriver, C.R. & Clow, C.L. (1980b). Phenylketonuria: epitome of human biochemical genetics. Part II. *New England Journal of Medicine*, 303, 1394–400.

Shaw, D., Macleod, P. M. & Applegarth, D. A. (1991). Recurrent abortion and amnio-acid abnormalities. *Journal of Inherited Metabolic Disease*, 14, 851.

Shimono, N., Ishibashi, H., Ikematsu, H., Kudo, J., Shirahama, M., Inaba, S., Maeda, K., Yamasaki, K. & Niho, Y. (1991). Fulminant hepatic failure during perinatal period in a pregnant woman with Wilson's disease. *Gastroenterologica Japonica*, 26, 69–73.

Taylor, E. S., Hagerman, D. D., Betz, G., Williams, K. L. & Grey, P. A. (1970). Estriol concentrations in blood during pregnancy. *American Journal of Obstetrics and Gynecology*, 108, 868–77.

Wald, N. J., Cuckle, H. S., Densem, J. W., Nanchahal, K., Canick, J. A., Haddou, J. E., Knight, G. J. & Palomaki, G. E. (1988). Maternal serum unconjugated estriol as an antenatal screening test for Down's syndrome. *British Journal of Obstetrics and Gynecology*, 95, 334–41.

Walshe, J. M. (1977). Pregnancy in Wilson's disease. *Quarterly Journal of Medicine*, 46, 73–83.

Walshe, J. M. (1986). The management of pregnancy in Wilson's disease treated with trientine. *Quarterly Journal of Medicine*, 58, 81–7.

White, C. W., Wiedermann, B. L. & Kirkland, R. T. (1981). Hereditary congenital nongoitrous hypothyroidism. *American Journal of Diseases of Children*, 135, 568–9.

6 Multifetal pregnancy reduction

LAUREN LYNCH

Incidence of multifetal pregnancies

The incidence of multifetal pregnancies has increased dramatically in industrialized countries throughout the world. This increase is mainly because of the widespread use of ovulation-induction agents and assisted reproduction techniques. In the US from 1972 to 1974 and 1985 to 1989 the rate of multifetal births defined as three or more livebirths increased by 113% among infants of white mothers and by 22% among infants of black mothers (Kiely, Kleiman & Kiely, 1992). The increase was particularly large in white women aged 30 to 34 years (152%) and 35 to 39 years and in more highly educated mothers. The rate of triplet livebirths increased by 156%, quadruplets by 356% and quintuplets and higher-order births by 182% between 1972 and 1989. In blacks, a modest increase in the rate of multifetal pregnancies was mostly a result of an upward shift in the maternal age distribution.

Similarly, there has been a marked increase in the number of triplets born in England and Wales since the late 1970s, as well as a four-fold increase in the number of higher-order multiple births, defined as four or more livebirths, between 1971 and 1985 compared with the 15 year period 1956–70 (Botting, Davies & MacFarlane, 1987). A survey of multifetal births in 1989 in the British Isles identified 143 triplets, 12 quadruplets and 1 quintuplet set (Levene, Wild & Steer, 1992). Of these, only 31% were conceived naturally, 34% had ovarian stimulation, 24% had *in vitro* fertilization (IVF) and 11% gamete intrafallopian transfer (GIFT). None of the quadruplet and quintuplet pregnancies were conceived spontaneously. Therefore, assisted reproduction is the major cause of triplets and higher-order multiple births in the British Isles.

Equivalent national data regarding the cause of multifetal pregnancies are not available in the United States because the US standard certificate of livebirth does not differentiate between spontaneous and induced gestations. However, in all recent published series in this country, the majority of multifetal pregnancies are a product of assisted reproduction, suggesting that this trend is true on a national level.

Natural history of multifetal pregnancies

Despite modern perinatal management, the rate of prematurity in multifetal pregnancies has not changed since the 1960s, but perinatal mortality rates have declined, probably secondary to improved neonatal care (Kiely *et al.*, 1992). In most published series of triplets, the average gestational age at delivery is consistently around 33 weeks (Table 6.1). Approximately 80–90% of patients deliver before 37 weeks, 20–30% before 32 weeks and 5–10% before 28 weeks. Perinatal mortality rates as low as zero have recently been reported but the average is 77 per 1000 livebirths. Very little information is available regarding the morbidity and long-term outcome of the survivors. Creinin *et al.* reported 13 triplet pregnancies with no perinatal deaths but some form of neonatal morbidity in 80% of the infants (Creinin, Katz & Laros, 1991). Complications included hyperbilirubinaemia in 51%, hypoglycaemia in 30%, respiratory distress syndrome in 28%, patent ductus arteriosus in 15% and intraventricular haemorrhage in 10%. Lipitz *et al.*

Table 6.1 *Natural history of triplet pregnancies*

Author	Years	No. of pregnancies	Mean (weeks)	Gestational age at delivery (weeks)		
				< 37 (%)	< 32 (%)	< 28 (%)
Itzkowic, 1979	1946–76	59	33	83	25	10
Holcberg *et al.*, 1982	1960–79	31	32	87	35	16
Syrop & Varner, 1985	1946–83	20	33	75	N/A	15
Australian IVF, 1988	1975–85	32	N/A	97	39	3
Newman *et al.*, 1989	1985–88	198	34	88	20	7[a]
Gonen *et al.*, 1990	1978–88	24	32	100	N/A	N/A
Boulot *et al.*, 1993	1985–91	48	34	53	15	2
Lipitz *et al.*, 1994	1984–92	106	33	92	24	N/A
Average			33	84	26	9

N/A, not available.

[a] Less than 29 weeks.

(1994) reported 106 triplet pregnancies delivered between 1984 and 1992. The mean gestational age at delivery was 33.5 weeks; 92% delivered before 37 weeks and 24% before 32 weeks. The perinatal and neonatal mortality rates were 109/1000 and 46/1000, respectively. Follow-up data for at least one year (range 1 to 6 years) were available for 52 surviving infants with birthweights of less than 1500 g. Six of the infants (12%) had severe neurological handicaps and 10 (20%) had mild disabilities, predominantly abnormalities of muscle tone or attention deficit disorder. One other publication including long-term outcome of surviving infants, authored by Gonen *et al.* (1990), included 24 triplets, 5 quadruplets and 1 quintuplet pregnancy. The incidence of respiratory distress syndrome was 41%, bronchopulmonary dysplasia 4%, retinopathy of prematurity 4%, and intraventricular haemorrhage 4%. Follow-up from 1 to 10 years, however, showed that among all the survivors only one was moderately handicapped.

The available data regarding the natural history of quadruplets are extremely limited (Table 6.2). The mean gestational age at delivery is approximately 31 weeks. Almost all patients with quadruplets deliver before 37 weeks, approximately half deliver before 32 weeks and one fifth deliver before 28 weeks. The perinatal mortality in the largest series was 67 per 1000 (Collins & Bleyl, 1990). Recently Elliot & Radin (1992)

reported 10 quadruplet pregnancies cared for in one perinatal practice with a mean gestational age at delivery of 32.5 weeks and no perinatal deaths.

Although most quadruplet neonates survive, there is very little information about the morbidity and long-term outcome. This information is sorely needed since the risk of severe prematurity is substantial and mortality figures may not tell the entire story. Lipitz *et al.* (1990) described the outcome of 11 pregnancies consisting of four or more fetuses: eight quadruplets, two quintuplets and one sextuplet. The overall perinatal mortality was 119/1000. Most of the surviving infants were followed for at least two years: 30% were found to have neurodevelopmental abnormalities, including 25% of surviving quadruplets. Most reports of pregnancies of five or more fetuses are anecdotal and meaningful statistics do not exist.

Multifetal pregnancies also pose maternal risks. Mothers carrying triplets have a 20% incidence of pregnancy-induced hypertension, 11–35% incidence of anaemia and 35% incidence of postpartum haemorrhage (Lynch & Berkowitz, 1991). Of the mothers carrying quadruplets, 30–90% develop pregnancy-induced hypertension, 25% develop anaemia and 20% experience postpartum haemorrhage (Lynch & Berkowitz, 1991; Elliot & Radin, 1992).

Table 6.2 *Natural history of quadruplet pregnancies*

Author	Years	No. of pregnancies	Mean (weeks)	Gestational age at delivery (weeks)		
				< 37 (%)	< 32 (%)	< 28 (%)
Vervliet *et al.*, 1989	1985–88	5	31	100	60	20
Lipitz *et al.*, 1990	1975–89	8	31	100	50	25
Gonen *et al.*, 1990	1978–88	5	30	100	N/A	N/A
Collins & Bleyl, 1990	1980–89	71	31	97	61	20
Elliot & Radin, 1992	1986–91	10	32	100	40	0
Average			31	99	53	16

N/A, not available.

Multifetal pregnancy reduction

Background

Multifetal pregnancies are at increased risk of preterm delivery and the magnitude of this risk is directly correlated with the number of fetuses within the uterus. Multifetal pregnancy reduction has been advocated as a way of reducing that risk. The initial report of first-trimester reductions of multifetal pregnancies was published in 1986. Dumez & Oury (1986) presented 15 multifetal pregnancies reduced to 4 singletons, 10 sets of twins and 1 set of triplets. At the time the report was written, nine patients had successfully delivered, four pregnancies were ongoing and two women had lost the entire pregnancy. The technique used by these authors was transcervical aspiration of one or more sacs under ultrasound guidance. The same year, Kanhai *et al.* (1986) reduced a quintuplet pregnancy to twins by thoracic puncture under ultrasound visualization. Our group (Berkowitz *et al.*, 1988) reported the first series of transabdominal multifetal pregnancy reductions. The first three procedures were performed by the transcervical aspiration method, but the third patient experienced intractable bleeding secondary to placental separation so the following nine patients were treated with transabdominal intrathoracic injection of potassium chloride.

Outcome

More recently, we have reported the outcome of 200 consecutive multifetal pregnancies reduced to a smaller number by transabdominal intrathoracic injection of potassium chloride (Berkowitz *et al.*, 1993). At the time of the procedure, 88 women had triplets, 89 had quadruplets, 16 had quintuplets, and seven had from six to nine fetuses. These pregnancies were reduced to 189 sets of twins, five sets of triplets, and six singletons. Reductions to triplets were done at the patient's request, and reductions to singletons were only done for medical indications. There were no cases of chorioamnionitis or other maternal complications attributable to the procedure. One hundred and eighty-one women delivered one or more liveborn infants after 24 weeks' gestation, and 19 (10%) lost their entire pregnancies prior to that time. The mean gestational age at delivery was 35.7 weeks. The mean age of gestation varied inversely with the initial number of fetuses, from 36.1 weeks for women who presented with triplets to 33.8 weeks for those who had six or more fetuses. There were two neonatal and one infant death. Of the complete pregnancy losses, 16 of the 19 occurred more than four weeks after the procedure. The loss rates were 8% for those who presented with three or four fetuses, 13% for those with five, and 43% for those with six or more. The actual percentage may not be representative in the group with six or more fetuses because there were only seven patients in this category. However, statistical analysis did find a significant trend towards higher loss rates in patients with five or more fetuses as compared with those with three or four.

Other authors have also published their experience with transabdominal reductions with similar results (Wapner *et al.*, 1990; Tabsh, 1993; Donner *et al.*, 1991).

Evans *et al.* (1993) recently compiled data on 463 transabdominal multifetal pregnancy reductions from several centres including our own. A success rate of 100% was observed. The total pregnancy loss rate was 4% at two weeks or less postprocedure, 5% at four weeks or less, and 16% at less than 24 weeks' gestation. The overall loss rate was related to the starting and the finishing number of fetuses. The loss rates were 7%, 15%, and 30% for patients presenting with triplets, quadruplets and quintuplets, respectively, and who were reduced to twins. The total loss rate was the lowest in patients reduced to twins (14%) compared with singletons (25%) and triplets (27%). The data on singletons must be interpreted with caution because most centres only reduced to singletons when other factors were present that would make a twin pregnancy too risky. Most of the procedures were performed between 8 and 12 weeks' gestation and there was no difference in loss rates by week. Eighty-four per cent of the patients delivered potentially viable infants of 24 weeks' gestation, 9% delivered between 29 and 32 weeks, and 7% between 24 and 29 weeks. The larger the starting and finishing number of fetuses, the earlier the ultimate delivery.

Based on ours and other series of transabdominal multifetal pregnancy reductions the following can be concluded: (i) the total pregnancy loss rate is correlated with the initial and the final number of fetuses; (ii) the proportion of losses related to the actual procedure cannot be assessed because the background loss rate is not known; (iii) gestational age at delivery is inversely correlated with the initial and final number of fetuses; (iv) gestational age at the time of the procedure within the 8 to 12 week window has no effect on pregnancy loss rates, but procedures performed after 12 weeks' gestation may be associated with higher rates of prematurity; (v) significant maternal complications have not been reported; and (vi) the risk of congenital anomalies in the survivors is not increased.

Transvaginal embryo aspiration (Itskowitz-Eldor *et al.*, 1992) or intrathoracic injection has also been utilized. Timor-Tritsch *et al.* (1993) reported 134 multifetal pregnancy reductions performed by transvaginal intrathoracic injection of potassium chloride. A corrected loss rate of 11% was observed. Three intrauterine infections occurred resulting in total pregnancy loss in one patient. The total pregnancy loss rate was similar whether the presenting or a non-presenting fetus was terminated.

At the present time it is unclear whether the transabdominal or transvaginal approach is superior (Evans *et al.*, 1994). Experience so far suggests that the risks of pregnancy loss are quite similar, although there might be a slightly higher risk of intrauterine infection after transvaginal reductions. Certain technical or clinical conditions would on occasion favour one approach over the other. For example, active vaginal infection would dictate a transabdominal approach, while extreme obesity or poor ultrasonic visualization would make the transvaginal approach safer.

Technique

The technique utilized at the Mount Sinai Medical Center has been described in detail elsewhere (Lynch *et al.*, 1990). Briefly, an ultrasound examination is performed before the procedure in order to identify the locations of all the fetuses, ascertain their viability, measure their crown–rump lengths, look for morphologic abnormalities and evaluate the chorionicity of the separating membranes. Separate placentas are obviously dichorionic. If the placentas are fused, the chorionicity must be determined by the ultrasonographic appearance of the dividing membrane. The difference in thickness between the thick dichorionic and thin monochorionic membranes is much more obvious during the first trimester than it is later in pregnancy. Furthermore, the presence of chorionic villi between the layers of a dichorionic membrane produces what has been called 'twin peak' (Finberg, 1992) or 'lambda sign' (Bessis & Papiernik, 1981), which is a triangular projection where the membrane originates from the placenta (Figs. 6.1 and 6.2). This finding clearly establishes the dividing membrane as dichorionic.

Whenever possible the fetus in the lowest sac is not terminated unless it has a detectable anomaly or appears to be a member of a monochorionic set of twins. A 22 gauge 9 cm needle is introduced under direct ultrasonographic visualization into the thorax of a fetus, and 2–3 mEq potassium chloride (2 mEq/ml concentration) is injected. If cardiac activity persists, more potassium chloride is injected. Cardiac standstill is observed for several minutes before the needle is removed. This procedure is then repeated for other fetuses if necessary. Usually separate percutaneous needle insertions are required to terminate each fetus. However, on occasion one of the fetuses to be terminated is located directly beneath another and two fetuses can be terminated with one needle insertion. Generally we avoid traversing the sac of a fetus with the needle unless this fetus is also going to be terminated. We do not terminate more than three fetuses at one visit; therefore, women with six or more fetuses have their procedures performed during two or more sessions, generally one week apart. One dose of a cephalosporin is given intravenously as prophylaxis before the procedure.

The transvaginal method as described by Timor-Tritsch *et al.* (1993) utilizes a spring-loaded device with a 21 gauge needle attached to the transvaginal probe. Alternatively, standard needles attached to the transvaginal probe can be manually inserted into the gestational sac and into the fetal thorax. Potassium chloride is injected in order to achieve asystole. Other authors have reported transvaginal needle embryo aspiration (Itskovitz-Eldor *et al.*, 1992).

Timing

Most multifetal pregnancies result from infertility treatment and are, therefore, identified early in the first trimester. If the procedure is performed too early, spontaneous loss of one or more fetuses is not allowed to occur. If performed too late, the risk of premature delivery may be greater (Evans *et al.*, 1993). Most centres performing transabdominal reduction do so at 10 to 12 weeks' gestation and those using the transvaginal

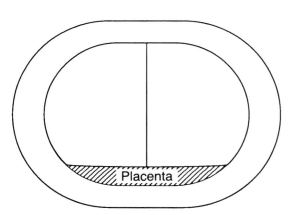

Monochorionic Membrane

Fig. 6.1 *Ultrasonographic appearance of dichorionic membrane with 'twin peak' sign.*

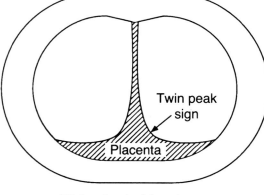

Dichorionic Membrane

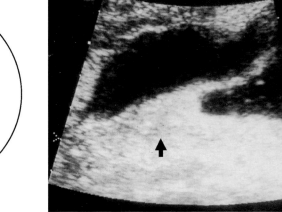

approach perform the procedures at nine to 10 weeks' gestation.

Initial number of fetuses

Most obstetricians would agree that multifetal pregnancy reduction is likely to be beneficial in pregnancies of four or more fetuses given the risks of extreme prematurity. Reduction of triplets is more controversial, mainly because neonatal survival has improved so dramatically since the 1960s. However, the rates of prematurity have not changed despite the advent of modern obstetrical tools such as outpatient contraction monitoring and tocolytics. Since the risk of preterm birth is unchanged but the rate of survival is higher, it is important to consider the morbidity and long-term outcome of the survivors. Unfortunately, there are very few pub-

lished data regarding the long-term follow-up of surviving triplets, as discussed earlier. However, six studies comparing the perinatal outcome of triplets with twins have recently been published and are summarized in Table 6.3. Five of them found a significant difference in gestational age at delivery and mean birthweight. Three found a significant difference in mean neonatal hospital stay. Of the five studies that included data on neonatal morbidity, two did not find any difference between the groups (Sassoon *et al.*, 1990; Porreco, Burke & Hendrix, 1991), and three did find significantly greater rates of neonatal morbidity in triplets (Seoud *et al.*, 1992; Boulot *et al.*, 1993; Lipitz *et al.*, 1994). Follow-up after the neonatal period was provided in two of these studies. Boulot *et al.* (1993) at six months' follow-up found one infant in each group with severe

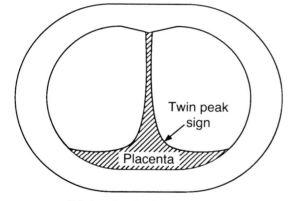

Dichorionic Membrane

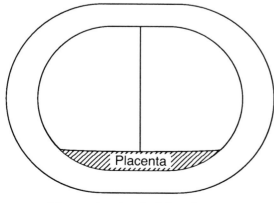

Monochorionic Membrane

Fig. 6.2 *Ultrasonographic appearance of monochorionic membrane.*

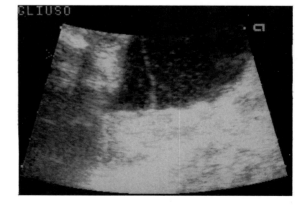

Table 6.3 *perinatal outcome of triplets compared with twins*

Author	Study groups	No. of patients	Mean GA at delivery (weeks)	Mean birthweight (g)	Mean neonatal hospital stay (days)	Perinatal mortality rate
Sassoon *et al*, 1990	Triplets	15	33*	1720*	29 ± 46*	95/1000
	Twins	15	36.6*	2475*	8.5 ± 11*	100/1000
Porreco *et al.*, 1991	Twins	11	35.7	2239	11.7 ± 13	0
	Twins, reduced from triplets	13	35.5	2727	12.7 ± 17	0
Seoud *et al.*, 1992	Triplets	13	31.8*	1666*	28.1 ± 16*	22/1000
	Twins	107	35.5*	2473*	8.9 ± 10*	72/1000
Macones *et al.*, 1993	Triplets	14	31.2*	1593*	N/A	210/1000*
	Twins, reduced from triplets	47	35.6*	2279*	N/A	30/1000*
	Twins	63	34.8	2292	N/A	40/1000
Boulot *et al.* 1993	Triplets	48	34.4*	1870*	31.3 ± 15*	59/1000
	Twins, reduced from triplets	32	36.7*	2340*	16.9 ± 13*	38/1000
Lipitz *et al.*, 1994	Triplets	106	33.5*	1780*	N/A	109/1000
	Twins, reduced from triplets	34	36.7*	2350*	N/A	48/1000

GA, gestational age. N/A, not available.
*, Statistically significant difference.

mental retardation and the others were deemed normal. Lipitz *et al.* (1994) followed 52 triplet infants weighing less than 1500 g at birth until at least one year of age and found that 12% had severe disabilities and 20% had mild disabilities. None of the four surviving twins with birthweights less than 1500 g had any disabilities. Pregnancy complications were more common in triplets than in twins in all studies. Interestingly, in the report by Boulot *et al.* (1993), 10% of women with triplets suffered life-threatening complications versus none in the twin group.

In summary, compared with twin pregnancies, triplets generally deliver at a significantly earlier gestational age, have a higher risk of low birthweight and have more complications in the neonatal period. However, it is not clear whether all this translates into higher rates of permanent disabilities. Patients with triplets should receive all the information available and the option of multifetal pregnancy reduction should be offered. The possibility that reducing the number of fetuses may decrease the rate of maternal complications should also be discussed.

Final number of fetuses

When multifetal pregnancy reduction was first introduced, most operators felt that reducing the number of fetuses to twins was optimal and refused to reduce multifetal pregnancies to a singleton unless there were other significant risk factors.

In about 2% of cases after multifetal pregnancy reduction to twins, one of the remaining fetuses will have a significant congenital anomaly or die *in utero*. If the pregnancy had been reduced to a singleton, the couple would have lost the entire pregnancy. Another disadvantage is that it is not clear whether reducing to a singleton

Table 6.4 *Relative risk for twins compared with singletons for very low birthweight, low birthweight, neonatal death, postnatal death and infant death*

	Relative risk[a]
Very low birthweight	10.0 (9.8–10.1)
Low birthweight	8.6 (8.6–8.7)
Neonatal death	7.1 (6.9–7.3)
Postneonatal death	2.8 (2.6–2.9)
Infant death	5.4 (5.3–5.6)

Modified from Powers & Kiely, 1994.
[a] Relative risk with 95% confidence intervals in parentheses.

Table 6.5 *Cerebral palsy prevalence in twins and singletons in three birthweight groups*

| | Birthweight (g) | | |
	<1500	1500–2499	≥ 2500
Twins			
No. with CP	12	4	4
CP prevalence[a]	68	3.5	2.4
95% CI	(37–118)	(1.1–9.7)	(0.8–6.5)
Singletons			
No. with CP	42	33	97
CP prevalence[a]	48	5.3	0.7
95% CI	(3.5–64)	(3.7–7.6)	(0.5–0.8)

Modified from Grether, Nelson & Cummins, 1993.
CI, confidence interval.
[a] per 1000 surviving 3 year olds.

increases the risk of pregnancy loss. In the data compiled by Evans *et al.* (1993), those patients reduced to one fetus had a significantly higher miscarriage rate than those reduced to twins. However, most centres participating in that study only performed pregnancy reductions to a singleton when there where other medical risk factors. This may have artificially increased the rate of pregnancy loss in this group.

There are several potential medical benefits of reducing to a singleton. There is a significant increase in the risk of very low birthweight, low birthweight, neonatal death, and infant death in twins compared with singletons (Table 6.4) (Powers & Kiely, 1994; Luke & Keith, 1992; Spellacy, Handler & Ferre, 1990).

The rate of permanent disabilities is also higher in twins compared with singletons. Recently, Grether *et al.* (1993) identified 2985 infants from 1537 twin pregnancies and 152 587 singletons born in 1983 to 1985 in four northern California counties and surviving to three years. Among 2985 twins, 20 children in 18 pairs had cerebral palsy. The prevalence was 6.7 per 1000 three-year-old twin children (95% confidence interval (CI) 4.2 to 11), 12 per 1000 twin pregnancies (95% CI, 7.2 to 19), and 1.1 per 1000 singletons (95% CI, 0.97 to 1.3). Twins were over-represented among very low birthweight infants but their risk of cerebral palsy was comparable with that of very low birthweight in

singletons (Table 6.5). Twins born weighing 2500 g or more had a cerebral palsy risk 3.6 times that of singletons of similar weight. The rate in unlike sex pairs was 13 per 1000; therefore, even in obligatory dichorionic pregnancies, the risk of cerebral palsy was increased. Although twin pregnancies produced a child with cerebral palsy 12 times more often than singleton pregnancies, the absolute risk is quite small and may not justify reducing a multifetal pregnancy to a singleton pregnancy.

In addition to the potential, albeit marginal, medical benefits of reducing to a singleton, other ethical, social, psychological, and financial considerations may be compelling reasons to comply with a patient's wish to have her pregnancy reduced from three or more fetuses to one. Although reducing a multifetal pregnancy to a singleton on demand may be disturbing to some people, present public policy in the USA would permit the whole pregnancy to be terminated before viability. In contrast, the selection procedure preserves at least some fetuses. This author's approach is to advise couples to reduce to twins unless other risk factors are present such as previous preterm delivery, incompetent cervix, and uterine anomalies. However, reduction to a singleton will be undertaken if, after extensive counselling, the couple still wishes to do so. For a more in-depth discussion of the ethical considerations of multifetal pregnancy reduction, the reader is referred to Chapter 22.

Psychological aspects

The emotional response of women suffering spontaneous pregnancy loss is characterized by feelings of bereavement and mourning which recede gradually over three months and generally persist no more than a year (Kennell, Slyter & Klaus, 1970; Borg & Lasker, 1988; Friedman & Gradstein, 1982). Typically, grief is re-experienced for several years on the anniversary of the fetal loss. Women who electively abort have been found to have acute emotional reactions as severe as those having a spontaneous miscarriage but do not grieve nearly as long (Kessler, 1979; Osterweis, Solomon & Green, 1984) and subsequently experience little regret about their decision (Notman & Nadelson, 1978).

Women who undergo multifetal pregnancy reduction are different from those having spontaneous or induced abortions. These are all patients who received infertility treatment, whose pregnancies are often desperately wanted, and who are now faced with the decision to terminate some fetuses to improve the outcome of the others. A natural consequence is that these patients sometimes feel they are choosing or 'selecting' which fetuses are to survive (Berkowitz & Lynch, 1990).

Because of these differences, our group sought to determine the acute and persistent psychological impact of multifetal pregnancy reduction (Schreiner-Engel et al., 1994). The first 100 women to undergo this procedure were invited to participate in a study assessing their emotional reactions and attitudes towards the procedure. Interviews were conducted at least six months after the completion of their pregnancies. The majority of women agreed that the reduction procedure was stressful, painful emotionally, and frightening. Mourning for the lost fetuses was reported by 70% of the women; but for most, grieving lasted only one month. Persistent depressive symptoms were mild, although moderately severe levels of sadness and guilt continue for many. Nevertheless, the overwhelming majority would make the same decision to have multifetal pregnancy reduction in a future pregnancy. Emotional reactions of patients who lost the entire pregnancy after the procedure differed little. We concluded that multifetal pregnancy reductions, although highly stressful psychologically, are well tolerated.

Prenatal care and perinatal outcome

The prenatal care of patients whose pregnancy has been reduced to twins should be no different than that of normal twins with the following exceptions. After first-trimester multifetal pregnancy reduction, second-trimester maternal serum alpha-fetoprotein (MSAFP) is consistently elevated (Grau et al., 1990; Lynch & Berkowitz, 1993). This elevation is primarily caused by the presence of a dead fetus or fetuses. Amniocentesis is not indicated in these cases, but ultrasound evaluation of the fetal anatomy should be considered since MSAFP cannot be used in these patients to screen for fetal defects. Clinically significant disseminated intravascular coagulopathy has never been reported after first-trimester procedures; therefore, monitoring of coagulation parameters is not necessary in these patients (Lynch & Berkowitz, 1993).

The perinatal outcome of pregnancies reduced to twins does not appear to be significantly different from that of pregnancies conceived as twins (Macones et al., 1993; Donner, de Maertellaer & Rodesch, 1992). The one exception may be a higher incidence of intrauterine growth retardation found by some (Macones et al., 1993) but not others (Donner et al., 1992).

Conclusion

Multifetal pregnancy reduction has emerged as a safe and widely accepted option for couples with pregnancies of three or more fetuses. Cumulative experience to date suggests that the transabdominal approach undertaken between 10 and 12 weeks' gestation is preferred. The fetal loss rates for patients presenting with triplets, quadruplets and quintuplets who underwent reduction to twins were 7%, 15% and 30%, respectively.

Patients experience grief which resolves in the majority of cases within one month of the procedure. Although multifetal reduction would appear to be of benefit for high-order gestations, the more logical approach would be prevention of their occurrence through the more judicious use of newer assisted reproductive technologies.

References

Australian In Vitro Fertilization Collaborative Group (1988). In-vitro fertilization pregnancies in Australia and New Zealand, 1979–1985. *Medical Journal of Australia*, 148, 429–36.

Berkowitz, R. L. & Lynch, L. (1990). Selective reduction: an unfortunate misnomer. *Obstetrics and Gynecology*, 75, 874.

Berkowitz, R. L., Lynch, L., Chitkara, U., Wilkins, I. A., Mehalek, K. E. & Alvarez, E. (1988). Selective reduction of multifetal pregnancies in the first trimester. *New England Journal of Medicine*, 318, 1043–7.

Berkowitz, R. L., Lynch, L., Lapinski, R. & Bergh, P. (1993). First trimester transabdominal multifetal pregnancy reduction: a report of 200 completed cases. *American Journal of Obstetrics and Gynecology*, 169, 17–21.

Bessis, R. & Papiernik, E. (1981). Echographic imagery of amniotic membranes in twin pregnancies. In *Twin Research*, Vol. 3: *Twin Biology and Multiple Pregnancy*, ed. L. Gedda & P. Parisi, pp. 183–7. New York: Alan R. Liss.

Borg, S. & Lasker, J. N. (1988). *When Pregnancy Fails: Families Coping with Miscarrage, Ectopic pregnancy, Stillbirth and Infant Death.* New York: Boston Beacon Press.

Botting, B. J., Davies, I. M. & Macfarlane, A. J. (1987). Recent trends in the incidence of multiple births and associated mortality. *Archives of Disease in Childhood*, 62, 941–50.

Boulot, P., Hedon, B., Pelliccia, G., Peray, P. & Laffargue, F. (1993). Effects of selective reduction in triplet gestation: a comparative study of 80 cases managed with or without this procedure. *Fertility and Sterility*, 60, 497–503.

Collins, M. S. & Bleyl, J. A. (1990). Seventy-one quadruplet pregnancies: management and outcome. *American Journal of Obstetrics and Gynecology*, 162, 1384–91.

Creinin, M., Katz, M. & Laros, R. (1991). Triplet pregnancy: changes in morbidity and mortality. *Journal of Perinatology*, 111, 207–12.

Donner, C., McGinnis, J. A., Simone, P. & Rodesch, F. (1991). Multifetal pregnancy reduction: a Belgian experience. *European Journal of Obstetrics, Gynecology, and Reproductive Biology*, 38, 183–7.

Donner, C., de Maertelaer, V. & Rodesch, F. (1992). Multifetal pregnancy reduction: comparison of obstetrical resullts with spontaneous twin gestations. *European Journal of Obstetrics, Gynecology, and Reproductive Biology*, 44, 181–4.

Dumez, Y. & Oury, J. (1986). Method for first trimester selective abortion in multiple pregnancy. *Contributions to Gynecology and Obstetrics*, 15, 50–3.

Elliott, J. P. & Radin, T. G. (1992) Quadruplet pregnancy: contemporary management and outcome. *Obstetrics and Gynecology*, 80, 421–4.

Evans, M. I., Dommergues, M., Wapner, R. J., Lynch, L., Dumez, Y., Goldberg, J. D., Zador, I. E., Nicolaides, K. H., Johnson, M. P., Golbus, M. S., Boulot, P. & Berkowitz, R. L. (1993). Efficacy of transabdominal multifetal pregnancy reduction: collaborative experience among the world's largest centers. *Obstetrics and Gynecology*, 82, 61–6.

Evans, M. I., Dommergues, M., Timor-Tritsch, I., Zador, I. E., Wapner, R. J., Lynch, L., Dumez, Y., Goldberg, J. D., Nicolaides, K. H., Johnson, M. P., Golbus, M. S., Boulot, P., Aknin, A. J., Monteagudo, A. & Berkowitz, R. L. (1994). Transabdominal versus transcervical and transvaginal multifetal pregnancy reduction: international collaborative experience of more than one thousand cases. *American Journal of Obstetrics and Gynecology*, 170, 902–9.

Finberg, H. J. (1992). The 'twin peak' sign: reliable evidence of dichorionic twinning. *Journal of Ultrasound in Medicine*, 11, 571–7.

Friedman, R. & Gradstein, B. (1982). *Surviving Pregnancy Loss*. Boston: Little Brown.

Gonen, R., Heyman, E., Asztalos, E. V., Ohlsson, A., Pitson, L. C., Shennan, A. T. & Milligan, J. E. (1990). The outcome of triplet, quadruplet, and quintuplet pregnancies managed in a perinatal unit: obstetric, neonatal and follow-up data. *American Journal of Obstetrics and Gynecology*, 162, 454–9.

Grau, P., Robinson, L., Tabsh, K. & Crandall, B. F. (1990). Elevated maternal serum alpha-fetoprotein and amniotic fluid alpha-fetoprotein after multifetal pregnancy reduction. *Obstetrics and Gynecology*, 76, 1042–5.

Grether, J. K., Nelson, K. B. & Cummins, S. K. (1993). Twinning and cerebral palsy: experience in four northern California counties, births 1983 through 1985. *Pediatrics*, 92, 854–8.

Holcberg, G., Biale, Y., Lewenthal, H. & Insler, V. (1982). Outcome of pregnancy in 31 triplet gestations. *Obstetrics and Gynecology*, 59, 472–6.

Itzkowic, D. (1979). A survey of 59 triplet pregnancies. *British Journal of Obstetrics and Gynaecology*, 86, 23–8.

Itskovitz-Eldor, J., Drugan, A., Levron, J., Thaler I. & Brandes J. M. (1992). Transvaginal embryo aspiration – a safe method for selective reduction in multiple pregnancies. *Fertility and Sterility*, 58, 351–5.

Kanhai, H. H., van Rijssel, E. J., Meerman, R. J. & Bennebroek-Gravenhorst, J. (1986). Selective termination in quintuplet pregnancy during first trimester. *Lancet*, i, 1447.

Kennell, J. H., Slyter, H. & Klaus, M. H. (1970). The mourning response of parents to the death of a newborn infant. *New England Journal of Medicine*, 283, 344–9.

Kessler, S. (1979). *Genetic Counseling: Psychological Dimensions*. New York: Academic Press.

Kiely, J. L., Kleinman, J. C. & Kiely, M. (1992). Triplets and higher-order multiple births: time trends and infant mortality. *American Journal of Diseases in Children*, 146, 862–8.

Levene, M. I., Wild, J. & Steer, P. (1992). Higher multiple births and the modern management of infertility in Britain. The British Association of Perinatal Medicine. *British Journal of Obstetrics and Gynaecology*, 99, 607–13.

Lipitz, S., Frenkel, Y., Watts, C., Ben-Rafael, Z., Barkai, G. & Reichman, B. (1990). High-order multifetal gestation – management and outcome. *Obstetrics and Gynecology*, 76, 215–18.

Lipitz, S., Reichman, B., Uval, J., Shalev, J., Achiron, R., Barkai, G., Lusky, A. & Mashiach, S. (1994). A prospective comparison of the outcome of triplet pregnancies managed expectantly or by multifetal reduction to twins. *American Journal of Obstetrics and Gynecology*, 170, 874–9.

Luke, B. & Keith L. G. (1992). The contribution of singletons, twins and triplets to low birth weight, infant mortality and handicap in the United States. *Journal of Reproductive Medicine*, 37, 661–6.

Lynch, L. & Berkowitz, R. L. (1993). Maternal serum alpha fetoprotein and coagulation profiles after multifetal pregnancy reduction. *American Journal of Obstetrics and Gynecology*, 169, 987–90.

Lynch, L & Berkowitz, R. L. (1991). Multifetal pregnancy reduction. *Ultasonography in Reproductive Medicine*, 2, 771–81.

Lynch, L., Berkowitz, R. L., Chitkara, U. & Alvarez, M. (1990). First-trimester transabdominal multifetal reduction: a report of 85 cases. *Obstetrics and Gynecology*, 75, 735–8.

Macones, G. A., Schemmer, G., Pritts, E., Weinblatt, V. & Wapner, R. J. (1993). Multifetal reduction of triplets to twins improves perinatal outcome. *American Journal of Obstetrics and Gynecology*, 169, 982–6.

Newman, R. B., Hamer, C. & Clinton Miller, M. (1989). Outpatient triplet management: a contemporary review. *American Journal of Obstetrics and Gynecology*, 161, 547–53.

Notman, M. T. & Nadelson, C. C. (ed.) (1978). The emotional impact of abortions. In *The Woman Patient*, 1st edn, pp. 173–9. New York: Plenum Press.

Osterweis, M., Solomon, F. & Green, M. (ed.) (1984). In *Bereavement: Reactions, Consequences and Care*. Washington, DC: National Academy Press.

Porreco, R. P., Burke, M. S. & Hendrix, M. L. (1991). Multifetal reduction of triplets and pregnancy outcome. *Obstetrics and Gynecology*, 78, 335–9.

Powers, W. F. & Kiely, J. L. (1994). The risk confronting twins: a national perspective. *American Journal of Obstetrics and Gynecology*, 170, 456–61.

Sassoon, D. A., Castro, L. C., Davis, J. L. & Hobel, C. J. (1990). Perinatal outcome in triplet versus twin gestations. *Obstetrics and Gynecology*, 75, 817–20.

Schreiner-Engel, P., Walther, V. N., Mindes, J., Lynch, L. & Berkowitz, R. L. (1995). First trimester multifetal pregnancy reduction: acute and persistent psychological reaction. *American Journal of Obstetrics and Gynecology*, 172, 541–7.

Seoud, M. F., Toner, J. P., Kruithoff, C. & Muasher, S. J. (1992). Outcome of twin, triplet, and quadruplet *in vitro* fertilization pregnancies: the Norfolk experience. *Fertility and Sterility*, 57, 825–34.

Spellacy, W. N., Handler, A. & Ferre, C. D. (1990). A case-control study of 1253 twin pregnancies from a 1982–1987 perinatal data base. *Obstetrics and Gynecology*, 75, 168–71.

Syrop, C. H. & Varner, M. W. (1985). Triplet gestation: maternal and neonatal implications. *Acta Geneticae Medicae et Gemmellologiae*, 34, 81–8.

Tabsh, K. A. (1993). A report of 131 cases of multifetal pregnancy reduction. *Obstetrics and Gynecology*, 82, 57–60.

Timor-Tritsch, I. E., Peisner, D. B., Monteagudo, A., Lerner, J. P. & Sharma, S. (1993). Multifetal pregnancy reduction by transvaginal puncture: evaluation of the technique used in 134 cases. *American Journal of Obstetrics and Gynecology*, 168, 799–804.

Vervliet, J., de Cleyn, K., Renier, M., Janssens, P., Buytaert, P., Gerris, J. & Delbeke, L. (1989). Management and outcome of 21 triplet and quadruplet pregnancies. *European Journal of Obstetrical and Gynecological Reproductive Biology*, 33, 61–9.

7 Respiratory distress syndrome
CAROLINE A. CROWTHER

Background

Infants born preterm are at high risk of developing respiratory distress syndrome (RDS) as a consequence of lung immaturity (Roberton, 1982). The earlier in gestation the delivery the greater this risk. At 29–30 weeks of gestation, the incidence of RDS in vaginal births is 64%, decreasing as age increases in two-weekly increments to 35%, 20%, 5% down to 0.8% at 37 weeks or more (Usher et al., 1971).

Worldwide RDS together with the sequelae of chronic lung disease remain the most common cause of infant mortality for infants weighing less than 1500 g at birth, as recent reports from the USA (Wegman, 1989) and Australia (Australian Bureau of Statistics, 1993) confirm. In addition, RDS and its sequelae are associated with considerable morbidity and high costs (Boyle et al., 1983; Doyle, Murton & Kitchen, 1989). Given this significant mortality and morbidity associated with RDS and the costs of hospital care, any intervention that reduces the frequency or severity of RDS, and thereby the inherent complications, is of great importance.

This chapter briefly reviews the regulation of fetal lung maturation and the rationale for antenatal treatment for the prevention of RDS. For combinations of hormones used to accelerate lung maturation, laboratory and animal evidence is reviewed followed by data from randomized clinical trials in humans, using glucocorticoids and thyrotrophin-releasing hormone (TRH) to prevent RDS. Wherever possible, a pooled analysis of comparable studies or meta-analysis is presented. The areas for future development are outlined and recommendations made for clinical practice and further research.

Lung development

The state of maturation of the fetal lung is the major determinant of whether the preterm infant will survive. Fetal lung development involves growth, maturation of lung structure and maturation of lung function (Liggins & Schellenberg, 1985). The regulation of lung development is under multihormonal control and is influenced by glucocorticoids, insulin, androgens, oestrogen, catecholamines, epidermal growth factor, transforming growth factor, prolactin, thyroid hormones and TRH and other factors (Gross, 1990). The actions of some of these agents will be reviewed briefly.

Gluococorticoids, the hormones most widely studied, accelerate most aspects of lung differentiation. Surfactant phospholipid synthesis is increased (Gross et al., 1983) as is the production of surfactant-associated proteins (Liley et al., 1989; Odom et al., 1988), which are required for the normal structure, function and metabolism of surfactant. Glucocorticoids also enhance fetal lung compliance (Rider et al., 1990).

Thyroid hormones, like glucocorticoids, increase surfactant phospholipids (Ballard, Hovey & Gonzales, 1984) through a receptor-mediated action, with tri-iodothyronine (T_3) being more potent than thyroxine (T_4). However, they do not increase the surfactant-associated proteins (Gross, 1990). Thyroid hormones do not readily cross the placenta, but after maternal administration, TRH does cross the placenta and stimulates the fetal pituitary to produce thyroid-stimulating hormone (TSH), which, in turn, stimulates fetal thyroid hormone release (Roti et al., 1981).

The polypeptide growth factor epidermal growth factor (EGF) has been shown to enhance surfactant phospholipid synthesis (Gross *et al.*, 1986) and increase surfactant-associated protein (SP), especially SP-A (Whitsett *et al.*, 1987). The role of other hormones considered to be involved in the regulation of fetal lung maturation, such as prolactin, oestrogen and α-interferon, is less certain (Gross, 1990).

Some agents appear to inhibit fetal lung maturation. These include transforming growth factor-β (TGF-β) (Whitsett *et al.*, 1987), insulin (Gross *et al.*, 1980) and androgens, which decrease phosphatidylcholine synthesis; this may explain the apparent delayed lung development in male fetuses (Torday, 1990).

Rationale for *in utero* treatment

RDS has been known to be associated with surfactant deficiency since Avery and Mead's classic paper in 1959 (Avery & Mead, 1959). Surfactant is produced and secreted by type II epithelial cells in the alveoli of the lung and is composed of a monolayer of phospholipid that stabilizes the alveoli and so prevents alveolae collapse at low volumes. Deficiency of surfactant results in RDS. In recent years, surfactant-replacement therapy has become available and when administered to the neonate as either a natural or a synthetic surfactant is effective in the prevention or treatment of RDS. Trials conducted to establish the effectiveness of surfactant replacement therapy have been reviewed recently by Soll & McQueen (1992).

The use of antenatal maternal administration of corticosteroids in women at risk of preterm delivery had been advocated many years prior to the availability of postnatal surfactant therapy (Liggins & Howie, 1972), based on the glucocorticoid action of increasing pulmonary surfactant synthesis and facilitating other mechanisms of lung maturation (Gross, 1990).

However, even when glucocorticoids are used, RDS remains a major problem, particularly if delivery occurs at a very early gestational age or within 24 hours of steroid administration. Attention, therefore, has focused on other agents involved in the regulation of lung maturation, such as TRH whose antenatal administration might be efficacious in accelerating lung maturation in the fetus at risk of preterm delivery (Liggins *et al.*, 1988a). The use of antenatally administered gluco-

corticoids and TRH to reduce the risk of neonatal respiratory disease will be reviewed in detail.

Antenatal administration of glucocorticoids before preterm delivery

Laboratory and animal studies

In 1969, Liggins reported that glucocorticoid infusion induced precocious lung maturation in lambs delivered prematurely. Survival was longer than for placebo-treated animals (Liggins, 1969). Liggins and colleagues applied this observation to human perinatal medicine in their now classic randomized placebo-controlled trial of antenatal betamethasone, given to women at risk of preterm delivery (Liggins & Howie, 1972). In the betamethasone-exposed babies born before 32 weeks, there was a reduction in the incidence of RDS and there was a reduction in neonatal mortality for babies born before 37 weeks' gestation.

Many studies have subsequently demonstrated that glucocorticoids accelerate, *in vitro* and *in vivo*, the physiological, biochemical and morphological maturation of the fetal lung. The mechanisms of action are complex, with differential effects on lung morphology and biochemistry that are likely to be dependent on gestational age (Brumley *et al.*, 1977).

Dose–response effects of corticosteroids on the induction of lung maturation in preterm rabbits have suggested that the beneficial effects of antenatal corticosteroids are not primarily the result of the induction of surfactant synthesis (Tabor *et al.*, 1991). There is an all or nothing response rather than a linear dose response. The increase in lung compliance suggests alterations in lung structure caused by changes in elastin and collagen composition. Such studies suggest corticosteroids improve and mature lung function by multiple pathways.

There is increasing evidence, from work with fetal sheep, that cortisol requires the presence of other hormones to induce lung maturation (Schellenberg *et al.*, 1988; Barker *et al.*, 1990). Cortisol given to the preterm ovine fetus induces many of the morphological and cellular features of lung parenchymal maturation but has minimal effects on the rough endoplasmic reticulum, Golgi apparatus and glycogen content of the type II cell necessary for full pulmonary parenchymal maturation (Kendall *et al.*, 1990). Again, synergism with cortisol catecholamines and T_3 appears important for these maturational effects (Van Golde, Batenburg & Robertson, 1988).

An elegant series of experiments by Schellenberg and colleagues (1988) investigated the hormonal interaction of cortisol, T_3, noradrenaline, prolactin and epidermal growth factor when given alone or in combination for 84 hours to fetal sheep at 124 days of gestation. Cortisol had minimal effect on lung maturation at less than 130 days of gestation. A combination of cortisol, prolactin and T_3, but not any combination of two hormones, increased both distensibility and stability to values obtained near full-term and significantly above values obtained with cortisol treatment alone. Similarly, alveolar-saturated phosphatidylcholine levels were higher after treatment with combinations of cortisol and T_3; cortisol, T_3 and prolactin; and cortisol and oestrogen than after cortisol treatment alone. The conclusion is that cortisol, T_3 and prolactin have a synergistic effect on the secretion of phospholipids in fetal lung and on the development of distensibility and stability in the ovine fetal lung.

Randomized trials of corticosteroids for the prevention of RDS

Since the first report of a clinical trial on the use of antenatal corticosteroids to enhance lung maturity by Liggins and Howie in New Zealand (1972), there are now a further 13 randomized controlled trials in the literature providing clinical outcomes spanning 20 years and involving over 3200 women and their infants (Block, Kling & Crosby, 1977; Morrison *et al.*, 1978; Pagageorgiou *et al.*, 1979; The Amsterdam Trial: Schutte *et al.*, 1979; Tauesch *et al.*, 1979; Doran *et al.*, 1980; Teramo, Hallman & Raivio, 1980; Collaborative Group on Antenatal Steroid Therapy, 1981; Schmidt *et al.*, 1984; Morales *et al.*, 1986; Gamsu *et al.*, 1989; Carlan *et al.*, 1991; Garite, Rumney & Briggs, 1992).

Meta-analysis of trials of corticosteroids prior to preterm delivery

These trials have been reviewed for the Cochrane Collaboration Database of Systematic Reviews, Pregnancy and Childbirth module by Crowley (1994a) (Fig. 7.1).

The type of corticosteroid administered in these trials varied from 24 mg betamethasone, 24 mg dexamethasone to 2 g hydrocortisone, a natural glucocorticoid. There are no randomized trial data suggesting one preparation or route of administration is more efficacious than another (Whitt *et al.*, 1976; Ballard & Ballard, 1979a).

Meta-analysis of the trials showed a marked reduction in the incidence of RDS in babies exposed to antenatal corticosteroids (odds ratio [OR] 0.49 45% CI 0.41–0.59) (Crowley, 1994a). This reduction in RDS, which is independent of gender, was evident in all the subgroups examined and is significant for babies who received optimal treatment (delivery 24 hours or after and within seven days or less of treatment) (OR 0.31 95% CI 0.23–0.42) and for babies who delivered at less than 31 weeks' gestation (OR 0.41 95% CI 0.27–0.62).

There was a suggestion of a beneficial effect with delivery within 24 hours of corticosteroid treatment (OR 0.72 95% CI 0.49–1.06) and treatment after 34 weeks but less than 37 weeks of gestation (OR 0.62 95% CI 0.29–1.30). The effect of antenatal corticosteroids on other non-respiratory neonatal morbidity showed a reduction in periventricular haemorrhage, (OR 0.36 95% CI 0.20–0.67), necrotizing enterocolitis (OR 0.32 95% CI 0.16–0.64) and early neonatal death (OR 0.60 95% CI 0.48–0.76). No effect is seen on the overall incidence of fetal death.

The are no data from randomized controlled trials as to whether or not the course of glucocorticoid therapy should be repeated if the woman remains undelivered but still at risk of preterm delivery.

The efficacy of antenatal corticosteroids at very early gestational ages continues to be a topic for debate with a widespread view that they are ineffective (Ballard *et al.*, 1979; Roberton, 1982). In the very preterm infant, there are likely to be different pathophysiological mechanisms responsible for neonatal respiratory disease, such as immature development of lung architecture in addition to surfactant deficiency, which is primarily responsible for the RDS in infants greater than 32 weeks.

There has only been one randomized trial reported to date that examines the outcome of very low birthweight infants after maternal antenatal corticosteroid therapy before 28 weeks' gestation (Garite *et al.*, 1992). Although no reduction in the incidence or severity of

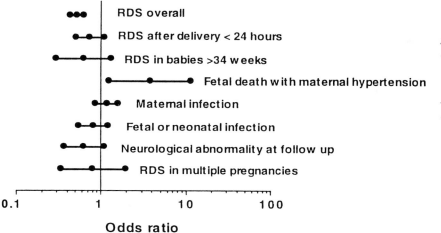

Fig. 7.1 *Overall effect of corticosteroids prior to preterm delivery in meta-analysis of 15 randomized controlled trials (after Crowley, 1994a). Graph shows odds ratios and 95% confidence intervals.*

RDS is seen in the betamethasone-exposed infants, there was a reduction in severe intraventricular haemorrhage (3% vs 25%) and a trend to a reduced stay in the neonatal intensive care unit. The power calculation for that study was based on showing a 50% reduction in RDS, whereas even a small reduction would be of clinical importance. Non-randomized studies examining the efficacy of corticosteroids in very preterm infants have shown promising results (Doyle *et al.*, 1986; Maher *et al.*, 1993). Until evidence is available from further trials, clinical practice should be guided by the current meta-analysis of the seven trials with data for infants born at less than 31 weeks' gestation, which shows a greater reduction in RDS (OR 0.41 95% CI 0.27–0.62) than observed for preterm infants as a whole (OR 0.49 95% CI 0.41–0.59) (Crowley, 1994a).

Preterm delivery in multiple pregnancy is a major cause of mortality and morbidity. The one trial with data for multiple pregnancies is the US Collaborative Group on Antenatal Steroid Therapy Study (Burkett *et al.*, 1986). This suggested reduced benefits from the use of antenatal corticosteroids in multiple pregnancy compared with singletons. Crowley (1989) considers a larger dose of corticosteroids may be necessary in multiple pregnancy and recommends a trial to establish the correct dose.

Potential risks

The beneficial effects of antenatal corticosteroids need to be balanced against any potential risks of treatment to mother or baby. The meta-analysis failed to show any increase in infection for the mother (OR 1.15 95% CI 0.84–1.57), fetus or neonate (OR 1.46 95% CI 0.78–2.72) either with intact membranes or after prelabour rupture of membranes (Crowley, 1994a). Potential suppression of maternal immunity with a corresponding increase in maternal and neonatal risk of infection is an often stated concern when using corticosteroids. A recent study assessing the effects of betamethasone on maternal cellular resistance to infection provided reassurance in that both specific and non-specific immune function remained intact in the mother after betamethasone administration (Cunningham & Evans, 1991).

Cases of pulmonary oedema (Stubblefield & Kitzmiller, 1980) have been reported in women receiving a combination of corticosteroids and tocolytic drugs, as has maternal death (Milliez, Blot & Surean, 1980). In all the randomized controlled trials, only two patients with pulmonary oedema are cited (Morales *et al.*, 1986), both in women who received corticosteroids and magnesium sulphate. The true estimate of risk for pulmonary oedema is, therefore, uncertain.

In women with hypertension, a subgroup analysis in the Auckland trial (Howie & Liggins, 1977) suggested an increased risk of fetal death with the use of antenatal corticosteroids. No fetal deaths were reported in the other two trials for which data are available (Collaborative Group on Antenatal Steroid Therapy, 1981; Gamsu *et al.*, 1989).

Concern has been expressed that corticosteroids might initiate hypertension in normotensive women or aggravate it in those with an already elevated blood pressure (Schneider *et al.*, 1989). Such an adverse effect cannot be ruled out on evidence available. Hypertensive disease remains a frequent indication for preterm delivery (Hewitt & Newnham, 1988) and the 48 hour postponement of delivery required to complete antenatal corticosteroid therapy may be unacceptable because of the maternal risks of pre-eclampsia. Further appropriately sized trials in the use of antenatal corticosteroids in women with hypertensive disease are warranted.

The efficacy of antenatal corticosteroids in women with diabetes mellitus is uncertain. Infants born to women with diabetes mellitus have a 5.6-fold increased risk of developing RDS than infants born to women without diabetes (Robert *et al.*, 1976). The 14 randomized controlled trials of antenatal corticosteroids included very few women with diabetes. If corticosteroids are used in women with diabetes mellitus, close supervision is necessary to avoid loss of diabetic control. There is the potential to do more harm than good (Crowley, 1989) and assessment within the context of a randomized controlled trial would seem appropriate with the necessary close supervision and possibility of needing insulin infusion remembered.

Corticosteroids, in addition to enhancing lung development and maturation, have effects on other fetal organs. Fetal body and breathing movements are reduced and fetal heart rate variability is transiently lowered in 46% of fetuses after maternal betamethasone administration (Mulder *et al.*, 1994). These effects occur within 48 hours from the commencement of treatment and return to normal when treatment is completed. These transient changes in biophysical variables after corticosteroid administration should be considered prior to delivery prompted by deterioration in biophysical scoring.

Long-term follow-up of infants exposed to antenatal corticosteroids

The most reliable evidence about possible long-term effects of antenatal corticosteroid administration comes from three trials that have published follow-up data on physical growth and development, namely a three year follow-up in the Collaborative Group on Antenatal Steroid Therapy (1984), a six year follow-up in the Auckland trial (MacArthur *et al.*, 1982) and a 10–12 year follow-up in the Amsterdam trial (Smolders-de-Haas, 1990). There is no evidence that antenatal corticosteroids adversely affect physical growth, development or psychometric testing. Indeed, there is the suggestion that corticosteroids may protect against neurological sequelae such as hemiparesis, diplegia and quadriplegia (OR 0.62 95% CI 0.36–1.08) (Crowley 1994a).

Meta-analysis of trials of corticosteroids after preterm prelabour rupture of the membranes

The use of antenatal corticosteroids given to women following preterm prelabour rupture of the membranes has been assessed in 11 randomized trials (Block *et al.*, 1977; Garite *et al.*, 1981; Collaborative Group on Antenatal Steroid Therapy, 1981; Schmidt *et al.*, 1984; Iams *et al.*, 1985; Nelson *et al.*, 1985; Morales *et al.*, 1986; Parsons *et al.*, 1988; Morales *et al.*, 1989; Cararach *et al.*, 1990; Carlan *et al.*, 1991). The trials have been reviewed for the Cochrane Collaboration Database of Systematic Reviews Pregnancy and Childbirth Module by Crowley (1994b).

Antenatal corticosteroids given to women with preterm prelabour rupture of the membranes is associated with a marked reduction in the incidence of RDS (OR 0.50 95% CI 0.38–0.66) without an increase in the risk of neonatal infection (OR 1.29 95% CI 0.74–2.26). The size of the reduction in RDS in this group is comparable to that seen in patients with intact membranes. Meta-analysis of trials with a combined policy of antenatal corticosteroids in women with prelabour premature rupture of the membranes followed by induction of labour after 48 hours shows no reduction in the incidence of RDS and a possible increased risk of neonatal infection (Crowley, 1994c) and fails to support such a policy.

Cost implications

Clearly antenatal corticosteroids, given to women at risk of preterm delivery can dramatically reduce the risk of RDS in their infants. The potential cost savings have been recognized ever since corticosteroids were first advocated (Johnson, Mason & Thompson, 1981; Avery, 1984; Mugford, Piercy & Chalmers, 1991). The cost of caring for babies with RDS is twice that of caring for babies of similar gestational age without RDS.

Recent estimates suggest that if antenatal steroids are used to prevent RDS, there is a 10% reduction in the costs of caring for infants born at less than 35 weeks' gestation (Mugford *et al.*, 1991). Mugford and colleagues estimated the potential reduction in neonatal costs by the use of antenatal corticosteroids could be as much as 8 million pounds a year in England and Wales, which is more than 1% of the total amount spent on the maternity services (Comptroller and Auditor General, 1990).

Randomized controlled trials confirm the efficacy of both synthetic surfactant and natural surfactant extracts for the prevention and treatment of RDS (Soll & McQueen, 1992). There is increasing animal experimental evidence (Ikegami *et al.*, 1987) and work from clinical studies (Farrel *et al.*, 1989; Jobe, Mitchell & Gunkel, 1993) that combined antenatal induction of lung maturation with corticosteroids and postnatal use of surfactant improves lung function and improves neonatal outcome compared with preterm newborns treated only with surfactant. There are no data from randomized trials assessing the possible additional benefits to infants receiving both corticosteroids and surfactant.

Management recommendations

Maternal antenatal corticosteroid administration as 24 mg betamethasone, 24 mg dexamethasone or 2 g hydrocortisone, to women at risk of preterm delivery substantially reduces the risk of RDS and other neonatal morbidity and mortality. There is no strong evidence of adverse effects of such a policy. Further trials in women with hypertensive disease and diabetes would provide evidence in these situations as to the efficacy of antenatal corticosteroids.

In spite of the strong evidence in favour of the use of antenatal corticosteroids, there is wide variation as to their use in clinical practice. Keirse (1984) reported only 33% of obstetricians in northern Belgium and the Netherlands routinely used antenatal corticosteroids. In the UK, in a survey of how obstetricians manage preterm labour, when asked about their use of glucocorticoids 18% responded never, 40% sometimes and only 42% frequently (Lewis *et al.*, 1980). Steroid usage remains as low as 20–23% even in more recent reports (Donaldson, 1992; The OSIRIS Collaborative Group, 1992). The differences in obstetric practice reflect the variation there is in interpretation of the efficacy and risks of antenatal corticosteroid treatment. Given the strong evidence from the systematic review of relevant randomized controlled trials of a substantial reduction in RDS, early neonatal mortality and other neonatal morbidity without an increase in maternal, fetal or neonatal infectious morbidity (Crowley, Chalmers & Keirse, 1990; Crowley 1993a) together with the reduction in duration of hospitalization and significant cost savings (Mugford *et al.*, 1991), maternal antenatal corticosteroid administration should be considered for all women at risk of preterm delivery.

Antenatal administration of TRH and glucocorticoids before preterm delivery

Laboratory and animal studies of TRH and thyroid hormones

Glucocorticoids, T_3 and prolactin have synergistic interactions in fetal sheep on the secretion of surfactant phospholipids and to improve lung stability and distensibility (Schellenberg *et al.*, 1988). The superadditive interactions on surfactant production had earlier been shown in lung explants in the rat (Gross & Wilson, 1982), the rabbit (Ballard *et al.*, 1984) and the human (Gonzales *et al.*, 1986). Not all studies, however, have been able to confirm a synergistic effect of T_3 with corticosteroids (Moya, Sanchez & Baudy, 1992).

Unfortunately, thyroid hormones and TSH fail to cross the placenta readily. However, TRH readily crosses the placenta. TRH is a tripeptide stimulating the release of TSH, which in turn stimulates fetal thyroid hormone production. Synthetic TRH, pyroglutamyl-histidyl-proline amide, is thought to be identical to endogenous TRH. TRH is present in many areas of the nervous system, including the hypothalamus, cerebellum, limbic system, nucleus tractus solitarius and the gastrointestinal tract (Kaplan, Grumbach & Aubert, 1976; Engler, Scanlon & Jackson, 1981). TRH is present in the fetal hypothalamus in the human from 10–12 weeks' gestation and concentrations increase with gestational age (Kaplan *et al.*, 1976).

Many effects of TRH infusion have been observed in several different animals. In relation to lung maturation, an increase in rabbits in the secretion of surfactant phospholipids, but not their synthesis, was observed (Rooney et al., 1979) together with morphological and functional maturation (Devaskar et al., 1987; Ikegami et al., 1987). In fetal sheep, lung stability and distensibility were increased and morphological lung maturation enhanced by cortisol and TRH but not by either agent alone (Liggins et al., 1988b). Alveolar phospholipids, as measured by phosphatidylcholine (Boshier et al., 1989), were increased with TRH or TRH plus cortisol (Liggins et al., 1988b), although this has not been a consistent finding (Ikegami et al., 1991). TRH and cortisol enhance β-adrenergic receptor binding and β-agonist effects are enhanced with TRH and cortisol in fetal sheep, although neither cortisol or TRH has this effect singly (Warburton et al., 1988).

TRH, in addition to increasing T_3, stimulates the secretion of prolactin and the combination of cortisol, T_3 and prolactin is more effective in increasing lung distensibility than cortisol and T_3 alone (Liggins et al., 1988b).

TRH can act as a central sympathetic neurotransmitter and some of its lung maturational effects may be mediated via the sympathetic nervous system (Liggins, 1993).

Around the time of birth, pulmonary fluid production is reduced and mechanisms for reabsorption stimulated, which facilitates clearance of lung fluid at birth. Both glucocorticoids and T_3 increase the synthesis in type II alveolar cells of atrial natriuretic factor, a peptide involved in decreasing lung fluid production (Matsubara et al., 1988).

Glucocorticoids and thyroid hormones do not always have synergistic actions. While dexamethasone stimulates fatty acid synthesis in fetal lung, thyroid hormones inhibit this effect (Rooney, Gobrau & Chu, 1986). Similarly in rats, glucocorticoids accelerate maturation of the antioxidant enzyme system (AOE) in the fetal lung whereas T_3 significantly delays it (Sosenko & Frank, 1987). Prenatal TRH administration in rats also significantly decreases pulmonary AOE levels in late gestation (Antigua, Sosenko & Frank, 1989; Rodriguez et al., 1991). Pulmonary AOE systems prevent cell injury by O_2 free radicals that are produced under normoxic metabolic conditions and in excess in hyperoxic states.

It is suggested that this negative effect of thyroid hormones on the AOE system may be potentially harmful to preterm infants exposed to thyroid hormones who require O_2 therapy. The suppression of AOE activity in the fetal lung by TRH administration occurs by negative regulation of AOE gene expression, which is most likely to be at the level of gene transcription rather than posttranscriptionally (Chen, Whitney & Frank, 1993).

Human studies of TRH and thyroid hormones

Roti and colleagues (1981) first demonstrated that TRH administered to women at term crossed the human placenta. They found that the fetal pituitary was responsive to TRH and that the endogenous TSH produced stimulated the fetal thyroid gland. The TRH was given 8–820 minutes before delivery and TSH, T_3 and T_4 were measured in cord bloods. An increase in fetal TSH lwas seen within 15 to 30 minutes of maternal TRH infusion, with a peak in fetal TSH levels at 40–60 minutes. Elevation in T_3 and T_4 were of slower onset with peak levels for T_3 and T_4 between 2 and 4 hours. This fetal responsiveness to maternally administered TRH has been confirmed in preterm infants by others (Moya et al., 1991; Thorpe-Beeston et al., 1991). Elevation in serum prolactin has also been reported in term (Moya, Mena & Heusser, 1986) and preterm infants (Moya et al., 1991), although not all studies in preterm infants (Roti et al., 1990) have been consistent.

In adults after intravenous administration of TRH, there is a prompt rise in TSH, T_3 and T_4. Snyder & Utiger (1972) showed that the maximal response in the adult occurred with a dose of 400 μg TRH. Increasing the dose of TRH further in healthy adults failed to result in increased stimulation or release of TSH. TRH, when given intravenously to adults, results in one or more side effects in up to two-thirds of subjects. These are usually mild and transitory lasting from 1–5 minutes (Anderson et al., 1971) and include nausea, urinary urgency, light headedness, facial flushing, metallic taste and a rise in blood pressure which may be dose related (Hall et al., 1976).

To try to determine the optimal dose of TRH to provide maximal pituitary stimulation for the fetus, Moya et al., (1986) administered to 26 pregnant women at term either 600 or 400 μg TRH 2 hours before elective caesarean section or 400 μg TRH 12 hours before operation. There was a control group of women too. Similar increases in cord blood TSH and T_3 levels were seen in the 600 and 400 µg groups when given 2 hours before caesarean section. No elevations in thyroid hormone levels were seen in the cord bloods in the group of infants exposed to TRH 12 hours before operation. At 6 hours following delivery, no differences in TSH or T_3 levels were seen between control infants and infants exposed to TRH. Therefore, a single dose of antenatal TRH in this report did not blunt the normal postnatal surge of TSH and T_3. In preterm fetuses between 26–34 weeks' gestation, maternal administration of 400 µg TRH prior to delivery resulted in elevation in TSH, T_3, T_4 and prolactin (Moya et al., 1991) in cord blood. However, the peak level of T_3 was slightly lower than in the term fetuses (Moya et al., 1986; Moya & Gross, 1993).

Given that the maximal response to TRH in the adult occurs with 400 µg (Snyder & Utiger, 1972) and that animal studies have reported maturational effects with administration of 20–40 µg/kg (Rooney et al., 1979; Tabor et al., 1990), the minimal dose of TRH in the mother to produce maximal fetal pituitary response is likely to be less than 200 µg TRH. Crowther et al. (1995), in a randomized study in 27 women, found that 200 µg TRH administered prior to preterm delivery produced similar elevations above controls in cord TSH levels as did 400 µg TRH.

Randomized trials of antenatal TRH and glucocorticoid administration prior to preterm delivery

Following the demonstration of synergism between glucocorticoids and TRH, Liggins and colleagues tested the use of 400 µg TRH 12 hourly for 48 hours in a placebo-controlled trial in women of 24–32 weeks' gestation at risk of delivering preterm. Initial interim results from a subgroup of 106 (40%) from the first 270 babies entered in the trial related to liveborn infants given at least three doses of TRH or placebo and who delivered between 24 hours and 11 days from trial entry (Liggins et al., 1988a).

Clear benefit was seen in this subgroup for the neonates exposed to TRH and glucocorticoids in utero prior to preterm birth between 24 and 31^6 weeks' gestation compared with neonates only exposed to antenatal glucocorticoids. Long-term ventilatory assistance (mean 477 days vs 303 days) and duration of oxygen therapy (mean 1443 days vs 1006 days) were about one-third less in the treated group than in the placebo group. No significant effects were observed on the early phase of RDS. TRH treatment was discontinued because of maternal hypertension in eight (7.6%) women.

Full results for the New Zealand trial have been published now (Knight et al., 1994). A total of 378 women entered the trial and delivered 418 babies. A reduction in the incidence of RDS (RR 0.52 95% CI 0.27–0.99) and a reduced need for O_2 at 36 weeks' gestation (RR 0.46 95% CI 0.22–0.95) was seen in the subgroup of 38.5% of the babies randomized to antenatal TRH who received three to four doses and who were born alive between 24 hours and 10 days from entry compared with the control babies exposed to glucocorticoids alone under the same conditions.

Since the initial report of Liggins et al. (1988a), there have been four further trials published, two from the USA (Morales et al., 1989; Ballard et al., 1992b), one from New Zealand (Knight et al., 1994) and one from Australia (ACTOBAT, 1995) (Table 7.1). To the best of our knowledge, there are three other trials reported in abstract form; from Argentina (Althabe et al., 1991; Ceriani Cernadas et al., 1992), Japan (Jikihara et al., 1990) and Chile (cited in Moya & Gross, 1993).

All the trials have had slightly different protocols. The majority have used 400 µg TRH but either given 8 hourly (Morales et al., 1989) or 12 hourly (Jikihara et al., 1990; Ballard et al., 1992b; Knight et al., 1994; Ceriani Cernadas et al., 1992; ACTOBAT, 1995) and for two (Ceriani Cernadas et al., 1992), four (Jikihara et al., 1990; Ballard et al., 1992b; Knight et al., 1994; ACTOBAT, 1995) or six (Morales et al., 1989) doses. Other trials (Althabe et al., 1991; ACTOBAT, 1995) have used 200 µg treatment doses. Some studies have presented the clinical outcome data for all mothers and babies recruited (Jikihara et al., 1990; Knight et al., 1994; ACTOBAT, 1995); the rest have reported outcome data for selected subgroups and it is not always clear as to whether these were prespecified analyses. Glucocorticoids were used in both study groups in all these trials, in keeping with the synergism shown in animal experimental work (Liggins et al., 1988b).

Morales and colleagues (1989) recruited 248 women

Table 7.1 *Randomized controlled trials of antenatal TRH together with glucocorticoids prior to preterm delivery*

Author	TRH (µg)	Placebo	Hourly	No. of treatments	No. of women	Percentage of babies outcomes reported
Morales *et al.*, 1989	400	No	8	6	248	35
Jikihara *et al*, 1990	400	No	12	4	124	100
Ballard *et al.*, 1992b	400	Yes	8	4	404	23–52
Ceriani Cernadas *et al.*, 1992	200	Yes	12	2	Uncertain	57
Knight *et al*, 1994	400	Yes	12	4	378	38.5
Campos, 1993[a]	400	Uncertain	8	4	Uncertain	Uncertain
ACTOBAT, 1995	200	Yes	12	4	1064	99.7

[a] Cited by Moya & Gross, 1993.

under 34 weeks' gestation with an L/S ratio of <2.0. Women randomized to TRH received 400 µg TRH 8 hourly for six doses. The control corticosteroid group did not have a placebo infusion. The 35% of babies delivered within one week from the start of therapy had a lower incidence of bronchopulmonary dysplasia (not defined in the paper) (8% vs 24% $p < 0.05$) and spent less time on respirators (mean 2.1 days vs 5.1 days $p < 0.05$) if exposed to antenatal TRH compared with controls. No differences in other neonatal morbidity were seen. Transient maternal side effects of nausea, flushing, hot flushes or palpitations were experienced by 35% of the women receiving TRH.

Ballard *et al.* (1992b) reported on 404 women (446 infants) in threatened preterm labour who were randomized <32 weeks' gestation to receive either 400 µg TRH 8 hourly for four doses or saline placebo. Both groups of women received corticosteroids. In a subgroup of 231 (52%) babies who delivered less than 10 days after entry, no differences were seen in the incidence of RDS, severe RDS or other neonatal morbidity between the study groups. In a further subgroup of 103 (23%) babies who were fully treated and weighed less than 1500 g at birth, the incidence of chronic lung disease (defined as a requirement for O_2 at 28 days) was less (44% vs 18% $p < 0.01$) in the TRH-exposed babies compared with the control group. Women given TRH in this study also experienced the side effects of nausea, vomiting and flushing more frequently than the placebo control group (17% vs 2% $p < 0.0001$). No women were

withdrawn from the study because of raised blood pressure.

Researchers in Argentina (Althabe *et al.*, 1991) initially reported the use of 200 µg TRH given 12 hourly for two doses to 52 women at risk of preterm delivery between 26 and 31 weeks' gestation; an update report was given by Ceriani Cernadas *et al.* (1992). In the subgroup of 57 babies born within 10 days from entry, no differences were seen in the incidence of RDS (27% vs 29%) in the TRH group compared with the controls, although a reduction in the mean duration of O_2 therapy and mean duration of ventilation was reported in the TRH group. In addition, in this subgroup analysed, no infant exposed to antenatal TRH needed O_2 at 28 days compared with the control group, where six infants did.

The Japanese trial (Jikihara *et al.*, 1990) used 400 µg TRH 8 hourly for four doses without a placebo. In 80 women between the gestational age of 23 and 26 weeks, the use of antenatal TRH reduced the incidence of RDS (33% vs 71%).

Interim data are available from the Chilean study by Campos and colleagues (cited in Moya & Gross, 1993) in which 400 µg TRH was used between 25–32 weeks' gestation. In a subgroup of babies who delivered within 48 hours of the last treatment, there was a reduction in the incidence of RDS in TRH-treated infants (20% vs 36%) compared with control infants.

In contrast to the above studies, the largest trial reported to date, the Australian multicentred AC-TOBAT study (ACTOBAT, 1995), failed to demonstrate any beneficial effect of antenatal TRH. In 1234 women at risk of preterm delivery between 24 and 31[6] weeks' gestation, centrally randomized to receive either 200 µg TRH 12 hourly or saline placebo, an increase in the incidence of RDS (RR 1.17 95% CI 1.00–1.36, $p = 0.05$) and the need for ventilation (RR 1.15 95% CI 1.01–1.31, $p = 0.04$) was found in babies exposed to antenatal TRH compared with the control babies. No benefit was seen in other neonatal morbidity with the use of TRH. In addition, women receiving TRH had a fourfold increased risk of nausea, a threefold increase in vomiting, a twofold increase in light headedness and a slightly increased risk of developing a rise in blood pressure $\geq 140/90$ mmHg compared with the women receiving placebo.

Other trials of the use of antenatal TRH, together with corticosteroids, are ongoing in the USA (R. A. Ballard, personal communication) with others planned in the Netherlands (J. Kok, personal communication) and the UK (D. Elbourne, personal communication). Some workers have criticized the applicability of the ACTOBAT results because it used a lower dose (200 mg) and frequency of administration (12 hourly) than most other studies (Ballard et al., 1995; Moya & Maturana, 1995). Future studies should, therefore, use 400 µg TRH (Crowther & Alfirec, 1995).

Only one small trial has been reported comparing TRH alone with TRH plus glucocorticoids and with placebo (Jackson et al., 1994). In 70 women with a singleton pregnancy and not in labour 24 hours after prelabour preterm rupture of the membranes, no differences were seen in any of the neonatal endpoints, but the study was too small to exclude a type II error.

Meta-analysis of trials of antenatal TRH and corticosteroids prior to preterm delivery

In total, over 2300 women have been entered into the seven trials comparing antenatal administration of TRH and glucocorticoids with glucocorticoids alone prior to preterm delivery. The majority of data available is interim or from subgroup analysis. The most reliable estimate of the effects of maternally administered antenatal TRH on the problems and sequelae of immaturity and, in particular, RDS are derived from overview or meta-analysis of the data from these randomized controlled trials.

The most recent update of the review of the trials of anatenatal TRH is found in the pregnancy and childbirth module of the Cochrane Database of Systematic Reviews (Crowther & Alfirevic, 1995). Only three trials have reported outcome data in full (Jikihara et al., 19940; Knight et al., 1994; ACTOBAT, 1995). No clear effect on mortality is shown, although there were slightly more deaths of TRH-treated babies. Combining death with need for O_2 did not suggest a beneficial effect of antenatal TRH. No differences were seen in the incidence of

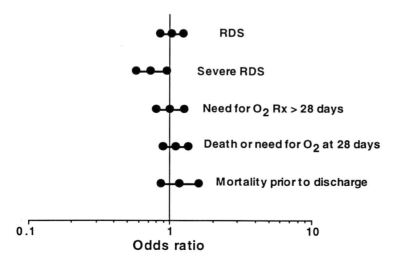

Fig. 7.2 *Effect of TRH and steroids versus steroids alone prior to preterm delivery in a meta-analysis of randomized controlled trials with complete neonatal outcome (after Crowther & Alfirevic, 1995). Graph shows odds ratios and 95% confidence intervals.*

RDS, although severe RDS was less common in the TRH-treated group.

Although promising therapeutic effects of antenatal TRH have been reported in babies delivering within 10 days of treatment, this represents a minority subgroup of babies entered. The majority of babies in the studies (44%) were born more than 10 days after trial entry and those receiving TRH had a poorer outcome.

Potential adverse effects of antenatal TRH

Data are few for maternal side effects from the trials to date, but those available show an increased risk of nausea, vomiting and light headedness in mothers given antenatal TRH compared with control mothers (OR 5.30 95% CI 2.72–10.32) (Crowther & Alfirevic, 1994).

There is a hypothesized risk of a rise in maternal blood pressure with TRH administration. Ballard *et al.* (1992b) reported a rise in maternal blood pressure of 20 mmHg in eight (4%) women given TRH compared with six (3%) control women (OR 1.40 95% CI 0.48–4.06). In the New Zealand trial, five (3%) mothers receiving TRH were withdrawn because of a transient rise in blood pressure compared with one (0.5%) mother, in the control group. In the Australian trial women in the TRH group were more likely to have a blood pressure $\geq 140/90$ mmHg during treatment than the control group (RR 1.29 95% CI 1.05–1.59). There is a belief but no supporting randomized trial data as yet that infusion of the maternal treatment dose of TRH over 20 minutes reduces the risk of elevation in blood pressure compared with a bolus dose. Peek *et al.* (1995) considered the 5–6 mmHg rise in mean arterial pressure with TRH infusion to be clinically insignificant in normotensive women but cautioned against TRH usage in women with severe pre-eclampsia, because of their significantly greater rise (mean 10–15 mmHg) during treatment.

The effect on neonatal thyroid status of more than one dose of TRH administered antenatally requires further detailed study, as pituitary thyroid axis suppression is a possibility. Ballard *et al.* (1992a), in infants exposed to 400 µg TRH 2–6 hours before delivery, showed a twofold increase or more in cord blood TSH, T_3 and prolactin and a 19% increase in T_4 compared with control infants. The response was similar after one, two, three or four doses of TRH. In infants delivered 13–36 hours after the last dose of TRH, cord blood TSH levels were decreased by 62% and T_3 levels by 54% compared with the control group. In these infants, all TSH, T_3 and T_4 levels were significantly lower at 2 hours of age in treated infants compared with the controls. It appears that in preterm infants exposed antenatally to maternally administered TRH initial increases in thyroid hormone and prolactin levels are followed by suppression of the pituitary–thyroid axis. Infants born during the early phase of suppression do not have the normal postnatal surge in thyroid hormones. The length and clinical significance of this suppression remains to be determined.

TRH is found in many areas of the nervous system, placenta (Shambaugh, Kubek & Wilber, 1979) and gastrointestinal tract (Fisher & Polk, 1989). TRH is rapidly degraded in tissues, although in pregnant women, this activity is reduced (Neary *et al.*, 1978). The ability of the human fetus to degrade TRH is considerably reduced compared with adults (Neary *et al.*, 1978). TRH receptors have been identified in the fetus with expression regulated by cell-specific post-transcriptional mechanisms (cited in de Zegher, Spitz & Devlieger, 1992) Cellular desensitization to TRH can occur by down regulation of the receptor by TRH either over time or by increasing dosages (Perlman & Gershengorn, cited in de Zegher *et al.*, 1992). Complete neuronal recovery from desensitization can take up to a week (Ogawa *et al.*, 1983). TRH acts via cell membrane receptor binding and a secondary messenger system believed to be inositol trisphosphate/diacylglycerol to increase intracellular calcium (Gershengorn, 1986).

Changes in fetal heart rate have been reported after TRH administration – both an increase (Ballard *et al.*, 1992b) and a decrease (Gyselaers *et al.*, 1992). The biophysical effects of TRH on the fetus warrant further study.

Long-term follow-up of infants exposed to TRH

Long-term follow-up of infants recruited to trials of antenatal TRH has still to be reported, as experience has been limited to date (Ballard *et al.*, 1993). It is important that such data are provided with as complete a follow-up as possible on all babies recruited to reduce bias.

Management recommendations

On the basis of the currently available evidence, antenatal TRH cannot be recommended for clinical practice. Further randomized controlled trials using 400 µg TRH are necessary to provide more reliable evidence on mortality and long-term morbidity (Crowther & Alfirevic, 1995). Studies to assess the effect of TRH therapy on the need for, and efficacy of, surfactant therapy are needed.

Intra-amniotic injections of T_3 and T_4 have been used to accelerate fetal lung maturation (Mashiach *et al.*, 1979) but there have been no randomized controlled trials reported of this invasive therapy and accurate estimates of the risks and benefits of such treatment are not available.

Intra-amniotic administration of exogenous surfactant has similarly been proposed and suggested to improve the pulmonary characteristics of the preterm rabbit pup (Galen *et al.*, 1992) and to improve the clinical respiratory course in baboons delivered prematurely (Galen *et al.*, 1993). There is a debate as to whether amniotically administered surfactant actually reaches the fetal lung, given the flux of lung fluid from lung to amniotic cavity. No randomized controlled trials or uncontrolled studies of this invasive therapy have been reported in humans to date, so the risks and benefits are unknown.

Conclusions

Antenatal corticosteroids given to the mother have proved effective in improving the outcome for the preterm infant by reducing the risk of RDS and neonatal mortality. This intervention should be routinely considered for all women expected to deliver before 34 weeks' gestation.

Other interventions such as antenatal TRH, which in initial studies suggest promise, need further evaluation by randomized controlled trials. On the available evidence, antenatal TRH cannot be recommended for clinical use outside the context of further trials.

The implications for future research are many. The efficacy of maternal antenatal corticosteroids at very early gestational ages and in women with hypertensive disease and diabetes needs to be established. There is

scope for comparison of different routes of glucocorticoid administration, different types of corticosteroid, different dose regimens and whether there is a need to repeat the course of corticosteroids if undelivered after 7–10 days. Whether a larger dose regimen is efficacious in multiple pregnancy should be studied.

Further placebo-controlled trials of 400 µg antenatal TRH are warranted to establish the efficacy and clarify the effects on mortality and long-term morbidity. Issues needing clarification are the optimal frequency of administration and the need for repetition of the treatment course if undelivered. The interaction of glucocorticoids, TRH and the use of surfactant warrants study.

References

ACTOBAT Study Group (1995). Australian collaborative trial of antenatal thyrotropin-releasing hormone (ACTOBAT) for prevention of neonatal respiratory disease. *Lancet*, 345, 877–82.

Althabe, F., Fustinana, C., Althabe, O. & Ceriani Cernadas, J. M. (1991). Controlled trial of prenatal betamethasone plus TRH vs betamethasone plus placebo for prevention of RDS in preterm infants. *Pediatric Research*, 29, 200A.

Anderson, M. S., Bowers, G., Kastin, A. J., Schalch, D. S., Schally, A.V., Snyder, P. J., Utiger, R. D., Wilber, J. F. & Wise, A. J. (1971). Synthetic thyrotropin releasing hormone. *New England Journal of Medicine*, 285, 1279–83.

Antigua, M. C. B., Sosenko, I. R. S. & Frank, L. (1989) Thyrotropin–releasing hormone (TRH) depresses antioxidant enzyme maturation in fetal rat lung. *Pediatric Research*, 25, 46A.

Australian Bureau of Statistics (1993). *Perinatal Deaths in Australia (1992)*. Canberra. Cat. No. 3304.0.

Avery, M. E. (1984). The argument for prenatal administration of dexamethasone to prevent respiratory distress syndrome. *Journal of Pediatrics*, 104, 240.

Avery, M. E. & Mead, J. (1959). Surface properties in relation to atelectasis and hyaline membrane disease. *American Journal of Diseases of Children*, 97, 517–23.

Ballard, P. L. & Ballard, R. A. (1979). Corticosteroids and respiratory distress syndrome: status 1979. *Pediatrics*, 63, 163–4.

Ballard, P. L., Ballard, R. A., Creasy, R. K., Padbury, J., Polk, D., Bracken, M., Moya, F. R. & Gross, I. (1992a). Plasma thyroid hormones and prolactin in premature infants and their mothers after prenatal treatment with thyrotropin–releasing hormone. *Pediatric Research*, 32, 673–8.

Ballard, R. A., Ballard, P. L., Creasy, R. K., Padbury, J., Polk, D. H., Bracken, M., Moya, F. R., Gross, I. & The TRH Study Group (1992b). Respiratory disease in very low birthweight infants after prenatal thyrotropin-releasing hormone and glucocorticoid. *Lancet*, 339, 510–15.

Ballard, R. A., Ballard, P. L., Creen, A. & Pinto-Martin, J. (1995). Thyrotropin releasing hormone for prevention of neonatal respiratory disease. *Lancet*, 345, 1572.

Ballard, R. A., Ballard, P. L., Granberg, J. P. & Sniderman, S. (1979b). Prenatal administration of betamethasone for prevention of respiratory distress syndrome. *Journal of Pediatrics*, 94, 97–101.

Ballard, P. L., Hovey, M. L. & Gonzales, L. K. (1984). Thyroid hormone stimulation of phosphatidylcholine synthesis in cultured fetal rabbit lung. *Journal of Clinical Investigation*, 74, 898–905.

Ballard, R., Piecuch, R., Leonard, C. & Behle, M. (1993). Effect of antenatal thyrotropin-releasing hormone (TRH) on the neurodevelopmental outcome of preterm infants. *2nd World Congress of Perinatal Medicine*, Rome, p. 358, Abstract 65.

Barker, P. M., Markiewicz, M., Parker, K. A., Walters, D. V. & Strang, L. B. (1990). Synergistic action of triiodothyronone and hydrocortisone on epinephrine-induced re-absorption of fetal lung liquid. *Pediatric Research*, 27, 588–91.

Block, M. F., Kling, O. R. & Crosby, W. M. (1977). Antenatal glucocorticoid therapy for the prevention of respiratory distress syndrome in the premature infant. *Obstetrics and Gynecology*, 50, 186–90.

Boshier, D. P., Holloway, H., Liggins, G. C. & Marshall, R. J. (1989). Morphometric analyses of the effects of thyrotropin releasing hormone and cortisol on the lungs of fetal sheep. *Journal of Developmental Physiology*, 12, 49–54.

Boyle, M. H., Torrance, G. W., Sinclair, J. C. & Harwood, S. P. (1983). Economic evaluation of neonatal intensive care of very low birthweight infants. *New England Journal of Medicine*, 308, 1330–7.

Brumley, G. W., Nelson, J. H., Schonberg, D. W. & Crenshaw, J. C. (1977). Whole and disaturated lung phosphatidycholine in cortisol treated intrauterine growth retarded and twin control lambs at different gestational ages. *Biology of the Neonate*, 31, 155–66.

Burkett, G., Bauer, C. R., Morrison, J. C. & Curet, L. B. (1986). Effect of prenatal dexamethasone administration on prevention of respiratory distress syndrome in twin pregnancies. *Journal of Perinatology*, 6, 304–8.

Cararach. V., Sentis, J., Botet, F. & De Los Rios, L. (1990). A multicentric prospective randomized study in premature rupture of membranes (PROM). Respiratory and infectious complications in the newborn. In *Proceedings of 12th European Congress of Perinatal Medicine*, Lyon, France, p. 216.

Carlan, S. J., Parsons, M., O'Brien, W. F. & Krammer, J. (1991). Pharmacologic pulmonary maturation in preterm premature rupture of membranes (SPO abstract 454). *American Journal of Obstetrics and Gynecology*, 164, 371.

Ceriani Cernadas, J. M., Fustinana, C., Althabe, F. & Althabe, O. (1992). Controlled trial of prenatal betamethasone (B) plus TRH for prevention of respiratory distress syndrome (RDS) *Pediatric Research*, 32, 738, A9.

Chen, Y., Whitney, P. L. & Frank, L. (1993). Negative regulation of antioxidant enzyme gene expression in the developing fetal rat lung by prenatal hormonal treatments. *Pediatric Research*, 33, 171–6.

Collaborative Group on Antenatal Steroid Therapy (1981). Effect of antenatal dexamethasone administration on the prevention of respiratory distress syndrome. *American Journal of Obstetrics and Gynecology*, 141, 276–87.

Collaborative Group on Antenatal Steroid Therapy (1984). Effects of antenatal dexamethasone administration in the infant: long-term follow-up. *Journal of Pediatrics*, 104, 259–67.

Comptroller and Auditor General (1990). *National Audit Office Report on the Maternity Services*, London: HMSO.

Crowley, P. (1989). Promoting pulmonary maturity. In *Effective Care in Pregnancy and Childbirth*, ed. I. Chalmers, M. W. Enkin & M. J. N. C. Keirse, pp. 746–64. Oxford: Oxford University Press.

Crowley, P. (1994a). Corticosteroids prior to preterm delivery. In *Pregnancy and Childbirth Module*, ed. M. J. N. C. Keirse, H. J. Renfrew, J. P. Neilson & C. Crowther. London: The Cochrane Database of Systematic Reviews, BMJ Publishing Group.

Crowley, P. (1994b). Corticosteroids after preterm prelabour rupture of membranes. In *Pregnancy and Childbirth Module*, ed. M. J. N. C. Keirse, H. J. Renfrew, J. P. Neilson & C. Crowther. London: The Cochrane Database of Systematic Reviews, BMJ Publishing Group.

Crowley, P. (1994c). Corticosteroids and induction of labour after PROM preterm. In *Pregnancy and Childbirth Module*, ed. M. J. N. C. Keirse, H. J. Renfrew, J. P. Neilson & C. Crowther. London: The Cochrane Database of Systematic Reviews, BMJ Publishing Group.

Crowley, P., Chalmers, I. & Keirse, M. J. N. C. (1990). The effects of corticosteroid administration before preterm delivery: an overview of the evidence from controlled trials. *British Journal of Obstetrics and Gynaecology*, 97, 11–25.

Crowther, C. A. & Alfirevic, Z. (1995). Antenatal thyrotropin-releasing hormone prior to preterm delivery. In *Pregnancy and Childbirth Module*, ed. M. J. N. C. Keirse, H. J. Renfrew, J. P. Neilson & C. Crowther. London: The Cochrane Database of Systematic Reviews, BMJ Publishing Group.

Crowther, C. A., Haslam, R. R., Hiller, J. E., McGee, T. & Robinson, J. S. (1991) Thyrotrophin releasing hormone (TRH) and lung maturation: does 200 mg TRH provide effective stimulation to the preterm fetal pituitary gland compared with 400 mg TRH. *American Journal of Obstetrics and Gynecology*, in press.

Cunningham, D. S. & Evans, E. E. (1991). The effects of betamethasone on maternal cellular resistance to infection. *American Journal of Obstetrics and Gynecology*, 165, 610–15.

Devaskar, U., Nitta, K., Szewczyk, K., Sadiq, F. & de Mello, D. (1987). Transplacental stimulation of functional and morphologic fetal rabbit lung maturation. Effect of thyrotropin-releasing hormone. *American Journal of Obstetrics and Gynecology*, 157, 460–4.

de Zegher, F., Spitz, B. & Devlieger, H. (1992). Prenatal treatment with thyrotrophin releasing hormone to prevent neonatal respiratory distress. *Archives of Disease in Childhood*, 67, 450–4.

Donaldson, L. J. (1992). Maintaining excellence: the preservation and development of specialised services. *British Medical Journal*, 305, 1280–4.

Doran, T. A., Swyer, P., MacMurray, B., Mahon, W., Enhorning, G., Bernstein, A., Falk, M. & Wood, M. M. (1980). Results of a double blind controlled study on the use of betamethasone in the prevention of respiratory distress syndrome. *American Journal of Obstetrics and Gynecology*, 136, 313–20.

Doyle, L. W., Kitchen, W. H., Ford, G. W., Rickards, A. L., Lissenden, J. V. & Ryan, M. M. (1986). Effects of antenatal steroid therapy on mortality and morbidity in very low birthweight infants. *Journal of Pediatrics*, 108, 287–92.

Doyle, L. W., Murton, L. J. & Kitchen, W. H. (1989). Increasing the survival of extremely immature (24 to 28 weeks gestation) infants – at what cost? *Medical Journal of Australia*, 150, 558–68.

Engler, D., Scanlon, M. F. & Jackson, I. M. D. (1981). Thyrotropin-releasing hormone in the systemic circulation of the neonatal rat is derived from the pancreas and other extraneural tissues. *Journal of Clinical Investigation*, 67, 800–8.

Farrell, E., Silver, R., Kimberlin, L., Wolf, E. & Duski, J. (1989) Impact of antenatal dexamethasone administration on respiratory distress syndrome in surfactant treated infants. *American Journal of Obstetrics and Gynecology*, 161, 628–33.

Fisher, D. A. & Polk, D. H. (1989). Development of the thyroid. *American Journal of Endocrinology and Metabolism*, 3, 627–57.

Galen, H. L. & Kuel, T. (1992) Effect of intra-amniotic administration of exosurf in preterm rabbit fetuses. *Obstetrics and Gynecology*, 80, 604–8.

Galen, H. L., Cipriani, C., Coalson, J., Bean, J., Collier, R. & Kuehl, T. (1993). Surfactant replacement therapy *in utero* for prevention of hyaline membrane disease in preterm baboon. *American Journal of Obstetrics and Gynecology*, 169, 817–24.

Gamsu, H. R., Mullinger, B. M., Donnai, P. & Dash, C. H. (1989). Antenatal administration of betamethasone to prevent respiratory distress syndrome in preterm infants: report of a UK multicentre trial. *British Journal of Obstetrics and Gynaecology*, 96, 401–10.

Garite, T. J., Freeman, R. K., Linzey, E. M., Braly, P. S. & Dorchester, W. L. (1981). Prospective randomized study of corticosteroids in the management of premature rupture of the membranes and the premature gestation. *American Journal of Obstetrics and Gynecology*, 141, 508–15.

Garite, T. J., Rumney, P. J. & Briggs, G. G. (1992). A randomized, placebo-controlled trial of betamethasone for the prevention of respiratory distress syndrome at 24 to 28 weeks' gestation. *American Journal of Obstetrics and Gynecology*, 166, 646–51.

Gershengorn, M. C. (1986). Mechanisms of thyrotropin-releasing hormone stimulation of pituitary hormone secretion. *Annual Review of Physiology*, 48, 515–26.

Gonzales, I. W., Ballard, P. L., Ertsey, R. & Williams, M. C. (1986). Glucocorticoids and thyroid hormones stimulate biochemical and morphological differentiation of human fetal lung in organ culture. *Journal of Clinical Endocrinology and Metabolism*, 62, 678–91.

Gross, I. (1990). Regulation of fetal lung maturation. *American Journal of Physiology*, 259, L337–44.

Gross, I., Ballard, P. L., Ballard, R. A., Jones, C. T. & Wilson, C. M. (1983). Corticosteroid stimulation of phosphatidylcholine synthesis in cultured fetal rabbit lung. Evidence for de novo protein synthesis mediated by glucocorticoid receptors. *Endocrinology*, 112, 829–37.

Gross, I., Dynia, D. W., Rooney, S., Smart, D. A., Warshaw, J. B., Sissom, J. F. & Hoalt, S. B. (1986). Influence of epidermal growth factor on fetal rat lung development *in vitro*. *Pediatric Research*, 20, 473–7.

Gross, I., Smith, E. J. W., Wilson, C. M., Maniscaleo, W. M., Ingleson, L. D., Brehier, A. & Rooney, S. (1980). The influence of hormones on the biochemical development of fetal rat lung in organ culture II insulin. *Pediatric Research*, 14, 834–8.

Gross, I. & Wilson, C.M. (1982). Fetal lung in organ culture – IV supra–additive hormone interactions. *Journal of Applied Physiology*, 52, 1420–5.

Gyselaers, W., Spitz, B., de Zegher, F., van Ballaer, P, Hanssens, M. & van Assche, F.A. (1992). Effects of thyrotropin-releasing hormone on fetal heart rate. *Lancet*, 339, 1417.

Hall, R., Amos, J., Garry, R. & Burton, R. L. (1976). Thyroid-stimulating hormone response to synthetic thyrotropin-releasing hormone in man. *British Medical Journal*, 2, 274–7.

Hewitt, B. & Newnham, J. P. (1988). A review of the obstetric and medical complications leading to the delivery of infants of very low birthweight. *Medical Journal of Australia*, 149, 234–42.

Howie, R. N. (1986) Pharmacological acceleration of lung maturation. In *Respiratory Distress Syndrome*, ed. C. A. Villee, D. B. Villee & J. Zuckerman, pp. 385–96. London: Academic Press.

Howie, R. N. & Liggins, G. C. (1977). Clinical trial of antepartum betamethasone therapy for prevention of respiratory distress in preterm infants. In *Preterm Labour*, ed. A. B. M. Anderson, R. W. Beard, J. M. Brudenell & P. M. Dunn, pp. 281–9. London: Royal College of Obstetrics and Gynaecology.

Iams, J. D., Talbert, M. L., Barrows, H. & Sachs, L. (1985). Management of preterm prematurely ruptured membranes: a prospective randomized comparison of observation vs use of steroids and timed delivery. *American Journal of Obstetrics and Gynecology*, 151, 32–8.

Ikegami, M., Jobe, A. H., Petenazzo, A., Seidner, S. R., Berry, D. B. & Ruffini, C. (1987). Effects of maternal treatment with corticosteroids, T_3, TRH and their combinations on lung function of ventilated preterm rabbits with and without surfactant treatments. *American Review of Respiratory Disease*, 136, 892–8.

Ikegami, M., Polk, D., Tabor, B., Lewis, J., Yamada, T. & Jobe, A. (1991). Corticosteroid and thyrotropin-releasing hormone effects on preterm sheep lung function. *Journal of Applied Physiology*, 70, 2268–78.

Jackson, D., Nageotte, M., Towers, C., Asrat, T., Freeman, R., Gardner, K., Rumney, P., Murray, K. & Briggs, G. (1994). Thyroid-releasing hormone (TRH) versus betamethasone or placebo in preterm ruptured membranes: a prospective randomized study (SPO Abstract 391). *American Journal of Obstetrics and Gynecology*, 170, 383.

Jikihara, H., Sawada, Y., Imai, S., Morishige, K., Taniguchi, I., Nohara, A., Lynn, G., Miyanishi, K., Shimizu, I., Sumida, H., Fujimura, M., Suehara, N. & Takeuchi, T. (1990). Maternal administration of thyrotropin-releasing hormone for prevention of neonatal respiratory distress syndrome. In *Proceedings of 6th Congress of the Federation of the Asia-Oceana Perinatal Societies*, Perth, Western Australia, Abstract A87.

Jobe, A. H., Mitchell, B. R. & Gunkel, J. H. (1993). Beneficial effects of the combined use of prenatal corticosteroids and postnatal surfactant on preterm infants. *American Journal of Obstetrics and Gynecology*, 168, 508–13.

Johnson, D. E., Mason, D. P. & Thompson, T. R. (1981). Effects of antenatal administration of betamethasone on hospital costs and survival of premature infants. *Pediatrics*, 68, 633–7.

Kaplan, S. L., Grumbach, M. M. & Aubert, M. C. (1976). The autogenesis of pituitary hormones and hypothalamic factors in the human fetus: maturation of central nervous system regulation of anterior pituitary function. *Recent Progress in Hormone Research*, 32, 101.

Keirse, M. J. N. C. (1984). Obstetrical attitudes to glucocorticoid treatment for lung maturation: time for a change? *European Journal of Obstetrics and Gynecology and Reproductive Biology*, 17, 247–55.

Kendall, J., Lakritz, J., Plopper, C. G., Richards, G. E. & Randall, G. C. B. (1990). The effects of hydrocortisone on lung structure in fetal lambs. *Journal of Developmental Physiology*, 13, 165–72.

Knight, D. B., Liggins, G. C. & Wealthall, S. R. (1994). A randomized, controlled trial of antepartum thyrotropin-releasing hormone and betamethasone in the prevention of respiratory disease in preterm infants. *American Journal of Obstetrics and Gynecology*, 171, 11–16.

Lewis, P. J., de Swiet, M., Boylan, P. & Bulpitt, C. J. (1980). How obstetricians in the United Kingdom manage preterm labour. *British Journal of Obstetrics and Gynaecology*, 87, 574–7.

Liggins, G. C. (1969). Premature delivery of fetal lambs infused with glucocorticoids. *Journal of Endocrinology*, 45, 515–23.

Liggins, G. C. (1993) TRH – how it may work. In *Proceedings of the Ross Laboratories Special Hot Topics Conference*, pp. 34–42. Washington, DC.

Liggins, G. C. & Howie, R. N. (1972). A controlled trial of antepartum glucocorticoid treatment for prevention of the respiratory distress syndrome. *Pediatrics*, 50, 515–25.

Liggins, G. C., Knight, D. B., Wealthall, S. R. & Howie, R. N. (1988a). A randomized, double-blind trial of antepartum TRH and steroids in the prevention of neonatal respiratory disease. In *Clinical Reproductive Medicine – The Liggins Years*. Auckland, New Zealand.

Liggins, G. C. & Schellenberg, J. C. (1985) Aspects of fetal lung development. In *The Physiological Development of the Fetus and the Newborn*, ed. C. T. Jones and P. W. Nathanielsz, pp.179–87. London: Academic Press.

Liggins, G. C., Schellenberg, J. C., Manzai, M., Kitterman, J. A. & Lee, C. C. (1988b). Synergisms of cortisol and thyrotropin releasing hormone in lung maturation in fetal sheep. *Journal of Applied Physiology*, 65, 1880–4.

Liley, H. G., White, R. T., Warr, R. G., Benson, B. J., Hawgood, S. & Ballard, P. L. (1989). Regulation of messenger RNAs from the hydrophobic surfactant proteins in human lung. *Journal of Clinical Investigation*, 83, 1191–7.

MacArthur, G., Howie, R. N., de Zoete, J. & Elkins, J. (1982). School progress and cognitive development of 6-year-old children whose mothers were treated antenatally with betamethasone. *Pediatrics*, 70, 99–105.

Maher, J., Goldenberg, R., Cliver, S., Davis, R. & Cooper, R. (1993). Corticosteroid efficacy in very premature infants (SPO Abstract A272). *American Journal of Obstetrics and Gynecology*, 167, 374.

Mashiach, S., Serr, D. M., Sack, J., Stern, E., Brish, M. & Goldman, B. (1979). The effect of intra-amniotic thyroxine administration on fetal lung maturity in man. *Journal of Perinatal Medicine*, 7, 161–70.

Matsubara, M., Mori, Y., Umeda, Y., Oikawa, S., Nakeizato, H. & Inada, M. (1988). A trial of naturetic peptide gene expression and its secretion.

Biochemical and Biophysical Research Communications, 156, 19–27.

Milliez, J., Blot, P. & Surean, C. (1980). A case report of maternal death associated with betamimetics and betamethasone administration in premature labour. *European Journal of Obstetrics and Gynecology and Reproductive Biology*, 11, 95–100.

Morales, W. J., Angel, J. L., O'Brien, W. F. & Knuppel, R. A. (1989). Use of ampicillin and corticosteroids in premature rupture of membranes: a randomized study. *Obstetrics and Gynecology*, 73, 721–6.

Morales, W. J., Diebel, N. D., Lazar, A. J. & Zadrozny, D. (1986). The effect of antenatal dexamethasone administration on the prevention of respiratory distress syndrome in preterm gestations with premature rupture of membranes. *American Journal of Obstetrics and Gynecology*, 154, 591–5.

Morrison, J. C., Whybrew, W. D., Bucovaz, E. T. & Schneider, J. M. (1978). Injection of corticosteroids into the mother to prevent neonatal respiratory distress syndrome. *American Journal of Obstetrics and Gynecology*, 131, 358–66.

Moya, F. R. & Gross, I. (1993). Combined hormonal therapy for the prevention of respiratory distress syndrome and its consequences. *Seminars in Perinatology*, 17, 267–74.

Moya, F. R. & Maturana, A. (1995). Thyrotropin releasing hormone for prevention of neonatal respiratory distress. *Lancet*, 345, 1572–3.

Moya, F., Mena, P., Foradori, A., Becerra, M., Inzunza, A. & Germain, A. (1991). Effect of maternal administration of thyrotropin releasing hormone on the preterm fetal pituitary-thyroid axis. *Journal of Pediatrics*, 119, 966–71.

Moya, F., Mena, P. & Heusser, F. (1986). Response of the maternal, fetal and neonatal pituitary thyroid axis to thyrotropin-releasing hormone. *Pediatric Research*, 20, 982–6.

Moya, F. R., Sanchez, I. & Baudy, D. (1992). Effects of betamethasone and thyroid hormones on fetal rat lung maturation *in vivo*. *Developmental Pharmacology and Therapeutics*, 18, 14–19.

Mugford, M., Piercy, J. & Chalmers, I. (1991). Cost implications of different approaches to the prevention of respiratory distress syndrome. *Archives of Disease in Childhood*, 66, 757–64.

Mulder, E. J. H., Derks, J. B., Zonneveld, M. F., Bruinse, H. & Visser, G. H. A. (1994). Transient reduction in fetal activity and heart rate variation after maternal betamethasone administration. *Early Human Development*, 36, 49–60.

Neary, J. T., Nakamura, C., Davies, I. J., Soodak, M. & Maloof, F. (1978). Lower levels of TRH-degrading activity in human sera and in maternal sera than in the serum of euthyroid, non-pregnant adults. *Journal of Clinical Investigation*, 62, 1–5.

Nelson, L. H., Meis, P. J., Hatjis, C. G., Ernest, J. M., Dillard, R. & Schey, H. M. (1985). Premature rupture of membranes: a prospective, randomized evaluation of steroids, latent phase, and expectant management. *Obstetrics and Gynecology*, 66, 55–8.

Odom, M. J., Snyder, J. M., Boggaram, V. & Mendelson, C. R. (1988). Glucocorticoid regulation of the major surfactant associated protein (SP-A) and its messenger ribonucleic acid and of morphological development of human lung *in vitro*. *Endocrinology*, 123, 1712–20.

Ogawa, N., Mizuno, S., Mukina, U. Tsukamoto, S. & Mori, A. (1983). Effect of chronic thyrotropin-releasing hormone (TRH) administration on TRH receptors and muscarinic cholinergic receptors in CNS. *Brain Research*, 263, 348–50.

OSIRIS Collaborative Group open study of infants at high risk of or with respiratory insufficiency – the role of surfactant (1992). Early versus delayed neonatal administration of a synthetic surfactant – the judgement of OSIRIS. *Lancet*, 340, 1363–9.

Oulton, M., Rasmusson, M., Yoon, R. Y. & Fraser, M. (1989). Gestational dependent effects of the combined treatment of glucocorticoids and thyrotropin-releasing hormone on surfactant production by fetal rabbit lung. *American Journal of Obstetrics and Gynecology*, 160, 961–7.

Papageorgiou, A. N., Desgranges, M. F., Masson, M., Colle, E., Shatz, R. & Gelfand, M. M. (1979). The antenatal use of betamethasone in the prevention of respiratory distress syndrome: a controlled double-blind study. *Pediatrics*, 63, 73–9.

Parsons, M. T., Sobel, D., Cummiskey, K., Constantine, L. & Roitman, J. (1988). Steroid, antibiotic and tocolytic vs no steroid, antibiotic and tocolytic management in patients with preterm PROM at 25–32 weeks. In *Proceedings of 8th Annual Meeting of the Society of Perinatal Obstetricians*, p. 44. Las Vegas, NV.

Peek, M. J., Bajoria R., Shennan, A. H., Dalzell, F., de Swiet, M. & Fisk, N. M. (1995). Hypertensive effect of antenatal thyrotropin releasing hormone in pre-eclampsia. *Lancet*, 345, 793.

Rider, E. D., Jobe, A. H., Ikegami, M., Yamada, T. & Sneider, S. (1990). Antenatal betamethasone dose effect in preterm rabbits studied at 27 days gestation. *Journal of Applied Physiology*, 68, 1134–41.

Robert, M. F., Neff, R. K., Hubell, J. P., Taeusch, H. W. & Avery, M. E. (1976). Association between maternal diabetes and the respiratory distress syndrome in the newborn. *New England Journal of Medicine*, 294, 357–60.

Roberton, N. R. C. (1982). Advances in respiratory distress syndrome. *British Medical Journal*, 284, 917–18.

Rodriguez, M. P., Sosenko, I. R. S., Antigua, M. C. B. & Frank, L. (1991). Prenatal hormone treatment with thyrotropin releasing hormone and with thyrotropin releasing hormone plus dexamethasone delays antioxidant enzyme maturation but does not inhibit a protective antioxidant enzyme response to hyperoxia in newborn rat lung. *Pediatric Research*, 30, 522–7.

Rooney, S., Gobrau, L. & Chu, A. J. (1986). Thyroid hormone opposes some glucocorticoid effects on glycogen content and lipid synthesis in developing fetal rat lung. *Pediatric Research*, 20, 545–50.

Rooney, S., Marino, P., Gobrau, L., Gross, I. & Warshaw, J. (1979). Thyrotropin-releasing hormone increases the amount of surfactant in lung lavage from fetal rabbits. *Pediatric Research*, 13, 623–5.

Roti, E., Gardini, E., Minelli, R., Bianconi, L., Alboni, A. & Braverman, L. E. (1990). Thyrotropin releasing hormone does not stimulate prolactin release in the preterm human fetus. *Acta Endocrinologica*, 122, 462–6.

Roti, E., Gnudi, A., Braverman, L. Robuschi, G., Emanuele, R., Bandini, P., Benassi, L., Pagliani, A. & Emerson, C. (1981). Human cord blood concentrations of thyrotropin, thyroglobulin and iodothyronines after maternal administration of thyrotropin releasing hormone. *Journal of Clinical Endocrinology and Metabolism*, 53, 813–17.

Schellenberg, J. C., Liggins, G. C., Manzai, M., Kitterman, J. A. & Lee, H. (1988). Synergistic hormonal effects on lung maturation in fetal sheep. *Journal of Applied Physiology*, 65, 94–100.

Schmidt, P. L., Sims, M. E., Strassner, H. T., Paul, R. H., Mueller, E. & McCart, D. (1984). Effect of antepartum glucocorticoid administration upon neonatal respiratory distress syndrome and perinatal infection. *American Journal of Obstetrics and Gynecology*, 148, 178–86.

Schneider, J. M., Morrison, J. C., Curet, L. B., Rao, A. V., Poole, K., Burkett, E., Anderson, G. D. & Rigatto, H. (1989). The use of corticosteroids to accelerate fetal lung maturity among parturients with hypertensive disorders. *Clinical and Experimental Hypertension in Pregnancy*, B8, 41–52.

Schutte, M. F., Treffers, P. E., Koppe, J. G., Breur, W. & Filedt Kok, J. C. (1979). The clinical use of corticosteroids for the acceleration of foetal lung maturity. *Nederlands Tijdschrift voor Geneeskunde*, 123, 420–7.

Shambaugh, G. III, Kubek, M. & Wilber, J.F. (1979) Thyrotropin-releasing hormone activity in the human placenta. *Clinical Endocrinology and Metabolism*, 3, 627–57.

Smolders-de Haas, H., Neuvel, J., Schmand, B., Treffers, P. E., Koppe, J. G. & Hoeks, J. (1990). Physical development and medical history of children who were treated antenatally with corticosteroids to prevent respiratory distress

syndrome: a 10- to 12-year follow-up. *Pediatrics*, 86, 65–70.

Snyder, P. J. & Utiger, R. D. (1972). Response to thyrotropin-releasing hormone (TRH) in normal man. *Journal of Clinical Endocrinology and Metabolism*, 34, 380–5.

Soll, R. F. & McQueen, M. C. (1992) Respiratory distress syndrome. In *Effective Care of the Newborn Infant*, ed. J. Sinclair & M Bracken, pp. 325–58. Oxford: Oxford University Press.

Sosenko, I. & Frank, L. (1987). Thyroid hormone depresses antioxidant enzyme maturation in fetal rat lung. *American Journal of Physiology*, 253, R592–8.

Stubblefield, P. G. & Kitzmiller, J. L. (1980). Maternal pulmonary oedema following combination treatment with betamimetics and high-dose steroids during pregnancy. In *Betamimetic Drugs in Obstetrics and Perinatology. Third Symposium on Betamimetic Drugs*, ed. H. Jung & G. Leinberti, p. 144. New York: Thieme Stratton.

Tabor, B., Ikegami, M., Jobe, A. H., Yamada, I. & Oetomo, S. B. (1990). Dose response of thyrotropin-releasing hormone on pulmonary maturation in corticosteroid-treated preterm rabbits. *American Journal of Obstetrics and Gynecology*, 163, 669–76.

Tabor, B., Rider, E. D., Ikegami, M., Jobe, A. H. & Lewis, J. (1991) Dose effects of antenatal corticosteroids for induction of lung maturation in preterm rabbits. *American Journal of Obstetrics and Gynecology*, 164, 675–81.

Taeusch, H. W. Jr, Frigoletto, F., Kitzmiller, J., Avery, M. E., Hehre, A., Fromm, B., Lawson, E. & Neff, R. K. (1979). Risk of respiratory distress syndrome after prenatal dexamethasone treatment. *Pediatrics*, 63, 64–72.

Teramo, K., Hallman, M. & Raivio, K. O. (1980). Maternal glucocorticoid in unplanned premature labor. *Pediatric Research*, 14, 326–9.

Thorpe-Beeston, J. G., Nicolaides, K. H., Felton, G., Butler, J. & McGregor, A. M. (1991). Maturation of the secretion of thyroid hormone and thyroid stimulating hormone in the fetus. *New England Journal of Medicine*, 324, 532–6.

Torday, J. S. (1990). Androgens delay human fetal lung maturation *in vitro*. *Endocrinology*, 126, 3240–4.

Usher, R. H., Allen, A. C. & McLean, F. (1971) Respiratory distress syndrome related to gestational age, route of delivery and maternal diabetes. *American Journal of Obstetrics and Gynecology*, 163, 558–660.

van Golde, L. M. G., Batenburg, J. J. & Robertson, B. (1988). The pulmonary surfactant system: biochemical aspects and functional aspects and functional significance. *Physiological Reviews*, 68, 374–455.

Warburton, D., Parton, L., Buckley, S., Cosico, L., Enn, S. G. & Saluma, T. (1988). Combined effects of corticosteroid, thyroid hormones and β-agonist on surfactant, pulmonary mechanics and β-receptor binding in fetal lamb lung. *Pediatric Research*, 24, 166–70.

Wegman, M. E. (1989). Annual summary of vital statistics. *Pediatrics*, 86, 835–47.

Whitt, G. G., Buster, J. E., Killan, A. P. & Scragg, W. H. (1976). A comparison of two glucocorticoid regimens for acceleration of fetal lung maturation in premature labour. *American Journal of Obstetrics and Gynecology*, 124, 479–82.

Whitsett, J. A., Weaver, T. E., Lieberman, M. A., Clark, J. C. & Daugherty, C. (1987). Differential effects of epidermal growth factor and transforming growth factor-β on synthesis of MR = 35 000 surfactant-associated protein in fetal lung. *Journal of Biological Chemistry*, 262, 7908–13.

8 Fetal infections

PHILLIP BENNETT AND UMBERTO NICOLINI

Introduction

Prenatal diagnosis of congenital infections, let alone their therapy, is one of the least established areas in fetal medicine. Screening policies vary greatly in different countries reflecting different perceptions of the relevance of a specific infection. The frequency of a given infection during pregnancy and the rate of transplacental passage, both largely dependent on the tests employed, is often unknown. Before 20 weeks' gestation, assay of specific IgM is an unreliable means of excluding infection, since the fetus is unable to produce measurable quantities of antibodies. Even later in gestation, the sensitivity of IgM in fetal blood may be as low as 28% in the diagnosis of infections such as toxoplasmosis. At birth, reliance on finding specific IgM in cord blood may underestimate the fetal infection rate, since fetal IgM synthesis might have occurred earlier in gestation and already ended. The presence of specific IgG in fetal blood simply reflects maternal levels, resulting from facilitated transplacental passage of IgG. The persistence of specific IgG antibodies at one year of age, however, does suggest intrauterine infection.

The application of the polymerase chain reaction (PCR) to detect the presence of an infectious agent's genome constitutes a significant improvement in the ability to assess the rate of fetal infection but, because of its high sensitivity, is prone to false positive results from maternal or environmental contamination, or to false negatives if strains of the microorganism exhibit significant genetic variability. The time elapsed from maternal infection to testing is crucial just as with isolation or culture of the infective agent from fetal tissues. With slow growing viruses, some weeks are needed for mater-nal viraemia, additional time for the infection to spread to the placenta and fetus and, finally, for the fetus to excrete the virus in the compartment being tested. However, if fetal blood is sampled, viraemia may be a transitional phase in the cycle of the infectious agent that might be missed.

Evidence of infection, however, does not imply fetal damage and/or long-term sequelae. It is not unexpected that, given the uncertainties about the true rate of fetal infection for any specific disease, the frequency of congenital anomalies is even less precisely assessed. The issue is further confused by several variables which interfere with the natural history of the congenital infection. Termination of pregnancy has been offered or requested since pre-natal diagnosis has become available, often following detection of infection rather than evidence of fetal lesions. Various treatments have become accepted in clinical practice without proper randomized trials.

The fetus may also become infected as a result of ascending infection, especially with bacteria after preterm prelabour rupture of the membranes. The fetus can also acquire infection vertically at the time of delivery, either bacterial, such as group B streptococcus or viral, such as human immunodeficiency virus. Fetal diagnosis is not so relevant here, where the focus is on accurate identification of those carrying the organisms and then institution of appropriate prophylactic therapies.

Rubella

The rubella virus is an RNA-containing togovirus with only one identified serotype (Banatvala & Best, 1990). Rubella is transmitted by respiratory droplets. Initial infection is via the respiratory tract to the cervical lymph nodes from where it is disseminated haematogenously. There is an incubation period of 14 to 21 days before development of the characteristic rash. Only 10% of adult infections are asymptomatic. Viraemia is present for about a week prior to the rash, during which the individual may experience lymphadenopathy, malaise and fever. The rash begins as pinpoint macular lesions on the face and trunk which then spreads to the extremities, coalescing to form erythematous maculopapules. Lesions may also be seen on the soft palate. The rash lasts for a few days although the associated lymphadenopathy may persist for several weeks. Infected individuals shed virus from the nasopharynx several days before onset of the rash until several days after its disappearance.

Diagnosis in the mother

Most cases of suspected maternal infection present either as contact with another affected individual, usually a child, or as a rash in the pregnant woman herself. Diagnosis is by demonstration of rising IgM titres, as a high antibody titre in a single sample is not diagnostic. If the presentation is as a contact with rubella, symptoms, if any, will not appear for 14 to 21 days and follow-up measurements of IgM titres will need to take this incubation period into consideration.

Anti-rubella antibodies detected by the haemagglutination inhibition test appear at the time of the appearance of the rash and become maximal seven to ten days later. Antibody titres measured by other techniques such as complement fixation or fluorescent antibodies become maximal several days later. Titres may remain elevated for years. Specific IgM antibodies may be detected within a few days of the development of the rash and remain detectable for between four and eight weeks, although there are isolated cases where IgM titres have remained elevated for over six months following primary infection (Sidle, 1985). False positives for anti-rubella IgM may occur in the presence of rheumatoid factor or infection by Epstein–Barr virus, CMV or parvovirus B19.

The congenital rubella syndrome

The congenital rubella syndrome (Gregg, 1941) comprises the classic triad of cataracts, deafness and con-

genital heart disease. Deafness is present in 70% of patients, cataracts in 30%, heart defects, most commonly patent ductus and pulmonary stenosis, in 20% and CNS defects in 20%. The earlier in pregnancy the infection occurs the more severe the syndrome, with cardiac and eye defects commonly caused by infection during organogenesis in the first eight weeks. The only defects found after infection in the second or third trimester are deafness and retinopathy, which may not affect vision. Affected neonates have a mortality of up to 20% and survivors may have significant handicap because of deafness, visual impairment and both motor delay and mental retardation.

Congenital infection occurs via transplacental transmission. With maternal infection in the first month following conception, congenital infection is found in 50% of neonates. This decreases to 25 and 10% with maternal infection in the second and third months and to less than 1% thereafter (Miller, Cradock-Watson & Pollock, 1982; Enders et al., 1988).

Management

Since virtually all cases of congenital rubella syndrome occur after infection in the first trimester of pregnancy, the only therapeutic option is termination of pregnancy. In most patients the demonstration of rising anti-rubella IgM titres in the first trimester would be sufficient grounds to offer termination. If the presentation is late after contact with rubella, if there is doubt about the diagnosis or if the parents are resistant to termination of pregnancy without proof that the fetus has been infected, attempts may be made to identify fetal infection directly. Viral isolation in amniotic fluid (Levin et al., 1974) is unfortunately limited by the time needed to grow and identify the virus and a high rate of false negatives (Alestig et al., 1974). Identification of anti-rubella antibodies in amniotic fluid has also proved unreliable (Cederqvist et al., 1977). The use of PCR to detect virus in amniotic fluid may possibly improve diagnosis by amniocentesis, although little information is yet available on its accuracy. Specific anti-rubella IgM may be demonstrated in fetal blood but not prior to 22 weeks. Daffos et al. (1984) first described fetal blood sampling for IgM titres, although one of six IgM-negative fetuses was infected at birth, possibly because fetal blood sampling had been performed too early.

Prevention

Immunity resulting from natural infection is lifelong and in areas without vaccination programmes most individuals acquire infection in childhood (Burke, Hinmann & Krugman, 1985). Seroconversion and lifelong immunity occurs in about 95% of vaccinated individuals (Morgan-Capner *et al.*, 1988). Immunization policies were introduced in the late 1960s/early 1970s. Over the next two decades, the prevalence of congenital rubella became lower under the herd immunization policy practised in the USA, where all male and female children are vaccinated, compared with the selective policy in the UK where seronegative teenage girls are vaccinated. The UK has, therefore, recently switched to immunizing all pre-school children.

Cytomegalovirus

Cytomegalovirus (CMV) is a DNA virus, and the largest of the herpes virus family. Human CMV is specific for human cells and will not infect other mammals. Although genetically homologous, there is considerable variation in viral DNA sequences so that restriction analysis can be used to trace routes of infection in epidemiological studies. Like all herpes viruses, infection then remains in a latent form and may be reactivated if the individual becomes immunocompromised. CMV infection causes the appearance of typical cytomegalic cells with characteristic intranuclear inclusions.

In post-natal life, CMV infection is almost always asymptomatic and subclinical. Occasional patients may report an influenza-like illness with fever, headache, sore throat, cervical lymphadenopathy, muscular pains and a transient rash. Very rarely signs of encephalitis or meningitis develop. CMV infection is more severe and prolonged in immunocompromised individuals (Stagno *et al.*, 1982a; 1986). It is not highly infectious but may be transmitted by intimate contact with an infected individual, either through saliva or sexual contact, or through blood transfusion or organ transplantation. CMV seropositivity is more common in lower socio-economic groups and among those who work with children. In the third world, CMV is almost always acquired during childhood and most adults are seropositive. In developed countries up to 50% of the population may escape infection until adulthood (Stagno *et al.*, 1982a).

Diagnosis in the mother

CMV can be isolated from a range of body fluids, although the most convenient and consistent source is urine. The standard diagnostic test is viral culture in human fibroblasts. Although the typical cytopathic effect may be seen after a few days, cultures need to be maintained for ⩾21 days to be certain that a result is negative. Serological methods such as fluorescence antibody tests and enzyme-linked immunoassays have the advantages of convenience and speed but the disadvantage of poor specificity and sensitivity. PCR has been used to amplify CMV-specific DNA in donated blood (Stanier *et al.*, 1992) and is beginning to be used in diagnosis from urine and amniotic fluid. Although PCR is highly sensitive, contamination may contribute to a high false positive rate whereas false-negatives may be caused by failure to extract DNA adequately from urine or amniotic fluid.

Maternal infection, being asymptomatic, is rarely diagnosed. Occasionally in the presence of symptoms the diagnosis may be made by detection of specific anti-CMV IgM in maternal serum. However, anti-CMV IgM may persist for up to 16 weeks following primary infection (Griffiths *et al.*, 1982) and detection of IgM in the first trimester may represent infection before conception. The diagnosis is more certain if seroconversion is demonstrated or if the index illness can be accurately timed to during the pregnancy.

Congenital CMV infection

CMV infection *in utero* is associated with a spectrum of fetal and neonatal disease. Ultrasound findings include fetal growth retardation, microcephaly and cerebral calcification. The most common findings in affected neonates include petechiae and thrombocytopenia in 60 to 80%, hepatosplenomegaly in 70% and jaundice in 55%, growth retardation in 40%, microcephaly in 40% and, more rarely, seizures, interstitial pneumonia and congenital deafness.

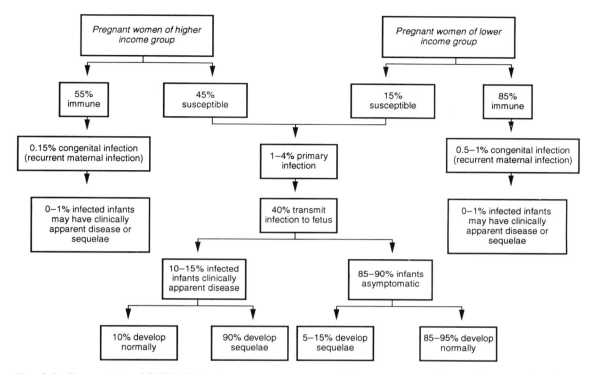

Fig. 8.1 *Characteristics of CMV infection in pregnancy. (Redrawn from Stagno and Whiteley, 1985).*

The principal method of perinatal transmission is transplacental. Infection during delivery, from vaginal secretions or maternal blood is rare, as is infection through breast-feeding (Stagno *et al.*, 1986). Although infants with congenital CMV infection shed virus in their urine and saliva, transmission to other infants, for example in neonatal units, is rare and isolation of congenitally infected infants is not indicated (Tookey & Peckham, 1992).

Transplacental transmission can occur during both a primary or a reactivation infection (Fig. 8.1). The rate of transmission is 40% in primary infections but less than 1% in reactivated infection (Stagno *et al.*, 1982b). In areas with a high rate of seropositivity, reactivation accounts for a high proportion of cases of congenital infection, such as in 30% of cases in the UK (Tookey & Peckham, 1992). Unlike other congenital infections there is no change in the risk of perinatal transmission or the severity of congenital disease at different gestational

ages. The most severe forms of congenital infection result from primary maternal infection, and reactivation virtually never causes severe congenital disease (Stagno *et al.*, 1982b). The incidence of congenital infection varies between 0.3 and 3% of live births. Of these, 5% will be symptomatic at birth, with a neonatal mortality of 30% and long-term handicap in all survivors. This includes developmental delay in up to 90%, hearing loss in 60% and neurological deficits including IQ (Peckham et al., 1987; Stagno *et al.*, 1986; Preece, Pearl & Peckham, 1984)

Diagnosis *in utero*

Prenatal diagnosis in the fetus is based upon ultrasound findings and the detection of viral particles in amniotic fluid or fetal blood. Ultrasonography may demonstrate hydrops fetalis or ascites, ventriculomegaly, intracranial calcification, bowel echodensity and growth retardation but is often normal in infected fetuses.

Isolation of CMV in amniotic fluid is the most reliable index of congenital infection. Five series reported 77 patients in which the indication for prenatal testing was a primary maternal CMV infection in the absence of fetal abnormalities detected by ultrasound (Hohlfeld *et al.*, 1991; Lynch *et al.*, 1991; Lamy *et al.*, 1992; Nicolini *et al.*, 1994). Thirty one fetuses were found infected, and five false diagnoses occurred in the 46 negative at prenatal testing. Approximately 40% of infected fetuses had negative virus-specific IgM, and 30% had normal haematological and biochemical findings at blood sampling. These results highlight the difficulties in counselling patients in whom a primary infection is diagnosed before viability. The rate of fetal infection is very high (47%), whereas the sensitivity of prenatal diagnosis, even with multiple tests, is <90%. One study, of amniocentesis before 21 weeks, found a false-negative rate of 45% using PCR, and a sensitivity of only 18% based on culture alone (Donner *et al.*, 1993). In one series, two false-negative cases, which occurred in the second half of pregnancy, were tested within a month of infection, whereas more than six weeks had elapsed from infection in the true positive diagnoses (Nicolini *et al.*, 1994). The effect of time on the reliability of prenatal diagnosis of CMV infection is not surprising, since the incubation period in post-transfusion CMV mononucleosis is three to six weeks. Additional causes for false-negative diagnoses may be viral load in amniotic fluid and variability of CMV strains. The former may be implicated in instances in which PCR confirms prenatal infection in the absence of a positive viral culture, whereas false-negative diagnoses caused by the latter could be reduced by use of more than one set of primers.

The timing of prenatal diagnosis remains a crucial variable in dealing with women at risk of congenital CMV. We, therefore, recommend amniocentesis for culture and/or PCR four to six weeks after documentation of primary maternal infection. Early testing allows the option of termination of pregnancy, but the risk of false-negative diagnoses increases with too short an interval from infection.

Fetal blood sampling has been suggested to have a role in indicating which infected fetuses have organ compromise, those with normal haematological and biochemical indices being less likely to have serious sequelae (Hohlfeld *et al.*, 1991). However, the occurrence of fetal changes may not coincide with serological or microbiological confirmation of infection (Nicolini *et al.*, 1994). In this perspective, serial prenatal testing

may have a role in infected fetuses at risk of sequelae who may be candidates for fetal therapy.

Management

If primary CMV with transplacental transmission in pregnancy is confirmed, there is a 10% chance of severe congenital disease, and termination of pregnancy should be offered. Recurrent disease carries a much lower risk of handicap and would probably not justify pregnancy termination. Attempts have been made to treat the infected fetus directly with anti-viral agents such as ganciclovir either through the mother (Einsele *et al.*, 1991) or directly to the fetus. Prenatally, serial intravascular administration of ganciclovir has been reported in a 27 week fetus with documented CMV infection, abnormal liver function tests and thrombocytopenia (Revello, Percivalle & Baldanti, 1993). During treatment, a dramatic decrease in viral load was observed in amniotic fluid, with normalization of the platelet count and γ-glutamyl transpeptidase levels (Fig. 8.2). The fetus died subsequently in labour, probably from unrelated causes, but there was no evidence of structural abnormalities or cerebral infection at post-mortem.

The low transplacental passage of ganciclovir together with its renal, hepatic and bone marrow toxicity present an obstacle to treating infected fetuses via the mother. While awaiting results of studies on the effectiveness of neonatal treatment with ganciclovir, intravascular, or intra-amniotic administration to the fetus needs to be restricted to selected cases with sufficient grounds to recommend fetal treatment rather than termination of pregnancy.

An alternative approach would be intra-amniotic treatment, since oral therapy in neonates has been shown to achieve adequate serum levels. We have tried this in one patient, in which intra-amniotic ganciclovir led to a huge reduction in fetal blood viral load, but no change in platelets or liver function (U. Nicolini, unpublished observations).

Prevention

Routine screening for CMV seropositivity is unlikely to be valuable since there is no vaccine available and little can be done to prevent infection in pregnancy in those who are seronegative. Those in high-risk groups for seroconversion, such as those who work with large numbers of young children, could be screened and then counselling about the need for hygiene and avoidance of intimate contact during pregnancy given to seronegatives (Alford *et al.*, 1990). Vaccines have been developed but are not in use because of concerns about their oncogenic potential and the risks of reactivation of the live attenuated virus used (Alford *et al.*, 1990).

Parvovirus B19

Parvovirus is a small, single-strand DNA virus of high infectivity transmitted through respiratory droplets. In childhood, infection presents as erythema infectiosum, also known as fifth disease. Approximately 50% of adults will have serological evidence of past infection and current immunity. In non-immune individuals, contact with an infected person carries a 20–50% risk of infec-

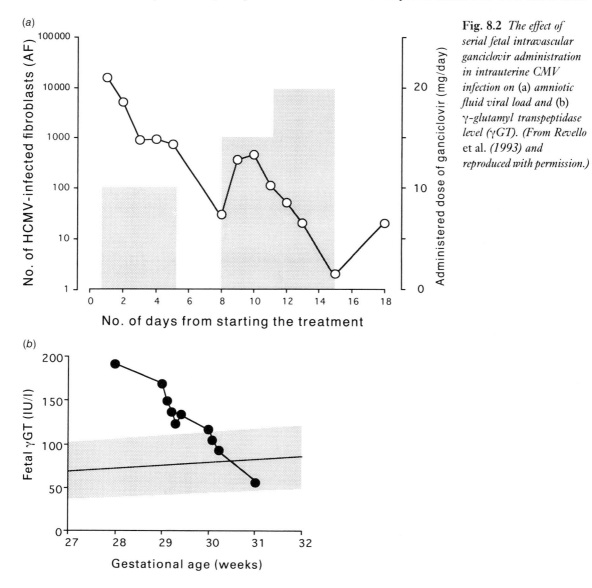

Fig. 8.2 *The effect of serial fetal intravascular ganciclovir administration in intrauterine CMV infection on* (a) *amniotic fluid viral load and* (b) *γ-glutamyl transpeptidase level (γGT). (From Revello et al. (1993) and reproduced with permission.)*

tion. Following the initial respiratory tract infection and viraemia, the virus replicates in erythroid precursor cells in the bone marrow. This causes a transient aplastic event which lasts up to 10 days and is self limiting with full recovery within three weeks. It is associated, however, with massive viral release and a transient heavy viraemia. The clinical incubation period is 4–20 days. The illness then develops as a sore throat, cold-like symptoms and a mild fever. After a few days, a bright erythematous macular rash develops on the face and then the trunk and limbs, and this persists for up to 10 days before fading. In most individuals the aplastic event is asymptomatic. Woolf *et al.* (1989) studied a community outbreak of parvovirus B19 and found that 29% of adults were asymptomatic, 44% reported a rash, 59% had cold-like symptoms and 48% developed a symmetrical polyarthropathy. Women appear to be more severely affected than men.

Although parvovirus B19 specifically affects the erythroid series, a transient decrease in neutrophils and platelet counts may also occur (Alestig *et al.*, 1974).

In vivo, parvovirus replicates only in precursors of red cells, while *in vitro* it can be propagated in bone marrow, peripheral blood and fetal liver. The reason for this specific tropism of parvovirus B19 has been elucidated by the recent finding that the virus binds to the P antigen, or globoside, which is present on the surface of erythrocytes, erythroblasts, megakaryocytes, endothelial cells, placenta, fetal liver and heart cells. The P blood group consists of two common antigens, P_1 and P, and a third rarer P^k antigen. Individuals lacking the P antigen on red cells and erythroid precursors seem immune to parvovirus B19, none of 17 subjects without the P antigen in a recent study having serological evidence of previous infection, compared with 47–71% in controls (Brown *et al.*, 1994).

Diagnosis in the mother

In the UK and in the USA, approximately 50% of pregnant women are not immune to B19. The rate of infection in pregnancy has not been clearly established but is probably about 1% and is subject to epidemics. Some 25% of infections in pregnancy will be asymptomatic and the majority of the others will be thought of as a cold or influenza.

There are no conventional cell culture methods for isolation of the virus although in specialist laboratories the virus can be grown in bone marrow or fetal liver cultures. Currently the virus is most reliably detected by dot-blot hybridization or PCR of parvovirus B19-specific DNA or by electron microscopy. The mainstay of diagnosis, however, remains serology. There is only one serotype and anti-B19 IgM appears in the serum at the onset of the illness and remains detectable for up to three months. The IgG response begins after seven days and persists, probably to confer life long immunity.

Congenital parvovirus B19 infection

The rate of transplacental passage is 33% from one study of 190 women with serologically confirmed infection in pregnancy (Public Health Laboratory Service Working Party on Fifth Disease, 1990). However, the true risks of fetal infection and perinatal loss cannot be assessed precisely, given the high frequency at which asymptomatic maternal infection occurs. In the two prospective studies of mainly symptomatic women, the percentage of live healthy neonates was from 84–95% (Public Health Laboratory Service Working Party on Fifth Disease, 1990; Rodis *et al.*, 1990). This contrasts with a 74% rate (seven hydropic fetuses and one fetal death from 22 maternal infections) in another study (Smoleniec *et al.*, 1994), although assessment of maternal infection was based on reported contact or the finding of hydrops on ultrasound.

There is no evidence that B19 is teratogenic. Although it may be associated with pregnancy loss in the first trimester, it is not, in general, a significant cause of early miscarriage. The most common presentation is hydrops fetalis in which severe anaemia, congestive heart failure and generalized fluid retention leads to fetal death. Hydrops without fetal anaemia has been documented and viral particles have been identified in fetal myocardium, suggesting that hydrops may be, at least in part, cardiogenic. The rate of fetal death following maternal infection has been estimated at 9% (Public Health Laboratory Service Working Party on Fifth Disease, 1990). The interval between maternal infection and fetal death is usually four to five weeks but may be up to 11 weeks.

Diagnosis *in utero*

Maternal infection, if suspected, may be confirmed by detection of specific anti-B19 IgM. The presence of IgG without IgM virtually excludes recent infection and indicates immunity. B19 infection forms an important part of the differential diagnosis of non-immune hydrops fetalis. Serological studies in the fetus are hindered by the poor fetal IgM response, although this lack of antibodies leads to a persistently high viral load in fetal blood. Viral particles can be seen with electron microscopy in fetal ascitic fluid or fetal blood (Naides & Weiner, 1989). The principle method of fetal diagnosis is, therefore, direct detection of viral particles using hybridization or PCR (Sheikh, Ernest & O'Shea, 1992). B19 virus can also be cultured from amniotic fluid, although the delay involved in amniotic fluid culture may reduce its clinical value.

Management

Most cases of transplacental B19 infection will present as unexplained hydrops fetalis. It is unlikely that a maternal infection in pregnancy will be diagnosed primarily unless it is part of an established epidemic. If maternal infection in pregnancy is documented, serial ultrasound scans are indicated to detect hydrops. When fetal hydrops related to parvovirus B19 is diagnosed, fetal blood sampling to detect anaemia and the need for intrauterine transfusions is indicated, as discussed in detail in Chapter 10.

Varicella-zoster

Varicella-zoster virus (VZV) infection causes chicken pox, a benign childhood illness. Infections in adults, particularly the immunocompromised, may cause serious pulmonary and central nervous complications. VZV is highly contagious. The incubation period is between 10 and 20 days before the onset of fever, malaise and the characteristic maculopapular rash. The rash resolves within four to six days. Immunity is then lifelong and chicken pox does not recur, although viral latency in the sensory nerve ganglia may give rise to herpes zoster or shingles when immunity is depressed. Ninety per cent of adults have immunity to VZV.

Diagnosis in the mother

Diagnosis in the mother is by serology. Both IgM and IgG antibodies appear between two and five days after the rash and peak at four weeks. IgM remains elevated for one or two months while IgG persists and confers lifelong immunity. Acute infection can be confirmed by demonstration of rising IgG titres or the presence of specific IgM.

Congenital varicella syndrome

The prevalence of VZV infection during pregnancy ranges from 0.7 to 3%. Transplacental transmission before 20 weeks is associated with the congenital varicella syndrome but this is very rare, accounting for only 30 reported cases worldwide (Cradock-Watson, 1990). The rate of intrauterine VZV infection is difficult to estimate. Using a combination of criteria, which included detection of specific IgM, persistence of high levels of VZV IgG antibodies, and specific lymphocyte transformation in response to VZV antigen, evidence of intrauterine infection was found in 21% of infants in a series of 43 pregnancies complicated by varicella, but in only 11% when maternal infection occurred in the first or second trimester (Paryani & Arvin, 1986). However, immunological response is far from a sensitive method to estimate the rate of transplacental infection, since only a minority of neonates with congenital varicella syndrome have specific IgM detectable, and discordance between the different immunological markers occurs frequently (Enders *et al.*, 1994).

The congenital varicella-zoster syndrome includes skin scarring with a dermatomal distribution with associated bone and muscle hypoplasia, microcephaly, mental retardation, bowel and bladder sphincter dysfunction, cataracts, microphthalmia and chorioretinitis. In three prospective and two cohort studies comprising 145 pregnant women exposed to VZV in the first trimester, the cumulative rate of varicella embryopathy was 2.8% (Pastuszak *et al.*, 1994). Another study identified only two patients with congenital varicella syndrome among 472 pregnant women who acquired infection in the first trimester, with no case of congenital varicella syndrome observed after 19 weeks' gestation (Enders *et al.*, 1994). Following maternal infection in the second half of gestation, however, a 1.7% frequency of herpes zoster in infancy or early childhood has been reported (Enders *et al.*, 1994).

Analysis of the congenital malformations in 27 infants born to mothers infected largely within the first 20 weeks of pregnancy, revealed dysfunctions attributable to encephalitis, and skin, musculoskeletal, peripheral and autonomic nervous system anomalies which exhibit a peculiar segmental pattern (Higa, Dan & Manabe, 1987). This suggests that the congenital malformations caused by the VZV may not be the direct effect of the primary viral infection, but the consequence of herpeszoster *in utero*. Therefore, embryopathy may result from intrauterine reactivation of the virus, an inadequate cell-mediated fetal immune response being the cause of the short latency between primary infection and the development of herpes zoster infection.

Affected infants generally die in infancy from recurrent pneumonia. Infection in latter pregnancy may be associated with herpes zoster in an otherwise healthy child.

Diagnosis *in utero* and management

In women who have been infected by VZV in the first half of gestation, serial ultrasound is used to detect the more obvious structural abnormalities such as limb hypoplasia, microcephaly and intrauterine growth retardation, although other serious features of varicella embryopathy, i.e. ocular and nervous system lesions, are unlikely to be diagnosed. In view of the high frequency of normal ultrasound findings, termination of pregnancy is rarely offered.

PCR, using primers which define a 221 bp region of the gene coding for the 44 kDa protein of VZV (Davison & Scott, 1986) has recently been used to diagnose prenatal infection in 4/13 fetuses tested in the first or second trimester (Nicolini *et al.*, 1995). A similar rate of maternal fetal transmission has been documented by detecting VZV IgM antibodies in 4/17 fetuses undergoing blood sampling after maternal infection in the first 20 weeks of pregnancy, although PCR analysis of VZV, done retrospectively on stored amniotic fluid and fetal blood, was negative in all cases (Liesnard *et al.*, 1994).

Given the high frequency of transplacental passage and the low rate of malformations, any role for invasive prenatal diagnosis in detecting the presence of the virus in fetal blood, amniotic fluid or chorionic villi would mainly be that of reassuring women whose fetuses tested negative.

Prevention

The use of prophylactic VZV immunoglobulin is recommended in non-immune pregnant women who are in contact with the disease (Department of Health, 1990). VZV immunoglobulin has not been proved to prevent congenital infection, and its use in mothers after the onset of the rash would seem of little benefit. Acyclovir is also indicated in infected immunocompromised pregnant women and in pregnant women with varicella pneumonia.

Maternal infection at around the time of delivery may lead to neonatal chicken pox. In mothers whose rash appears between five days before and two days after delivery, the neonatal disease may be severe with a fatality rate of up to 30% (Gershon, 1975). Prophylactic VZV immunoglobulin is recorrected for neonates delivered in this window. Infants who are infected outside this high-risk period generally have a mild self-limiting illness. There is no risk of transplacental transmission from maternal herpes zoster.

Toxoplasmosis

Toxoplasma gondii is a unicellular protozoan parasite. The cat is the primary host and reservoir of *T. gondii*. Cats initially acquire the infection from birds or rodents, with viable parasites forming oocysts in the gut, which are then shed in the faeces for the next one to three weeks. These are not infectious until sporulation takes place about three days later, after which they remain in the soil for a year or more, from where they may be transported by insects onto fruit or vegetables. Infected cats develop immunity but may shed small numbers of oocysts on re-infection.

Humans become infected through contaminated meat, fruit or vegetables, or from contact with cat faeces.

Toxoplasma cysts may be found in pork or lamb but rarely in beef or chicken. Toxoplasma cysts in meat may be destroyed by freezing or by cooking until the meat changes colour. Unwashed fruit or vegetables may also transmit the parasite, but again, these are destroyed by freezing or boiling. Cat owners may be at increased risk of infection, as are gardeners or children who play in soil in which a cat may have buried its infected faeces.

The incidence of infection shows marked geographical variation. In areas with high prevalence the majority of individuals show seroconversion by age 20. In low-prevalence areas such as the UK, the annual seroconversion rate is less than 1% and less than 20% of pregnant women show serological evidence of previous infection. The differences in prevalence may result from both climate and variations in eating habits. Seropositivity is highest in areas like Central Africa, with warm, moist climates where the oocysts survive longer in the soil, and in France, where the preference is for undercooked or raw meat.

Human infection with *T. gondii* is often asymptomatic or subclinical. After an incubation period of 9 to 10 days, vague flu-like symptoms such as fatigue, headache and fever may appear, together with lymphadenopathy, and are frequently misdiagnosed as a cold, influenza or infectious mononucleosis. Symptoms usually persist for a few days, although in those with immunodeficiency infection may lead to multiorgan damage. Ocular infection with *T. gondii* is an important cause of blindness worldwide and accounts for up to 70% of cases of chorioretinitis. The primary lesion is a focal necrotizing retinitis, which later becomes a well-demarcated pigmented scar, these being found in clusters. Following initial infection, the proliferative tachyzoites are present in the blood stream and lymphatics and may be carried to any organ and infect any nucleated cell. Once a cell has become infected, the tachyzoites rapidly replicate, destroy the host cell and go on to infect adjacent cells producing a region of focal necrosis. Once immunity has developed, the progression of infection stops but the organisms are not completely eradicated. The form of the organism changes to that of the slowly replicating bradyzoite, forming well-demarcated cysts in infected tissues, especially muscle, brain and retina. These remain indefinitely and may lead to reactivation of infection if immunity is impaired.

The incidence of infection in pregnancy depends upon the number of women who enter pregnancy without previous infection and the prevailing infection risk. In France, although only 30% of women are sero-negative at antenatal booking, the high rate of infection gives rise to an incidence of infection in pregnancy of 3 per 1000. In the UK, 85% of pregnant women are at risk of infection but the lower *a priori* risk produces an incidence of only 2 infections per 1000 pregnancies.

Diagnosis in the mother

The initial IgM antibody response appears about five days after infection, to peak at one month. Although titres then decrease, IgM may remain detectable in some individuals years after primary infection. IgG antibodies appear several weeks after the IgM response, reaching a maximum up to six months later. The high IgG titre may persist for several years and although it may then gradually decline, IgG antibodies are generally detectable lifelong. The most reliable indication of maternal toxoplasmosis is seroconversion on IgG testing, confirmed by the presence of IgM. Ideally comparison should be made with preconception or early pregnancy samples. With the presence of IgM during the index pregnancy, testing of preconception samples will often show that IgM was present before the pregnancy and that there is, therefore, no risk to the fetus. Unfortunately early samples are usually not available. The presence of IgM without IgG in a single sample is likely to be the result of recent infection. More commonly, both IgM and IgG are found and diagnosis will then require a second sample 21 days later to demonstrate rising titres, usually defined as a four dilution increase in specimens assayed in parallel (e.g. 1:2 to 1:32).

A number of methods for measuring anti-toxoplasma antibodies are available. The Sabin Feldman dye test is the traditional method but is limited to laboratories in which living parasites can be generated. The test depends upon the damage caused by IgG antibodies to toxoplasma which then allows the uptake of dye. The IgG indirect fluorescent antibody test (IFAT) is more readily performed in laboratories which cannot grow the parasite and its results are broadly comparable to those of the dye test. The indirect haemagglutination test measures a subset of antibodies different to those of the

IFAT, become positive later in the disease history and remains positive for longer. Since it is often negative in the early stages, it is inaccurate in the diagnosis of primary infection. High levels of IgG may prevent accurate measurement of IgM antibodies and false positives may be caused by antibodies to systemic lupus or rheumatoid disease. Enzyme-linked immunosorbant assays (ELISA), which are easier to perform by automated methods, are available for both IgG and IgM detection and show good correlation with other tests.

Congenital toxoplasma infection

During the parasitaemia phase of maternal infection, large numbers of toxoplasma infect the placenta, which then acts as a reservoir for subsequent fetal infection which may occur at any time if maternal infection is not treated. The risk of transmission to the fetus increases as pregnancy advances. Desmonts and Couvreur (1974) showed that, without treatment, the risk of vertical transmission rose from 25% in the first trimester to 54% in the second and 65% in the third trimester. More recent data suggest that the gradient may be even steeper with only a 10% risk in the first trimester rising to 90% in the third (Remington & Desmonts, 1990). The severity of fetal damage shows a gradient in the reverse direction. Infection before the third trimester is associated with a 25% risk of severe congenital toxoplasmosis, the most hazardous time being between 10 and 24 weeks (Desmonts, 1982), while infection in the third trimester is associated with subclinical disease in 90% of patients (Remington & Desmonts, 1990; Foulon *et al.*, 1990). Infection in the first trimester is, therefore, unlikely to cause congenital toxoplasmosis, but if it does it will be severe. In contrast, infection in the third trimester nearly always causes congenital disease, but of the mildest form. The ability of the immune system to contain old toxoplasma infection within tissue cysts and the central role of the placenta in fetal transmission means that there is no risk of fetal infection in women infected before conception.

The congenital toxoplasma syndrome consists of hydrocephalus, intracranial haemorrhage, convulsions and chorioretinitis. Other reported features include hepatitis, pneumonia, myositis and myocarditis. Infants who have one or more of these signs at birth have a poor prognosis. Up to 85% will be mentally retarded, 75% will have epilepsy and over half will suffer from major visual impairment (Eichenwald, 1960). The outlook for infants born without signs is considerably better; mild neurological damage may be seen in 10–30%, mostly hearing deficits and developmental delay (Roberts & Frenkel, 1990). If untreated, however, the majority of mildly affected infants will develop chorioretinitis, which may not become apparent until adulthood (Koppe, Loewer-Sieger & de Roever-Bonnet, 1986; Remington & Desmonts, 1990).

In areas with screening for congenital toxoplasmosis most cases will be identified by the new appearance of anti-toxoplasma antibodies in a previously seronegative woman. Since maternal infection is frequently asymptomatic or subclinical, most cases in areas without screening programmes will not be identified in the antenatal period. Occasionally, toxoplasma infection may be suspected following an influenza-like illness in the mother or if fetal ventricular dilatation, hydrocephalus or cerebral calcification are seen on ultrasound. There may also be an association between toxoplasma infection and fetal growth retardation. If toxoplasma infection in pregnancy is suspected, investigations are performed to determine, firstly whether the mother is genuinely infected and, secondly, whether transplacental transmission has taken place.

Diagnosis *in utero*

Ideally diagnosis is made by identification of specific IgM in fetal blood or identification of toxoplasma parasites in either fetal blood or amniotic fluid. The high risk of fetal damage following infection in the first trimester makes the identification of transplacental transfer of great importance. Fetal blood sampling is technically more difficult prior to 20 weeks and the fetus is unable to mount an IgM response before this time. Delaying identification of transplacental transmission until after 20 weeks is problematic in many countries with a legal bar to termination once fetal viability has been reached. Toxoplasma parasites may be identified in some 60% of patients where transplacental transmission has occurred before 16 weeks (Daffos *et al.*, 1988). Several methods are available for the identification of toxoplasma parasites. Inoculation into mice is very sensitive but results take up to six weeks. Tissue culture inoculation produces results in five days but is less sensitive. Toxoplasma parasites may also be detected using mono- or polyclonal antibodies (Remington & Desmonts, 1990). PCR may also be used, which has the advantage of speed and sensitivity and does not require viable parasites (Dupouy-Camet et al., 1992).

Diagnosis after 20 to 22 weeks may be easier, since fetal blood sampling can then be done for the detection of anti-toxoplasma IgM in fetal blood in addition to identification of parasites. The detection of anti-toxoplasma IgM antibodies in fetal blood depends upon gestational age. Before 24 weeks only 10% of affected fetuses have demonstrable IgM, increasing to 30% between 25 and 30 weeks and over 60% after 30 weeks. Toxoplasma parasites will be identified in fetal blood in 70% of affected patients (Daffos et al., 1988). There are a number of non-specific signs of fetal toxoplasma infection in fetal blood, which although not independently diagnostic, may help to support the diagnosis, including abnormal liver function tests, thrombocytopenia, leucocytosis eosinophilia and changes in the lymphocyte CD4:CD8 ratio (Foulon et al., 1990). Daffos et al. (1988) have shown that using a combination of these methods over 90% of infected fetuses can be identified in utero.

The use of PCR on amniotic fluid to detect congenital toxoplasma infection has been demonstrated to be 100% sensitive when compared with traditional tests in fetal blood (Hohlfeld et al., 1994). Furthermore, evidence of eosinophilia, thrombocytopenia, increased levels of γGT, and of total IgM in fetal blood is not predictive of the severity of lesions in infected fetuses (Hohlfeld et al., 1994). Therefore, prenatal diagnosis should now rely on the less invasive and more timely procedure of amniocentesis. The shift from fetal blood sampling should reduce the number of procedure-related losses. However, the risk of fetal infection based on PCR is only 7.4% overall, lower than 10% in the first trimester, and between 10 and 20% from 14–22 weeks' gestation (Hohlfeld et al., 1994). After that stage, no case of ventricular dilatation was diagnosed among 154 women despite fetal infection rates of 26–67%.

Management

Termination of pregnancy should be offered where transplacental transmission in the first or early second trimester is demonstrated or strongly suspected since the risk of several congenital disease is as high as 25%. After 20 weeks, there is virtually no risk of severe congenital disease.

Drug treatment has two aims: the first to prevent transplacental transmission where it is not already suspected, the second to treat the already infected fetus to reduce the severity of congenital disease. When infection in pregnancy is suspected, spiramycin therapy should be started while investigations are still in progress and stopped if these prove negative. The usual dose in pregnancy is 1 g t.d.s. Spiramycin is a macrolide antibiotic which is relatively free of side effects and has no teratogenic activity. It concentrates in tissues, producing a concentration in the placenta five times that in maternal serum, although fetal blood concentrations will probably not reach the therapeutic range (Forestier et al., 1987).

If laboratory investigations suggest fetal infection, anti-parasitic therapy is then indicated to limit fetal damage. The most commonly used combination is pyrimethamine and sulphadiazine, both folic acid antagonists which prevent toxoplasma replication by interference with DNA synthesis. Their combined activity is eight times greater than would be expected from their individual effects. Experience with their use in malaria prophylaxis in pregnancy has shown that there is no risk of teratogenesis although spiramycin therapy may be used as a precaution in the first trimester. Pyrimethamine is given in a dose of 1 mg/kg/day and sulphadiazine in a dose of 50–100 mg/kg per day, both in four divided doses. Treatment is given in cycles alternating three weeks of combined therapy with three weeks of spiramycin therapy until delivery. Their principle side effect is bone marrow depression. Maternal blood counts should be monitored weekly and the mother given 10 mg/day folinic acid.

Berrebi et al. (1994) recently reported a low risk of neurological impairment in congenitally infected infants. Of 206 women with toxoplasma infection from 8–26 weeks' gestation who were treated with spiramycin plus, if fetal blood was positive for toxoplasma exposure, pyrimethamine, there were seven fetal losses resulting from complications of fetal blood sampling, three intra-uterine deaths with severe toxoplasmosis, and 27 live-births with proven congenital infection. All infected infants, either symptomatic or with clinical abnormalities at birth, had normal neurological examinations at 15–71 months of age. They concluded that termination need not be offered if serial fetal ultrasounds were normal and anti-parasitic treatment given.

There is little doubt that the awareness of the problem of congenital toxoplasmosis, which ensued among obstetricians in some countries since the late 1970s, has prevented the birth of seriously handicapped infants but has also led to a number of healthy fetuses lost because of invasive procedures or terminated following diagnosis of infection without evidence of damage.

Whether the low frequency of congenital anomalies and the low risk of sequelae among infected infants can be attributed to maternal treatment has also been debated (Jeannel *et al.*, 1990), and studies on the effectiveness of treating toxoplasma infections in pregnant women have produced mixed results (Henderson *et al.*, 1984).

Neonates who are known to be congenitally infected, either because of prenatal diagnosis or because of signs at birth, should be treated with alternating three weekly courses of pyrimethamine, sulphadiazine and folic acid, and spiramycin, for the first year of life. It is less clear whether infants in whom infection is suspected but not proven should be treated with such a toxic regimen and some paediatricians prefer to use spiramycin therapy alone. Development of an IgM response may be delayed by treatment. The persistence of IgG antibodies beyond the 10th month of post-natal life indicates congenital infection. Since ocular disease may manifest itself or worsen at any time, close ophthalmology supervision of congenitally infected individuals should continue into adulthood.

Prevention

Pregnant women should be educated to reduce their risk of acquiring toxoplasma. Fruit and raw vegetables should be washed thoroughly and cooked adequately. Direct contact with cat faeces should be avoided and gloves worn when gardening.

The enthusiasm with which programmes of screening for toxoplasmosis in pregnancy have been embraced in some countries has probably been justified by the general consensus that the condition is severe, reasonably frequent, treatable, and diagnosis of fetal infection feasible with a relatively low risk; if the fetus is infected, the risk of damage is so serious that termination of pregnancy can be offered. All these assumptions have been recently questioned (Royal College of Obstetricians and Gynaecologists, 1992), with the exception of the possibility of pre-natal diagnosis, which is nowadays indeed safer and more reliable. Therefore, in the 1990s, while pressure from the media and consumers' associations is mounting, there is probably less support for toxoplasmosis screening in pregnancy than in the past.

Syphilis

Syphilis is caused by infection with *Treponema pallidum*, an anaerobic spirochaete principally transmitted by sexual contact. Although no longer endemic, its incidence has increased steadily since the early 1970s. After an incubation period of 10 to 90 days, the primary chancre appears on the cervix or vaginal wall, a small painless ulcer with local lymphadenopathy which heals in three to six weeks. In one third of patients, there will be full recovery and serology will become negative. In the remainder, secondary syphilis will manifest at between two and six months as a maculopapular rash, condylomata lata, iritis, alopecia and generalized lymphadenopathy. These signs will resolve by six weeks and the patient will enter the latent phase during which there may be recurrence of the signs of secondary syphilis. In one third of patients, tertiary syphilis will develop after several decades. This is characterized by gumma formation, aortic aneurysm and valve damage, central nervous involvement and eye damage.

Diagnosis in the mother

Diagnosis in the mother is serological. Treponemal infection causes both specific anti-treponemal antibodies and non-specific antibodies which cross-react with cardiolipin. The VDRL (Venereal Disease Reference Laboratory) test is a screening test for non-specific antibodies which becomes positive early in the course of an infection. The TPHA (*T. pallidum* haemagglutination) test is more specific but may not be positive in the early stages of the disease. A positive VDRL result should then be confirmed using a specific test of which the FTA (fluorescent treponemal antibody) is probably the best. Tests for specific IgM have been developed, but their usefulness is limited by cross-reactivity to rheumatoid factor and from competition from excess IgG. Maternal screening according to WHO recommendations should use both the VDRL and the TPHA test. If either of these is positive then a diagnosis of syphilis may be made on clinical grounds together with identification of spirochaetes in material from lesions. The screening tests may remain positive after treated disease.

Congenital syphilis

The rate of transplacental transmission to the fetus decreases from over 80% in the first year of untreated infection to virtually nil after five years. In an untreated mother with early syphilis, 30% of fetuses will die *in utero*, 30% will die in the neonatal period and the remainder will develop late symptomatic syphilis. At birth, 60% of affected neonates will have no clinical signs of congenital syphilis and will be detected only by positive serology. Clinical features do not usually develop until at least two weeks after birth. The earliest sign is rhinitis with organisms detected in the discharge, followed by formation of macular or papular erythema around the mouth and anus and on the palms and soles. In some neonates, hepatosplenomegaly may be detected. In those infants who are clinically unaffected at birth, manifestations of late congenital syphilis will develop between the ages of five and early adulthood. The most common manifestation is keratitis with variable visual impairment. Bone and joint lesions occur in some 20% of patients. Juvenile general paralysis and juvenile tabes dorsalis occur in less than 1% of patients. Sensory deafness may have its onset at any time but often occurs in adulthood rather than in childhood. The lesions of congenital syphilis may heal to leave classical stigmata including saddle-shaped nasal deformity, teeth deformities and eye and ear defects.

Diagnosis in the fetus

The risks to the fetus with active maternal infection are so high that separate investigation of whether the fetus is infected is not usually indicated. There are no serological techniques for diagnosis in the fetus, although background examination for spirochaetes can be performed on amniotic fluid (Wendel *et al.*, 1991).

Management

Any woman with a positive screen for syphilis should be considered infected unless both prior treatment and sequential serological antibody titres (VDRL or RPR) show an appropriate response. To aid in treating her fetus, penicillin is preferred because of the spirochaetes' extreme sensitivity to the drug, its ease of transplacental passage and its effectiveness in lowering the risk of multiorgan inflammation. In primary or early latent phase syphilis, a single dose of 2.4 million units of benzathine penicillin intramuscularly is indicated (Centers for Disease Control Guidelines, 1988). In the late latent phase or in syphilis of unknown duration, 2.4 million units of benzathine penicillin should be given intramuscularly each week for three doses.

If given during the first trimester, penicillin should prevent fetal infection. Administered after the first three months, penicillin usually cures the fetal infection; however, a 14% failure rate has been reported. Serological antibody titres must be determined monthly so that further treatment can be given if needed. The CDC also encourages ultrasonic assessment of fetal growth. Even after receiving transplacental therapy, an infant should be treated if there is any physical evidence of disease, reactive CSF-VDRL, abnormal CSF finding, quantitative serological antibody titre four fold higher than the mother's, or positive FTW-ABS IgM antibody.

In cases of penicillin allergy, alternative antibiotics are undesirable during pregnancy. Tetracycline and doxycycline are contraindicated, and erythromycin is unappealing because of its slow transplacental passage and high risk of failure to cure infection in the fetus. The Centers for Disease Control recommends that all patients allergic to penicillin be desensitized for the treatment of syphilis in pregnancy, as shown in Table 8.1

Table 8.1 *Centers for Disease Control Recommendations for oral densensitization of penicillin allergy in pregnant patients with syphilis*

Dose[a]	Penicillin V elixir (units/ml)	Amount[b]		Cumulative dose (units)
		ml	units	
1	1 000	0.1	100	100
2	1 000	0.2	200	300
3	1 000	0.4	400	700
4	1 000	0.8	800	1 500
5	1 000	1.6	1 600	3 100
6	1 000	3.2	3 200	6 300
7	1 000	6.4	6 400	12 700
8	10 000	1.2	12 000	24 700
9	10 000	2.4	24 000	48 700
10	10 000	4.8	48 000	96 700
11	80 000	1.0	80 000	176 700
12	80 000	2.0	160 000	336 700
13	80 000	4.0	320 000	656 700
14	80 000	8.0	640 000	1 296 700

Source: Wendel *et al.*, 1985. Reproduced with the permission of the author.

[a] Interval between doses, 15 minutes; elapsed time, 3 hours and 45 minutes; cumulative dose, 1.3 million units.

[b] The specific amount of drug was diluted in approximately 30 ml of water and then given orally.

(Wendel *et al.*, 1985). The infant should be routinely treated with one dose of benzathine penicillin.

Ascending fetal bacterial infection

During pregnancy, the fetus is protected from ascending infection from the maternal genital tract by the cervical mucus plug, the intact fetal membranes and the amniotic fluid, which itself has anti-bacterial properties. Although fetal infection may occur despite these barriers, the major risks to the fetus are following rupture of the fetal membranes and during vaginal delivery. Abnormal genital tract infection may lead to pre-term labour or to premature membrane rupture. When these are associ-

ated with chorioamnionitis, the risk of neonatal infection is high and efforts to prolong pregnancy may increase this risk.

Pre-term labour and membrane rupture

There is a clear association between pre-term labour and infection. Mothers are more likely to have puerperal sepsis and infants are more likely to have infections following pre-term labour (Daikoku *et al.*, 1981; Bouton, Klein & Lane, 1965). There is a strong epidemiological association between pre-term delivery and infection (Bennett & Fisk, 1993). Most cases of clinically overt chorioamnionitis associated with pre-term labour are caused by ascending infection following pre-term premature rupture of membranes, although there is evidence for an ascending route for microbial invasion with intact membranes (Romero *et al.*, 1989).

The mechanism of pre-term prelabour rupture of membranes (PPROM) is not clearly understood. While prematurely ruptured membranes are not generally weaker when tested for bursting strength, they do appear to be thinner at the site of rupture (Artal *et al.*, 1976). PPROM is associated with a similar history in previous pregnancies. It may result from abnormal membrane structure, cervical incompetence or uterine distension (Naeye & Peters, 1980). It is likely that infection is major aetiological factor. Naeye and Peters (1980) reported that among 6613 women who delivered before 37 weeks, the incidence of genital tract infection was three times greater in those whose membranes ruptured before rather than during labour, suggesting that infection was a cause and not the effect of membrane rupture. Where infection is the primary cause of PPROM, labour usually ensues. Where infection is not initially present, membrane rupture may then place the fetus at risk of ascending infection.

Diagnosis

In both pre-term labour and PPROM, chorioamnionitis may not be clinically obvious. Earlier clinical signs include fetal tachycardia, maternal tachycardia and pyrexia. Uterine tenderness and foul vaginal discharge are later signs. Fetal septicaemia may not necessarily be associated with other abnormalities of the cardiotocograph. Maternal leukocytosis (15 000/mm³) is common

(Gibbs & Duff, 1991). The results of culture of a high vaginal swab may not be available until after delivery but, where available, a Gram stain may be valuable in demonstrating the presence of gonococci or streptococci.

The role of amniocentesis in the diagnosis of amnionitis associated with either pre-term labour or PROM is uncertain. Only one study has prospectively examined the usefulness of amniocentesis in PPROM (Cotton *et al.*, 1984), finding no benefit, although amniocentesis continues to be a part of the management of both PPROM and pre-term labour in some centres.

The use of an elevation in maternal serum C-reactive protein (CRP) as an early indicator of chorioamnionitis is complicated by the overlap between CRP levels in infected and non-infected pregnancy and to differences in the indices of infection (Fisk *et al.*, 1987).

Management

There is a clear difference in the management of patients with pre-term labour in which there are clinical signs of infection and those in which infection is not apparent. There is currently no evidence that antibiotic therapy is of benefit in uncomplicated pre-term labour (Crowley, 1995). Where there is a strong suspicion that intra-amniotic infection is present, delivery should be allowed to take place as quickly as possible in the interests of both mother and baby, irrespective of fetal maturity. The controversy as to whether antibiotics should be given to the mother before delivery has not been resolved by any controlled studies. The principle argument against antibiotic treatment for the mother is that it may lead to resistant infection in the neonate and to difficulties in culturing organisms from the fetus. The one randomized controlled trial of maternal antibiotics for intrapartum infection (McCredie Smith, Jennison & Langley, 1956) failed to show a significant advantage but is now 30 years old. Two more recent retrospective studies have addressed this question. Sperling, Ramamurthy and Gibbs (1987) found that the incidence of neonatal sepsis was significantly lower in mothers treated with antibiotics in the intrapartum period rather than post-partum. Gilstrap *et al.* (1988) also found a lower incidence of neonatal sepsis with intrapartum treatment compared with post-partum or no treatment. Neither study found differences in the rates of maternal infection but they do suggest that early administration of antibiotics leads to a reduction in neonatal sepsis and an improvement in survival.

PPROM without the onset of labour has long been the obstetricians enigma, with management options finely balanced between the risks of prematurity and the risks of infection. It has been calculated (Goldenberg *et al.*, 1984) that the chance of survival without major handicap increases by 3% per day between 23 and 30 weeks. Use of antibiotics may eradicate the original causative organism or may act as a prophylaxis for ascending infection. Thirteen randomized controlled trials have been the subject of meta-analysis (Crowley, 1994) showing a significant reduction in the risk of pre-term delivery following PPROM if prophylactic antibiotics are used. There were also significant reductions in the rates of maternal sepsis and neonatal infections, in particular pneumonia (Fig. 8.3). The heterogeneity of these trials makes recommendations of the type and duration of antibiotic treatment impossible and until further trials have explored this issue individual clinicians will need to select their own regimen.

Group B streptococcus

Group B streptococcal infection, acquired during vaginal delivery, remains a significant cause of neonatal morbidity and mortality both at term and pre-term. Group B streptococcal colonization is significantly associated with both pre-term labour and PPROM. Randomized controlled trials of intrapartum antibiotics in patients known to be colonized show a clear reduction in neonatal colonization rates and neonatal sepsis rates (Fig. 8.3) although there are currently insufficient numbers to show a decrease in perinatal mortality (Smaill, 1994). Intrapartum vaginal chlorhexadine washing (Smaill, 1995a) has not been proved to eradicate maternal colonization or prevent neonatal colonization.

The principal dilemma in current practice is the identification of patients at risk. Screening of the pregnant population is complicated by large geographical variation in colonization and vertical transmission rates. Furthermore, a patient identified at screening may not be colonized later in their pregnancy while a negative patient may become colonized near term. Universal screening or antepartum antibodies in colonized patients has not currently been proved beneficial in reducing neonatal disease (Smaill, 1995b).

The contribution of group B streptococcus towards perinatal mortality, the efficacy of intrapartum antibiotics and the occurrence of disease in low-risk patients are persuasive arguments for screening, despite the lack of data to support universal screening. Attitudes towards screening vary worldwide, largely depending on the frequency of neonatal disease, but also very markedly within countries. For instance, in the USA, the American College of Pediatrics (1992) recommends routine screening at 26 to 28 weeks, whereas the American College of Obstetricians and Gynecologists (1992) advocates selective identification of those in high-risk groups.

At the very least, vaginal microbiological examination to detect group B streptococcus should be performed in patients with PPROM, pre-term labour or chorioamnionitis and antibiotics given to those who are colonized. The low risk of adverse effects suggests that intrapartum antibiotics should also be given to any patient previously identified as carrying group B streptococcus at any time during their pregnancy.

Human immunodeficiency virus

It is estimated that there are 4.5 million cases of AIDS and approximately 20 million people infected with the HIV virus worldwide. In the USA <18% of AIDS patients in 1994 were women, for whom AIDS is now the fourth most common cause of death at age 25–44 years (Horton 1995). One study found a frequency of HIV positivity of 1/10000 in Swedish women attending abortion and antenatal clinics from 1987 to 1991 (Lindgren *et al.*, 1993), but up to 1 in 500 women may be infected in other areas within developed countries (Ades *et al.*, 1991). Worldwide, Sub-Saharan Africa has the highest prevalence although more recently the epidemic has spread in southern Asia, in which the greatest number of new infections is expected in the next decade.

HIV is a single-stranded RNA retrovirus that binds the CD4 receptor of its target cells. Once it enters the cell, double-stranded DNA is synthesized by reverse transcriptase. The circular DNA is integrated into the host DNA and viral RNA and messenger RNA produced, thus initiating viral protein synthesis. HIV grows mainly in lymphocytes, monocytes-macrophages and some bone marrow precursor cells. The HIV virion has a

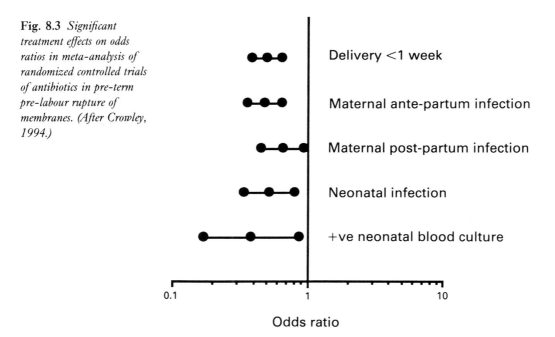

Fig. 8.3 *Significant treatment effects on odds ratios in meta-analysis of randomized controlled trials of antibiotics in pre-term pre-labour rupture of membranes. (After Crowley, 1994.)*

Delivery <1 week

Maternal ante-partum infection

Maternal post-partum infection

Neonatal infection

+ve neonatal blood culture

0.1   1   10

Odds ratio

diameter of approximately 100 nm, with a lipid envelope surrounding a cylindrical core which contains a helical nucleocapsid. The major surface proteins are gp120 and gp41, while the core proteins are p18 and p24. The HIV genome has long terminal repeats at both ends and contains at least eight genes.

Maternal infection

Several years can elapse from the time of HIV infection to the development of immunodeficiency-dependent infections and/or malignant disorders. During this period, the virus is not quiescent but active viral replication occurs in the lymphoid system, with rapid turnover of CD4 lymphocytes. This has led to the proposal that the term AIDS be abandoned in favour of 'advanced HIV disease' to underline the continuum between infection and the first appearance of opportunistic infections (Lifson, 1994).

Although the rate of progression of AIDS is similar in both sexes, the pattern of the initial illness differs in women, recurrent vaginal candidosis and pelvic inflammatory disease being the most common reasons for referral. Given the non-specific nature of symptoms,

HIV-infected women tend to have the diagnosis made at a later stage of the disease (Melnick *et al.*, 1994). This is of major concern since the incidence of AIDS is increasing faster in women than in men, and mother-to-child transmission is responsible for the vast majority of infections in children. Early diagnosis allows the initiation of aggressive prophylaxis for opportunistic infections and anti-retroviral therapy, while the identification of pregnant women with HIV infection is a prerequisite for prevention of vertical transmission.

HIV does not appear to be teratogenic or produce any specific congenital syndrome.

Screening

In the late 1980s, it was recommended that prenatal HIV testing be offered to women who acknowledge a risk behaviour for HIV infection, but approximately one third of HIV-positive women would be missed by such a policy, even if all at-risk patients accepted testing (Lindgren *et al.*, 1993; Barbacci, Repke & Chaisson, 1991). More recently, the Centers for Disease Control (1989) recommended that 'all pregnant women are routinely counselled and encouraged to be tested for HIV

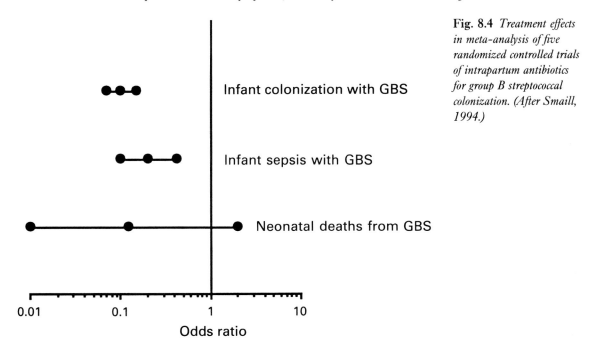

Fig. 8.4 *Treatment effects in meta-analysis of five randomized controlled trials of intrapartum antibiotics for group B streptococcal colonization. (After Smaill, 1994.)*

infection' and that 'HIV testing of pregnant women and their infants should be voluntary' (Horton, 1995). This statement contrasts with calls for mandatory screening of all pregnant women, which, besides contradicting one of the principles of bioethics, the right of autonomy of all patients, would be of doubtful success, since it might drive women most at risk away from screening. The offer of voluntary testing has repeatedly been shown to yield high acceptance rates, around 90%.

The costs of routine screening are considerable. In a population with a low prevalence of HIV infection, US$96 000 was the estimated cost of identifying one infected pregnant woman (Lindgren *et al.*, 1993). Nevertheless, several benefits arise from diagnosis of HIV infection in pregnancy.

Prophylaxis

Pregnancy itself does not appear to accelerate progression of HIV disease, but the finding of a CD4 cell count $<200/\mu$l is associated with an 8% and 18% chance of developing *Pneumocystis carinii* pneumonia within 6 and 12 months, respectively, which carries a mortality of 5–20% (Phair *et al.*, 1990). Primary prophylaxis, usually with trimethoprim–sulphamethoxazole, or pentamidine, is recommended for pregnant women, similar to the routine for non-pregnant individuals. Pentamidine, if administered by aerosol, has little systemic absorption, and no untoward fetal/neonatal effect should be expected. Trimethoprim–sulphamethoxazole, in contrast, readily crosses the placenta and may produce neonatal jaundice through displacement of unconjugated bilirubin from the albumin-binding site. However, in view of the high risk of morbidity and mortality of *P. carinii* pneumonia, and the lack of clear advantages brought by new therapeutic options, such as clindamycin with primaquine, dapsone with trimethoprim, atovoquone and trimetrexate (Sepkowitz & Armstrong, 1995), withholding therapy in pregnancy is not justified (Sperling & Stratton, 1992). Maternal neutropenia and megaloblastic anaemia resulting from an anti-folate effect may occur with trimethoprim–sulphamethoxazole, and folic acid supplementation is indicated unless a regimen of a low dose three times a week prophylaxis is adopted (Ruskin & LaRiviere, 1991).

Prevention of vertical transmission

In HIV-infected women, the chance of vertical transmission to the child varies in different populations. Whereas rates as high as 30% have been found in Africa, the most recent publication of the European Collaborative Study reported that paediatric HIV infection, as defined by the presence of HIV antibodies beyond 18 months, the onset of AIDS or the detection of virus or antigen on two or more occasions, occurred in 16.2% (95% CI = 13.9–18.5) of 1012 mother–child pairs (European Collaborative Study, 1994). There were no differences between the participating centres nor changes with time, but transmission appeared more common in the presence of a CD4 count $<700/\mu$l, p24 antigenaemia or breast-feeding (European Collaborative Study, 1992). In Europe, maternal age, parity and the use of intravenous drugs were not significantly related to the risk of having a congenitally infected child, while in South Africa multiparity seems the most significant risk factor (Moodley *et al.*, 1994).

Caesarean section

Both in Europe and Africa, caesarean section, whether emergency or elective, appeared to lower by half the rate of vertical transmission (European Collaborative Study, 1992; Moodley *et al.*, 1994). This, together with the observations that vaginally delivered second-born twins have a lower risk (Goedert *et al.*, 1991) and that only a minority of neonates later found to be infected have detectable virus, suggests that a significant percentage of cases of vertical transmission occur at delivery through exposure to vaginal and/or cervical secretions. The European Collaborative Study estimated that 12 caesarean sections need to be performed in order to prevent infection in one infant (European Collaborative Study, 1992). Since infectious morbidity is more prevalent and more severe in HIV-infected women, a policy of elective caesarean section needs careful evaluation, even without considering the additional costs. Vaginal lavage with HIV-inactivating agents, such as nonoxynol-9, benzalkonium chloride and chlorhexidine, might constitute an alternative approach although as yet of unproven efficacy (Newell & Peckham, 1994).

Zidovudine

The ACTG 076 study (Connor *et al.*, 1994) has opened a further perspective in reducing maternal–child HIV transmission. This randomized placebo-controlled study enrolled 477 infected women with a CD4 cell count >200/μl, and found that women who received zidovudine (AZT) antenatally (100 mg orally five times a day, and an intravascular bolus of 2 mg/kg over 1 hour, followed by a 1 mg/kg per hour infusion) and whose children also received zidovudine (2 mg/kg, four times a day for six weeks) had a 67.5% (95% CI = 40.7–82.1) reduction in the risk of HIV transmission compared with women who received placebo.

Zidovudine, after phosphorylation by intracellular kinases to the active form (zidovudine triphosphate), inhibits retroviral reverse transcriptase, which results in inhibition of HIV-1 replication *in vitro* and a transient reduction of viral load *in vivo*. Nevertheless, the Concorde trial did not show any benefit over three years if the treatment was initiated immediately in adult infected individuals compared with treatment delayed until the development of symptomatic disease (Concorde Coordinating Committee, 1994). This may be explained by the changes which occur in serum viral RNA following the initial administration of zidovudine. While HIV-1 RNA and p24 antigen fall in the serum within one to two days of treatment, the levels start to return to pretreatment values within weeks, and the reverse transcriptase gene develops mutations which are associated with drug resistance within months (Loveday *et al.*, 1995). It is, therefore, likely that the success of the ACTG 076 is related to the shorter duration of treatment needed in order to reduce the viral load to which the fetus is exposed. In this perspective, if exposure at the time of delivery is confirmed to be the main prognostic variable, even shorter courses of treatment may be effective.

Conclusions

Optimal screening and management strategies for infections transmitted transplacentally and ascendingly/intrapartum remain controversial, although in the latter group some consensus is beginning to emerge from randomized controlled trials.

The principles of managing transplacental infection are to confirm maternal exposure and then to assess the chance and severity of fetal infection and fetal affliction, either from the natural history and/or from invasive testing. Drug therapy has a role in reducing the fetal consequences of infection in toxoplasmosis and syphilis. Anti-microbials appear to have no role in rubella and parvovirus infection, although the latter is successfully treated by intrauterine transfusion.

Randomized controlled trials demonstrate a clear role for antibiotics antepartum in preventing ascending infection in pre-term premature rupture of the membranes and intrapartum in preventing neonatal transmission in carriers of group B streptococcus. Zidovudine is currently recommended to reduce vertical transmission of HIV, based on the results of a single randomized controlled trial.

References

Ades, A., Parker, S., Berry, T., Holland, F. J., Davison, C. F., Cubitt, D., Hjelm, M., Wilcox, A. H., Hudson, C. N., Briggs, M., Tedder, R. S. & Peckham, C. S. (1991). Prevalence of maternal HIV-1 infection in Thames regions: results from anonymous unlinked neonatal testing. *Lancet*, 337, 1562–5.

Alestig, K., Bartsch, F. K., Nilsson, A. & Strannegard, O. (1974). Studies of amniotic fluid in women infected with rubella. *Journal of Infectious Diseases*, 129, 79–81.

Alford, C. A., Stagno, S., Pass, R. F. & Britt, W. J. (1990). Congenital and perinatal cytomegalovirus infections. *Review of Infectious Diseases*, 12, S745–53.

American Academy of Obstetrics and Gynecology (1992). Group B streptococcal infections in pregnancy. *ACOG Technical Bulletin*, 170, 1–5.

American Academy of Pediatrics (1992). Guidelines for prevention of group B streptococcal infection by chemoprophylaxis. Committee on Infectious Diseases and Committe on Fetus and Newborn. *Pediatrics*, 90, 775–8.

Artal, R., Sokal, R. J., Neuman, M., Burstein, A. H. & Stokjov, J. (1976). The mechanical properties of prematurely and non–prematurely ruptured membranes. *American Journal of Obstetrics and Gynecology*, 125, 655–9.

Banatavala, J. E. & Best, J. M. (1990). Rubella. In *Topley and Wilson's Principles of Bacteriology, Virology and Immunology*, 8th edn, vol. 4, ed. L. Collier & M. Timbery. London: Edward Arnold.

Barbacci, M., Repke, J. T. & Chaisson, R. E. (1991). Routine prenatal screening for HIV infection. *Lancet*, 337, 709–11.

Bennett, P. R. and Fisk, N. M. (1993). Chorioamnionitis and pre-term delivery. In *Infectious Diseases: Challenges for the 1990s, Baillière's Clinical Obstetrics and Gynaecology*, 7. ed. G. L. Gilbert, pp. 25–43. London: W.B.Saunders.

Berrebi, A., Kobuch, W. E., Bessieres, M. H., Bloom, M. C., Rolland, M., Sarramon, M. F., Roques, C. & Fournie, A. (1994). Termination of pregnancy for maternal toxoplasmosis. *Lancet*, 344, 36–9.

Bouton, K., Klein, S. & Lane, R. (1965). Septicemia in premature infants. *American Journal of Diseases of Children*, 110, 29–41.

Brown, K. E., Hibbs, J. R., Gallinella, G., Anderson, S. M., Lehman, E. D., McCarthy, P. & Young, N. S. (1994). Resistance to parvovirus B19 infection due to lack of virus receptor (erythrocyte P antigen). *New England Journal of Medicine*, 330, 1192–6.

Burke, J. P., Hinmann, A. R. & Krugman, S. (1985). International symposium on prevention of congenital rubella syndrome. *Review of Infectious Disease*, 7, 174S–7S.

Cederqvist, L. L., Zervoudakis, I. A., Ewool, L. C., Senterfit, L. B. & Litwin, S. D. (1977). Prenatal diagnosis of congenital rubella. *British Medical Journal*, 1, 615.

Centers for Disease Control (1988). Guidelines for the prevention and control of congenital syphilis. *Morbidity and Mortality Weekly Report*, 37, S1–S13.

Centers for Disease Control (1989). Risks associated with human parvovirus B19 infection. *Morbidity and Mortality Weekly Report*, 38, 81–97.

Concorde Coordinating Committee, Concorde (1994). MRC/ANRS randomised double-blind control trial of immediate and deferred zidovudine in symptom free HIV infection. *Lancet*, 343, 871–81.

Connor, E. M., Sperling, R. S., Gelber, R., Kiselev, P., Scott, G., O'Sullivan, M. J., van Dyke, R., Bey, M., Shearer, W., Jacobson, R. L., Jimenez, E., O'Neill, E., Bazin, B., Defraissy, J.-F., Culnane, M., Coombs, R., Elkins, M., Moye, J., Stratton, P. & Balsley, J. (1994). Reduction of maternal–infant transmission of human immunodeficiency virus type 1 with zidovudine treatment. *New England Journal of Medicine*, 331, 1173–80.

Cotton, D. B., Hill, L. M., Strassner, H. T., Platt, L. D. & Ledger, W. J. (1984). Use of amniocentesis in pre-term gestation with ruptured membranes. *Obstetrics and Gynecology*, 63, 38–43.

Cradock-Watson, J. E. (1990). Varicella zoster virus infection during pregnancy. In *Current Topics in Clinical Virology*, ed. M. Kapner. London: Public Health Laboratory Service.

Crowley, P. (1994). Antibiotics for pre-term prelabour rupture of membranes. In *Pregnancy and Childbirth Module*, ed. M. J. N. C. Keirse, M. J. Renfew, J. P. Neilson & C. Crowther. London: The Cochrane Database of Systematic Reviews, BMJ Publishing Group.

Crowley, P. (1995). Antibiotics in pre-term prelabour with intact membranes. In *Pregnancy and Childbirth Module*, ed. M. J. N. C. Keirse, M. J. Renfew, J. P. Neilson & C. Crowther. London: The Cochrane Database of Systematic Reviews, BMJ Publishing Group.

Daffos, F., Forestier, F., Capella-Pavlovsky, M., Thulliez, P., Aufrant, C., Valenti, D. & Cox, W. L. (1988). Prenatal management of 746 pregnancies at risk for congenital toxoplasmosis. *New England Journal of Medicine*, 318, 5, 271–5.

Daffos, F., Forestier, F., Grangeot-Keros, L., Capella-Pavlovsky, M., Lebon, P., Chartier, M. & Pillot, J. (1984). Prenatal diagnosis of congenital rubella. *Lancet*, 2, 1–3.

Daikoku, N. H., Kaltreider, F. D., Khouzami, V. A., Spence, M. & Johnson, J. W. (1981). Premature rupture of membranes and spontaneous pre-term labor: maternal endometritis risks. *Obstetrics and Gynecology*, 59, 13–20.

Davison A. J. & Scott J. E. (1986). The complete DNA sequence of varicella zoster virus. *Journal of Genetic Virology*, 67, 1759–818.

Department of Health, Welsh Office, Scottish Home and Health Department (1990). *Immunisation against Infectious Disease.* London: HMSO.

Desmonts G. (1982). Toxplasmosae aquicitae de la femme enceinte. *Lyon Medical*, 248, 114–23.

Desmonts G. & Couvreur J. (1974). Congenital toxoplasmosis. A prospective study of 378 pregnancies. *New England Journal of Medicine*, 290, 1110–16.

Donner C., Liesnard C., Content J., Busine A., Aderca J. & Rodesch F. (1993). Prenatal diagnosis of 52 pregnancies at risk for congenital cytomegalovirus infection. *Obstetrics and Gynecology*, 82, 481–6.

Dupouy-Camet, J., Bougnoux, M. E., Lavareda de Souza, S., Thulliez, P., Dommergues, M., Mandelbrot, L., Ancelle, T., Tourte-Schaefer, C. & Benarous, R. (1992). Comparative value of polymerase chain reaction and conventional biological tests for the prenatal diagnosis of congenital toxoplasmosis. *Annales de Biologie Clinique Paris*, 50, 315–19.

Eichenwald, H. F. (1960). A study of congenital toxoplasmosis. In *Human Toxoplasmosis*, ed. J. C. Simm. Copenhagen: Williams and Wilkins.

Einsele, H., Eininger, G., Steidle, M., Vallbracht, A., Mueller M., Schmidt, H., Saal, J. G., Waller, H. D. & Mueller, C. A. (1991). Polymerase chain reaction to evaluate anti-viral therapy for cytomegalovirus. *Lancet*, 338, 1170–2.

Enders, G., Miller, E., Cradock-Watson, J., Bolley, I. & Ridehalgh, M. (1994). Consequences of varicella and herpes zoster in pregnancy: prospective study of 1739 cases. *Lancet*, 343, 1548–51.

Enders, G., Nickerl-Pacher, U., Miller, E. & Cradock-Watson, J. E. (1988). Outcome of confirmed periconceptual maternal rubella. *Lancet*, 1, 1445–7.

European Collaborative Study (1992). Risk factors for mother-to-child transmission of HIV-1. *Lancet*, 339, 1007–12.

European Collaborative Study (1994). Caesarean section and risk of vertical transmission of HIV-1 infection. *Lancet*, 343, 1464–7.

Fisk, N. M., Fysh, J., Child, A. G., Gatenby, P. A., Jeffrey, H. & Bradfield, A. H. (1987). Is C-reactive protein really useful in pre-term premature rupture of the membranes. *British Journal of Obstetrics and Gynaecology*, 94, 1159–64.

Forestier, F., Daffos, F., Rainaut, M. & Desnottes, J. F. & Gaschard, J. C. (1987). Suivi therapeutique foetomaternel de la spiromycine en cour de grossesse. *Archives Francais de pediatrie*, 44, 539–44.

Foulon, W., Naissens, A., Mahler, T., de Waele, M., de Catte, L. & de Meuter, F. (1990). Prenatal diagnosis of congenital toxoplasmosis. *Obstetrics and Gynecology*, 76, 5, 769–72.

Gershon, A. A. (1975). Varicella in mother and infant. Problems old and new. In *Infections of the Fetus and Newborn Infant*, vol. III, ed. S. Krugman & A. A. Gershon. New York: Liss.

Gibbs, R. S. & Duff, P. (1991). Progress in pathogenesis and management of clinical intra-amniotic infection. *American Journal of Obstetrics and Gynecology*, 164, 1317–26.

Gilstrap, L. C., Leveno, K. J., Cox, S. M., Burris, J. S., Mashburn, M. & Rosenfeld, C. R. (1988). Intrapartum treatment of acute chorioamnionitis: impact on neonatal sepsis. *American Journal of Obstetrics and Gynecology*, 159, 579–83.

Goedert, J. J., Duliege, A. M., Amos, C. I., Felton, S. & Biggar, R. J. (1991). High risk of HIV-1 infection for first-born twins. The International Registry of HIV-exposed twins. *Lancet*, 338, 1471–5.

Goldenberg, R. L., Nelson, K. G., Davis, R. O. & Koski, J. (1984). Delay in delivery: influence of gestational age and duration of delay on perinatal outcome. *Obstetrics and Gynecology*, 64, 480–4.

Gregg, N. M. (1941). Cataract following german measles in the mother. *Transactions of the Ophthalmic Society of Australia*, 3, 34–6.

Griffifths, P. D., Stagno, S., Pass, R. F., Smith, R. J. & Alford, C. A. (1982). Infection with cytomegalovirus during pregnancy: specific IgM antibodies as a marker of recent primary infection. *Journal of Infectious Diseases*, 145, 647–53.

Henderson, J. B., Beattie, C. P., Hale, E. G. & Wright, J. (1984). The evaluation of new services: possibilities for preventing congenital toxoplasmosis. *International Journal of Epidemiology*, 13, 65–72.

Higa, K., Dan, K. & Manabe, H. (1987). Varicella-zoster virus infections during pregnancy: hypothesis concerning the mechanisms of congenital malformations. *Obstetrics and Gynecology*, 69, 214–22.

Hohlfeld, P., Daffos, F., Costa, J. M., Thulliez, P., Forestier, F. & Vidaud, M. (1994). Prenatal diagnosis of congenital toxoplasmosis with a polymerase-chain-reaction test on amniotic fluid. *New England Journal of Medicine*, 331, 695–9.

Hohlfeld, P., Via, Y., Maillard-Brignon, C., Vaudaux, B. & Fawer, C. L. (1991). Cytomegalo-virus fetal infection: prenatal diagnosis. *Obstetrics and Gynecology*, 78, 615–18.

Horton, R. (1995). Women as women with HIV. *Lancet*, 345, 531–2.

Jeannel, D., Costagliola, D., Niel, G., Hubert, B. & Danis, M. (1990). What is known about the prevention of congenital toxoplasmosis? *Lancet*, 336, 359–61.

Koppe, J. G., Loewer-Sieger, D. H. & de Roever-Bonnet, H. (1986). Results of a 20-year follow-up of the congenital toxoplasmosis. *Lancet*, 1, 254–6.

Lamy, M. E., Mulongo, K. N., Gadisseux, J. F., Lyon, G., Gaudy, V. & van Lierde, M. (1992). Prenatal diagnosis of fetal cytomegalovirus infection. *American Journal of Obstetrics and Gynecology*, 166, 91–4.

Levin, M. J., Oxman, M. N., Moore, M. G., Daniels, J. B. & Scheer, K. (1974). Diagnosis of congenital rubella *in utero*. *New England Journal of Medicine*, 290, 1187–8.

Liesnard, C., Donner, C., Brancart, F. & Rodesch, F. (1994). Varicella in pregnancy. *Lancet*, 344, 950–1.

Lifson, A. R. (1994). Preventing AIDS: have we lost our way? *Lancet*, 343, 1306–8.

Lindgren, S., Bohlin, A. B., Forsgren, M., Arneborn, M., Ottenblad, C., Lidman, K., Anzen, B., von Sydow, M. & Bottiger, M. (1993). *Lancet*, 307, 1447–51.

Loveday, C., Kaye, S., Tenant-Flowers, M., Semple, M., Ayliffe, U., Weller, I. V. & Tedder, R. S. (1995). RNA serum-load and resistent viral genotypes during early zidovudine therapy. *Lancet*, 345, 820–4.

Lynch, L., Daffos, F., Emanuel, D. Giovangrandi, Y., Meisel, R., Forestier, F., Cathomas, G. & Berkowitz, R. L. (1991). Prenatal diagnosis of cytomegalovirus infection. *American Journal of Obstetrics and Gynecology*, 165, 714–18.

McCredie Smith, J. A., Jennison, R. F. & Langley, F. A. (1956). Perinatal infection and perinatal death: clinical aspects. *Lancet*, 2, 903–6.

Melnick, S. L., Sherer, R., Louis, T. A., Hillman, D., Rodriguez, E. M., Lackman, C., Capps, L., Brown, L. S., Carlyn, M., Korvick, J. A. & Deyton, L. (1994). Survival and disease progression according to gender of patients with HIV infection: the Terry Beirn Community Programs for Clinical Research on AID. *Journal of the American Medical Association*, 272, 1915–21.

Miller, E., Cradock-Watson, J. E. & Pollock, T. M. (1982). Consequences of confirmed maternal rubella at successive stages of pregnancy. *Lancet*, 2, 781.

Moodley, D., Bobat, R. A., Coutsoudis, A. & Coovadia, H. M. (1994). Caesarean section and vertical trasnmission of HIV-1. *Lancet*, 334, 338.

Morgan-Capner, P., Wright, J., Miller, C. L. & Miller, E. (1988). Surveillance of antibody to measles, mumps and rubella by age. *British Medical Journal*, 297, 770–2.

Naeye, R. L. & Peters, E. C. (1980). Causes and consequences of premature rupture of fetal membranes. *Lancet*, 1, 192–4.

Naides, S. J. & Weiner, C. P. (1989). Antenatal diagnosis and palliative treatment of non immune hydrops fetalis secondary to fetal parvovirus B19 infection. *Prenatal Diagnosis*, 9, 105–14.

Newell, M. L. & Peckham, C. S. (1994). Working towards a European strategy for intervention to reduce vertical transmisison of HIV. *British Journal of Obstetrics and Gynaecology*, 101, 192–6.

Nicolini, U., Kustermann, A., Tassis, B., Fogliani, R., Galimberti, A., Percivalle, E., Grazia-Revello, M. & Gerna, G. (1994). Prenatal diagnosis of congenital human cytomegalovirus infection. *Prenatal Diagnosis*, 14, 903–6.

Nicolini, U., Kustermann, A., Zoppini, C., Tassis, B., Della Morte, M. & Colucci, G. (1995). Prenatal diagnosis of varicella infection. *Prenatal Diagnosis*, in press.

Paryani, S. G. & Arvin, A. M. (1986). Intrauterine infection with varicella-zoster virus after maternal varicella. *New England Journal of Medicine*, 314, 1542–6.

Pastuszak, A. L., Levy, M., Schick, B., Zuber, C., Feldkamp, M., Gladstone, J., Bar-Levy, F., Jackson, E., Donnenfeld, A., Meschino, W. & Koren, G. (1994). Outcome after maternal varicella infection in the first 20 weeks of pregnancy. *New England Journal of Medicine*, 330, 901–5.

Peckham, C. S., Johnson, C., Ades, A., Pearl, K. & Chin, K. S. (1987). Early acquisition of cytomegalovirus infection. *Archives of Disease in Childhood*, 62, 780–785.

Phair, J., Munoz, A., Deteils, R., Kaslow, R., Rinaldo, C. & Saah, A. (1990). The risk of *Pneumocystis carinii* pneumonia among men infected with human immunodeficiency virus type 1. *New England Journal of Medicine*, 322, 1607–8.

Preece, P. M., Pearl, K. N. & Peckham, C. S. (1984). Congenital cytomegalovirus infection. *Archives of Disease in Childhood*, 59, 1120.

Public Health Laboratory Service Working Party on Fifth Disease (1990). Prospective study on human parvovirus B19 infection in pregnancy. *British Medical Journal*, 300, 1166–70.

Remington, J. S. & Desmonts, G. (1990). Toxoplasmosis. In *Infectious Diseases of the Fetus and Newborn Infant*, 3rd edn, ed. J. S. Remington & J. O. Klein, pp. 89–120. Philadelphia: W. B. Saunders.

Revello, M. G., Percivalle, E. & Baldanti, F. (1993). Prenatal treatment of congenital human cytomegalovirus infection by fetal intravascular administration of gancyclovir. *Clinical and Diagnosis Virology*, 1, 61–7.

Roberts, T. & Frenkel, J. K. (1990). Estimating income losses and other preventable costs caused by congenital toxoplasmosis in people in the United States. *Journal of American Veterinarian Medical Association*, 196, 249–56.

Rodis, J. F., Quinn, D. L., Gary, G. W., Anderson, L. J., Rosengren, S., Cartter, M. L., Campbell, W. A. & Vintzileos, A. M. (1990). Management and outcomes of pregnancies complicated by human B19 parvovirus infection: a prospective study. *American Journal of Obstetrics and Gynecology*, 163, 1168–71.

Romero, R., Sirtori, M., Oyarzun, E., Avila, C., Mazor, M., Callahan, R., Sabo, V., Athanassiadis, A. P. & Hobbins, J. C. (1989). Infection and labor. V. Prevalence, microbiology, and clinical significance of intra-amniotic infection in women with pre-term labor and intact membranes. *American Journal of Obstetrics and Gynecology*, 161, 817–24.

Royal College of Obstetricans and Gynaecologists (1992). *Prenatal Screening for Toxoplasmosis in the UK. Report of a Multidisciplinary Working Group.* London: Royal College of Obstetricians and Gynaecologists.

Ruskin, J. & LaRiviere, M. (1991). Low dose co-trimoxazole for prevention of *Pneumocystis carinii* pneumonia in human immunodeficiency virus disease. *Lancet*, 337, 468–71.

Sepkowitz, K. A. & Armstrong, D. (1995). Treatment of opportunistic infections in AIDS. *Lancet*, 346, 588–9.

Sheikh, A. U., Ernest, J. M. & O'Shea, M. (1992). Long-term outcome in fetal hydrops from parvovirus B19 infection. *American Journal of Obstetrics and Gynecology*, 167, 337–41.

Sidle, N. (1985). *Rubella in Pregnancy*. London: SENSE.

Smaill, F. (1994). Intrapartum antibiotics for group B streptococcus colonisation. In *Pregnancy and Childbirth Module*, M. J. N. C. Keirse, M. J. Renfrew, J. P. Neilson & C. Crowther. London: The Cochrane Database of Systematic Reviews, BMJ Publishing Group.

Smaill, F. (1995a). Vaginal chlorhexadine for maternal colonisation with group B streptococcus. In: *Pregnancy and Childbirth Module*, ed. M. J. N. C. Keirse, M. J. Renfrew, J. P. Neilson & C. Crowther. London: The Cochrane Database of Systematic Reviews, BMJ Publishing Group.

Smaill, F. (1995b). Antepartum antibiotics for group B streptococcus colonisation. In *Pregnancy and Childbirth Module*, ed. M. J. N. C. Keirse, M. J. Renfrew, J. P. Neilson & C. Crowther. London: The Cochrane Database of Systematic Reviews, BMJ Publishing Group.

Smoleniec, J. S., Pillai, M., Caul, E. O. & Usher, J. (1994). Subclinical transplacental parvovirus B19 infection: an increased fetal risk? *Lancet*, 343, 1100–1.

Sperling, R. S., Ramamurthy, R . S. and Gibbs, R. S. (1987). A comparison of intrapartum versus immediate post-partum treatment of intra-amniotic infection. *Obstetrics and Gynecology*, 70, 861–5.

Sperling, R. S. & Stratton, P. (1992). Treatment options for human immunodeficiency virus-infected pregnant women. *Obstetrics and Gynecology*, 79, 443–8.

Stagno, S., Pass, R. F., Cloud, G., Britt, W. J., Henderson, R. E., Walton, P. D., Veren, D. A., Page, F. & Alford, C. A. (1986). Primary cytomegalovirus infection in pregnancy: incidence, transmission to fetus, and clinical outcome. *Journal of the American Medical Association*, 256, 1904–8.

Stagno, S., Pass, R. F., Dworsky, M. E. & Alford, C. A. (1982a). Maternal cytomegalovirus infection and perinatal transmission. *Clinical Obstetrics and Gynecology*, 25, 563–76.

Stagno, S., Pass, R. F., Dworsky, M. E., Henderson, R. E., Moore, E. G., Walton, P. D. & Alford, C. A. (1982b). Congenital cytomegalovirus infection: the relative importance of primary and recurrent maternal infection. *New England Journal of Medicine*, 306, 945–9.

Stagno, S. & Whitley, R. J. (1985). Herpes virus infections of pregnancy. I: Cytomegalovirus and Epstein Barr virus infections. *New England Journal of Medicine*, 313, 1270–4.

Stanier, P., Kitchen, A. D., Taylor, D. L. & Tyms, A. S. (1992). Detection of human cytomegalovirus in peripheral mononuclear cells and urine samples using PCR. *Molecular Cell Probes*, 6, 51–8.

Tookey, P. A. & Peckham, C. S. (1992). Cytomegalovirus. In *Congenital Perinatal and Neonatal Infections*, ed. A. Greenhough, J. Osborne & S. Sutherland, pp. 49–61. London: Churchill Livingstone.

Wendel, G. D. Jr, Sanchez, P., Peters, M. T., Harstad, T. W., Potter, L. L. & Norgaard, M. V. (1991). Identification of *T. pallidum* in amniotic fluid and fetal blood from pregnancies complicated by congenital syphilis. *Obstetrics and Gynecology*, 78, 890–5.

Wendel, G. D. Jr, Stark, B. J., Jamison, R. B., Molina, R. D. & Sullivan, T. J. (1985). Penicillin allergy and desensitization in serious infections during pregnancy. *New England Journal of Medicine*, 312, 1229–32.

Woolf, A. D., Campion, G. V., Chishick, A., Wise, S., Cohen, B. J., Klouda, P. T., Caul, D. & Dieppe, P. A. (1989). Clinical manifestations of human parvovirus B19 adults. *Archives of Internal Medicine*, 149, 1153–6.

9 Intrauterine growth restriction

BRIAN J. TRUDINGER AND SHELLEY ROWLANDS

Any circumstance interfering with fetal well being can be expected to affect fetal growth. In fact, fetal growth and development is such an integral part of a successful pregnancy that any alteration represents a threat to fetal health. The factors responsible for normal fetal growth include both the genetic and biological potential of the individual and a number of modulating and regulating influences. The circumstance of growth failure or constraint is rarely simple absence of one of these influences. Far more commonly, intrauterine growth restriction (IUGR) is the result of failure of supply of oxygen and nutrients. The small fetus may also be the result of a reduced growth potential.

These concepts are fundamental to fetal therapy for disorders of growth. The use of a 'growth' promoting factor is futile if the supply of oxygen and nutrients is inadequate or the lowered potential size is being achieved.

Fetal growth

Normal fetal growth

Growth and development of the embryo and fetus is unquestionably complex. It is determined by two major factors: (i) *genetic*, the genome of the embryo or fetus, and (ii) *environmental*, maternal, fetal and/or placental factors that alter the expression of the fetal genome.

Currently it is believed that growth and development of the embryo and fetus is regulated by the genome turning on and off genes specific to it at specific stages of development. Environmental factors then operate on this process. Macromolecules promoting cell adhesion, growth, multiplication and differentiation are expressed at critical periods of development to regulate this process. Extracellular matrix molecules influencing cell shape, proliferation and migration have been described along with intercellular recognition molecules expressed on cell membranes, and peptide growth factors have been recognized. It is likely that growth-inhibitory factors exist to balance growth-promoting factors. Major defects in genetic structure such as trisomy 18 may alter fetal growth but very minor variations in DNA sequence could produce the same growth impairment through an effect on genes encoding growth factors and related macromolecules.

Concept of IUGR

For 50 years it has been known that some babies were small because they failed to grow rather than because they were born early (McBurney, 1947). Therefore, fetuses failed to achieve their full genetic size or biological potential as a result of a retarded growth rate. The importance of this is the association with fetal death *in utero* or adverse outcome. The terms small for gestational age (SGA) and small for dates were developed to quantify this problem. Infants whose birthweight was less than the tenth centile were referred to as SGA and regarded as victims of retarded fetal growth. This statistical approach oversimplified the problem. Some infants in the lowest tenth centile were biologically small and so achieving their full potential; others with birthweight above this arbitrary cut off had stopped growing, but their weight had not yet dropped to the tenth centile limit. It is not possible to know the true biological potential or size of a fetus or newborn. The grouping

SGA does, however, concentrate many fetuses who have not achieved this potential and so remains as a useful concept despite its limitations.

Recognition of IUGR implies a preceding period of inadequate growth sufficient that the deficit between observed and expected size has reached a recognizable or measurable threshold. The factors restricting growth may vary in the extent to which they affect growth. The most complete or severe restriction could result in fetal demise before there is time to recognize growth failure. In contrast, mild restriction may affect growth but not other aspects of fetal well being. Failure of growth is then one sign of possible fetal compromise. There is a spectrum of consequences beyond interference with growth associated with deprivation of oxygen and nutrients. These outcomes depend upon the time of onset and severity of the insult. Manifestations may be seen in the antenatal period, in labour, in the early neonatal period and later in childhood. Intrauterine fetal death may occur. Studies of large groups of 'unexplained stillbirths' reveal a large proportion to be small for dates (Williams *et al.*, 1982). In labour, fetal distress and perinatal asphyxia are more common. In the neonatal nursery, the problems of hypoglycaemia, renal failure and necrotizing enterocolitis may all be seen in addition to hypoxic ischaemic encephalopathy consequent upon asphyxia. Polycythaemia, thrombocytopenia and hypocalcaemia may all occur. Long-term developmental assessment in childhood indicates that neurodevelopmental deficit is a possibility, especially in the preterm infant that is also SGA (Fitzhardinge & Steven, 1972). Follow-up studies have shown that the risk of neurological deficit is greater the earlier the onset of IUGR (Fancourt *et al.*, 1976) and the greater the immaturity at birth. The small fetus born at term appears to have little risk of poor neurological outcome in the absence of hypoxaemia. Catch-up growth in the first year of life also indicates a good outcome (Babson, Behrman & Lessel, 1970; Low *et al.*, 1979). The potential benefits of fetal therapy, therefore, carry beyond fetal size to all of these manifestations.

Patterns of fetal growth

The time of occurrence or onset of the factor affecting fetal growth may be used to divide cases of fetal growth retardation into two broad groups: low growth potential and loss of growth support. In the case of low growth potential, the biological potential is reduced and growth disturbance affects fetal size from early pregnancy. This includes both fetal anomalies such as aneuploidy and early acquired disease such as congenital rubella. Growth progresses at a normal velocity but at a lower level throughout pregnancy. Preterm delivery does not benefit such fetuses. Loss of growth support implies a restriction of oxygen and nutrient supply, which no longer matches requirements. This is a later phenomenon and results in growth failure at the end of pregnancy. Vascular disease may cause this. Such fetuses no longer being adequately nourished may benefit from early delivery.

The period around 30 weeks is normally a time of rapid weight increase (high growth velocity) while a relative slowing occurs over the last few weeks of pregnancy. However, this growth pattern is different if length is used as the growth parameter, as peak growth velocity occurs earlier at 20 weeks (Tanner, 1978). The increase in weight is contributed to by fat deposition in the third trimester. A factor operating from the first trimester will affect both weight and length, resulting in an infant in whom weight and length are reduced by equal proportions. Such babies are short for dates as well as light for dates and may be described as symmetrically growth retarded. Using ultrasound biparietal diameter measurements, Campbell (1974) referred to this group as 'low growth profile'. If the process adversely affects growth after 27 weeks then most of the length growth is already accomplished but weight growth will be affected, resulting in an infant with a disproportionately greater decrease in weight than length. This situation has been described as asymmetrical IUGR. If the restriction operates over only the last three or four weeks of pregnancy, then length is normal, and muscle mass is also relatively normal. Weight loss might even occur as the infant uses fat stores. These infants are long and thin.

Aetiology of IUGR

The causes of IUGR are broadly divided into two groups. The genetically determined growth potential of the fetus exists at conception. The optimum expression of this is dependent upon the availability of oxygen and nutrients via the placenta.

Altered biological potential

Up to 40% of birthweight variation may be genetically determined. The chromosomally abnormal fetus is likely to be small. The average weight, defined as percentage weight relative to normal at term, of fetuses with Turner syndrome (84%), trisomy 13 (80%), trisomy 18 (62%), and trisomy 21 (80-90%) is reduced. Low birthweight is also present with chromosomal deletions and triploidy (Polani, 1974). Many major non-chromosomal malformations are also associated with IUGR. Anencephalic fetuses are usually growth retarded, even allowing for the lack of cerebral tissue, as are those with renal agenesis. Fetal infection, typified by rubella, but indeed including all of the TORCH group of organisms, may present in this way. Worldwide, however, malaria is probably the most important infective cause of low birthweight through infestation of the placenta (McGregor, Wilson & Billewicz, 1983). Therapeutic drugs may produce IUGR, usually in association with an embryopathy. They include antiepileptics and anticoagulants. Possibly the immunosuppressive agents cyclophosphamide and azathioprine affect growth. High-dose irradiation also affects fetal growth. In addition, maternal smoking and alcohol addiction affect fetal growth, although the mechanisms are not well defined.

Failure of supply

IUGR is widely held to result from inadequate supply of oxygen and nutrients. In this sense it is the result of environmental factors. The concept of growth support through the provision of oxygen and nutrients was proposed by Gruenwald *et al.* (1967) who directed attention to growth failure in late pregnancy if supply was inadequate. Failure of growth can be regarded in part as an adaptive response by the fetus to conserve vital nutrients for essential metabolic processes.

A variety of medical disorders in the mother may lead to fetal growth restraint. They have been explained in terms of failure of supply. The most frequent group centres on pregnancy hypertension whether primary to pregnancy or aggravated by pregnancy in a mother with an underlying cause, such as essential hypertension, renal disease and autoimmune disorders. In these conditions, the small arteries of the placental bed are believed to be affected by vascular disease. Other maternal diseases are far less frequent but include chronic respiratory illness, especially if associated with hypoxaemia, and heart disease, especially cyanotic congenital heart lesions. Anaemia *per se* is an unlikely cause of fetal undergrowth unless the haemoglobin is below 6 g/dl. The haemoglobinopathies may be associated with placental infarction as a result of sickling in the placental bed. Chronic inflammatory bowel disorders may also be associated. Recurrent antepartum haemorrhage in the first or second trimester is strongly associated. Both chorioangioma of the placenta and single umbilical artery have also been associated.

Maternal nutrition is important in communities with inadequate intake. Protein and caloric restriction may constrain growth in the third trimester, as reported after the Dutch famine and the Leningrad siege in World War II. Preconceptual nutritional status appears important, as the degree of fetal undergrowth is much greater after the protracted under nutrition in Leningrad than after the shorter duration deprivation in Holland. It remains uncertain whether it is inadequate intake of calories or deficiency of a specific substrate such as protein or minerals which is important. A variety of supplementation studies in developing countries show an increase in birthweight, although the effects do depend upon basal diet (Rush, 1982). Oxygen may also be an important nutrient and it is well known that mean birthweight at higher altitudes is less than at sea level.

It has not been established which particular substrates might maximize benefits for the fetus but the major fetal substrates are glucose, amino acids and lactate. Glucose is the main source of carbon and energy for the growing fetus and accounts for 50–70% of oxidative fuel requirements and 20% of caloric requirements in fetal sheep (Battaglia & Meschia, 1978). Blood glucose levels in the normally grown fetus are lower than in the mother and glucose is transported across the placenta by facilitated diffusion. Glucose uptake is proportional to the maternal–fetal concentration gradient (Hay *et al.*, 1984). This relationship appears to be lost in the growth-retarded fetus (Char & Creasy, 1977). Some growth-retarded fetuses have been shown to be hypoglycaemic (Soothill, Nicolaides & Campbell, 1987; Phillips *et al.*, 1968). *In vivo* studies in growth-retarded sheep have shown that placental utilization of glucose is also reduced. Glucose uptake across the placenta is reduced, thus fetal supply is decreased (Owens, Falconer &

Robinson, 1987; Oh *et al.*, 1975; Nitzan, Orloff & Schulman, 1979).

Amino acids are a major source of carbon and nitrogen for fetal growth and account for approximately 20% of fetal requirements (Battaglia & Meschia, 1978). The growth-retarded human fetus has lowered serum amino acid levels compared with the normally grown fetus (Soothill *et al.*, 1992; Cetin *et al.*, 1988). Some of these are probably essential amino acids that cannot be synthesized by the fetus. Some non-essential amino acids are increased in the growth-retarded fetus, probably as a result of increased utilization or tissue breakdown (Soothill, Ajayi & Nicolaides, 1992). Changes occur in amino acid metabolism, and in late pregnancy the fetus begins to lose amino acids back across the placenta. There appears to be selective loss of alanine and branched amino acids (Owens, 1991). Studies of growth-retarded pigs have shown that those with a smaller placenta and decreased placental blood flow have diminished transfer of amino acids (Saintonge & Rosso, 1981). The specific amino acids most likely to limit growth have not been established.

Lactate is the third major fetal substrate. Fetal lactate synthesis is high relative to uptake from the placenta (Sparks *et al.*, 1982) and IUGR and fetal distress are associated with high fetal lactate concentrations (Owens *et al.*, 1987; Sabata *et al.*, 1973). For these reasons' lactate has not been used as a fetal nutrient supplement. Fructose is another potential fetal nutrient; however severe fetal metabolic acidosis has been reported following maternal fructose infusion in labour (Pearson & Shuttleworth, 1971) and studies have not been pursued.

Placental insufficiency

Placental lesion

The concept of a primary placental pathology underlying fetal deprivation is often debated. It is important because it underlies the rationale for the more common approaches to therapy. Central to the idea of small fetal size through growth restraint or loss of growth support is the relationship between the fetus and its placenta. The term 'placental insufficiency' has long existed in the language of the obstetrician to define the situation of fetal deprivation resulting in IUGR, death *in utero*, distress in labour and the associated neonatal problems.

Their pathogenesis, however, is not well understood and this makes a rational base for therapy difficult. There is a view that changes in uteroplacental and umbilical placental circulations in IUGR are secondary to maternal disease. An alternate view, to which the authors subscribe, is that disease in the placenta can both constrain the fetus and produce a maternal syndrome. The placenta is fetal tissue and it has been questioned whether the fetus determines its placenta and hence the uterine placental bed, or is it the uterine circulation which constrains the fetus (Rankin & McLaughlin, 1979).

During pregnancy, the uterine spiral arteries which open into the placental bed undergo well-described changes. Cytotrophoblast invades the decidual and inner myometrial segment of these vessels and transforms the muscular walls into fibrinoid tubes (Brosens, Robertson & Dixon, 1972). It is postulated that these changes allow for the high blood flow to the placental bed. In pre-eclampsia, there appears to be a failure of trophoblast migration into the myometrial segments of the spiral arteries in the second trimester. The decidual arteries later show changes of acute atherosis. Thrombosis may occur in these damaged arteries. Haemorrhage and infarction in the placental bed and placenta may follow. These same changes have been described in association with IUGR in non-hypertensive pregnancies. It was attractive to link the changes seen in the spiral arteries with the idea of IUGR consequent upon fetal constraint, as advocated by Gruenwald *et al.* (1967). A reduction in uterine blood flow has long been postulated as part of the uteroplacental insufficiency associated with pre-eclampsia and IUGR and was easily attributed to these pathological changes. Indirect measures of uteroplacental blood flow were reported by studying the clearance of radio-labelled [23]Na injected into the placental bed (Browne & Veall, 1953) and by measuring uterine blood flow with xenon radioisotopes (Kaar *et al.*, 1980). These methods, though not suited to wide application, suggested a decrease in flow.

Doppler ultrasound

Doppler ultrasound offers a non-invasive technique for studying both the fetal umbilical placental and maternal uteroplacental circulations. The blood flow velocity waveform (FVW) of the insonated vessel is analysed using indices shown to reflect the resistance downstream in the peripheral vascular bed (Trudinger, 1987).

The umbilical placental circulation has been most studied. In high-risk pregnancy, between two-thirds and three-quarters of fetuses subsequently born SGA exhibit high-resistance systolic diastolic ratio or pulsatility index (Trudinger *et al.*, 1991). Among SGA fetuses as well as those appropriate for gestational age, those with high indices exhibited more neonatal morbidity than those with a normal study. The high-resistance umbilical FVW pattern is associated with a reduced population of small <90 μm diameter arteries in the tertiary villi of the placenta (Giles, Trudinger & Baird, 1985) and obliterative changes in the remaining vessels (Fok *et al.*, 1990). The same FVW changes have been produced by embolization of the umbilical circulation (Trudinger *et al.*, 1987). This evidence is in keeping with the concept that the placental lesion produces the fetal effects. The placental lesion is detected by Doppler studies in some two-thirds of SGA fetuses. Serial umbilical Doppler studies indicate that those fetuses with an increasing index of resistance, indicating progressive vessel obliteration, exhibit the most morbidity. Why this process of vessel obliteration is established in the umbilical placenta circulation remains to be determined.

As mentioned above, conventional belief has it that the fetus is deprived by an inadequate uteroplacental circulation. While this is a possibility, recent Doppler studies (Bewley, Cooper & Campbell, 1991) suggest that fewer than 20% of subsequent SGA fetuses are associated with a high-resistance pattern in the uterine artery FVW. The umbilical FVWs are more sensitive than uterine FVWs in predicting fetal condition (Trudinger, Giles & Cook, 1985). These findings neither support nor refute the suggestion that the reduced uterine circulation may be a consequence rather than a cause of the umbilical placental vascular lesion.

Some SGA fetuses exhibit normal umbilical and uterine Doppler studies. It is attractive to postulate that this group represents the genetically small fetuses with low growth potential in whom growth in pregnancy continues although size is reduced. The decline in resistance indices on serial umbilical Doppler studies reflects continuing placental growth. Neonatal morbidity in this group is less than the abnormal umbilical group (Trudinger *et al.*, 1991).

Placental mosaicism

A further dimension has been added by the demonstration of confined placental mosaicism (Kalousek, 1994) in which the genetic identity between the fetus and placenta is broken. It is present in up to 2% of pregnancies and presumed to result from a mitotic error before implantation. In such circumstances, there is a higher probability of unexplained intrauterine fetal death, IUGR or perinatal mortality.

It has been suggested that the mosaicism within the placenta results in abnormal function and possibly vasculature. This is relevant to the question of umbilical blood flow as a high frequency of abnormal Doppler studies have been reported in association with aneuploidy (Trudinger, 1991).

The mosaicism may not only be confined to the placenta but may be generalized to cell lineages in the embryo/fetus. Placental mosaicism may be confined to the trophoblast or the chorionic stroma. This latter form may be present in otherwise unexplained fetal death or growth restriction. This problem has been further extended by the identification of uniparental disomy in the diploid fetus associated with abnormal fetal growth, and the suggestion of fetal rescue from a trisomy situation by loss of one of the trisomic chromosomes (Engel, 1993).

Principles of therapy for fetal growth retardation

Three general approaches have been taken to promote fetal growth in the presence of growth failure: (i) therapy aimed at reversing the pathological lesion of placental insufficiency, such as aspirin and fish oil; (ii) increased supply of oxygen and nutrients to the fetus; (iii) measures used to increase uterine blood flow.

Treating maternal diseases underlying fetal constraint may improve fetal growth, although this has not been shown by randomized trials. It is noteworthy that trials of antihypertensive medication demonstrate no improvement in fetal weight. No therapeutic measures which alter fetal growth potential have been described in human pregnancy, although DNA diagnosis and manipulation, particularly in the large group of fetuses with reduced growth potential, is clearly an area for future study.

Therapies directed against the vascular lesion of placental insufficiency

Aspirin

Rationale

Clinical trials of low-dose aspirin to prevent maternal hypertension and fetal growth retardation have a common rationale. Reduced uteroplacental perfusion (Nylund *et al.*, 1983), uteroplacental arterial thrombosis resulting in placental infarction (Altshuler, Russell & Ermocilla, 1975) and abnormal platelet behaviour (Wallenburg & Rotmans, 1982) have in turn been associated with abnormal interactions between platelet and vessel wall with evidence of endothelial cell injury (Rodgers, Taylor & Roberts, 1988) and an imbalance in the prostacyclin thromboxane production with a shift to thromboxane release by various tissues (Walsh, 1985). The vasospasm, ischaemia and thrombosis associated with pre-eclampsia (for review see Dekker & Sibai, 1993) were attributed to thromboxane, which promotes vasoconstriction and platelet aggregation. All these phenomena are described in the maternal uteroplacental circulation. It is the purpose of therapy with low-dose aspirin to affect platelet behaviour and prevent or reduce thromboxane release. In the maternal compartment, low-dose aspirin was shown to reduce thromboxane release in relation to prostacyclin, its natural antagonist (Sibai *et al.*, 1989; Benigni *et al.*, 1989; Schiff *et al.*, 1989). This change in eicosanoid balance was associated with the conversion of a positive (pressor) angiotensin infusion-sensitivity response to a negative response (Spitz *et al.*, 1988).

The authors have questioned whether the beneficial effects of low-dose aspirin therapy are the result of its actions in the maternal uteroplacental bed. When patients were selected on the basis of umbilical placental pathology, as defined by umbilical Doppler studies, aspirin was shown to increase fetal and placental weight. Mothers with hypertension were excluded (Trudinger *et al.*, 1988). Platelet consumption was demonstrated in the fetal circulation in association with abnormal umbilical Doppler study (Wilcox & Trudinger, 1991). The mothers of these fetuses were also angiotensin sensitive and conversion to the angiotensin-refractory state of normal pregnancy was associated with fetal benefit

(Cook & Trudinger, 1991). More recently, maternal platelet angiotensin binding, which correlates with angiotensin sensitivity, has been shown to be more associated with abnormal fetal umbilical Doppler values than with maternal pre-eclampsia (Baker, Basheer & James, 1994). Aspirin crosses from the maternal to the fetal circulation, as demonstrated across the isolated perfused human placental cotyledon (Jacobson *et al.*, 1991). It differentially affects thromboxane production by umbilical placental vessels (Thorp, Walsh & Brath, 1988). The reduction in production by whole villi is the result an effect on the villous core rather than on the trophoblast compartments (Nelson & Walsh, 1989).

Pharmacology

The major action of aspirin (acetylsalicylic acid) is to inhibit the cyclooxygenase enzyme, which results in a decrease in the production of both prostacyclin and thromboxane. Aspirin is deacetylated to salicyclic acid, which is active especially on the lipoxygenase pathways and also may promote platelet adhesion. However, salicylates at levels achieved in the human do not inhibit cyclooxygenase. The aspirin effect is, therefore, different from the salicylate effect. Aspirin is absorbed from the small intestine and is de-esterified in the liver. Little or no aspirin emerges from the liver when a low dose, less than 100 mg, is taken. In such circumstances, however, there will be effective aspirin levels in the portal circulation (Pedersen & Fitzgerald, 1984). The rapid de-esterification of aspirin after uptake from the gut means that in the adult the level falls approximately 50% in 20 minutes. There is little fetal aspirin effect in mothers taking less than 100 mg, but a full effect with a maternal dose of 500 mg (Ylikorkala *et al.*, 1986). These studies have been confirmed (Benigni *et al.*, 1989; Forestier, Daffos & Rainaut, 1985). The available evidence indicates that there is no aspirin effect on fetal platelet activity at maternal doses of 50 to 75 mg (Sibai *et al.*, 1989). In the fetus, the decline in blood levels is slower than those in the mother. As aspirin reacts irreversibly with its receptors, the duration of the effect of aspirin is determined by the rate at which new receptor molecules are synthesized. Endothelium appears capable of replacing cyclooxygenase within 4 hours, but platelets, which are anucleate, cannot synthesize new enzymes and are, therefore, inactivated for their life span (about 10 days). This is the basis for the belief that low-dose aspirin will inhibit platelet cyclooxygenase with no significant effect on the systemic vascular endothelium. Maternal platelets are exposed to aspirin in the portal circulation, whereas in the fetus the site of exposure is probably the systemic circulation. Aspirin reduces thromboxane production in human placental arteries by 60–80%, whereas prostacyclin production is reduced by only 25% (Thorp *et al.*, 1988).

Adverse effects

The safety of aspirin in pregnancy was shown by the Collaborative Perinatal Project (Slone *et al.*, 1976) in which 5128 women heavily exposed to aspirin in the first 17 weeks of pregnancy, and 9736 with intermediate exposure, were compared with 35 418 women who did not take aspirin. The data collected before birth included 3152 malformations, but neither any single malformation type nor total numbers of malformations were greater in either of the aspirin-treated groups in comparison with the control group. This refutes the suggestion of teratogenic effects raised from rat studies and seemingly supported by uncontrolled human observations (Turner & Collins, 1975).

Aspirin has well-known effects on coagulation and bleeding. Both platelets and endothelial cells are affected by it. Platelet aggregation in response to ADP is reduced, but platelets are not prevented from adhering to the endothelium. If enough platelets adhere, then other stimulants of aggregation will be released, which can provoke aggregation. This is especially likely if the endothelium is disrupted. Bleeding time may not be affected by aspirin. In pregnancy, there are reports of increases in antepartum and postpartum haemorrhage among aspirin takers (Turner & Collins, 1975). It has been pointed out, however, that these data were probably collected from patients with a very high aspirin intake. No evidence of maternal haemorrhage has been reported from trials of low-dose aspirin in pregnancy, with the exception of one trial (Sibai *et al.*, 1993).

In the fetus or neonate, low-dose maternal aspirin is not associated with prolongation of prothrombin time whereas high doses may be (Earle, 1961). There are reports of an increase in intracranial haemorrhage in the fetus or neonate in association with maternal aspirin intake (Rumack *et al.*, 1981; Stuart *et al.*, 1982). This finding has been challenged because the data related to the study of preterm infants, in whom this complication occurs frequently, because there was no control group and because the dosage of aspirin was high. No increase in intracranial haemorrhage was noted in either the large Collaborative Perinatal Project or the many trials of low-dose aspirin therapy in pregnancy. The fact that aspirin in doses of ≤75 mg has little effect on platelet thromboxane production also questions the validity of the data on adverse haemorrhagic outcomes.

There have also been concerns about premature closure of the ductus arteriosus. In the fetal lamb, aspirin causes ductal constriction (Rudolph, 1981), although the high dose used (90 mg/kg fetus) renders the significance of this uncertain. Echocardiographic studies of fetuses exposed to indomethacin demonstrated narrowing of the ductus arteriosus during the exposure (Moise *et al.*, 1988). This effect has also been observed with other prostaglandin synthetase inhibitors. However, aspirin was shown to be a far less potent constrictor on a molar basis in animal experiments. The significance of this observation in clinical practice is uncertain. There is no excess of newborn pulmonary hypertension in the Collaborative Perinatal Project (Shapiro *et al.*, 1976) or the human trials of low-dose aspirin for pre-eclampsia or fetal growth retardation, while the trials with indomethacin for preterm labour (Niebyl & Witter, 1986) similarly do not demonstrate such cases.

Since low-dose aspirin is associated with very low levels in the maternal systemic circulation, secretion in breast milk and transmission to the newborn is unlikely (de Swiet & Fryers, 1990).

Therapeutic approaches

The concept of placental insufficiency as a disease with a maternal syndrome of pre-eclampsia and a fetal syndrome of IUGR unites the various approaches to therapy with low-dose aspirin. Three strategies have been advocated: (i) treat all primiparous women (universal therapy); (ii) treat women identified by a predictive factor or test; (iii) treat at the earliest manifestation of disease.

In principle, universal therapy demands that the drug (aspirin) is free of adverse side effects since a large number of women with normal pregnancies will be treated. The risk benefit ratio is maximal for risk and minimal for benefit and, therefore, this approach is difficult to justify if significant benefits are not clearly evident. The theoretical concerns of low-dose aspirin to the mother are antepartum haemorrhage and bleeding at delivery. In the fetus, a risk of cerebral haemorrhage and premature closure of the ductus arteriosus leading to pulmonary hypertension have been suggested (see above). These have not emerged in the trials done to date, but caution should apply to the adoption of this approach.

The use of disease predictors to guide preventative therapy has exposed our limited ability to identify a high-risk group (Uzan, Haddad & Breart, 1994). Past history is of little value in a condition affecting first pregnancies. Laboratory parameters such as uric acid, platelet count, microalbuminuria, fibronectin and atrial natriuretic peptide assay become abnormal only at the onset of disease, limiting the opportunity for primary prevention. The angiotensin-sensitivity test is too elaborate to apply universally. Measurement of plasma volume lacks sensitivity. Data on determining who to treat by measurements of human chorionic gonadotrophin (hCG) and a-fetoprotein are not yet available (Wenstrom *et al.*, 1994).

The use of aspirin at the earliest manifestation of disease shifts the focus of therapy from prevention to early treatment. This may in fact be the correct approach. One disadvantage is that it is unlikely to be applicable to acute fulminant cases where rapid progression of disease denies the opportunity for therapy, and it may not work because irreversible pathology has already occurred.

The trials

The published randomized controlled trials of low-dose aspirin therapy in pregnancy are summarized in Table 9.1. It is very difficult to analyse the data presented in these studies and achieve a clear conclusion. The smaller directed studies in which a specific high-risk pregnancy indicator was used for patient selection do point to benefit in terms of a reduced incidence of proteinuric pregnancy-induced hypertension (pre-eclampsia) and of an increase in birthweight, suggesting improved fetal growth. However, the more recently performed larger trials, and in particular the CLASP study (1994), do not show benefit to mother or fetus.

Notwithstanding this, they do confirm the safety of low-dose aspirin therapy in pregnancy. Any attempt at meta-analysis (Fig. 9.1) is rendered difficult by large differences in patient selection criteria and treatment regimens, particularly the inclusion of large numbers of patients primarily at risk of pre-eclampsia. The Cochrane database concludes (Collins, 1994) 'the results of available trials do not support the widespread routine prophylactic or therapeutic use of antiplatelet therapy in pregnancy amongst all women judged to be at risk of pre-eclampsia or IUGR'. This is a necessarily cautious and conservative interpretation of the data. The studies that demonstrated improved fetal weight used a 150 mg dose. This is relevant in the context of the pharmacokinetics and possible site of action of aspirin. The authors have presented evidence that the action in the umbilical placental and fetal circulation is paramount (Trudinger, 1993). This would account for the varying fetal benefit of the other studies in which a lower dose of aspirin was used, too low in fact to act on the fetal compartment. The authors' trial also noted a 30% increase in placental weight, suggesting the possibility of placental repair in the aspirin-treated group (Trudinger *et al.*, 1988).

The available information on low-dose aspirin therapy does not support treatment of the total obstetric population. It highlights the need to evaluate further high-risk markers for IUGR and maternal pre-eclampsia. Further trials are warranted. Dosage may be important and requires further investigation. Treatment of late-established disease would appear to be of little value.

Omega-3 unsaturated fatty acids

The use of fish oil or eicosapentanoic acid (EPA) as a therapy to promote fetal growth and prevent hypertension followed the same rationale as aspirin. EPA is a competitive antagonist to arachidonic acid, the precursor of thromboxane and prostacyclin. The thromboxane produced by incorporating EPA is the inactive TXA_3. In contrast, PGI_3 has platelet disaggregatory and vasodilatory effects. The result of therapy is, therefore, a shift in prostacyclin/thromboxane balance to prostacyclin effects. To achieve this, however, high doses of EPA are necessary, such as 6 to 10 g per day, and this presents

Table 9.1 *Randomized controlled trials of low-dose aspirin therapy*

Study	Inclusion criteria	Dosage (mg)	No. treated/controls
Beaufils *et al.*, 1985	Poor obstetric history	ASA 150, dipyridamol 300	48/45
Wallenburg *et al.*, 1986	Positive AIST	ASA 60	23/23
Benigni *et al.*, 1989	Poor obstetric history	ASA 60	17/16
Schiff *et al.*, 1989	Positive rollover	ASA 100	34/31
Trudinger *et al.*, 1988	Abnormal umbilical Doppler	ASA 150	22/24
McParland *et al.*, 1990	Abnormal uterine Doppler	ASA 75	48/52
Uzan *et al.*, 1991	Poor obstetric history	ASA 150, ASA 150 + dipyridamol 225	156/73
Viinnika *et al.*, 1993	Poor obstetric history		1014/104
CLASP, 1994	Risk PE 12–32 wks IUGR	ASA 60	4810/4821
Italian Study, 1993	Post/present obstetric/ medical history	ASA 50	583/523
NICHHD (Sibai *et al.*, 1993)	Nulliparas	ASA 60	1570/1565
Hauth *et al.*, 1993	Nulliparas	ASA 60	302/302

ASA, acetyl salicylic acid; AIST, angiotensin infusion sensitivity test.

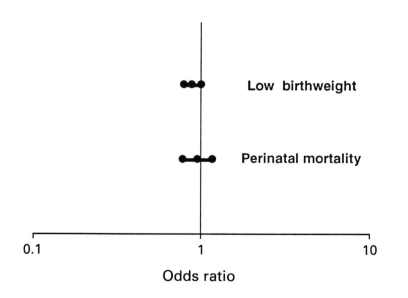

Fig. 9.1 *Meta-analytical odds ratios for the effect of antiplatelet agents for IUGR and pre-eclampsia (after Collins, 1994).*

problems of tolerance. In a Danish population with a diet rich in fish oil, prolonged pregnancy has been noted (Olsen, 1992). A trial of 3 g EPA daily in women with a previous complicated pregnancy did not show benefit in terms of size at birth (Bulstra-Ramakers, Huisjes & Visser, 1994). In analysis of these results, the authors acknowledged that the level of supplementation may have been too low and arachidonic acid intake may also need to be restricted. Similar results have also been reported more recently (Onwude *et al.*, 1995).

Increased supply of oxygen and nutrients to the fetus

Nutrient supplementation

IUGR appears, in part, to be caused by the inadequate flow of nutrients from mother to fetus. There are recent reports of successful treatment of fetal growth retardation using total parenteral nutrition in severe maternal undernutrition (Herbert *et al.*, 1986). Reports of the success of maternal supplementation for the growth-retarded fetus where there is an absence of maternal undernutrition have, however, differed. No dramatic effect on fetal growth with maternal supplementation is expected unless the mother is significantly malnourished (Rush, 1992).

Three routes of supplementation have been examined: maternal, amniotic fluid and direct fetal.

Maternal supplementation
In 1971, Beischer and colleagues began treating pregnant women with low urinary oestriol excretion with intravenous dextrose, fructose, amino acids and fats. Intravenous 25% dextrose and 20% fructose was given to 473 women (Beischer, 1978). This was followed by a fall in the proportion of women with low oestriols from 21% to 10%, and a fall in perinatal mortality rate. However, there was no increase in fetal size or the proportion of infants with birthweights less than the tenth centile. This study has been criticized because of the poor correlation between oestriol excretion and fetal growth (Campbell & Kurjak, 1972) and because no estimates of fetal size or growth were given (Harding & Charlton, 1990). It is not possible to differentiate the

women who may have benefited from bed rest alone, because of the lack of controls. The effect of improved perinatal care during the seven year period of the treatment may be significant. Sabata *et al.* (1973) studied the effects of intravenous glucose given to women in labour with SGA babies by comparing their cord and neonatal blood metabolites with those from women with SGA babies who were not infused. In the fetuses of infused mothers, blood glucose was elevated and remained elevated for three days following delivery. Sixty women with small-for-dates babies in the third trimester of pregnancy were then treated with daily infusions of 10% glucose (Sabata *et al.*, 1985). A significant acceleration of fetal growth and increase in mean birthweight (2712 g) was noted.

Three recent studies have reported on maternal amino acid supplementation in IUGR. Chimura *et al.* (1982) treated 131 women with reduced maternal symphysis–fundal height and fetal biparietal diameter with therapy 'mainly consisting of amino acids'. The incidence of SGA infants in the treated group was 26% compared with 44.5% in non-treated patients. The effect of maternal intravenous infusions of glucose and amino acid was studied by another group (Mesaki, Kubo & Iwasaki, 1980) in 20 women diagnosed by ultrasound at 30 weeks as having a growth-retarded fetus: nine were treated with 10% glucose (500 ml) and 12% amino acids (200 ml) daily until delivery, while the other 11 served as controls. They found a significant difference in mean birthweight between the treated and non-treated groups (2996 ±92 g, 2490 ±65 g, respectively). Xu (1993) carried out a comparative prospective study on the use of a commercially available parenteral combination of lipid, carbohydrate and amino acids, versus amino acid infusion alone, as treatment for patients with intrauterine growth retardation and found the incidence of SGA to be reduced in the combination supplement group compared with the amino acid group (2820 g vs 2656 g). He concluded that this supplement is an effective treatment for intrauterine growth retardation.

Animal studies have shown that reduced fetal growth rate induced by maternal undernutrition is corrected by refeeding of ewes (Mellor, 1983; Mellor & Murray, 1982). However, if the period of maternal undernutrition exceeded 21 days, diminished growth rates did not reverse.

Amniotic fluid supplementation

Amniotic fluid is a potential route for supplementation. It normally contains a number of fetal nutrients, including glucose, amino acids and lactate. Amniotic fluid is digested and absorbed by the second-trimester fetus and provides 0.2–0.3 g protein/kg per day, and 10–30 calories/day in the third-trimester fetus. Amniotic fluid nutrients may also be absorbed by the placenta and cord. Studies of amniotic fluid protein in the human (Gitlin et al., 1972) found that two-thirds of the protein in amniotic fluid is cleared each day, 80% by swallowing, the remainder by other mechanisms. The volume of amniotic fluid swallowed tended to vary directly with the volume of amniotic fluid in the cavity. Studies in monkeys (Pitkin & Reynolds, 1975) showed that the animals swallowed and digested amniotic fluid protein and that the resultant amino acids were utilized by the fetus in protein synthesis. This is estimated to provide 10–15% of fetal nitrogen requirements. Mulvihill et al. (1985) used fetal rabbits to show that amniotic fluid infusions of dextrose and/or amino acids resulted in a significant increase in serum and gastric glucose levels and that fetal growth had a linear relationship with non-protein calories infused. Size did not correlate with glucose concentrations. Supplementation with amino acids in addition to dextrose resulted in an increase in fetal measurements, although this was not statistically significant. No excess mortality or morbidity was noted. During the third trimester, the fetal intestine is able to absorb glucose and fructose, as seen by increasing levels of serum glucose following administration of carbohydrates into the duodenum of chronically catheterized fetal lambs (Char & Rudolph, 1979). This gives further support for the role of amniotic fluid supplementation.

There are no controlled studies available for intra-amniotic supplementation in humans and relatively few reported cases. The question has recently been reviewed (Harding & Charlton, 1990). Three reports are noted. The diagnosis of IUGR was based on decreased oestriol excretion and a small fetal biparietal diameter. Small portions (50 ml or 250 ml) of amino acid solutions were repeatedly infused. One study reported an increase in oestriol excretion in four of five women and all fetuses delivered were appropriately grown and in good condition. The second study reported an increase in oestriol excretion in four women and normalization of an abnor-mal CTG in one woman (the cohort number was not stated). The last study reported on five patients: out of five babies, two died in utero, one did well though this was thought to be unrelated to treatment, and two had improved oestriol excretion and biparietal diameter growth following treatment. No conclusions can reasonably be drawn from these reports.

Harrison and Villa (1982) developed an animal model for transamniotic fetal feeding (TAFF) in rabbits. Charlton and Johengen (1985) provided support for TAFF since they were able to reverse the effects of experimentally created IUGR by intragastric infusions of nutrients in fetal lambs. Increased somatic growth in fetal rabbits with IUGR has been reported (Buchmiller et al., 1994) with the use of transamniotic fetal feeding with dextrose or dextrose with amino acids.

Direct fetal supplementation

Direct supplementation of the fetus is the other treatment route. Experience with human fetuses is limited although there is a single report of a 33 week growth-retarded fetus being given amino acid and vitamins intraperitoneally (Saling, 1987). The infant was delivered spontaneously following nine days of treatment and was of normal size. However, there was no evidence to show that the infusion affected growth rate.

Animal studies have examined direct fetal feeding. Fetuses, growth retarded by maternal dietary restriction in the last three weeks of pregnancy, were infused with glucose and amino acid intragastrically (Charlton & Johengen, 1985). Compared with controls and animals who were growth retarded but not supplemented, the supplemented animals were close in size to the control group with similar brain–body ratios. Placental size, although less than controls, was greater than that in the non-supplement group.

Direct intravenous fetal feeding has only been studied in animals. In fetal lambs in whom IUGR had been induced by placental embolization, intravenous supplementation with glucose and amino acids resulted in the same birthweight in the controls and supplemented group (Charlton & Johengen, 1985; 1987). The difference in birthweight between supplemented and non-supplemented experimental groups correlated positively with the amount of supplement received. Placental weight was maintained in the supplemented group and umbilical blood flow was better than in the non-supplemented group. The specific nutritional factors responsible were not identified.

Safety

The safety of maternal supplementation has been questioned. Infusing mothers of normal human fetuses with glucose may result in the fetus becoming acidotic within a few hours (Lawrence *et al.*, 1982). Shelley, Bassett & Milner (1975) showed hyperglycaemia in hypoxic fetal lambs results in metabolic acidosis. Duodenal infusion of glucose or lactose in fetal lambs results in a rise in glucose or lactose in serum but a decrease in pH (Charlton & Rudolph, 1979). Similarly a decrease in pH occurs in human growth-retarded fetuses given glucose directly (Nicolini *et al.*, 1990). Philipps *et al.* (1984) studied the effects of hyperglycaemia on oxygen consumption in sheep and found an increase in fetal glucose may lead to an obligatory increase in fetal oxygen consumption, which would result in a decrease in fetal pO^2 and pH (Charlton & Johengen, 1985). Similar changes may occur in the human fetus (Benny, Legge & Aickin, 1978). MacMahon, Frampton & Yardley (1990) showed that even moderate maternal supplementation could result in high fetal concentrations of phenylalanine.

Practical problems also arise. Maternal infusion requires the placement of a central venous catheter. Access to the amniotic cavity may be made difficult by oligohydramnios, often present with IUGR. The problem of long-term direct access to the fetus has been recently addressed (Hedrick *et al.*, 1993). Infection, regardless of the route chosen, is a potential problem and entry into the amniotic cavity or fetus directly carries with it a risk of preterm labour. Cord accidents are also a risk.

Oxygen

Fetal growth is dependent upon adequate placental function for the delivery of nutrients and oxygen to the fetus. Decreased uteroplacental blood flow also results in decreased oxygen supply to the placenta (O'Shaughnessy, 1981). This may in turn impair the placental capacity to transfer glucose (Lumley & Wood, 1967) and amino acids (Longo, Yuen & Gusseck, 1973) to the fetus. It is also noteworthy that placental transfer of glucose and amino acid analogues correlates with maternal blood flow in fetuses with spontaneous and experimentally induced IUGR (Nitzan *et al.*, 1979; Saintonge & Rosso, 1981). This emphasizes the interrelationship between oxygen and nutrient supply.

Many chromosomally and structurally normal SGA fetuses are hypoxaemic and acidaemic (Soothill *et al.*, 1987). A reduction in uterine blood flow has been shown to result in fetal hypoxia and contribute to IUGR (Moll, 1973). The hypoxia may be related to a decrease in uteroplacental blood flow, inadequate umbilical blood flow or uterine umbilical perfusion balance inequality. Irrespective of cause, maternal oxygen supplementation has been attempted to improve fetal condition and prolong gestation. Nicolaides *et al.* (1987) administered 55% humidified oxygen by face mask chronically to five women (four singleton and one twin pregnancy) diagnosed as having growth-retarded fetuses (i.e. chromosomally normal, oligohydramnios, abdominal circumference below the fifth centile and abnormal umbilical Doppler waveforms). These patients were selected from a larger group of mothers with IUGR tested with humidified oxygen for 10 minutes. Only those fetuses demonstrated to respond to maternal oxygenation (increase in pO_2 on repeat fetal blood sampling) were admitted for continuous oxygen therapy. Five of six babies survived; the fetus that died *in utero* was the only one unable to increase its pO_2 into the normal range following initial maternal oxygenation. Gestation was prolonged (mean 38 days, range 5–63 days). Delivery was prompted by bleeding from a placenta praevia in one patient, worsening pre-eclampsia in two patients and failure to continue to respond to treatment in two patients (as measured by CTGs, Doppler FVW analysis and biophysical profiles). There was no evidence that maternal oxygen worsened fetal hypoxia or induced hypercapnia and acidosis. The authors concluded that three groups could be identified: those who increased fetal pO_2 to greater than normal levels and in whom oxygen therapy is contraindicated, those who increase oxygen to normal range and may benefit from oxygen therapy, and those who do not respond to oxygen and who may represent a group too severe to benefit. A limitation of this type of study is that fetal blood sampling is required to identify and diagnose these different groups.

More recently, Battaglia *et al.* (1992) have conducted a prospective randomized study of 36 pregnant women diagnosed as having a growth-retarded fetus between 26 and 34 weeks' gestation. Seventeen were treated with 55% humidified oxygen for 24 hours per day and 19 with bed rest alone. Fetal blood sampling was performed on entry and umbilical cord blood taken at delivery. Umbilical Doppler waveform analysis was performed on entry and at intervals thereafter. The mean treatment time was 10.1 days (±3.4) but gestation was not significantly increased in the treatment over the control group. Indications for delivery were the same in both groups; there was one intrauterine death in the untreated group. All liveborn infants in both groups were delivered by caesarean section. There was no significant difference in birthweight between treated and untreated groups. Significant improvement in Doppler waveform was observed in the treated group. Perinatal mortality rate in the treated group was 29% compared with 68% in the untreated group. The authors concluded that some benefit from maternal oxygenation was seen, as evidenced by improved fetal condition, but that an increase in placental transfer of nutrients did not occur as growth velocity was unaffected.

The effects of maternal hyperoxia on the behaviour and activity in growth-retarded fetuses has been examined (Gagnon, Hunse & Vijan, 1990). Although the fetuses displayed a sustained increase in fetal breathing, there was no change in the rate of gross body movement, fetal heart rate, or fetal heart rate variability when compared with normal-growth infants. This finding contrasted to previous reports of increased fetal body movements during and following maternal hyperoxia (Ruedrich, Devoe & Searle, 1989). The abnormalities in fetal heart rate and gross body movement associated with growth retardation may be related to altered central nervous system development and this may not be reversible with maternal administration of oxygen at the time of diagnosis. This is clearly an important issue.

Studies of oxygen supplementation to maternal ewes carrying a moderately growth-retarded fetus (Harding, Owens & Robinson, 1992) have shown that restoration of fetal pO^2 to normal is possible but is not seen in the most severe IUGR. Fetal oxygen consumption did not increase, which questions any benefit to the fetus of this practice. Cessation of supplementation was followed by a period of deterioration in fetal oxygenation. Although the previously cited reports in humans (Nicolaides *et al.*, 1987; Battaglia *et al.*, 1992) did not report this deterioration, the question of safety was not directly addressed and is yet to be answered. As stated above, there exists an inter-relationship between oxygen and nutrients. It is likely that there is need for normal supply of both before normal uptake and utilization is possible.

Physical methods to improve placental perfusion

It is clear that fetal growth is dependent upon adequate uteroplacental perfusion, as experimental reduction of placental blood flow induces growth retardation (Nitzan, 1979; Buchmiller *et al.*, 1994; Charlton & Johengen, 1987). A number of workers have studied ways of increasing placental blood flow to the growth-retarded fetus. Simple bed rest in the left lateral position results in increased uterine blood flow (Green, Duhring & Smith, 1965).

Abdominal decompression was first proposed by Heynes in 1959 as a method of overcoming the resistance of the abdominal wall to forward movement of the uterus during labour in an effort to optimize the forces of labour, reduce pain and enhance uteroplacental blood flow. A plastic suit worn over a rigid frame was designed to allow the pressure around the abdomen to be decreased by up to 100 mmHg. The suit was fed via a high-pressure pump, through which the patient controlled the decompression. Pressure was maintained for 15 seconds in each minute over 30 minutes or when contractions occurred during labour. Evidence was sought that abdominal decompression increased blood flow through the intervillous space by using intravenously injected radioisotopes and a collimated scintillation counter to scan the placenta and monitor blood flow rate (Coxon & Haggith, 1971). A 30% increase in count rate over the placenta during decompression with a simultaneous reduction of flow to the head and lower limbs was reported.

Three studies used abdominal decompression as treatment (Hofmeyr, Metrikin & Williamson, 1990) during pregnancies complicated by IUGR. All reported an increase in birthweight compared with controls. Meta-analysis of these studies (Hofmeyr, 1989) showed a decrease in the perinatal mortality rate. The only randomized double-blind trial of abdominal decompression (Coxon et al., 1973) did not find it helpful for preventing pre-eclampsia and there was no difference in birthweight between high- and low-decompression groups. Twice weekly 30 minute treatments of negative pressure 20 on 70 mmHg for 15 seconds every minute were used. In fact, the high-decompression group were found to have lighter placentas.

There are now case reports of abdominal decompression for prevention of growth retardation in high-risk pregnancies. Shimonovitz (1992) reported on its successful use for three women with poor obstetric histories previously complicated by IUGR, hypertension and poor fetal outcomes. Two of the three did not require antihypertensive treatment during their treated pregnancies. All commenced treatment prior to 15 weeks' gestation and all gave birth to normally grown babies at 38 to 39 weeks. It is not possible to discount the effect of rest in bed with these cases; however, one patient used the suit at home for her second successful pregnancy following the first reported one.

Conclusion

The management of IUGR has traditionally depended upon identification *in utero* and delivery when growth failure and/or fetal compromise is confirmed. The concept of therapy to improve fetal growth or reverse the pathogenic process is still relatively new and may depend more upon addressing the pathological mechanism of placental insufficiency rather than simply adding fetal growth factors or treating associated maternal disease. The majority of work has centred on aspirin to alter prostacyclin/thromboxane balance. Although meta-analysis of randomized controlled trials does not support routine use of low-dose aspirin in the prevention of growth restriction, trials employing a higher dose of 150 mg suggest a beneficial effect on fetal growth. There is currently no evidence to support transplacental supplementation with oxygen or nutrients, while supplementation methods that bypass the placenta would appear to be beyond our present technical limits.

References

Altshuler G., Russell P. & Ermocilla R. (1975). The placental pathology of small-for-gestational-age infants. *American Journal of Obstetrics and Gynecology*, 121, 351–9.

Babson, S. G., Behrman, R. E. & Lessel, R. (1970). Fetal growth. Liveborn birthweights for gestational age of white middle class infants. *Pediatrics*, 45, 937–44.

Baker, P. N., Basheer, T. & James D. K. (1994). Maternal platelet angiotensin II binding and fetal Doppler umbilical artery flow waveforms. *British Journal of Obstetrics and Gynaecology*, 101, 1009–10.

Battaglia, C., Artini, P. G., D'Ambrogio, G., Galli, P. A., Segre, A. & Genazzani, A. R. (1992). Maternal hyperoxygenation in the treatment of intrauterine growth retardation. *American Journal of Obstetrics and Gynecology*, 167, 430–5.

Battaglia, F. C. & Meschia, G. (1978). Principle substrates of fetal metabolism. *Physiological Reviews*, 58, 499–523.

Beaufils, M., Donsimoni, R., Uzan, S. & Colau J. C. (1985). Prevention of pre-eclampsia by early antiplatelet therapy. *Lancet*, 1, 840–2.

Beischer, N. A. (1978). Treatment of fetal growth retardation. *Australia and New Zealand Journal of Obstetrics and Gynaecology*, 18, 28–33.

Benigni, A., Gregorini, G., Frusca, T., Chiabrando C., Ballerini, S., Valcamonico, A., Orisio, S., Piccinelli, A., Pinciroli, V., Fanelli, R., Gastaldi, A. & Remuzzi, G. (1989). Effect of low-dose aspirin on fetal and maternal generation of thromboxane by platelets in women at risk for pregnancy-induced hypertension. *New England Journal of Medicine*, 21, 357–62.

Benny, P. S., Legge, M. & Aickin, D. R. (1978). The biochemical effects of maternal hyperalimentation during pregnancy. *New Zealand Medical Journal*, 88, 283–5.

Bewley, S., Cooper, D. & Campbell, S. (1991). Doppler investigation of uteroplacental blood flow resistance in the second trimester: a screening study for pre-eclampsia and intrauterine growth retardation. *British Journal of Obstetrics and Gynaecology*, 98, 871–9.

Brosens, I., Robertson, W. B. & Dixon, H. G. (1972). The role of the spiral arteries in the pathogenesis of pre-eclampsia. In *Obstetrics and Gynecology Annual*, ed. R. Wynn, pp.177–91. New York: Appleton Century Crofts.

Browne, J. C. & Veall, N. (1953). The maternal placental blood flow in normotensive and hypertensive women. *Journal of Obstetrics and Gynaecology of the British Empire*, 60, 141–7.

Buchmiller, T. L., Kim, C. S., Chopourian, L. & Fonkalsrud, E. W. (1994). Transamniotic fetal feeding: enhancement of growth in a rabbit model of intrauterine growth retardation. *Surgery*, 116, 36–41.

Bulstra-Ramakers, M. T. E. W., Huisjes, H. J. & Visser, G. H. A. (1994). The effects of 3 g eicosapentanoic acid daily on recurrence of intrauterine growth retardation and pregnancy induced hypertension. *British Journal of Obstetrics Gynaecology*, 102, 123–6.

Campbell, S. (1974). Assessment of fetal development by ultrasound. *Clinics in Perinatology*, 1, 507.

Campbell, S. & Kurjak A. (1972). Comparison between urinary oestrogen assay and serial cephalometry in assessment of fetal growth retardation. *British Medical Journal*, 4, 336–40.

Cetin, I., Marconi, A. M., Bozzetti, P., Sereni, L. P., Corbetta, C., Pardi, G. & Battaglia, F. C. (1988). Umbilical amino acid concentrations in appropriate and small for gestational age infants: a biochemical difference present *in utero*. *American Journal of Obstetrics and Gynecology*, 158, 120–6.

Char, V. C. & Creasy, R. K. (1977). Glucose and oxygen metabolism in normally oxygenated and spontaneously hypoxemic fetal lambs. *American Journal of Obstetrics and Gynecology*, 127, 499–504.

Char, V. C. & Rudolph, A. M. (1979). Digestion and absorption of carbohydrates by the fetal lamb *in utero*. *Pediatric Research*, 13, 1018–23.

Charlton, V. & Johengen, M. (1985). Effects of intrauterine nutritional supplementation on fetal growth retardation. *Biology of the Neonate*, 48, 125–42.

Charlton, V. & Johengen, M. (1987). Fetal intravenous nutritional supplementation ameliorates the development of embolisation-induced growth retardation in sheep. *Pediatric Research*, 22, 55–61.

Chimura, T., Funayama, T., Mitsui, T. & Kaneko, N. (1982). Effect of infusion therapy on intrauterine fetal growth retardation. *Acta Obstetrica Gynaecologica Japonica*, 34, 551–8.

CLASP (Collaborative Low-dose Aspirin Study in Pregnancy) Collaborative Group (1994). CLASP: a randomized trial of low-dose aspirin for the prevention and treatment of pre-eclampsia among 9364 pregnant women. *Lancet*, 343, 619–29.

Collins, R. (1994). Antiplatelet agents for IUGR and pre-eclampsia. In *Pregnancy and Childbirth Module*, ed. M. J. N. C. Keirse, M. J. Renfrew, J. P. Neilson & C. Crowther. London: Cochrane Database of Systematic Reviews, BMJ Publishing Group.

Cook, C. M. & Trudinger, B. J. (1991). Maternal angiotensin sensitivity and fetal Doppler umbilical artery flow waveforms. *British Journal of Obstetrics and Gynaecology*, 98, 698–702.

Coxon, A., Fairweather, D. V. I., Smyth, C. N., Frankenberg, J. & Vessey M. (1973). A randomized double blind clinical trial of abdominal decompression for the prevention of pre-eclampsia. *Journal of Obstetrics and Gynaecology of the British Commonwealth*, 80, 1081–5.

Coxon, A. & Haggith, J. W. (1971). The effects of abdominal decompression on vascular haemodynamics in pregnancy and labour. *Journal of Obstetrics and Gynaecology of the British Commonwealth*, 78, 49–54.

Dekker, G. A. & Sibai, B. M. (1993). Low-dose aspirin in the prevention of pre-eclampsia and fetal growth retardation: rationale, mechanisms and clinical trials. *American Journal of Obstetrics and Gynecology*, 168, 214–27.

de Swiet, M. & Fryers, G. (1990). The use of aspirin in pregnancy. *Journal of Obstetrics and Gynaecology*, 10, 467–82.

Earle, R. J. (1961). Congenital salicylate intoxication: report of a case. *New England Journal of Medicine*, 265, 1003–4.

Engel, E. & Delozier-Blanchet, C. (1991). Uniparental disomy, isodisomy and imprinting: probable effects in man and strategies for their detection. *American Journal of Medical Genetics*, 40, 432–9.

Fancourt, R., Campbell, S., Harvey, D. & Norman, A. P. (1976). Follow-up study of small-for-dates babies. *British Medical Journal*, i, 1435–7.

Fitzhardinge, P. M. & Steven, E. M. (1972). The small-for-dates infant. II. Neurological and intellectual sequelae. *Pediatrics*, 50, 50–7.

Fok, R. Y., Pavlova, Z., Benirschke, K., Paul, R. H. & Platt, L. D. (1990). The correlation of arterial lesions with umbilical artery Doppler velocimetry in the placental of small for dates pregnancies. *Obstetrics and Gynecology*, 75, 578–83.

Forestier, F., Daffos, F. & Rainaut, M. (1985). Pre-eclampsia and prostaglandins. *Lancet*, i, 1268.

Gagnon, R., Hunse, C. & Vijan, S. (1990). The effect of maternal hyperoxia on behavioural activity in growth-retarded fetuses. *American Journal of Obstetrics and Gynecology*, 183, 1894–9.

Giles, W. B., Trudinger, B. J. & Baird, P. J. (1985). Fetal umbilical artery flow velocity waveforms and placental resistance: pathological correlation. *British Journal of Obstetrics and Gynaecology*, 92, 31–8.

Gitlin, D., Kumate, J., Morales, C., Noriega, L. & Arevalo N. (1972). The turnover of amniotic fluid protein in the human conceptus. *American Journal of Obstetrics and Gynecology*, 113, 632–45.

Green, J. W., Duhring, J. L. & Smith K. (1965). Placental function tests. A review of methods available for assessment of the fetoplacental complex. *American Journal of Obstetrics and Gynecology*, 92, 1030–58.

Gruenwald, P., Funakawa, H., Mitani, S., Nishimura, T. & Takeuchi, S. (1967). Influence of environmental factors of foetal growth in man. *Lancet*, i, 1026–9.

Harding, J. E. & Charlton, V. (1990). Experimental nutritional supplementation for intrauterine growth-retardation. In *The Unborn Patient*, ed. M. R. Harrison, M. S. Golbus & R. A. Filly, pp. 598–613. Philadelphia: W. B. Saunders.

Harding, J. E., Owens, J. A. & Robinson, J. S. (1992). Should we try to supplement the growth-retarded fetus? A cautionary tale. *British Journal of Obstetrics and Gynaecology*, 99, 707–10.

Harrison, M. R. & Villa, R. L. (1982). Transamniotic fetal feeding I. Development of an animal model: continuous amniotic infusion in rabbits. *Journal of Pediatric Surgery*, 17, 376–80.

Hauth, J. C., Goldenberg, R. L., Parker, R. C., Phillips, J. B., Copper, R. L., DuBard, M. B. & Cutter, G. R. (1993). Low-dose aspirin therapy to prevent pre-eclampsia. *American Journal of Obstetrics and Gynecology*, 168, 1083–93.

Hay, W. W., Sparks, J. W., Wilkening, R. B., Battaglia, F. C. & Meschia, G. (1984). Fetal glucose uptake and utilisation as functions of maternal glucose concentration. *American Journal of Physiology*, 246, E237–42.

Hedrick, M. H., Jennings, R. W., MacGillvray, T. E., Rice, H. E., Flake, A. W., Adzick, N. S. & Harrison, M. R. (1993). Chronic fetal vascular access. *Lancet*, 32, 1086–7.

Herbert, N. P., Seeds, J. W., Bowes, W. A. & Sweeney, C. A. (1986). Fetal growth response to parenteral nutrition in pregnancy: a case report. *Journal of Reproductive Medicine*, 31, 264–6.

Heynes, O. S. (1959). Abdominal decompression in the first stage of labour. *Journal of Obstetrics and Gynaecology of the British Empire*, 66, 220–8.

Hofmeyr, G. J. (1989). Abdominal decompression during pregnancy. In *Effective Care in Pregnancy and Childbirth*, ed. I. Chalmers, M. Enkin & M. J. N. C. Keirse, pp. 647–52. Oxford: Oxford University Press.

Hofmeyr, G. J., Metrikin, D. C. & Williamson, I. (1990). Abdominal decompression: new data from a previous study. *British Journal of Obstetrics and Gynaecology*, 97, 547–8.

Italian Study of Aspirin in Pregnancy (1993). Low-dose aspirin in prevention and treatment of intrauterine growth retardation and pregnancy-induced hypertension. *Lancet*, 341, 396–400.

Jacobson, R. L., Brewer, A., Eis, A., Siddiqi, T. A. & Myatt, L. (1991). Transfer of aspirin across the perfused human placental cotyledon. *American Journal of Obstetrics and Gynecology*, 165, 939–44.

Kaar, K., Jouppila, P., Kaikka, J., Luotola, H., Toivanen, J. & Rekonon, A. (1980). Intervillous blood flow in normal and complicated late pregnancy measured by means of an intravenous 133Xe method. *Acta Obstetricia et Gynecologica Scandinavica*, 59, 7–10.

Kalousek, D. K. (1994). Current topic: confined placental mosaicism and intrauterine fetal development. *Placenta*, 15, 219–30.

Lawrence, G. F., Brown, V. A., Parsons, R. J. & Cooke, I. D. (1982). Fetomaternal consequences of high dose glucose infusion during labour. *British Journal of Obstetrics and Gynaecology*, 89, 27–32.

Longo, L. D., Yuen, P. & Gusseck, D. J. (1973). Anaerobic, glycogen-dependent transport of amino acids by the placenta. *Nature*, 243, 531–3.

Low, J. A., Galbraith, R. S., Muir, D., Killen, H., Karchmar, J. & Campbell, D. (1979). Intrauterine growth retardation: a preliminary report of long term morbidity. *American Journal of Obstetrics and Gynecology*, 130, 534–45.

Lumley, J. M. & Wood, C. (1967). Influence of hypoxia on glucose transport across the human placenta. *Nature*, 216, 403–4.

MacMahon, R. A., Frampton, R. J. & Yardley, R. W. (1990). Effect on the fetus of infusing a commercial amino acid preparation into a pregnant sheep. *Biology of the Neonate*, 57, 231–7.

McBurney, R. D. (1947). Undernourished full term infant: case report. *Western Journal of Surgery, Obstetrics and Gynecology*, 55, 363.

McGregor, I. A., Wilson, E. & Billewicz, W. Z. (1983). Malaria infection of the placenta in The Gambia, West Africa: its incidence and relationship to stillbirth, birthweight and placental weight. *Transactions of the Royal Society of Tropical Medicine and Hygiene*, 77, 223–44.

McParland, P., Pearce, J. M. & Chamberlain, G. V. (1990). Doppler ultrasound and aspirin in recognition and prevention of pregnancy-induced hypertension. *Lancet*, i, 1552–5.

Mellor, D. J. (1983). Nutritional and placental determinants of fetal growth rate in sheep and consequences for the newborn lamb. *British Veterinary Journal*, 139, 307–24.

Mellor, D. J. & Murray, L. (1982). Effects on the rate of increase in fetal girth of refeeding ewes after short periods of severe under-nutrition during late pregnancy. *Research in Veterinary Science*, 32, 377–82.

Mesaki, N., Kubo, T. & Iwasaki, H. (1980). A study of the treatment for intrauterine growth retardation. *Acta Obstetrica Gynaecologica Japonica*, 32, 879–85.

Moise, K. J., Huhta, J. C., Sharif, D. S., Ou, C. M., Kirshon, B., Wasserstrum, N. and Cano, L. (1988). Indomethacin in the treatment of premature labor. *New England Journal of Medicine*, 319, 327–31.

Moll, W. (1973). Placental function and oxygenation in the fetus. *Advances in Experimental Medicine and Biology*, 37, 1017–26.

Mulvihill, S. J., Albert, A., Synn, A. & Fonkalsrud, E. W. (1985). *In utero* supplemental fetal feeding in an animal model: effects on fetal growth and development. *Surgery*, 98, 500–5.

Nelson, D. M & Walsh, S. W. (1989). Aspirin differentially affects thromboxane and prostacylin production by trophoblast and villous core compartments of human placental villi. *American Journal of Obstetrics and Gynecology*, 161, 1593–98.

Nicolaides, K. H., Campbell, S., Bradley, R. J., Bilardo, C. M., Soothill, P. W. & Gibb, D. (1987). Maternal oxygen therapy for intrauterine growth retardation. *Lancet*, i, 942–5.

Nicolini, U., Hubinont, C., Santolaya, J., Fisk N. M. & Rodeck, C. H. (1990). Effects of fetal intravenous glucose challenge in normal and growth-retarded fetuses. *Hormone and Metabolic Research*, 22, 426–30.

Niebyl, J. R. & Witter, F. R. (1986). Neonatal outcome after indomethacin treatment for preterm labour. *American Journal of Obstetrics and Gynecology*, 155, 747–9.

Nitzan, M., Orloff, S. & Schulman, J. D. (1979). Placental transfer of analogs of glucose and amino acids in experimental intrauterine growth retardation. *Pediatric Research*, 13, 100–3.

Nylund, L., Lunell, N. O., Lewander, R. & Sarby, B. (1983). Uteroplacental blood flow index in intrauterine growth retardation of fetal or maternal origin. *British Journal of Obstetrics and Gynaecology*, 90, 16–20.

Oh, W., Omori, K., Hobel, C. J., Erenberg, A. & Emmanouilides, G. C. (1975). Umbilical blood flow and glucose uptake in lamb fetus following single umbilical artery ligation. *Biology of the Neonate*, 26, 291–9.

Olsen, S., Sorensen, J. D., Secher, N. L., Hedegaard, M., Henriksen, T. B., Hansen, H. S. & Grant, A. (1992). Randomized controlled trial of effect of fish oil supplementation on pregnancy duration. *Lancet*, 339, 1003–7.

Onwude, J. L., Lilford, R. J., Hjartardottir, H., Staines, A. & Tuffnell, D. (1995). A randomized double blind placebo controlled trial of fish oil in high-risk pregnancy. *British Journal of Obstetrics and Gynaecology*, 102, 95–100.

O'Shaughnessy, R. W. (1981). Uterine blood flow and fetal growth. In *Fetal Growth Retardation*, ed. F. A. van Assche & W. B. Robertson, pp. 101–16. Edinburgh: Churchill Livingstone.

Owens, J. A. (1991). Endocrine and substrate control of fetal growth: placental and maternal influences and insulin-like growth factors. *Reproduction, Fertility and Development*, 3, 501–7.

Owens, J. A., Falconer, J. & Robinson, J. S. (1987). Effect of restriction of placental growth on fetal and utero-placental metabolism. *Journal of Developmental Physiology*, 9, 225–38.

Pearson, J. F. & Shuttleworth, R. (1971). The metabolic effects of a hypertonic fructose infusion on the mother and fetus during labor. *American Journal of Obstetrics and Gynecology*, 111, 259–65.

Pedersen, A. K. & Fitzgerald, G. A. (1984). Dose related kinetics of aspirin. *New England Journal of Medicine*, 311, 1206–11.

Philipps, A. F., Porte, P. J., Stabinsky, S., Rosenkrantz, T. S. & Raye, J. R. (1984). Effects of chronic fetal hyperglycemia upon oxygen consumption on the ovine uterus and conceptus. *Journal of Clinical Investigation*, 74, 279–86.

Phillips, L., Lumley, J., Paterson, P. & Wood, C. (1968). Fetal hypoglycemia. *American Journal of Obstetrics and Gynecology*, 102, 371–7.

Pitkin, R. & Reynolds, W. A. (1975). Fetal ingestion and metabolism of amniotic fluid preterm. *American Journal of Obstetrics and Gynecology*, 123, 356–63.

Polani, P. E. (1974). Chromosomal and other genetic influences on birthweight variation. In *Size at Birth. CIBA Foundation Symposium No. 27*, pp. 127–160. Amsterdam: Elsevier.

Rankin, J. H. G. & McLaughlin, M. K. (1979). The regulation of placental blood flows. *Journal of Developmental Physiology*, 1, 3–30.

Rodgers, G. M., Taylor, R. N. & Roberts, J. M. (1988). Pre-eclampsia is associated with a serum factor cytoxic to human endothelial cells. *American Journal of Obstetrics and Gynecology*, 159, 908.

Rudolph, A. M. (1981). Effects of aspirin and acetaminophen in pregnancy and in the newborn. *Archives of Internal Medicine*, 141, 353–63.

Ruedrich, D. A., Devoe, L. D. & Searle, N. (1989). Effects of maternal hyperoxia on the biophysical assessment of fetuses with suspected intrauterine growth retardation. *American Journal of Obstetrics and Gynecology*, 161, 188–92.

Rumack, C. M., Guggenheim, M. A., Rumack, B. H., Peterson, R. G., Johnson, M. L. & Braithwaite, W. R. (1981). Neonatal intracranial hemorrhage and maternal use of aspirin. *Obstetrics and Gynecology*, 58, 52S–56S.

Rush, D. (1982). Effects of changes in protein and caloric intake during pregnancy on the growth of the human fetus. In: *Effectiveness and Satisfaction in Antenatal Care Clinics: Developmental Medicine Series*, ed. M. Enkin & I. Chalmers, pp. 92–113. London: Spastics International Medical Publications.

Rush, D. (1992). The effects of changes in protein and calorie intake during pregnancy on the growth of the human fetus. In *Effective Care in Pregnancy and Childbirth*, ed. I. Chalmers, M. Enkin & M. J. N. C. Keirse, pp. 255–80. Oxford: Oxford University Press.

Sabata, V., Paul, K., Zezulokova, J. & Dittrichova, J. (1985). The effect of prenatal therapy in pregnancies with small for dates fetuses on the psychoneurologic development of the infant. In *Prevention of Physical and Mental Congenital Defects. Part B: Epidemiology, Early Detection and Therapy and Environmental Factors*, ed. M. Maros, pp. 249–65. New York: Alan R. Liss.

Sabata, V., Znamenacek, K., Pribylova, H. & Melichar, V. (1973). The effect of glucose in the prenatal treatment of small-for-dates fetuses. *Biology of the Neonate*, 22, 78–86.

Saintonge, J. & Rosso, P. (1981). Placental blood flow and transfer of nutrient analogs in large, average and small guinea pig litter mates. *Pediatric Research*, 15, 152–6.

Saling, E. (1987). Versuch einer neuen kompensatorischen Versorgung des hypotrophen feten. *Geburtshilfe Frauenheilkunde*, 47, 90–2.

Schiff, E., Peleg, E., Goldenberg, M., Rosenthal, T., Ruppin, E., Tamarkin, M., Barkai, G., Ben-Baruch, G., Yahal, I., Blankstein, J., Goldman, B. & Maschiach, S. (1989). The use of aspirin to prevent pregnancy-induced hypertension and lower the ratio of thromboxane A_2 to prostacyclin in relatively high-risk pregnancies. *New England Journal of Medicine*, 321, 351–6.

Shapiro, S., Siskind, V., Monson, R. R., Heinonen, O. P., Kaufman, D. W., & Slone D. (1976). Perinatal mortality and birthweight in relation to aspirin taken during pregnancy. *Lancet*, 1, 1375–6.

Shelley, H. J., Bassett, J. M. & Milner, R. D. G. (1975). Control of carbohydrate metabolism in the fetus and newborn. *British Medical Bulletin*, 31, 37–43.

Shimonovitz, S., Yagel, S., Zacut, D., Ben–Chetrit, A., Celnikier, D. H. & Ron, M. (1992). Intermittent abdominal decompression: an option for prevention of intrauterine growth retardation. *British Journal of Obstetrics and Gynaecology*, 99, 691–5.

Sibai, B. M., Caritis, S. N., Thom E., Klebanoff, M., McNellis, D., Rocco, L., Paul, R. H., Romero, R., Witter, F., Rosen, M. Depp, R. and the National Institute of Child Health and Human Development Network of Maternal–Fetal Medicine Units (1993). Prevention of pre-eclampsia with low-dose aspirin in healthy, nulliparous pregnant women. *New England Journal of Medicine*, 329, 1213–18.

Sibai, B. M., Mirro, R., Chesney, C. M. & Leffler C. (1989). Low-dose aspirin in pregnancy. *Obstetrics and Gynecology*, 74, 551–7.

Slone, D., Siskind, V., Heinonen, O. P., Monson, R. R., Kaufman, D. W. & Shapiro, S. (1976). Aspirin and congenital malformations. *Lancet*, i, 1373–5.

Soothill, P. W., Ajayi, R. A. & Nicolaides, K. N. (1992). Fetal biochemistry in growth retardation. *Early Human Development*. 19, 91–7.

Soothill, P. W., Nicolaides, K. H. & Campbell, S. (1987). Prenatal asphyxia, hyperlacticaemia, hypoglycaemia and erythoblastosis in growth-retarded fetuses. *British Medical Journal*, 297, 1051–3.

Sparks, J. W., Hay, W. W., Bonds, D., Meschia, A. & Battaglia F. C. (1982). Simultaneous measurements of lactate turnover rate and umbilical lactate uptake in the fetal lamb. *Journal of Clinical Investigation*, 70, 179–92.

Spitz, B., Magness, R. R., Cox, S. M., Brown, C. E., Rosenfeld, C. R. & Grant, N. F. (1988). Low-dose aspirin. 1. Effect on angiotensin II pressor responses and blood prostaglandin concentrations in pregnant women sensitive to angiotensin II. *American Journal of Obstetrics and Gynecology*, 159, 1035–43.

Stuart, M., Gross, S. J., Elrad, H. & Graeber, J. (1982). Effects of acetyl salicylic acid ingestion on maternal and neonatal haemostasis. *New England Journal of Medicine*, 307, 909–12.

Tanner J. M. (1978). *Fetus into Man: Growth from Conception to Maturity*, pp. 40–2. London: Open Books, and Boston, Mass: Harvard University Press.

Thorp, J. A., Walsh, S. W. & Brath P. C. (1988). Low-dose aspirin inhibits thromboxane, but not prostacyclin production by human placental arteries. *American Journal of Obstetrics and Gynecology*, 159, 1381–4.

Trudinger, B. J. (1987). The umbilical circulation. *Seminars in Perinatology*, 11, 311–13.

Trudinger, B. J. (1991). Doppler ultrasound studies and fetal abnormality. In *Antenatal Diagnosis of Fetal Abnormalities*, ed. J. O. Drife & D. Donnai, pp.113–25. London: Springer-Verlag.

Trudinger, B. J. (1993). Pregnancy hypertension – a disease of fetus or mother? *Journal of Nephrology*, 6, 55–6.

Trudinger, B. J., Cook, C. M., Giles, W. B., Ng, S., Fong E., Connelly, A. & Wilcox W. (1991). Fetal umbilical artery velocity waveforms and subsequent neonatal outcome. *British Journal of Obstetrics and Gynaecology*, 99, 378–84.

Trudinger B. J., Cook C. M., Thompson R. S., Giles W. B. & Connelly A. (1988). Low-dose aspirin therapy improves fetal weight in umbilical placental insufficiency. *American Journal of Obstetrics and Gynecology*, 159, 681–5.

Trudinger, B. J., Giles, W. B. & Cook, C. M. (1985). Flow velocity waveforms in the maternal uteroplacental and fetal umbilical placental circulation. *American Journal of Obstetrics and Gynecology*, 152, 155–63.

Trudinger, B. J., Stevens, D., Connelly, A., Hales, J. R. S., Alexander, G., Bradley, L., Fawcett, A. & Thompson R. S. (1987). Umbilical artery flow velocity waveforms and placental resistance: the effects of embolization of the umbilical circulation. *American Journal of Obstetrics and Gynecology*, 157, 1443–9.

Turner, G. & Colins E. (1975). Fetal effects of regular salicylate ingestion in pregnancy. *Lancet*, ii, 338–9.

Uzan S., Beaufils M., Breart G., Bazin, B., Capitant, C. & Paris, J. (1991). Prevention of fetal growth retardation with low-dose aspirin: findings of the EPREDA trial. *Lancet*, 337, 1427–31.

Uzan S., Haddad, B. & Breart, G. (1994). Uteroplacental doppler and aspirin therapy in the prediction and prevention of pregnancy complications. *Ultrasound in Obstetrics and Gynecology*, 4, 342–9.

Viinikka, L., Hartikainen-Sorri, A. L., Lumme, R., Hiilesmaa, V. & Ylikorkala O. (1993). Low-dose aspirin in hypertensive pregnant women: effect on pregnancy outcomes and prostacyclin-thromboxane balance in mother and newborn. *British Journal of Obstetrics and Gynaecology*, 100, 809–15.

Wallenburg, H. C. S., Dekker, A., Makovitz, J. W. & Rotmans, P. (1986). Low-dose aspirin prevents pregnancy-induced hypertension and pre-eclampsia in angiotensin-sensitive primigravidae. *Lancet*, i, 840–2.

Wallenburg, H. C. S. & Rotmans, P. (1982). Enhanced reactivity of the platelet thromboxane pathway in normotensive and hypertensive pregnancies with insufficient fetal growth. *American Journal of Obstetrics and Gynecology*, 144, 523–8.

Walsh, S. W. (1985). Pre-eclampsia: an imbalance in placental prostacyclin and thromboxane production. *American Journal of Obstetrics and Gynecology*, 152, 335–40.

Wenstrom, K. D., Owen, J., Boots, L. R. & DuBard, M. B. (1994). Elevated second trimester human chorionic gonadotrophin levels in association with poor pregnancy outcome. *American Journal of Obstetrics and Gynecology*, 171, 1038–41.

Wilcox, G. R. & Trudinger, B. J. (1991). Fetal platelet consumption: a feature of placental insufficiency. *Obstetrics and Gynecology*, 77, 616–21.

Williams, R. L., Creasy, R. K., Cunningham, G. C., Hawes, W. E., Norris, F. D. & Tashiro, M. (1982). Fetal growth and perinatal viability in California. *Obstetrics and Gynecology*, 59, 624–32.

Xu, Y. (1993). Ensure treatment for intrauterine
·growth retardation. Chung-Kuo, Hsuch Ko Hsuch
Yuan Hsuch Pao, *Acta Academiae Medicinae Sinicae* ,
15, 63–6.

Ylikorkala, O., Makila, U. M., Kaapa, P. & Viinikka,
L. (1986). Maternal ingestion of acetyl salicyclic
acid inhibits fetal and neonatal prostacyclin and
thromboxane in humans. *American Journal of
Obstetrics and Gynecology*, 155, 345–9.

Part three

Treatment of established disease

10 Anaemia

KENNETH J. MOISE, JR AND BERND SCHUMACHER

Introduction

The infusion of donor red cells into the fetal circulation in cases of haemolytic disease of the fetus/newborn (HDN) represents one of earliest attempts at *in utero* therapy for the human fetus. Initial efforts to gain access to the fetal circulation utilized hysterotomy with placement of catheters into the fetal femoral artery (Freda & Adamsons, 1964), saphenous vein (Asensio, Figueroa Longo & Pelgrina, 1966) or internal jugular vein (Asensio, Figueroa Longo & Pelgrina, 1968). A less radical approach was proposed by Liley (1961) when he introduced the concept of infusing red cells into the fetal peritoneal cavity. The more recent advance of ultrasound-guided intravascular transfusion has brought fetal transfusion into the realm of a widely accepted and successful technique. Although red cell alloimmunization today remains the primary indication for intrauterine transfusion of red cells, fetal anaemia secondary to parvovirus infection and fetomaternal haemorrhage has also been treated with this modality.

Red cell alloimmunization

Aetiology

Alloimmunization to red cell antigens typically occurs in a woman of reproductive potential at the time of a pregnancy-related event. Several key factors play a role in determining whether a woman will develop red cell antibodies. The particular antigen involved is of some importance, the rhesus D (RhD) antigen being one of the most immunogenic of the antigen systems on the red cell. The volume of incompatible red cells that enters the maternal circulation also plays a role in determining whether there will be an immune reaction. However, studies in male volunteers have shown that as little as 0.1 ml of red cells may be sufficient to alloimmunize some individuals (Zipursky & Israels, 1967). We have experienced one case in which the patient was thought to have developed antibodies during intravenous drug use from sharing syringes with her partner prior to her first pregnancy. An ABO incompatibility between the mother and her fetus is felt to offer some protection. In this situation, the mother is typically blood type O and the fetus type A or B. Maternal anti-A or anti-B antibodies will usually remove the fetal red cells from circulation prior to recognition of the Rh antigen by the immune system. Clearly, the development of Rh immune globulin has prevented the great majority of cases of Rh disease. However, cases of antepartum sensitization and inadvertent omission of Rh immune globulin administration after delivery continue to occur. A recent study in Scotland revealed that two-thirds of alloimmunized cases were secondary to antepartum sensitization while an additional 13% were caused by failure to administer Rh immune globulin for the usual obstetric indications (Hughes *et al.*, 1994). In addition to the Rh antigen, more than 43 other red cell antigens have been implicated in haemolytic disease of the newborn (Weinstein, 1982, see Table 10.1). The antigen–antibody interactions that produce severe fetal disease necessitating intrauterine transfusion are, however, limited in number. Often the D antibody is found in conjunction with other Rh antibodies (c, C, E, e) of weaker titre. Two other antibodies that cause severe *in utero* disease are c and Kell. Duffy (FyA), Kidd (JkA, JkB) and E on

Table 10.1 *Antibodies associated with haemolytic disease of the newborn*

Blood group system	Antigen	Blood group system	Antigen
Rhesus	D	Public antigens	Yt^a
	C		Lan
	c		En^a
	E		Ge
	e		Jr^a
			Co^a
Kell	K		Co^3
	k		Wright^b
Duffy	Fy^a	Private antigens	Batty
			Becker
Kidd	Jk^a		Berrens
	Jk^b		Biles
			Evans
MNSs	M		Gonzales
	N		Good
	S		Heibel
	s		Hunt
			Jobbins
Lutheran	Lu^a		Radin
	Lu^b		Rm
			Ven
Diego	Di^a		Wright^a
	Di^b		Zd
Xg	Xg^a		
P	PP$_1$P^k		

Modified from Weinstein, L. (1982); reprinted with permission from the American Association of Blood Banks.

exceptionally rare occasions will cause severe fetal anaemia.

Incidence

Most centres involved in surveillance of infants affected by Rh haemolytic disease of the newborn have included all newborns with a positive direct Coombs' test as minimum evidence of disease. In the USA, the Centers for Disease Control reported an incidence of 10.6 cases per 10 000 total births in 1986 (Chavéz, Mulinare & Edmonds, 1991). Regional variations were noted, with the southwest region of the country having the highest incidence of 14.4/10 000 total births. A similar study in the Scottish population between 1985 and 1990 revealed an incidence of 53.5 cases per 10 000 total births (Hughes *et al.*, 1994). Rates of alloimmunization were reported to have stabilized in both studies.

Red cell alloimmunization to non-RhD antibodies continues to be a problem, since prophylactic immune globulin is not available to prevent these cases. The majority of cases of Kell sensitization in the USA are secondary to incompatible red cell transfusions since blood is not routinely crossmatched for the Kell antigen. In England, Caine *et al.* (1986) found 127 cases of Kell alloimmunization in 127 076 pregnancies (0.1%). Thirteen of the Kell- sensitized pregnancies resulted in an affected fetus or newborn. Two intrauterine deaths and one neonatal death occurred. Solola and coworkers (1983) reviewed seven previous series of Rh-positive pregnant patients screened for irregular red cell antibodies and noted 400 cases of irregular antibodies in the 131 898 patients, for an overall incidence of 1:330. Thirty infants in the series required exchange transfusions for HDN.

Perinatal losses secondary to Rh disease appear to be on the decline. Data from England and Wales indicate that the rate has declined from 18.4 per 10 000 live births in 1977 to 1.5 per 10 000 live births in 1989 (Hussey & Clarke, 1991). During this same time period, the perinatal loss rate secondary to other red cell antibodies remained stable at 0.45 per 10 000 live births.

Genetics

The genetics of the Rh red cell antigen system has been the subject of widespread speculation since the proposal by Race (1944) that three loci were responsible for the D, C and E antigens. Weiner (1943) alternatively proposed that a single gene encoded for all three antigens. In 1991, Colin and coworkers (1991) reported the successful cloning of the human D locus. The gene encoding for the D antigen appears to consist of 10 exons on the short arm of the first chromosome (see Fig. 10.1). In a subsequent publication, this group demonstrated the presence of only one additional gene, which encodes for the C/c and E/e red cell antigens through alternative splicing of a primary mRNA transcript (Mouro *et al.*, 1993). Like the D gene, the C/E gene is also 10 exons in length and is 96% homologous in its base pair sequences to the D gene. The E and e alleles differ from the D gene by a single base pair whereas the C and c alleles differ by six base pairs. This has led some to conclude that these genes appear to have evolved from the duplication of a common ancestral gene (Chérif Zahar *et al.*, 1990).

Individuals that are serologically typed as Rh negative were at first thought to have a gene deletion. This is consistent with the blood banking observation that no anti-serum for the 'd' antigen has been identified. More recent studies have noted that some 'Rh-negative' Black individuals may have an internal deletion of the D gene (Carritt, Steers & Avent, 1994). Other individuals that are serologically Rh negative have been found to have deletions of exons 7 through 9 or a stop codon in exon 5.

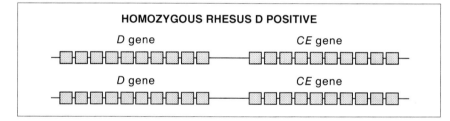

Fig. 10.1 *RhD gene locus on chromosome 1. (Reproduced from Van den Veyver* et al. *(1995); with permission from the C.V. Mosby Company.)*

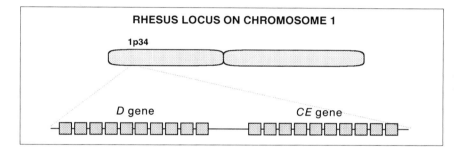

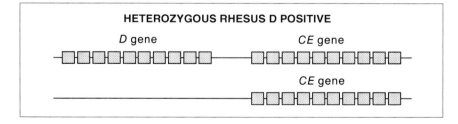

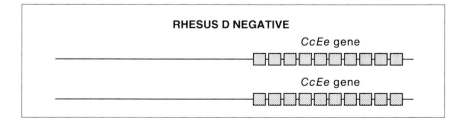

Preliminary investigation has identified at least eight different epitopes of the RhD antigen (Lomas *et al.*, 1989; Mouro *et al.*, 1994). Exons 4, 5, and 6 of the D gene appear critical for the reactivity of the majority of these (Mollison, 1994).

The fetus inherits the Rh gene in an autosomal dominant fashion. Although sophisticated DNA techniques have not yet been developed to determine a homozygous or heterozygous state, serology can be used to derive the paternal genotype in the great majority of cases. Since the genes for the C and E antigens are closely linked to the D locus, serology can be used to determine the remaining four antigens. Population studies are then used to determine the heterozygous or homozygous state at the D locus. A heterozygous genotype occurs in approximately 55% of Caucasian males. Half the offspring of such a couple will be Rh negative and escape the harmful effects of the maternal anti-D antibody.

Paternal genotype testing for other red cell antigens is more straightforward. In the case of the Kell antigen, 92% of males will be Kell negative; only Kell-negative unaffected offspring can, therefore, be expected. The remaining 8% of males will be Kell positive; 97% of these will be heterozygous while 3% will be homozygous. In the case of the little c antigen, 80% of males will be positive for the antigen and 60% will be heterozygous.

Diagnosis of fetal anaemia

Antibody quantification

An indirect Coombs' test should be obtained in all pregnant patients at their first prenatal visit. If an antibody that has been associated with HDN is then identified, an assessment of the amount of antibody present should be undertaken. In England, anti-D levels are measured and compared with an international standard and reported as international units/ml (IU/ml). In North America, maternal antibody titres are used to assess the degree of risk for fetal disease. Previous titre determinations by saline or albumin methods are outdated since they measure maternal IgM levels. Today, the anti-human globulin titre, i.e. indirect Coombs', a measure of the maternal IgG response, should be employed. A critical titre is defined as the titre at which

there is a significant risk of fetal hydrops. Although the actual titre will vary with institution, methodology and incidence of hydrops, most centres will use a titre value between 8 and 32 (dilution: 1:8 and 1:32) as their definition of a critical value. Once a patient is found to have this titre, invasive fetal testing is indicated. An anti-D antibody level of greater than 4 IU/ml has been recommended as the threshold to initiate amniocentesis (Bowell *et al.*, 1982). Nicolaides and Rodeck (1992) advised that fetal blood sampling to detect anaemia be reserved for pregnancies with a maternal anti-D concentration of >15 IU/ml.

Maternal in vitro *assays*

Since an indirect Coombs' titre is little more than a screening test for fetal haemolytic disease, several authors have investigated other maternal assays. Quantification of the actual amount of anti-D antibody has proved burdensome and added little to the accuracy of the prediction of fetal anaemia (Morley, Gibson & Eltringham, 1977). Considerable interest has been shown in *in vitro* assays that attempt to mimic the fetal conditions producing red cell haemolysis. Typically, maternal serum is mixed with adult red cells heterozygous for the involved antigen. These sensitized cells are then subjected to various types of effector cell such as macrophages, monocytes or lymphocytes. The degree of haemolysis or the activation of the effector cell is then quantified. The three tests most often studied in cases of red cell alloimmunization are the antibody-dependent cell-mediated cytotoxicity (ADCC) assay, the monocyte monolayer assay (MMA) and the monocyte chemiluminescence (CL) test.

In the ADCC assay, the release of ^{51}Cr from sensitized red cells is used as a measure of the *in vitro* destruction caused by mononuclear cells. The percentage of total monocytes involved in adherence or phagocytosis of sensitized red cells is assessed by microscopic examination in the MMA test. The CL assay utilizes the photoactivity of the substance luminol as a measure of the activation of monocytes when exposed to sensitized red cells. Urbaniak *et al.* (1984) were the first to study the ADCC in 11 pregnancies complicated by Rh alloimmunization. The authors concluded that the test could correctly identify those patients with high antibody titres associated with satisfactory neonatal outcomes. They suggested that the ADCC assay could avert the need for amniocentesis in alloimmunized pregnancies. This finding was substantiated by Nance and coworkers (1989) using the MMA in 16 pregnant patients with Rh alloimmunization. The authors found the MMA to be superior to amniocentesis for bilirubin determination in predicting the need for neonatal transfusion. Based on these data, we undertook a multicentred study to assess the usefulness of the MMA in the prediction of fetal anaemia detected by ultrasound-guided fetal blood sampling (FBS) of the fetus (Moise *et al.*, 1995a). In a series of 63 patients, the percentage of monocytes involved in phagocytosis was similar in antigen-negative, nonanaemic and in anaemic, antigen-positive fetuses. We concluded that the MMA was not useful in forecasting the need for intrauterine transfusion. Recently, Nance's group (Sacks *et al.*, 1993) have reported their further experience with the MMA and concluded that the test has little merit over surveillance with indirect Coombs' titres in the alloimmunized pregnancy. In the largest series of alloimmunized patients reported to date, Hadley *et al.* (1991) compared four different functional assays in predicting the need for neonatal transfusion. Both the maternal ADCC and CL tests drawn within eight weeks of delivery correctly differentiated neonates requiring exchange transfusion from those that were unaffected or only mildly affected. Clearly the ADCC and CL assays deserve further study regarding their role in the management of red cell alloimmunization in pregnancy. Unfortunately, most investigations to date have concentrated on the need for neonatal transfusion as a measure of haemolytic disease. The presence of fetal anaemia would appear to be a more applicable measure of disease severity in deciding if these assays are clinically useful. Should an *in vitro* test be found that correlates closely with fetal haematocrit, serial amniocenteses and FBS could be avoided.

Ultrasound

Ultrasound has played a key role in the improved survival of the fetus affected by maternal red cell alloimmunization. It can be used to establish the correct gestational age, since parameters such as the normal fetal haematocrit and amniotic fluid bilirubin levels are based on gestational age. It is an invaluable imaging modality to provide needle guidance for such procedures as amnio-

centesis, FBS and intrauterine transfusion. Unfortunately, its use in the diagnosis of fetal anaemia is relatively limited until overt fetal hydrops is present. Although some investigators have advocated the use of serial ultrasound examinations to detect signs of impending hydrops, Nicolaides *et al.* (1988) were unable to correlate fetal haematocrit with such parameters as increased placental thickness or increased umbilical vein diameter. Since the liver and spleen serve as sources of extramedullary haematopoiesis in response to fetal anaemia, these organs have been studied in the prediction of fetal anaemia. Two studies (Vintzileos *et al.*, 1986; Roberts, Mitchell & Pattison, 1989) have proposed that an increase in fetal liver dimensions is a good predictor of anaemia. Oepkes and coworkers (1993) measured the fetal splenic perimeter with ultrasound and noted that splenomegaly was present in all non-hydropic, anaemic fetuses. Splenomegaly predicted a haemoglobin deficit in excess of 5 standard deviations from the norm for gestational age with a sensitivity of 93%. However, several hydropic fetuses failed to exhibit splenomegaly. Another line of investigation for the non-invasive prediction of fetal anaemia is based on animal data indicating that fetal blood velocities in various circulatory beds increase secondary to an elevated cardiac output and a decline in blood viscosity (Fan *et al.*, 1980). Doppler ultrasound has been used to study blood velocities in fetal vessels, such as the umbilical vein (Warren, Gill & Fisher, 1987), descending thoracic aorta (Rightmire *et al.*, 1986), common carotid artery (Bilardo, Nicolaides & Campbell, 1989) and middle cerebral artery (Vyas, Nicolaides & Campbell, 1990). Unfortunately, the prediction of fetal haematocrit in these studies was disappointing.

Amniocentesis for OD_{450} measurements

Until the advent of FBS, measurement of amniotic fluid bilirubin was the primary means for determining the severity of fetal anaemia in haemolytic disease. Liley (1961) obtained amniotic fluid from 101 Rh-sensitized pregnancies between 27 and 41 weeks' gestation. Analysis of amniotic fluid from unaffected pregnancies revealed that the spectral absorption curve between 365 and 550 nm was approximately linear with a peak centred at 450 nm representing bilirubin. Liley derived the ΔOD_{450} value by subtracting the reading at 450 nm

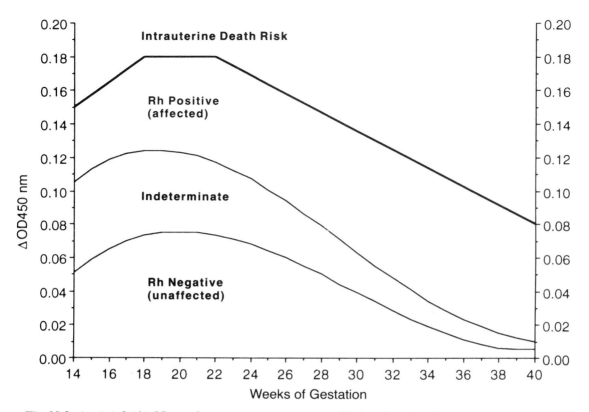

Fig. 10.2 *Amniotic fluid ΔOD_{450} value management zones based on gestational age. (Reproduced from Queenan et al. (1993); with permission from the C.V. Mosby Company.)*

from a line drawn between the spectral readings at 365 and 550 nm. He then used his data to delineate three zones related to gestational age. Values for ΔOD_{450} in the lower zone indicated a fetus with mild or no haemolytic disease while those in the upper zone indicated severe haemolytic disease with fetal death probable in 7 to 10 days. The Liley curve became the cornerstone of management for the pregnant patient with red cell alloimmunization. As neonatal survival at early gestational ages improved, 'modified' Liley curves were created by extrapolating the Liley zones backward to assess ΔOD_{450} values prior to 27 weeks of gestation. Nicolaides *et al.* (1986a) correlated fetal haematocrits obtained by FBS in 59 Rh-sensitized pregnancies between 18 and 25 weeks with ΔOD_{450} values from a 'modified' Liley curve. These authors found that 70% of anaemic fetuses had ΔOD_{450} values in the mid zone and

would, therefore, have been misdiagnosed as being only moderately affected. This single investigation led many centres to lose faith in amniocentesis as a useful tool for predicting fetal disease at early gestations. Queenan *et al.* (1993) published normal ΔOD_{450} values between 14 and 40 weeks' gestation based on 520 unaffected pregnancies (see Fig. 10.2). A further analysis of 163 amniotic fluid samples in 75 alloimmunized pregnancies resulted in the development of four new zones of management: an 'Rh-negative, unaffected' zone, an 'indeterminate' zone, a 'Rh-positive, affected' zone and an 'intrauterine death risk' zone. The authors recommended serial amniocenteses in the lower three zones and intrauterine transfusion or early delivery in the uppermost zone. Although these data have not been confirmed prospectively, a retrospective analysis of one centre's data has been undertaken using the Queenan graph. Fernandez *et al.* (1993) analysed all alloimmunized pregnancies and found that 14 antigen-positive fetuses had initial ΔOD_{450} values in the unaffected zone. Four of these fetuses required intrauterine transfusions and one required neonatal exchange transfusion. Unfortunately, the authors did not report how many of these 14 pregnancies involved alloimmunization to red cell antigen systems other than the RhD antigen.

Fetal blood sampling

Since its introduction by Daffos *et al.* (1983), FBS has come to play a major role in the treatment of haemolytic disease of the fetus. The technical aspects of this procedure are addressed in Chapter 2. Fetuses with severe anaemia do not appear to tolerate puncture of the umbilical vessels as well as fetuses with normal haematocrits and, therefore, a higher fetal mortality can be expected in these cases. Despite the risks associated with this procedure, direct access to the fetal circulation has provided new opportunities in the treatment of HDN. Normal values for fetal haematocrit (Leduc *et al.*, 1990), reticulocyte count (Nicolaides, Thilaganathan & Mibashan, 1989) and bilirubin (Weiner, 1992) have been determined. If paternal genotype testing for the particular red cell antigen involved in maternal alloimmunization reveals a heterozygous state, FBS can be used to obtain the blood type of the fetus. In half such cases, the specific antigen will be absent from the fetal red cells and the fetus will, therefore, be unaffected. In this situation, the fetus would no longer be at risk and further maternal or fetal testing is unnecessary. Although an attractive alternative to serial amniocenteses in pregnancies where the fetus may in fact be Rh negative, this approach is not without risk. If the placenta is located on the anterior wall of the uterus, the only access to the umbilical cord insertion for FBS may be directly through the placenta. An anamnestic response of the maternal immune system secondary to disruption of chorion villi with leakage of fetal cells into the maternal circulation has been reported in such situations (Nicolini *et al.*, 1988). This could lead to a worsening of fetal haemolytic disease in the 50% of patients where the fetal blood type is positive for the involved red cell antigen (MacGregor, Silver & Sholl, 1991). Therefore, if one is undertaking FBS for fetal blood typing, the placenta should be avoided and if necessary a floating loop of umbilical cord targeted.

Amniocentesis for fetal blood typing

Following the initial description of the RhD gene, Bennett *et al.* (1993) devised a series of DNA primers to be used in the diagnosis of the fetal Rh status. Utilizing the powerful technology of the polymerase chain reaction (PCR), 15 fetuses undergoing chorion villus biopsy and an additional 15 fetuses undergoing amniocentesis were correctly assessed for their Rh antigen status. These authors demonstrated the usefulness of this technique by averting the need for FBS for fetal blood typing in two of five patients in which the results of the DNA analysis were available to the clinician (Fisk *et al.*, 1994). More recently this group's updated experience with 135 amniocenteses was presented (Lighten *et al.*, 1995). One sample failed to amplify in the PCR reaction; 98 RhD-positive samples were confirmed by serology after the birth of these infants. In 36 cases where the PCR results indicated an RhD-negative fetus, two neonates were subsequently found to be RhD positive. In one, the fetus succumbed to hydrops fetalis at 28 weeks of gestation; the second fetus required neonatal exchange transfusions. Repeat PCR analysis after birth yielded an RhD positive result in both cases. These results would indicate a 1.5% false-negative rate for PCR analysis of amniotic fluid for RhD typing.

Williams *et al.* (1993) reported only one error when Bennett's primers were retrospectively used to type 347 stored samples of amniotic fluid. The one fetus that was incorrectly typed as Rh negative was felt to be the result of contamination of the amniotic fluid sample with maternal cells. We recently have developed our own set of DNA primers at Baylor College of Medicine (Van den Veyver *et al.*, 1995). Unlike previous strategies, we have elected to use a nested set of primers that does not incorporate exon 10 of the Rh gene but instead utilizes exon 7. To date, 108 amniotic fluid samples have been analysed in a prospective fashion. Two samples failed to amplify and no results were available. One hundred RhD-positive and six RhD-negative samples were confirmed by neonatal serology. Rossiter *et al.* (1994) have utilized a third set of primers and analysed 25 adult blood samples, including five weak D variants and one D mosaic. Their PCR technique agreed with serological testing in all cases. The authors went on to utilize their technique to analyse amniotic fluid samples from three ongoing pregnancies. One of the three fetuses was found to be Rh negative, obviating invasive studies.

More recently, several investigators have raised concerns regarding the accuracy of these PCR techniques in determining the fetal Rh status. Simsek (1994) evaluated 200 blood samples whose phenotype was known through standard serological testing. Three samples were incorrectly diagnosed as Rh positive when their corresponding serology revealed an Rh-negative blood type; two samples were misdiagnosed as Rh negative when their serology revealed an Rh-positive blood type. Simsek tested their own set of DNA primers and noted no errors in diagnosis. These discrepancies are likely to be the result of variations in the structure of the original gene proposed by Chérif-Bahir *et al.* (1990). Carritt and coworkers (1994) have reported that some patients who are serologically Rh negative may retain significant portions of the *D* gene. Such a case was detected in the Black race where the retention of exon 10 of an internally deleted *D* gene yielded a normal PCR product (Blunt, Daniels & Carritt, 1994). Additional examples include Rh-negative individuals with deletions of exons 7 through 9 or a stop codon in exon 5. Finally, in some individuals, RhD genes lacking certain exons may retain the capacity for a Rh-positive result with serological testing.

These discrepancies between serological typing and typing with DNA primer technology have important clinical implications. If a fetus is incorrectly typed as Rh positive using PCR, further invasive testing might be wrongly pursued by the physician. In the worst case scenario, an Rh-negative fetus could be lost when FBS is undertaken to assess the fetal haematocrit. In the case of a false-negative diagnosis, an Rh positive fetus mistyped as Rh negative, appropriate management would not be undertaken and a fetus could succumb to anaemia *in utero*. Currently, the DNA technology must be carefully utilized and not accepted as the gold standard for fetal typing when the father is heterozygous. Analysing paternal blood to confirm that a specific set of primers is accurate for detecting the presence of the RhD antigen would be one affirmative strategy. An alternative approach has been suggested by Bennett *et al.* (1994) and involves the use of multiple primer sets in a multiplex PCR reaction.

Spence and coworkers (1995) have pursued this diagnostic approach. Using two sets of primers, one specific for exons 4 and 5 and the other specific for exon 10 of the RhD gene, they correctly determined the RhD status of 50 fetuses by amniocentesis.

Fetal blood typing by maternal cell sorting

Clearly, a non-invasive technique for determining the fetal blood type would negate the risks of fetal loss and enhanced sensitization associated with fetal blood sampling or amniocentesis. Lo and coworkers (1993) were the first to study maternal blood for the presence of RhD-positive DNA of fetal origin. The technique proved accurate in detecting an RhD-positive fetus in 8 of 10 cases; one RhD-negative fetus yielded an RhD-positive result. More recently, fetal cell sorting from the maternal circulation correctly determined the fetal blood RhD type in 12 cases (Geifman-Holtzman *et al.*, 1995).

Diagnostic approach

With the advent of these new technologies, several diagnostic protocols are now available for the management of red cell alloimmunization in pregnancy. The spectrum of protocols ranges from the least invasive, utilizing only ultrasound, to a management scheme employing only FBS.

One approach advocates that serial ultrasounds be employed until overt hydrops fetalis is detected (U. Nicolini, personal communication). In this investigator's experience with fetuses requiring intrauterine transfusion, hydrops was not associated with increased perinatal mortality. This led to the recommendation that intrauterine transfusion should only be undertaken when early fetal ascites can be detected by ultrasound.

Other centres have abandoned amniocentesis as a useful tool for predicting fetal disease. Using haematocrit, reticulocyte count and direct Coombs' results obtained at FBS, Weiner *et al.* (1991) at the University of Iowa have described four patterns for the prediction of fetal anaemia (see Table 10.2). This algorithm was tested prospectively in 44 pregnancies at their centre (Weiner & Wenstrom, 1994). Two cases of unexpected neonatal anaemia occurred in the series. Further review revealed that one case was incorrectly managed according to their protocol secondary to an incorrect assessment of the fetal reticulocyte count.

At Baylor College of Medicine, we have chosen to follow a middle of the road approach (Fig. 10.3). Ultrasound is utilized as a surveillance tool but all efforts are made to detect fetal anaemia prior to the onset of overt hydrops. Amniocentesis is used as the initial step in invasive fetal testing as it has been associated with fewer

Table 10.2 *University of Iowa management scheme for red cell alloimmunization in pregnancy*

Haematocrit	Reticulocyte count	Direct Coombs' test	Interval for FBS (weeks)	Interval for ultrasound (weeks)	Comments
Normal	Normal	Negative–trace	–	4	If initial titre < 128, repeat titre in 4 weeks; if titre doubles, repeat FBS
Normal	Normal or decreased	1+ to 2+	5–6	2	Do not repeat FBS after 32 weeks; deliver at term
Normal	Elevated	3+ to 4+	2	1	Repeat FBS through 34 weeks if haematocrit stable; deliver after pulmonary maturity
<2 SD	Any	Any	1–2	1	Repeat FBS if haematocrit remains >30%; deliver after pulmonary maturity
<30%	Any	Any	–	–	Intrauterine transfusion

Modified from Weiner *et al.* (1991); reprinted with permission from the American Association of Blood Banks.

fetal complications than FBS. Paternal serotype and genotype testing are undertaken early in the course of evaluation. If the father is Rh negative, the fetus will be unaffected and further testing is not warranted if paternity is assured. In cases with a Rh positive father, maternal titres are repeated at monthly intervals until a critical titre is reached (16 at our institution). If the father is heterozygous, amniocentesis can be offered to determine fetal blood type. In cases of a homozygous paternal genotype or a fetus found to be Rh positive, serial amniocenteses are initiated at 26 to 27 weeks of gestation to determine ΔOD_{450} values. Repeat amniocenteses are performed at 10 to 14 day intervals until a ΔOD_{450} in the eightieth percentile of the 'Rh positive, affected' zone is noted. FBS is then performed with blood readied for intrauterine transfusion if the fetal haematocrit is found to be less than 30%.

In the pregnant patient whose previous child required either intrauterine transfusions or exchange transfusions after birth, a more aggressive management scheme is used at our institution. Titres are not used to guide management as their ability to predict fetal disease in a subsequent pregnancy has been questioned. Serial ultrasounds are initiated at 16 weeks' gestation and repeated every two weeks. At 20 to 22 weeks' gestation, an initial amniocentesis is performed and ΔOD_{450} values plotted on the Queenan curve. A decision to undertake intrauterine transfusion follows similar guidelines as the first affected pregnancy.

The management of Kell alloimmunization deserves special mention. Bowman *et al.* (1992) found that only 5% of live offspring born to sensitized Kell-negative women were affected by HDN. This is not unexpected in view of the fact that 91% of paternal blood typing will reveal a Kell-negative status. Early paternal testing for the Kell antigen will, therefore, eliminate the great majority of cases. Maternal antibody titres as low as 8 have been associated with hydrops fetalis (Bowman *et al.*, 1992). We, therefore, have reduced the critical titre for invasive testing in cases of Kell alloimmunization from 16 to 8 at our centre. With the successful cloning of the Kell gene, PCR primers for fetal blood typing by amniocentesis have been recently developed (N. M. Fisk, personal communication). Although FBS has been routinely used to determine the fetal antigen status in cases of a heterozygous paternal genotype, amniocentesis will probably gain widespread use for this indication in the near future. If the fetus is found to be Kell positive or, alternatively, if the father of the fetus is found to be homozygous for Kell, further invasive testing is problematic. Two investigations have compared Kell-affected fetuses to matched Rh-affected fetuses and noted a reduced haematopoietic response in association with the Kell-positive fetus (Vaughan *et al.*, 1994; Weiner & Wildness, 1995). In addition, Vaughan *et al.* (1994) noted lower ΔOD_{450} values associated with Kell antibodies. Other authors have also reported cases of low ΔOD_{450} values in association with severe fetal anaemia in Kell alloimmunization (Berkowitz, Beyth & Sadovsky, 1982; Barss *et al.*, 1985). These findings have led to proposals to use FBS as the sole means for evaluating fetal disease in Kell-sensitized pregnancies (Vaughan *et al.*, 1994). One should be cautious in using the algorithm of Weiner & Wenstrom (1994) to decide the need for further testing in these patients. Suppressed reticulocytosis in these pregnancies would lead to

erroneous conclusions regarding the need for subsequent FBS. In contrast, Bowman *et al.* (1992) have found amniotic fluid analysis to be 83% accurate for predicting fetal disease and have suggested that amniocentesis should remain the first line of invasive testing in these pregnancies. FBS is recommended when δOD_{450} values exceed the 65th percentile of the mid zone of a modified Liley curve. At our centre, we have chosen to follow Bowman's recommendations in the management of these pregnancies.

Because of the infrequency of the majority of other Rh antibodies (C, c, E, e) and other non-RhD red cell antibodies, diagnostic protocols are notably lacking from the literature. In these cases, we typically follow our algorithm for Rh disease.

Fig. 10.3 *Baylor College of Medicine management scheme for newly diagnosed red cell alloimmunization in pregnancy. (Modified from Moise, 1994.)*

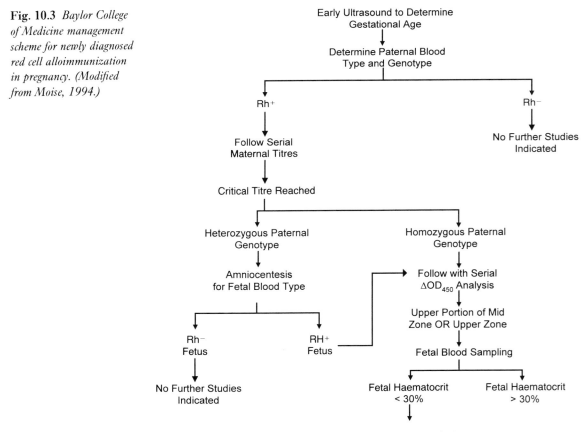

Intrauterine transfusion

Technique

The first successful treatment for haemolytic disease of the fetus was described by Liley (1963) when he introduced the technique of intraperitoneal transfusion (IPT). No further modifications in technique occurred until 1981. In that year, Rodeck et al. (1981) described the intravascular transfusion of the fetus by directing a needle into chorionic plate vessels under visualization through a fetoscope. The following year, a group in Denmark reported the intravascular transfusion (IVT) of a fetus by umbilical venous puncture under ultrasound guidance (Bang, Bock & Trolle, 1982). By 1986, two schools of thought had emerged regarding the optimal method for IVT. A group of investigators at Yale proposed an exchange intravascular technique similar to that used to treat HDN in the neonate (Grannum et al., 1986). Another group of researchers at Mt Sinai in New York advocated a direct transfusion technique similar to that used by the Danish investigators (Berkowitz et al., 1986). As more experience was gained with the two techniques, the direct IVT became more widely adopted by many centres because it had a shorter procedure time. Interest in IVT led to a virtual abandonment of the IPT by most centres treating red cell alloimmunization.

Prior to the advent of the IVT, it was generally accepted that the hydropic fetus appeared unable to absorb red cells effectively from its abdominal cavity after IPT (Lewis et al., 1973). Harman et al. (1990) compared the experience at one referral centre with IVT and IPT techniques with historical controls and demonstrated a marked improvement in survival of the hydropic fetus treated with IVT. It, therefore, appears that the IVT is advantageous in the hydropic fetus.

The routine use of only IVT as the method of intrauterine transfusion in the non-hydropic but anaemic fetus remains the topic of considerable debate. Complications not previously described in fetuses treated with IPT have been reported after IVT. Especially concerning is a case report of an unexplained porencephalic cyst after the procedure (Dildy et al., 1991). In addition, serial haematocrits from fetuses transfused with IVTs alone revealed a marked decline between procedures (Berkowitz et al., 1986). In order to avoid this problem, we began to evaluate whether a combined

IPT/IVT technique would result in a more stable fetal haematocrit between intrauterine transfusions (Moise et al., 1989a). Our technique involved administering enough packed red cells (haematocrit: 75–85%) by IVT to achieve a final fetal haematocrit of 35–40%. A standard IPT was then undertaken. Our hypothesis was that the intraperitoneal infusion of blood would serve as a reservoir allowing the slow absorption of red cells between procedures. Four transfusion techniques in 19 fetuses were compared. A combined direct IVT/IPT achieved a more stable fetal haematocrit compared with direct IVT alone: resulting in a decline in haematocrit of 0.01% per day between transfusions compared with a decline of 1.14% per day. Nicolini et al. (1989) also studied this technique. A final fetal haematocrit of 40% was achieved by IVT. The volume of blood (V ml) used for the IPT was calculated from the formula :

$$V = \frac{V_{IVT}\,(H_{post\text{-}IPT} - H_{post\text{-}IVT})}{(H_{post\text{-}IVT} - H_{pre\text{-}IVT})}$$

where V_{IVT} is the volume of IVT; $H_{post\text{-}IPT}$ is the final haematocrit desired post-IPT; $H_{pre\text{-}IVT}$ and $H_{post\text{-}IVT}$ are the values at the start of IVT and after IVT, respectively.

Assuming complete absorption of the blood infused into the peritoneal cavity, a theoretical final haematocrit of 50 to 60% was used by these investigators to determine the volume for the IPT. Although the decline in haematocrit per day was identical for IVT and IVT/IPT, the combined procedure achieved a significantly longer interval between transfusions and also maintained a higher initial fetal haematocrit at subsequent transfusion.

The endpoint for the completion of an intrauterine transfusion varies considerably. Most centres use a target haematocrit to decide when a transfusion is completed. Advocates of direct IVT will usually transfuse to a final value of 50 to 65%. This will allow for a reasonable interval between procedures based on a projected decline in haematocrit of 1% per day. However, one should be cautious in transfusing the fetus to nonphysiological values of haematocrit. Welch et al. (1994) demonstrated that a marked rise in whole blood viscosity is associated with fetal haematocrits above 50%. At our centre, we perform an IVT with a final target haematocrit of 35 to 40%. The volume of red blood cells to be transfused is calculated by first estimating the fetoplacental volume (FPC) (Mandelbrot et al., 1988). This volume (in ml) is equal to 1.046 + ultrasound-estimated fetal weight (in g × 0.14). The volume (in ml) to be transfused is:

$$V = \frac{FPC \ (H_{post\text{-}IVT} - H_{pre\text{-}IVT})}{H_{transfuse}}$$

where $H_{transfuse}$ is the haematocrit of the transfused blood.

A standard IPT is then undertaken (volume of blood to be transfused (ml) = (gestational age in weeks − 20)) (Bowman, 1978). Because the blood in the peritoneal reservoir will be absorbed over a 7 to 10 day period, fetal hyperviscosity can be prevented while maintaining a stable haematocrit between procedures. Subsequent intrauterine transfusions are scheduled at 14 day intervals until suppression of fetal erythropoiesis is noted on Kleihauer–Betke (K–B) stains. This usually occurs by the third intrauterine transfusion. Thereafter, the interval for repeat procedures can be determined based on the decline in haematocrit for the individual fetus, usually a three to four week interval.

The severely anaemic fetus at 18 to 24 weeks' gestation is less able to adapt to complete correction of its anaemia. Monitoring of the umbilical venous pressure during IVT has been found useful in such cases (Hallak et al., 1992). An increase of greater than 10 mmHg predicted fetal death within 24 hours after transfusion with a sensitivity of 80%. Radunovic et al. (1992) noted a 37% mortality within 72 hours of IVT in fetuses presenting with severe anaemia and hydrops. Based on their data, these authors recommended that, in the severely anaemic fetus, the final post-transfusion haematocrit after IVT should not exceed a value of 25% or a fourfold increase from the pretransfusion value. At our centre, we have chosen to use the umbilical venous pressure to determine when to conclude an IVT in a very anaemic fetus in the early second trimester. Periodic evaluation of the pressure is undertaken and the procedure concluded when the change in pressure approaches 10 mmHg. A second IVT is performed within 48 hours to correct the fetal haematocrit into the normal range; the third procedure is scheduled in 7 to 10 days. Thereafter, repeat transfusions are undertaken based on fetal haematocrits and K–B stains.

Another important development in the field of fetal transfusion has been the use of fetal paralysis during the procedure. Prior to this modification, fetal movement often resulted in injury to fetal viscera during IPT or umbilical cord damage during IVT. Fetal paralysis was first introduced by de Crespigny et al. (1985) in Australia. Initial use in the USA involved the intramuscular injection of (d)-tubocurarine into the fetal thigh under ultrasound guidance (Moise et al., 1987). Later, pancuronium bromide was used intravascularly (Moise et al., 1989b). More recently, short-acting agents such as atracurium besylate and vecuronium bromide have been utilized (Bernstein et al., 1988; Daffos et al., 1988). These latter agents do not appear to cause the fetal tachycardia and loss of short-term heart rate variability associated with pancuronium (Pielet et al., 1988). A vecuronium dose of 0.1 mg/kg ultrasound-estimated fetal weight produces immediate cessation of fetal movement after intravascular injection at the start of the intrauterine transfusion. Fetal paralysis can be expected for 1 to 2 hours. We have observed no untoward effects in neonates treated in this manner.

When IPTs were used as the sole means of in utero therapy, fetuses were routinely delivered at 32 weeks' gestation. Hyaline membrane disease and the need for neonatal exchange transfusions for the treatment of hyperbilirubinaemia were common. As experience with IVT became widespread, pregnancies were delivered at later gestational ages. Most authorities will now perform the final transfusion at up to 35 weeks' gestation, with delivery anticipated at 37 to 38 weeks. After a viable gestational age is attained, performing the transfusion in immediate proximity to the labour and delivery suite appears prudent so that operative delivery can be undertaken if fetal distress should occur.

In the past, O-negative, CMV-negative, allogeneic red blood cells were used as the primary source of blood for intrauterine transfusion. Patient concern regarding the transmission of human immunodeficiency virus (HIV) has led some to use maternal blood for intrauterine transfusion. Advantages include the availability of fresh blood and the decreased chance for sensitization to new red cell antigens if some of the transfused blood escapes back into the maternal circulation. In a series of 21 patients, up to 6 units of blood per patient were harvested for intrauterine transfusion (Gonsoulin et al.,

Table 10.3 *Literature review of intravascular intrauterine transfusions*

Authors	Technique	No. of patients	No. of survivors (total)	No. of survivors (hydrops)	No. of survivors (no hydrops)
Moise *et al.*, 1994	IVT/IPT	20	19	10	9
Weiner *et al.*, 1991	IVT	48	46	11	35
Rodeck *et al.*, 1991	IVT/IPT	18	16	16	0
Harman *et al.*, 1990	IVT	44	40	18	22
Pattison *et al.*, 1989	IVT	20	18	1	17
Poissonnier *et al.*, 1989	IVT/IPT	107	84	29	55
Lemery *et al.*, 1989	IVT	15	10	2	8
Nicolini *et al.*, 1989	IVT/IPT	30	25	NA	NA
Ronkin *et al.*, 1989	IVT	8	8	2	6
Parer *et al.*, 1988	IVT	5	4	NA	NA
Barss *et al.*, 1988	IVT/IPT	13	11	4	7
Orsini *et al.*, 1988	IVT	15	10	4	6
Grannum *et al.*, 1988	IVT	26	21	16	5
Socol *et al.*, 1987	IVT	3	3	3	0
Berkowitz *et al.*, 1986	IVT	8	6	2	4
Nicolaides *et al.*, 1986	IVT	18	17	10	7
Doyle *et al.*, 1986	IVT	8	5	0	5
DeCrespigny *et al.*, 1985	IVT	4	3	1	2
Bang *et al.*, 1982	IVT	1	1	1	0
Totals		411 (hydrops: 175) (no hydrops: 201)	347 (84%)	130 (74%)	188 (94%)

IVT, intravascular transfusion; IVT/IPT, combined intravascular and intraperitoneal transfusions; NA, not available.

1990). Supplementation with prenatal vitamins, folate and ferrous sulphate prevented maternal anaemia in all cases. No serious maternal or fetal effects were noted. The mother should undergo routine donor screening for syphilis, HIV, HTLV-1 and hepatitis B and C. The red cells are washed to remove the offending antibody, tightly packed to achieve a final haematocrit of 75 to 85% and then filtered through a leukocyte pore filter. Because the mother and fetus will share HLA antigens at many loci, the possibility of a graft-versus-host reaction must be considered. In order to avoid this complication, the maternal red cells are irradiated with 2500 Gy of external beam radiation. If the mother has antibody to the CMV virus, the blood may still be used as

the dormant CMV virus resides in the white blood cells that have been removed by the filtering process. On some occasions, an ABO incompatibility may be detected between the mother and her fetus after the initial FBS. We have used maternal blood in two such cases with no deleterious effects observed in the fetus. Follow-up at three years of age in one of these infants revealed anti-A and anti-B titres that were appropriate for age.

Survival

The survival rate after IVT varies with institution and experience. A review of the published series can be found in Table 10.3. An overall survival for 411 fetuses was 84%. Hydropic fetuses fared more poorly with a survival of 74% compared with 94% in their non-hydropic counterparts. A recent survey of 1087 IVTs undertaken in 389 fetuses at 16 centres in the USA and Canada revealed a survival rate for non-hydropic fetuses of 90% and a survival of 82% in hydropic fetuses (*Proceedings of the Fourth International Conference on Percutaneous Fetal Umbilical Blood Sampling*; October, 1989; Philadelphia, Pennsylvania).

Follow-up (short and long term)
Previous studies of infants treated with IPT alone revealed birthweights that were lower than matched controls (Binks, Lind & McNay, 1973). In contrast, a recent study by Roberts *et al.* (1993) revealed that fetuses treated with IVT demonstrated catch-up growth *in utero*. Birthweights in transfused fetuses were comparable to matched controls.

Immediate follow-up studies of infants treated with IVTs *in utero* have revealed a need for 'top-up' transfusions in the early months of life. Typically, these infants are born with a virtual absence of reticulocytes, with a red cell population consisting mainly of transfused red cells containing adult haemoglobin. Exchange transfusions for hyperbilirubinaemia are rarely necessary. However, at one month of age these infants often require a simple transfusion because of symptoms associated with anaemia. In our own series of 36 infants that had undergone intrauterine transfusions, 50% required top-up transfusions at a mean age of 38 days (range: 20 to 68 days) (Saade *et al.*, 1993). Of these, 11 of the 15 fetuses required only one transfusion while two fetuses required two transfusions and an additional two needed three transfusions. Newborns that required a late transfusion had a lower reticulocyte count at their last intrauterine transfusion, longer duration between their lowest fetal reticulocyte count and delivery, higher umbilical cord haemoglobin level at delivery and a higher percentage of adult red cells on cord K–B stain at delivery. Studies of these infants indicate erythroid hypoplasia of the bone marrow accompanied by low levels of circulating erythropoietin and reticulocytes (Koenig *et al.*, 1989). Therapeutic trials of exogenous erythropoietin to prevent the need for neonatal transfusions are currently in progress in this group of infants. Although the primary mechanism for the poor erythropoietin response is not understood, the low reticulocytosis is felt to be the result of high bone marrow levels of anti-D antibody. Since these infants do not require exchange transfusions in the immediate neonatal period, the passively acquired maternal antibody remains elevated in the neonatal circulation for at least six weeks. Because of this phenomenon, weekly haematocrit and reticulocyte determinations are recommended for the first one to two months of life in these infants (Millard *et al.*, 1990). One proposed criterion for transfusion includes a haemoglobin <5 to 6 g/dl in the symptom-free infant. In addition, any infant with symptoms related to anaemia, such as poor weight gain, lethargy or feeding difficulties, should be transfused.

Only one study has been published to date regarding the long-term neurological evaluation of fetuses successfully treated by IVT (Doyle *et al.*, 1993). In a series of 38 infants followed for two years, 35 of the children were noted to be developing normally. In the three remaining infants, no direct complications of IVT were felt to account for their abnormal development. Follow-up evaluations of fetuses treated with IPTs have revealed a higher incidence of inguinal hernias in males and an increased incidence of umbilical hernias in females compared with matched siblings (White *et al.*, 1978).

Alternative therapies
Oral administration of promethazine and Rh-positive cell fragments have been attempted in order to reduce the maternal anti-D response; however, both approaches did not prove effective (Gudson & Witherow, 1973; Gold *et al.*, 1983). Plasmapheresis has been successful in lowering antibody levels but fails to negate the need for intrauterine transfusions (Graham-Pole, Barr & Willoughby, 1977). This technique may have some application in the patient with a very high antibody titre associated with a history of recurrent pregnancy loss prior to 20 weeks of gestation. Its use may allow the pregnancy to continue until intrauterine transfusion becomes technically possible. The use of hyperimmune globulin (ivIgG) has been reported in two series. Chitkara *et al.* (1990) administered 1.0 g/kg ivIgG weekly in five patients with severe Rh and Kell alloimmunization. Despite the use of ivIgG, two to six intrauterine transfusions were required in these fetuses. More recently, Marguiles *et al.* (1991) administered a dose of 0.4 g/kg ivIgG every 15 to 21 days to 24 pregnant

women with severe Rh alloimmunization. The subjects were divided into three groups based on gestational age at the onset of therapy: group 1, <20 weeks; group 2, 20 to 28 weeks; group 3,>28 weeks. Only three fetal deaths occurred in groups 1 and 2; all were hydropic at the time of initiation of therapy. No fetus in the study developed hydrops during therapy. Thirteen patients had a previous pregnancy complicated by a fetal or neonatal death secondary to HDN. Only three fetal deaths occurred in these same patients treated with ivIgG in the study. The authors concluded that the use of ivIgG prior to 28 weeks' gestation was an effective method of treatment of severe Rh alloimmunization except in cases of hydrops fetalis. The exact mechanism by which ivIgG may work has yet to be elucidated (see Chapter 11). The large amount of exogenous IgG may saturate the Fc receptors of the placenta making the transfer of anti-D ineffective. Alternatively, pooled ivIgG may cross the placenta and suppress the fetal reticuloendothelial system. Both studies of ivIgG treatment for severe red cell alloimmunization in pregnancy revealed a decrease in maternal antibody titres during therapy. This may indicate a negative feedback effect through an anti-idiotype mechanism on the β-lymphocyte cell line that produces anti-D antibody.

Future therapy

Current therapy for red cell alloimmunization in pregnancy involves the use of intrauterine transfusion to alleviate fetal anaemia until the developing infant is mature enough to be removed from the hostile maternal environment. It is doubtful that improved survival can be achieved with additional advances in the technique of intrauterine transfusion. Alternative advances in the treatment of red cell alloimmunization must be sought.

One option for the sensitized patient with a history of repetitive fetal loss secondary to red cell alloimmunization and a heterozygous paternal genotype may involve the use of *in vitro* fertilization (Van den Veyver *et al.*, 1995). The cloning of the human Rh gene will allow blastocyst biopsy to be employed to determine the blood type of the developing embryo. Through this technique of preimplantation diagnosis, only Rh-negative embryos would then be transferred back into the uterus, guaranteeing an unaffected fetus.

In the case of a homozygous paternal genotype, preimplantation diagnosis would not be useful. Allo-immunization to paternal leukocyte antigens may have a role in the treatment of these patients. Anti-HLA antibodies formed in this manner may serve to block the Fc receptor-mediated functions of fetal monocytes and thereby inhibit the destruction of anti-D-sensitized fetal red blood cells. A total of 15 patients have been reported where the maternal ADCC assay, an *in vitro* test of antibody–antigen interaction, or a past history of a severely affected fetus should have predicted a severely affected fetus in a subsequent pregnancy (Dooren *et al.*, 1992; 1993; Eichler *et al.*, 1995). In all cases, the Rh-positive neonate survived with little or no intervention. Another attempt at immunomodulation of the maternal anti-D response may include the use of anti-idiotype antibodies. Both of these modalities are currently under investigation at our institution in a unique rabbit model for haemolytic disease of the newborn (Moise *et al.*, 1995b).

Parvovirus infection

Maternal infection with human parvovirus B19 has been associated with hydrops fetalis. The diagnostic evaluation of an exposed patient is illustrated in detail in Chapter 8.

Fetal infection is felt to occur during a window of 4 to 6 weeks after maternal infection, although hydrops has been reported as late as 12 weeks. Maternal infection prior to 20 weeks' gestation seems to represent the time period when the fetus is most susceptible to the development of hydrops. This may be secondary to the rapidly increasing red cell mass and the short half life of fetal red cells. Serial ultrasounds to check for the presence of hydrops fetalis should be performed on a weekly basis once maternal infection has been confirmed. These are continued for a total period of 10 to 12 weeks. Clearly some fetuses develop mild anaemia with recovery of their bone marrow before the development of overt hydrops. For this reason, FBS should be reserved for those cases complicated by hydrops fetalis. When hydrops is noted, donor red cells should be prepared and FBS performed. Fetal blood typically reveals a negative direct Coombs', anaemia, occasional thrombocytopenia, inappropriately low reticulocyte count, normal serum bilirubin levels, elevated total IgM and elevated hepatic enzymes (Peters & Nicolaides, 1990). Because there may be associated thrombocytopenia, our current practice is to have donor platelets readily available for concomitant transfusion if needed.

Several authors have reported spontaneous resolution of hydrops secondary to fetal parvovirus infection (Humphrey, Magoon, O'Shaugnessy, 1991; Pryde *et al.*, 1992). If a reticulocyte count performed on fetal blood before the first intrauterine transfusion reveals an elevated value, a second intrauterine transfusion is unwarranted as recovery of the fetal bone marrow is ongoing.

In some cases, non-immune hydrops may be found at the time of a routine ultrasound and the pregnant patient has an ambiguous history of exposure to parvovirus. Since maternal confirmatory testing may require a significant delay in treatment, proceeding with FBS appears to be a reasonable approach. If fetal anaemia is confirmed, intrauterine transfusion is performed. Maternal and fetal tests for confirmation of parvovirus would then dictate the need for subsequent transfusions.

A total of 10 fetuses are reported to have undergone treatment for confirmed parvovirus infection (Schwartz *et al.*, 1988; 1990; Peters & Nicolaides, 1990; Sahakian *et al.*, 1991; Soothill, 1990). All presented with hydrops and underwent IVT with an 80% rate of survival. Seven fetuses were transfused a single time, two fetuses twice and one fetus three times. As in the case in the fetus with immune hydrops, severe fetal anaemia should be corrected with serial transfusions at short intervals of one to seven days. An increase in the fetal reticulocyte count signals a recovery of the fetal bone marrow and negates the need for further transfusions. Experience with the anaemic Rh-positive fetus undergoing intrauterine transfusions would indicate that further transfusions may suppress fetal erythropoiesis and lead to fetal dependence on serial procedures to maintain the haematocrit. Congenital red cell aplasia, resulting in one death at nine months of age and transfusion dependency in two, has been reported in three infants with intrauterine parovirus infection who underwent repeated transfusions (Brown *et al.*, 1994). We, therefore, use a final fetal haematocrit of 30% as the endpoint for transfusion. Non-immune hydrops secondary to parvovirus infection may require several weeks before resolution after the fetal haematocrit has normalized.

Follow-up of infants transfused for parvovirus infection has revealed normal neonatal outcomes. Based on this limited data, IVT should be strongly considered as a therapeutic option in cases of fetal parvovirus infection in association with hydrops fetalis.

Fetomaternal haemorrhage

Significant fetomaternal haemorrhage is the aetiology of fetal mortality in 1 in 1000 births and fetal morbidity in 1 in 800 deliveries (Renaer, van de Putte & Vermylen, 1976). The use of intrauterine transfusion to treat this entity has been recently described in seven cases. In four, the patient presented with a chief complaint of decreased fetal movement, and subsequent fetal monitoring revealed a sinusoidal heart rate pattern (Fisher *et al.*, 1990; Rouse & Weiner, 1990; Elliot, 1991). In the remaining three patients, hydrops fetalis was noted as an incidental finding at the time of a routine ultrasound (Cardwell, 1988; Thorp *et al.*, 1992; Montgomery, Belfort & Adam, 1995). The maternal K–B stain was positive in all patients. A single intrauterine transfusion was performed in three patients, two procedures were undertaken in another three patients, and five procedures were undertaken in the remaining patient. Prolongation of pregnancy was achieved in three patients. In the first patient, an IPT at 21 weeks was successful in reversing hydrops fetalis with delivery of a normal infant at 38 weeks' gestation (Cardwell, 1988). Thorp *et al.* (1992) performed two IVTs at 26 and 27 weeks' gestation. Hydrops fetalis was noted to resolve and a normal infant was delivered at 39 weeks' gestation. In our own case, the fetus underwent five intrauterine transfusions beginning at 27 weeks' gestation (Montgomery *et al.*, 1995). A caesarean delivery of a 1740 g infant at 30 weeks was necessary because of chorioamnionitis. The infant was noted to have an initial haematocrit of 57% and experienced an uneventful neonatal course. In the other reported cases, fetal bradycardia or the return of decreased fetal movement necessitated delivery by caesarean section. Samplings in three of these fetuses revealed a falling haematocrit secondary to continued fetomaternal haemorrhage. It would, therefore, appear that the use of intrauterine transfusion in the treatment of fetomaternal haemorrhage may prove beneficial in selected cases involving extreme prematurity.

Conclusion

The dawn of successful fetal therapy began with the intraperitoneal infusion of red blood cells into the anaemic fetus affected by Rh alloimmunization. Major refinements in technique have now allowed for direct infusion of red cells into the fetal vascular space, with survival rates approaching 85%. Additional applications of intrauterine transfusion to patients with severe fetal anaemia secondary to fetomaternal haemorrhage and fetal parvovirus infection have also proved successful.

References

Asensio, S. H., Figueroa Longo, J. G. & Pelegrina, I. A. (1966). Intrauterine exchange transfusion. *American Journal of Obstetrics and Gynecology*, 95, 1129–33.

Asensio, S. H., Figueroa Longo, J. G. & Pelegrina, I. A. (1968). Intrauterine exchange transfusion. A new technique. *Obstetrics and Gynecology*, 32, 350–5.

Bang, J., Bock, J. E. & Trolle, D. (1982). Ultrasound-guided fetal intravenous transfusion for severe rhesus haemolytic disease. *British Medical Journal*, 284, 373–4.

Barss, V. A., Benacerraf, B. R., Frigoletto, F. D., Greene, M. F., Penso, C., Saltzman, D. H., Nadel, A., Heffner, L. J., Scherl, J. E. & Doubilet, P. M. (1988). Management of isoimmunized pregnancy by use of intravascular techniques. *American Journal of Obstetrics and Gynecology*, 159, 932–7.

Barss, V. A., Benacerraf. B. R., Greene, M. F., Phillippe, M. & Frigoletto, F. D. (1985). Sonographic detection of fetal hydrops. *Journal of Reproductive Medicine*, 30, 893–4.

Bennett, P. R., Kim, C. L., Colin, Y., Warwick, R. M., Chérif Zahar, B., Fisk, N. M. & Cartron, J.-P. (1993). Prenatal determination of fetal RhD type by DNA amplification following chorion villus biopsy or amniocentesis. *New England Journal of Medicine*, 329, 607–10.

Bennett, P., Warwick. R. & Cartron J.-P. (1994). Reply to letter to the editor: prenatal determination of fetal RhD type. *New England Journal of Medicine*, 330, 795–6.

Berkowitz, R. L., Beyth Y. & Sadovsky, E. (1982). Death *in utero* due to Kell sensitization without excessive elevation of the ΔOD_{450} value in amniotic fluid. *Obstetrics and Gynecology*, 60, 746–9.

Berkowitz, R. L., Chitkara, U., Goldberg, J. D., Wilkins, I., Chervenak, F. A. & Lynch, L. (1986). Intrauterine intravascular transfusions for severe red blood cell isoimmunization: ultrasound-guided percutaneous approach. *American Journal of Obstetrics and Gynecology*, 155, 574–81.

Bernstein, H. H., Chitkara, U., Plosker, H., Gettes, M. & Berkowitz, R. L. (1988). Use of atracurium besylate to arrest fetal activity during intrauterine intravascular transfusions. *Obstetrics and Gynecology*, 72, 813–16.

Bilardo, C. M., Nicolaides, K. H. & Campbell S. (1989). Doppler studies in red cell isoimmunization. *Clinics in Obstetrics and Gynecology*, 32, 719–27.

Binks, A. S., Lind, T. & McNay, R. A. (1973). Effects of rhesus haemolytic disease upon birthweight. *Journal of Obstetrics and Gynaecology of the British Commonwealth*, 80, 301–4.

Blunt, T., Daniels, G. & Carritt, B. (1994.) Serotype switching in a partially deleted RhD gene. *Vox Sanguinis*, 67, 397–401.

Bowell, P., Wainscoat J. S., Peto, T. E. & MacKenzie, Gunson, H. H. (1982). Maternal anti-D concentrations and outcome in rhesus haemolytic disease of the newborn. *British Medical Journal*, 285, 327–9.

Bowman, J. M. (1978). The management of Rh-isoimmunization. *Obstetrics and Gynecology*, 52, 1–16.

Bowman, J. M., Pollock, J. M., Manning, F. A., Harman, C. R. & Menticoglou, S. (1992). Maternal Kell blood group alloimmunization. *Obstetrics and Gynecology*, 79, 239–44.

Brown , K. E., Green, S. W., Antunez de Mayolo, J., Ballanti, J. A., Smith S. D., Smith, T. J. & Young, N. S. (1994). Congenital anaemia after transplacental B19 parovirus infection. *Lancet*, 343, 895–6.

Caine, M. E. & Mueller-Heubach, E. (1986). Kell sensitization in pregnancy. *American Journal of Obstetrics and Gynecology*, 154, 85–90.

Cardwell, M. S. (1988). Successful treatment of hydrops fetalis caused by fetomaternal hemorrhage. *American Journal of Obstetrics and Gynecology*, 158, 131–2.

Carritt, B., Steers, F. J. & Avent, N. D. (1994). Prenatal determination of fetal RhD type. *New England Journal of Medicine*, 344, 205–6.

Chavéz, G. F., Mulinare, J. & Edmonds, L. D. (1991). Epidemiology of Rh haemolytic disease of the newborn in the United States. *Journal of the American Medical Association*, 265, 3270–4.

Chérif Zahar, B., Bloy, C., Le Van Kim, C., Blanchard, D., Bailly, P., Hermand, P., Salmon, C., Cartron, J.-P. & Colin, Y. (1990). Molecular cloning and protein structure of a human group Rh polypeptide. *Proceedings of the National Academy of Science, USA*, 87, 6243–7.

Chitkara, U., Bussel, J., Alvarez, M., Lynch, L., Meisel R. L. & Berkowitz, R. L. (1990). High-dose intravenous gamma globulin: does it have a role in the treatment of severe erythroblastosis fetalis? *Obstetrics and Gynecology*, 76, 703–8.

Colin, Y., Chérif Zahar, B., Le Van Kim, C., Raynal, V., van Huffel, V. & Cartron, J. P. (1991). Genetic basis of the RhD positive and RhD negative blood group polymorphism as determined by Southern analysis. *Blood*, 78, 2747–52.

Daffos, F., Capella-Pavlovsky, M. & Forestier, F. (1983). A new procedure for fetal blood sampling *in utero*: preliminary results of 53 cases. *American Journal of Obstetrics and Gynecology*, 146, 985–7.

Daffos, F., Forestier, F., Mac Alesse, J., Aufrant, C., Mandelbrot, L., Cabanis, E. A., Iba-Zizen, M.T., Alfonso, J. M. & Tamaraz, J. (1988). Fetal curarization for prenatal magnetic resonance imaging. *Prenatal Diagnosis*, 8, 311–4.

de Crespigny, L., Robinson, H. P., Quinn, M., Doyle, L., Ross, A. & Cauchi, M. (1985). Ultrasound-guided fetal blood transfusion for severe rhesus isoimmunization. *Obstetrics and Gynecology*, 66, 529–32.

Dildy, G. A., Smith, L. G., Moise, K. J., Cano, L. E. & Hesketh D. E. (1991). Porencephalic cyst: a complication of fetal intravascular transfusion. *American Journal of Obstetrics and Gynecology*, 165, 76–8.

Dooren, M. C., Kuijpers, R. W., Joekes, E. C., Huiskes, E., Goldschmeding, R., Overbeeke, E. C., von dem Borne, A. E., Engelfriet, C. P. & Ouwehand, W. H. (1992). Protection against immune hemolytic disease of newborn infants by maternal monocyte-reactive IgG alloantibodies (anti-HLA-DR). *Lancet*, 339, 1067–70.

Dooren, M. C., van Kamp, I. L., Kanhai, H. H., Gravenhorst, J. B., von dem Borne, A. E. & Engelfriet, C. P. (1993). Evidence of the protective effect of maternal FcR-blocking IgG alloantibodies HLA-DR in Rh D-hemolytic disease of the newborn. *Vox Sanguinis*, 66, 55–8.

Doyle, L. W., Cauchi, M., de Crespigny, L. C. Robinson, H., Barrie, J., Young, J. & Quinn, M. A. (1986). Fetal intravascular transfusion for severe erythroblastosis: effects on hematology and survival. *Australian and New Zealand Journal of Obstetrics and Gynecology*, 26, 192–5.

Doyle, L. W., Kelley, E. A., Rickards, A. L., Ford, G. W. & Callanan, C. (1993). Sensorineural outcome at 2 years for survivors of erythroblastosis treated with fetal intravascular transfusions. *Obstetrics and Gynecology*, 81, 931–5.

Eichler, H., Zieger, W., Neppert, J., Kerowgan, M., Melchert, F. & Goldmann, S. F. (1995). Mild course of fetal RhD hemolytic disease due to maternal alloimmunisation to paternal HLA class I and II antigens. *Vox Sanguinis*, 68, 243–7.

Elliot, J. P. (1991). Massive fetomaternal hemorrhage treated by fetal intravascular transfusion. *Obstetrics and Gynecology*, 78, 520–3.

Fan, F.-C., Chen. R. Y., Schuessler, G. B. & Chien, S. (1980). Effects of hematocrit variations on regional hemodynamics and oxygen transport in the dog. *American Journal of Physiology*, 238, H545–52.

Fernandez, C. O., Wendel, P. J. & Brown C. L. (1993). Rh immunization: an evaluation of a proposed new clinical management protocol. *41st Annual Meeting of the Society for Gynecologic Investigation*. Chicago, Illinois.

Fisher, R. L., Kuhlman, K., Grover, J., Montgomery, O. & Wapner, R. J. (1990). Chronic, massive fetomaternal hemorrhage treated with repeated fetal intravascular transfusions. *American Journal of Obstetrics and Gynecology*, 162, 203–4.

Fisk, N. M., Bennett, P., Warwick, R. M., Letsky, E. A., Welch, R., Vaughan, J. & Moore, G. (1994). Clinical utility of fetal RhD typing in alloimmunized pregnancies by means of polymerase chain reaction on amniocytes or chorionic villi. *American Journal of Obstetrics and Gynecology*, 171, 50–4.

Freda, V. J. & Adamsons, K. (1964). Exchange transfusion *in utero*: report of a case. *American Journal of Obstetrics and Gynecology*, 89, 817–21.

Geifman-Holtzman, O., Bernstein, I. M., Berry, S. M. & Bianchi, D. W. (1995). Prenatal diagnosis of fetal rhesus (Rh) C, D, E type by polymerase chain reaction (PCR). *American Journal of Obstetrics and Gynecology*, 172, 265.

Gold, W. R., Queenan, J. T., Woody, J. & Sacher, R. A. (1983). Oral desensitization in Rh disease. *American Journal of Obstetrics and Gynecology*, 146, 980–1.

Gonsoulin, W. J., Moise, K. J., Milam, J. D., Sala, J. D., Weber, V. W. & Carpenter, R. J. (1990). Serial maternal blood donations for intrauterine transfusion. *Obstetrics and Gynecology*, 75, 158–62.

Graham-Pole, J., Barr, W. & Willoughby, M. L. (1977). Continuous-flow plasmapheresis in management of severe rhesus disease. *British Medical Journal*, i, 1185–8.

Grannun, P. A., Copel, J. A., Moya, F. R., Scioscia, A. L., Robert, J. A., Winn, H. N., Coster, B. C., Burdine, C. B. & Hobbins, J. C. (1988). The reversal of hydrops fetalis by intravascular intrauterine transfusion in severe isoimmune fetal anemia. *American Journal of Obstetrics and Gynecology*, 158, 914–19.

Grannum, P. A., Copel, J. A., Plaxe, S. C., Scioscia, A. L. & Hobbins, J. C. (1986). In utero exchange transfusion by direct intravascular injection in severe erythroblastosis fetalis. *New England Journal of Medicine*, 314, 1431–4.

Gudson, J. P. & Witherow, C. (1973). Possible ameliorating effects of erythroblastosis by promethazine hydrochloride. *American Journal of Obstetrics and Gynecology*, 117, 1101–8.

Hadley, A. G., Kumpel, B. M., Leader, K. A., Poole, G. D. & Fraser, I. D. (1991). Correlation of serologic, quantitative and cell-mediated functional assays of maternal alloantibodies with the severity of haemolytic disease of the newborn. *British Journal of Haematology*, 77, 221–8.

Hallak, M., Moise, K. J. & Hesketh, D. E., Cano, L. E. & Carpenter, R. J. (1992). Intravascular transfusion of fetuses with rhesus incompatibility: prediction of fetal outcome by changes in umbilical venous pressure. *Obstetrics and Gynecology*, 80, 286–90.

Harman, C. R., Bowman, J. M., Manning, F. A. & Menticoglou, S. M. (1990). Intrauterine transfusion–intraperitoneal versus intravascular approach: a case-control comparison. *American Journal of Obstetrics and Gynecology*, 162, 1053–9.

Hughes, R. G., Craig, J. I., Murphy, W. G. & Greer, I. A. (1994). Causes and clinical consequences of Rhesus (D) haemolytic disease of the newborn: a study of a Scottish population. *British Journal of Obstetrics and Gynaecology*, 101, 297–300.

Humphrey, W., Magoon, M. & O'Saughnessy, R. (1991). Severe non-immune hydrops secondary to parvovirus B19 infection: spontaneous reversal *in utero* and survival of a term infant. *Obstetrics and Gynecology*, 78, 900–2.

Hussey, R. M. & Clarke, C. C. (1991). Deaths from Rh haemolytic disease in England and Wales in 1988 and 1989. *British Medical Journal*, 303, 445–6.

Koenig J. M., Ashton R. D., DeVore G. R. & Christensen, R. D. (1989). Late hypogenerative anemia in Rh haemolytic disease. *Journal of Pediatrics*, 115, 315–18.

Leduc, L., Moise, K. J., Carpenter, R. J. & Cano, L. E. (1990). Fetoplacental blood volume estimation in pregnancies with Rh alloimmunization. *Fetal Diagnosis and Therapy*, 5, 138–46.

Lemery, D., Urbain, M. F., van Lieferinghen, P., Micorek, J. C. & Jacquetin B. (1989). Intrauterine exchange transfusion under ultrasound guidance. European Journal of *Obstetrics and Gynecology and Reproductive Biology*, 33, 161–8.

Lewis, M., Bowman, J. M., Pollock, J. & Lowen, B. (1973). Absorption of red cells from the peritoneal cavity of an hydropic twin. *Transfusion*, 13, 37–40.

Lighten, A., Overton, T., Sepulveda, W., Warwick, R. M., Fisk, N. M. & Bennett, P. R. (1995). Accuracy of prenatal determination of RhD type status by polymerase chain reaction using amniotic cells in RhD-negative women. *American Journal of Obstetrics and Gynecology*, 173, 1182–5.

Liley, A. W. (1961). Liquor amnii analysis in the management of the pregnancy complicated by rhesus sensitization. *American Journal of Obstetrics and Gynecology*, 82, 1359–70.

Liley, A. W. (1963). Intrauterine transfusion of foetus in haemolytic disease. *British Medical Journal*, ii, 1107–9.

Lo, Y.-M. D., Bowell, P. J., Selinger, M., Mackenzie, I. Z., Chamberlain, P., Gillmer, M. D., Littlewood, T. J., Fleming, K. A. & Wainscoat J. S. (1993). Prenatal determination of the fetal RhD status by analysis of peripheral blood of rhesus negative mothers. *Lancet*, 341, 1147–8.

Lomas, C., Tippett, P., Thompson, K. M., Melamed, M. D., Hughes Jones, N. C. (1989). Demonstration of seven epitopes on the Rh antigen D using human monoclonal anti D antibodies and red cells from D categories. *Vox Sanguinis*, 57, 261–4.

MacGregor, S. N., Silver, R. K. & Sholl, J. S. (1991). Enhanced sensitization after cordocentesis in a rhesus-isoimmunized pregnancy. *American Journal of Obstetrics and Gynecology*, 165, 382–3.

Mandelbrot, L., Daffos, F., Forestier, F., MacAleese, J. & Descombey, D. (1988). Assessment of fetal blood volume for computer assisted management of *in utero* transfusion. *Fetal Therapy*, 3, 60–6.

Margulies, M., Voto, L. S., Mathet, E. & Margulies, M. (1991). High dose intravenous IgG for the treatment of severe Rhesus alloimmunization. *Vox Sanguinis*, 61, 181–9.

Millard, D. D., Gidding, S. S., Socol, M. L., MacGregor, S. N., Dooley, S. L., Ney, J. A. & Stockman, J. A. (1990). Effects of intravascular, intrauterine transfusion on prenatal and postnatal hemolysis and erythropoiesis in severe fetal isoimmunization. *Journal of Pediatrics*, 117, 447–54.

Moise, K. J. (1994). Changing trends in the management of red cell alloimmunization in pregnancy. *Archives of Pathology and Laboratory Medicine*, 118, 421–8.

Moise, K. J., Carpenter, R. J., Deter, R. L., Kirshon, B. & Diaz, S. F. (1987). The use of fetal neuromuscular blockade during intrauterine procedures. *American Journal of Obstetrics and Gynecology*, 157, 874–9.

Moise, K. J., Carpenter, R. J., Kirshon, B., Deter, R. L., Sala, J. D. & Cano, L. E. (1989a). Comparison of four types of intrauterine transfusion: Effect on fetal hematocrit. *Fetal Therapy*, 4, 126–37.

Moise, K. J., Deter, R. L., Kirshon, B., Adam, K., Patton, D. E. & Carpenter, R. J. (1989b). Intravenous pancuronium bromide for fetal neuromuscular blockade during intrauterine transfusion for red cell alloimmunization. *Obstetrics and Gynecology*, 74, 905–8.

Moise, K. J., Perkins, J. T., Sosler, S. D., Brown, S. J., Saade, G., Carpenter, R. J., Thorp, J. A., Ludomirski, A., Wilkins, I. A., Grannum, P. A. & Copel, J. (1995a). The predictive value of maternal serum testing for the detection of fetal anemia in red cell alloimmunization. *American Journal of Obstetrics and Gynecology*, 172, 1003–9.

Moise, K. J., Rodkey, L. S., Saade, G. R., Duré, M., Dorman, K., Mayes, M. & Graham, A. (1995b). An animal model for hemolytic disease of the fetus and newborn. II. Fetal effects in New Zealand rabbits. *American Journal of Obstetrics and Gynecology*, 173, 747–53.

Mollison, P. L. (1994). The genetic basis of the Rh blood group system. *Transfusion*, 34, 539–41.

Montgomery, L. D. , Belfort, M. A. & Adam, K. (1995). Massive feto-maternal hemorrhage treated with serial combined intravascular and intra-peritoneal fetal transfusions. *American Journal of Obstetrics and Gynecology*, 172, 234–5.

Morley, G., Gibson, M. & Eltringham, D. (1977). Use of discriminant analysis in relating maternal anti-D levels to the severity of haemolytic disease of the newborn. *Vox Sanguinis*, 32, 90–8.

Mouro, I., Colin, Y., Chérif Zahar, B., Cartron, J.-P. & Le Van Kim, C. (1993). Molecular genetic basis of the human Rhesus blood group system. *Nature Genetics*, 5, 62–5.

Mouro, I., Le Van Kim, C., Rouillac, C., van Rhenen, D. J., Le Pennec, P. Y., Bailly, P., Cartron, J. P. & Colin, Y. (1994). Rearrangements of the blood group RhD gene associated with the DVI category phenotype. *Blood*, 83, 1129–35.

Nance, S. J., Nelson, J. M., Horenstein, J., Ardnt, P. A., Platt, L. A. & Garratty, G. (1989). Monocyte monolayer assay: an efficient noninvasive technique for predicting the severity of hemolytic disease of the newborn. *American Journal of Clinical Pathology*, 92, 89–92.

Nicolaides, K. H., Fontanarosa, M., Gabbe, S. G. & Rodeck, C. H. (1988). Failure of ultrasonographic parameters to predict the severity of fetal anemia in rhesus isoimmunization. *American Journal of Obstetrics and Gynecology*, 158, 920–6.

Nicolaides, K. H., Rodeck, C. H., Mibashan, R. S. & Kemp, J. R. (1986a). Have Liley charts outlived their usefulness? *American Journal of Obstetrics and Gynecology*, 155, 90–4.

Nicolaides, K. H., Soothill, P. W., Rodeck, C. H. & Clewell, W. (1986b). Rh disease: intravascular fetal blood transfusion by cordocentesis. *Fetal Therapy*, 1, 185–92.

Nicolaides, K. H., Thilaganathan, B. & Mibashan, R. S. (1989). Cordocentesis in the investigation of fetal erythropoiesis. *American Journal of Obstetrics and Gynecology*, 161, 1197–2000.

Nicolini, U., Kochenour, N. K., Greco, P., Letsky, E. A., Johnson, R. D., Contreras, M. & Rodeck, C. H. (1988). Consequences of fetomaternal haemorrhage after intrauterine transfusion. *British Medical Journal*, 297, 1379–81.

Nicolini, U., Kochenour, N. K., Greco, P., Letsky, E. & Rodeck, C. H. (1989). When to perform the next intra-uterine transfusion in patients with Rh allo-immunization: combined intravascular and intraperitoneal transfusion allows longer intervals. *Fetal Therapy*, 4, 14–20.

Oepkes, D., Meerman, R. H., Vandenbussche, F. P., van Kamp, I. L., Kok, F. G. & Kanhai, H. H. (1993). Ultrasonographic fetal spleen measurements in red blood cell alloimmunized pregnancies. *American Journal of Obstetrics and Gynecology*, 69, 121–8.

Orsini, L. F., Pilu, G., Calderoni, P., Zucchini, S., Tripoli, N., Pittalis, M. C., Brondelli, L., Gabrielli, S., Sermasi, G. & Bovicelli, L. (1988). Intravascular intrauterine transfusion for severe erythroblastosis fetalis using different techniques. *Fetal Therapy*, 3, 50–9.

Pattison, N. & Roberts, A. (1989). The management of the severe erythroblastosis fetalis by fetal transfusion: survival of transfused adult erythrocytes in the fetus. *Obstetrics and Gynecology*, 74, 901–4.

Peters, M. T. & Nicolaides, K. H. (1990). Cordo-centesis for the diagnosis and treatment of human fetal parvovirus infection. *Obstetrics and Gynecology*, 75, 501–4.

Pielet, B. W., Socol, M. L., MacGregor, S. N., Dooley, S. L. & Minogue, J. (1988). Fetal heart rate changes after fetal intravascular treatment with pancuronium bromide. *American Journal of Obstetrics and Gynecology*, 159, 640–3.

Poissonnier, M. H., Brossard, Y., Demedeiros, N, Vassileva, J., Parnet, F., Larsen, M., Gosset, M., Chavinie, J. & Huchet, J. (1989). Two hundred intrauterine exchange transfusions in severe blood incompatibilities. *American Journal of Obstetrics and Gynecology*, 161, 709–13.

Pryde, P. G., Nugent, C. E., Pridjian, G., Barr, M., & Faix, R. G. (1992). Spontaneous resolution of nonimmune hydrops fetalis secondary to human parvovirus B19 infection. *Obstetrics and Gynecology*, 79, 859–61.

Queenan, J. T., Tomai, T. P., Ural, S. H. & King, J. C. (1993). Deviation in the amniotic fluid optical density at a wavelength of 450 nm in Rh-immunized pregnancies from 14 to 40 weeks' gestation: a proposal for clinical management. *American Journal of Obstetrics and Gynecology*, 168, 1370–6.

Race, R. R. (1944). An 'incomplete' antibody in human serum. *Nature*, 153, 771–2.

Radunovic, N., Lockwood, C. J., Alvarez, M., Plecas, D., Chitkara, U. & Berkowitz, R. L. (1992). The severely anemic and hydropic isoimmmune fetus: changes in fetal hematocrit associated with intra-uterine death. *Obstetrics and Gynecology*, 79, 390–3.

Renaer, M., Van de Putte, I. & Vermylen, C. (1976). Massive fetomaternal hemorrhage as a cause of perinatal mortality and morbidity. *European Journal of Obstetrics and Gynecology and Reproductive Biology*, 6, 125–40.

Rightmire, D. A., Nicolaides, K. H., Rodeck, C. H. & Campbell S. (1986). Fetal blood velocities in Rh isoimmunization: relationship to gestational age and to fetal hematocrit. *Obstetrics and Gynecology*, 68, 233–6.

Roberts, A., Grannum, P., Belanger, K., Pattison, N. & Hobbins, J. (1993). Fetal growth and birthweight in isoimmunized pregnancies after intravenous intrauterine transfusion. *Fetal Diagnosis and Therapy*, 8, 407–11.

Roberts, A. B., Mitchell, J. M. & Pattison, N. S. (1989). Fetal liver length in normal and isoimmunized pregnancies. *American Journal of Obstetrics and Gynecology*, 161, 42–6.

Rodeck, C. H., Kemp, J. R., Holman, C. A., Whitmore, C. A., Karnicki, J. & Austin, M. A. (1981). Direct intravascular fetal blood transfusion by fetoscopy in severe Rhesus isoimmunization. *Lancet*, i, 625–7.

Ronkin, S., Chayen, B., Wapner, R. J., Blocklinger, A., Davis, G., Roberts, N. & Hux, C. H. (1989). Intravascular exchange and bolus transfusion in the severely isoimmunized fetus. *American Journal of Obstetrics and Gynecology*, 160, 407–11.

Rossiter, J. P., Blakemore, K. J., Kickler, T. S., Kasch, L. M., Khouzami, A. N., Pressman, E. K., Sciscione, A. C. & Kazazian, H. H. (1994). The use of polymerase chain reaction to determine fetal RhD status. *American Journal of Obstetrics and Gynecology*, 171, 1047–51.

Rouse, D. & Weiner, C. (1990). Ongoing fetomaternal hemorrhage treated by serial fetal intravascular transfusions. *Obstetrics and Gynecology*, 76, 974–5.

Saade, G. R., Moise, K. J., Belfort, M. A. , Hesketh, D. E. & Carpenter, R. J. (1993). Fetal and neonatal hematologic parameters in red cell alloimmunization: predicting the need for late neonatal transfusions. *Fetal Diagnosis and Therapy*, 8, 161–4.

Sacks, D. A., Nance, S. J., Garratty, G., Petrucha, R. A., Zhorenstein, J. & Fotheringham, N. (1993). Monocyte monolayer assay as a predictor of severity of hemolytic disease of the fetus and newborn. *American Journal of Perinatology*, 10, 428–31.

Sahakian, V., Weiner, C. P., Naides, S. J., Williamson, R. A. & Scharosch, L. L. (1991). Intrauterine transfusion treatment of nonimmune hydrops fetalis secondary to human parvovirus B19 infection. *American Journal of Obstetrics and Gynecology*, 164, 1090–1.

Schwartz, T. F., Nerlich, A. & Roggendorf, M. (1990). Parvovirus B19 infection in pregnancy. *Behring Institute Mitteilungen*, 85, 69–73.

Schwarz, T. F., Roggendorf, M., Hottenträer, B., Deinhardt, F., Enders, G., Gloning, K.P., Schramm, T. & Hansmann, M. (1988). Human parvovirus B19 infection in pregnancy. *Lancet*, 1, 655–7.

Simsek, S., Bleeker, P. M. & van dem Borne, A. E. (1994). Prenatal determination of fetal RhD type. *New England Journal of Medicine*, 330, 795–6.

Socol, M. L., MacGregor, S. N., Pielet, B. W., Tamura, R. K. & Sabbagha, R. E. (1987). Percutaneous umbilical transfusion in severe rhesus isoimmunization: resolution of fetal hydrops. *American Journal of Obstetrics and Gynecology*, 157, 1369–75.

Solola, A., Sibai, B. & Mason, J. M. (1983). Irregular antibodies: an assessment of routine prenatal screening. *Obstetrics and Gynecology*, 61, 25–30.

Soothill, P. (1990). Intrauterine blood transfusion for non-immune hydrops fetalis due to parvovirus B19 infection. *Lancet*, 335, 121–2.

Spence, W. C., Maddalena, A., Demers, D. B. & Bick, D. P. (1995). Molecular analysis of the RhD genotype in fetuses at risk for RhD hemolytic disease. *Obstetrics and Gynecology*, 85, 296–8.

Thorp, J. A. , Cohen, G. R., Yeast, J. D., Perryman, D., Welsh, C., Honssinger, N., Stephenson, S. & Hedrick, J. (1992). Nonimmune hydrops caused by massive fetomaternal hemorrhage and treated by intravascular transfusion. *American Journal of Perinatology*, 9, 22–4.

Urbaniak, S. J., Greiss, M. A. , Crawford, R. J. & Fergusson M. C. (1984). Prediction of the outcome of rhesus haemolytic disease of the newborn: additional information using an ADCC assay. *Vox Sanguinis*, 46, 323–9.

Van den Veyver, I. B., Chong, S. S., Cota, J., Bennett, P. R., Fisk, N. M., Handyside, A. H., Cartron, J.-P., Kim, C. L., Colin, Y., Snabes, M. C., Moise, K. J. & Hughes, M. R. (1995). Single cell analysis of the rhesus D blood type for use in preimplanation diagnosis in the prevention of severe hemolytic disease of the newborn. *American Journal of Obstetrics and Gynecology*, 172, 533–40.

Vaughan, J. I., Warwick, R., Letsky, E., Nicolini, U., Rodeck, C. H. & Fisk, N. M. (1994). Erythropoietic suppression in fetal anemia because of Kell alloimmunization. *American Journal of Obstetrics and Gynecology*, 171, 247–52.

Vintzileos, A. M., Campbell, W. A., Storlazzi, E., Mirochnick, M. H., Escoto, D. T. & Nochimson, D. J. (1986). Fetal liver ultrasound measurements in isoimmunized pregnancies. *Obstetrics and Gynecology*, 68, 162–7.

Vyas, S., Nicolaides, K. H. & Campbell, S. (1990). Doppler examination of the middle cerebral artery in anemic fetuses. *American Journal of Obstetrics and Gynecology*, 162, 1066–8.

Warren, P. S., Gill, R. W. & Fisher, C. C. (1987). Doppler flow studies in rhesus isoimmunization. *Seminars in Perinatology*, 11, 375–8.

Weiner, C. P. (1992). Human fetal bilirubin levels and fetal hemolytic disease. *American Journal of Obstetrics and Gynecology*, 166, 1449–54.

Weiner, C. P. & Wenstrom, K. D. (1994). Outcome of alloimmunized fetuses managed soley by cordocentesis but not requiring antenatal transfusion. *Fetal Diagnosis and Therapy*, 9, 233–8.

Weiner, C. & Wildness, J. (1995). Decreased erythropoiesis and hemolysis in Kell hemolytic disease. *American Journal of Obstetrics and Gynecology*, 172, 277.

Weiner, C. P., Williamson, R. A., Wenstrom, K. D., Sipes, S. L., Grant, S. S. & Widness, J. A. (1991). Management of fetal hemolytic disease by cordocentesis I. Prediction of fetal anemia. *American Journal of Obstetrics and Gynecology*, 165, 546–53.

Weinstein, L. (1982). Irregular antibodies causing hemolytic disease of the newborn: a continuing problem. Clinics in *Obstetrics and Gynecology*, 25, 321–32.

Welch, R., Rampling, M. W., Anwar, A., Talbert, D. G. & Rodeck, C. H. (1994). Changes in hemorheology with fetal intravascular transfusion. *American Journal of Obstetrics and Gynecology*, 170, 726–32.

White, C. A., Goplerud, C. P., Kisker, C. T., Stehbens, J. A., Kitchell, M. & Taylor, J. C. (1978). Intrauterine fetal transfusion, 1965–1976, with an assessment of the surviving children. *American Journal of Obstetrics and Gynecology*, 130, 933–42.

Wiener, A. S. (1943). Genetic theory of the Rh blood types. *Proceedings of the Society of Experimental Biology in Medicine*, 54, 316–9.

Williams, J., Baker, J., Dildy, G. & Ward, K. (1993). Rhesus D blood typing of the fetus at risk for isoimmunization using DNA from amniotic fluid. *41st Annual Meeting of the Society for Gynecologic Investigation*. Chicago, Illinois.

Zipursky, A. & Israels, L. G. (1967). The pathogenesis and prevention of Rh immunization. *Canadian Medical Association Journal*, 97, 1245–57.

11   Fetal thrombocytopenia

HELEN KELSEY AND CHARLES RODECK

Introduction

Fetal and neonatal thrombocytopenia (TP) predisposes to haemorrhage in the perinatal period. Neonatal TP, if severe ($<50 \times 10^9$/l), may lead to bleeding and/or death. Intracerebral haemorrhage (ICH) is the most serious complication, leading to death or to permanent neurological sequelae. Although delivery is a time of major risk for ICH in the thrombocytopenic fetus, there is evidence that ICH can occur *in utero* as early as 20 weeks' gestation (Bussel, McFarland & Berkowitz, 1990; Herman *et al.*, 1986). This may result in porencephaly or fetal loss (Friedman & Aster, 1985). Fetal anaemia may result from visceral haemorrhage (Kaplan, Dehan & Tchernia, 1992).

Megakaryocytes are found from 12 weeks' gestation in the fetal liver and lung. The platelet count in the normal fetus increases with gestation, reaching the normal adult range at about 18 weeks (Daffos *et al.*, 1988; Gruel *et al.*, 1986; Millar *et al.*, 1985; Van den Hof & Nicolaides, 1990). The finding of a low platelet count in the fetus or neonate warrants further investigation.

The incidence of TP, defined as $<150 \times 10^9$/l, in neonates has been found to be 4.1% (Burrows & Kelton, 1988), with 0.15% having counts $<10 \times 10^9$/l (Burrows & Kelton, 1988). A higher incidence of 25 to 40% is noted in special care baby units with 3% $<50 \times 10^9$/l (Kaplan *et al.*, 1992). Immune destruction of fetal and neonatal platelets by passively acquired maternal antibodies is an important cause of TP in an otherwise well infant. Other causes of TP are usually associated with an obvious clinical picture. This chapter will be concerned with the passive immune fetal and neonatal TPs, alloimmune and autoimmune.

Immunology of fetal thrombocytopenias

The neonatal TP caused by passively acquired maternal antibodies, although transient, is often severe. In addition, the fetus is frequently thrombocytopenic before delivery. In order to cause fetal and neonatal TP, the antibody must cross the placenta and so be of the IgG class. Autoantibodies may also be associated with maternal TP. The maternal history and platelet count is important in evaluating the cause of fetal or neonatal TP in a normal pregnancy. A family history of fetal TP among maternal female relatives is also valuable in possible cases of alloimmune TP (Bussel *et al.*, 1991a).

Platelet antigens

Several types of maternal antibody may give rise to fetal TP. These are defined by the antigens with which they interact as alloantibodies, isoantibodies or autoantibodies. An individual forms alloantibodies when exposed to alloantigens which they themselves do not carry, usually through transfusion of blood products or pregnancy. Rh antibodies are well-known examples. Isoantibodies are formed as a result of exposure to isoantigens, antigens that are congenitally absent from the individual who forms the isoantibody. Again exposure is through transfusion or pregnancy, e.g. antibodies to congenitally absent platelet surface glycoproteins in Glanzmann's thrombasthenia and Bernard Soulier syndrome. Alloantibodies and isoantibodies do not interact with the platelets of the individual producing the antibodies, since their platelets do not bear the antigens. In contrast, autoantibodies interact with antigens present on the host platelets. These antibodies interact with platelet surface glycoproteins (GP) (McMillan *et al.*, 1987) such as GP IIb/IIIa and GP Ib as well as phospholipids, glycosphingolipids and membrane proteins present on host platelets (von dem Borne & Ouwehand, 1986). As well as crossing the placenta and affecting the fetal platelet count, autoantibodies interact with maternal platelets and may cause maternal TP.

Platelet surface glycoproteins

The platelet surface bears a number of glycoproteins which have an important role in platelet–platelet and platelet–extracellular matrix interactions vital in haemostasis and the maintenance of endothelial integrity. Immunologically, they are important since the different polymorphic epitopes recognised as platelet-specific antigens are found on a number of the platelet surface GPs (Williamson *et al.*, 1992). On the platelet surface, the GP IIb/IIIa complex acts as the major receptor for fibrinogen, essential in platelet adhesion and aggregation. There are approximately 40 000–50 000 copies of GP IIb/IIIa on the platelet surface and it is, therefore, a relatively strong immunogen. It is absent or dysfunctional in Glanzmann's thrombasthenia (Caen, 1989), an autosomally inherited disorder characterized by a bleeding tendency. Other important GPs are GP Ia/IIa and GP Ic/IIa, which act as receptors for collagen, fibronectin and laminin. In contrast to IIb/IIIa, there are only 2000 copies of Ia/IIa on the platelet surface, which has implications both for the laboratory detection of the antigens/antibodies on GP Ia/IIa and for the severity of the related TP. GP I/IX acts as the major von Willebrand factor receptor and is absent in Bernard Soulier syndrome (Berndt, Fournier & Castaldi, 1989), a disorder characterized by TP and a bleeding tendency. The GP location of the platelet-specific antigens are shown in Fig. 11.1.

Platelet alloantigens

These can be divided into two groups: specific alloantigens found only on the platelet surface (von dem Borne & Ouwehand, 1989) and common alloantigens shared with other blood and tissue cells.

Platelet-specific antigens

The human platelet-specific antigens are bi-allelic polymorphisms involving the platelet surface GPs. Inherited in a codominant autosomal fashion, there is generally a high-frequency (a) and a low-frequency (b) allele. Until recently, systems were frequently named according to the initials or name of the propositus in which they were first described (Kekomaki, Raivio & Kero, 1992; Kekomaki *et al.*, 1993; Kiefel *et al.*, 1988; Kuijpers *et al.*, 1993; McFarland *et al.*, 1993, Shibata *et al.*, 1986). This has led to more than one name being assigned to one antigen system, and a new international system of nomenclature of human platelet antigens (HPAs) has been recognised (von dem Borne & Decary, 1990). To date HPAs 1 to 5 have been recognised (Table 11.1). In addition, at least seven other alloantigens have been described (Williamson *et al.*, 1992) which may yet be designated as recognised HPAs. The majority of HPAs are located on the GPIIb/IIIa complex, three HPAs and four of the other antigens, and generally result from a single amino acid difference in the GP sequence. The genetic basis for the five recognised HPAs and several of the other antigens such as Mo and Sr^a has been elucidated, all involving a single point mutation in the DNA coding for the GPs involved. This allows for platelet phenotyping by molecular methods (Johnson *et al.*, 1993; Kuijpers *et al.*, 1991; McFarland *et al.*, 1991; Metcalfe & Waters, 1993; Williamson *et al.*, 1992) including polymerase chain reaction (PCR) amplification of platelet mRNA or leucocyte/amniocyte DNA followed by allele-specific oligonucleotide probing (Johnson *et al.*, 1993; McFarland *et al.*, 1991) or PCR amplification with sequence specific primers (Metcalfe & Waters, 1993). Clinically these techniques have been used for the investigation of suspected cases of neonatal alloimmune TP as well as for the phenotyping of the fetus at risk of alloimmune TP (Johnson *et al.*, 1993; McFarland *et al.*, 1991, Metcalfe & Waters, 1993; Williamson *et al.*, 1992). This is in contrast to often cumbersome serological techniques which may be difficult to interpret especially in the presence of HLA antibodies.

Common alloantigens

There are broadly two groups of these antigens: the complex carbohydrate structure of the ABO blood group

Fig. 11.1 *Platelet membrane glycoproteins showing locations of the HPAs 1–5.*

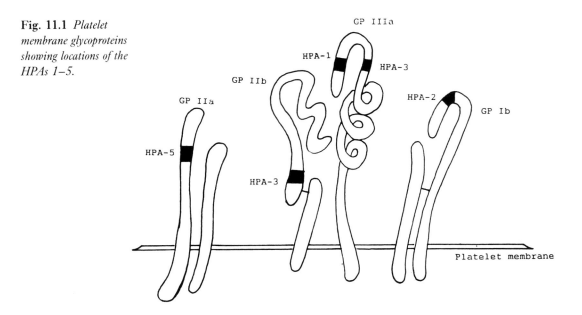

system and antigens of the Le, I and P systems, and the glycoprotein antigens of the HLA system. The origin of the latter is unclear. Although a proportion are endogenously produced by the megakaryocyte and platelet, a proportion are also absorbed onto the platelet surface from plasma, as occurs with the blood group antigens (Dunstan & Simpson, 1985).

Only class I HLA antigens are expressed on the platelet surface; HLA-C antigen expression is weak (Mueller-Eckhardt *et al.*, 1980), whereas expression of HLA-A and HLA-B antigens is more variable (Liebert, Aster & Izatkowski, 1977). The role of HLA and ABO antibodies in alloimmune TP is not clear; HLA antibodies have been demonstrated to interfere with fetal platelet transfusion therapy (Murphy *et al.*, 1993) and have been described as being responsible for fetal alloimmune TP (Omshi *et al.*, 1992). However, HLA antibodies are commonly found in the sera of pregnant women and their presence may complicate the detection of platelet-specific antibodies (von dem Borne & Ouwehand, 1989).

Alloimmune thrombocytopenia

Fetal and neonatal TP can result from the transplacental action of maternal alloantibodies directed against antigens on fetal platelets. This was first recognised 40 years ago (Harrington *et al.*, 1953; Pearson *et al.*, 1964), but with recent advances in the knowledge of platelet antigens and in serological and molecular techniques for their detection, management aspects of fetal alloimmune TP (FAITP) have become clearer. In comparison to the red cell equivalent, Rh alloimmunization, maternal alloimmunization against platelet antigens can result in fetal TP during the first pregnancy, the first born being affected in 50% of patients (Bussel *et al.*, 1988b; Mueller-Eckhardt *et al.*, 1989a; Reznikoff-Etievant *et al.*, 1983). FAITP is uncommon, affecting 1 in 678–5000 births (Blanchette *et al.*, 1990; Burrows & Kelton, 1988; Pearson *et al.*, 1964), but TP can be profound and permanent neurological sequelae may result from intracerebral bleeding in 15 to 35% of affected babies (Bussel *et al.*, 1988b; de Vries *et al.*, 1988; Kaplan *et al.*, 1992; Mueller-Eckhardt *et al.*, 1989a), with death occurring in 7–10% (Bussel *et al.*, 1988b; Kaplan *et al.*, 1992). The effects may, therefore, be devastating. After an initial affected pregnancy there is an 83% chance of subsequent pregnancies being affected, but with accurate paternal genotyping this risk can be more accurately predicted in individual patients (Lipitz *et al.*, 1992). Progress in antenatal diagnosis and management means that intervention may be planned with the aim of preventing antenatal and perinatal haemorrhage.

Table 11.1 *Human platelet antigen systems: glycoprotein locations and frequencies in the Caucasian population*

Antigen system	Antigens	Other names	Glycoprotein location (GP)	Gene frequency	Phenotype frequency (%)
HPA-1	HPA-1a	Zw[a], Pl[A1]	GP IIIa	0.85	1a/1a: 72
	HPA-1b	Zw[b], Pl[A2]		0.15	1a/1b: 26
					1b/1b: 2
HPA-2	HPA-2a	KO[b],	GP Ib	0.92	2a/2a: 85
	HPA-2b	KO[a], Sib[a]		0.08	2a/2b: 14
					2b/2b: 1
HPA-3	HPA-3a	Bak[a], Lek[a]	GP IIb	0.61	3a/3a: 37
	HPA-3b	Bak[b], Lek[b]		0.39	3a/3b: 48
					3b/3b: 15
HPA-4	HPA-4a	Pen[a], Yuk[b]	GP IIIa	0.99	4a/4a: >99
	HPA-4b	Pen[b], Yuk[a]		0.01	4a/4b: <1
					4b/4b: <1
HPA-5	HPA-5a	Br[b], Zav[b]	GPIa	0.89	5a/5a: 1
	HPA-5b	Bra, Zav[a]		0.11	5a/5b: 19
		Hc[a]			5b/5b: 80
HPA-6	HPA-6a	Sr[a]	GP IIIa		
HPA-7	HPA-7a	Mo	GPIIIa		
	HPA-7b				

Pathogenesis and serology

Anti-HPA-1a is the most frequently implicated antibody in FAITP in the Caucasian population (Mueller-Eckhardt *et al.*, 1989a). The HPA-1b antigen is rare in the Japanese population, in which HPA-4 is the most frequently implicated antibody system (Shibata *et al.*, 1986). HPA-1a-negative women (i.e. HPA-1b homozygotes) are over represented in reported series of suspected neonatal alloimmune TP (NAITP), accounting for 42% of mothers in one large series of 348 suspected cases (Mueller-Eckhardt, 1989a). Anti-HPA-1a was found in 74% of these HPA-1a-negative women, either alone or with HLA antibodies or other platelet-specific antibodies. Among the HPA-1a-positive mothers with affected infants, antibodies were detected much less often, anti-HPA-5b being the most frequent, in 4.4%. Antiplatelet antibodies, including

HLA anti-bodies, were found in only 5.9% of HPA-1a-positive, compared with 84% of HPA-1a-negative women. Overall, anti-HPA-1a accounts for 78 to 90% of serologically defined cases of NAITP, followed by anti-HPA-5b, detected in 19%. Other antibody specificities account for 3% of serologically defined cases (Mueller-Eckhardt *et al.*, 1989a; Reznikoff-Etievant, 1988; von dem Borne & Ouwehand, 1989; Bettaieb *et al.*, 1991).

Of suspected cases, 48–60% remain serologically undefined (Mueller-Eckhardt *et al.*, 1989a; Reznikoff-Etievant, 1988). This includes patients where HPA-1a incompatibility is clearly involved, in which up to 20% of such cases have no detectable antibody (Kaplan *et al.*, 1988; Reznikoff-Etievant, 1988). In some patients, antibodies may develop post-natally. Others may be antibody negative because of lack of sensitivity of the antibody detection method (Mueller-Eckhardt *et al.*, 1989a), or because of incompatibility of an as-yet-undefined platelet antigen system. A number of cases of suspected NAITP were attributed to anti-HPA-5b (Kaplan *et al.*, 1991) after a retrospective study of stored sera.

The role of nonplatelet-specific antibodies is less clear. HLA antibodies and IgG anti-A and anti-B react with their antigens on the platelet surface, and may interfere with the detection of underlying platelet-specific alloantibodies in maternal serum. Evidence for a role of anti-A or anti-B is circumstantial (Mueller-Eckhardt *et al.*, 1989a). HLA antibodies, however, can interfere with fetal platelet transfusion therapy (Murphy *et al.*, 1993), and in a number of patients have been the only alloantibodies detectable (Omshi *et al.*, 1992). Fetal HLA antigens are present in the placenta, and maternal HLA antibodies directed against fetal antigens are usually absorbed by the placenta and so do not cross into the fetus in sufficient quantities to cause fetal disease. In such cases, the presence of an antibody against a private platelet antibody cannot be excluded (Kekomaki *et al.*, 1992; Kuijpers *et al.*, 1993).

Although FAITP is a rare condition, HPA incompatibility is not infrequent. Considering alloimmunization by HPA-1a alone, with the frequency of the HPA-1b homozygous phenotype being 2%, then approximately 1 in 50 pregnancies will be incompatible for the HPA-1a antigen and potentially at risk for alloimmunization. The observed frequency of HPA-1a alloimmunization of 0.06% (Blanchette *et al.*, 1990), is much less than this. In a recent prospective study of 5000 pregnant women (Blanchette *et al.*, 1990), 80 (1.6%) were HPA-1a negative, of whom 50 were followed prospectively through pregnancy. Three formed anti-HPA-1a, two during pregnancy and one post-partum. Only one neonate was thrombocytopenic. Therefore, 6% of HPA-1a-negative women became alloimmunized – an incidence of 1 in 1666 pregnancies in the population overall. The incidence of alloimmune TP (AITP) was less than this, 1 in 5000. Therefore, alloimmunization is not an inevitable consequence of an incompatible pregnancy and fetal TP is not the inevitable consequence of alloimmunization. The reasons for these observations are not clear but may relate to antigen load or immunogenicity.

The development of HPA-1a alloantibodies is related to the HLA phenotype. MHC class II antigen HLA-DR3 is found in 60–80% responders compared with

16–20% non-responders (Reznikoff-Etievant *et al.*, 1983). There is a 100% coincidence of the HLA DRw52 antigen and cases of NAITP caused by anti-HPA-1a (de Waal *et al.*, 1986). Of the three sub-specificities of HLA-DRw52 antigen (a, b and c), HLA-DRw52a was found in 100% of the responders, compared with 28–35% in the normal population and up to 30% in non-responders (Decary *et al.*, 1991). Elucidation of the molecular basis of the immune response to HPA-1a would be valuable in the assessment of the risk of immunization, particularly in prospective screening programmes. HLA typing with reference to the DRw52 locus particularly should form part of the assessment of HPA-1a-negative women with regard to the risk both of immunization and of AITP. An association between immunization to HPA-5b and HLA-DRw6, which is included in the supertypic antigen DRw52, has also been demonstrated (Mueller-Eckhardt *et al.*, 1989b).

Clinical features

The majority of cases are detected on clinical presentation and since neonates and pregnant women are not routinely screened for TP and alloantibodies, respectively, milder, asymptomatic cases may go unrecognised. The first pregnancy is often affected (Mueller-Eckhardt *et al.*, 1989a; Reznikoff-Etievant, 1988). Therefore, in the absence of an antenatal screening programme (Flug, Karpatkin & Karpatkin, 1994), the condition is often unsuspected until the birth of a first child with ICH.

Maternal antibodies cross the placenta as early as 14 weeks, and platelet-specific antigens are expressed on fetal platelets from at least 18 weeks' gestation (Gruel *et al.*, 1986). TP has been known to occur by 18 weeks, with platelet counts as low as $15 \times 10^9/1$ at this stage (Murphy *et al.*, 1993) and as low as $5 \times 10^9/1$ at 20 weeks' gestation (Reznikoff-Etievant, 1988). Untreated, the TP is stable or, more often, progressive through pregnancy (Bussel *et al.*, 1988a; Kaplan *et al.*, 1988). Spontaneous remission is unlikely. The finding of a normal platelet count at 22 weeks does not preclude development of significant TP later on (Bussel *et al.*, 1988a, Kaplan *et al.*, 1988). At birth TP may be profound ($<10 \times 10^9/l$) or the platelet count may fall post-natally, often reaching a nadir between days 2 and 5. In NAITP caused by anti-HPA-1a, 89–95% of platelet counts are $<30 \times 10^9/l$ in the first hours of life (Kaplan *et al.*, 1992; Mueller-Eckhardt *et al.*, 1989a). The finding of a platelet count of $\geq 50 \times 10^9/l$ at the end of this period indicates a relatively good prognosis.

Clinically, the neonate may be asymptomatic (13–59%), exhibit superficial purpura (18–65%) or have evidence of more severe bleeding, either visceral or intracerebral (22–23%) (Kaplan *et al.*, 1992; Mueller-Eckhardt *et al.*, 1989a). The mortality rate overall is 1–2% (Bussel *et al.*, 1988a), with a rate of 6–10% in infants suffering ICH. ICH occurs in 10–30% of infants. Although the perinatal period is particularly high risk for ICH, 23–50% (Bussel *et al.*, 1988b; Kaplan *et al.*, 1992; Mueller-Eckhardt *et al.*, 1989a; Reznikoff-Etievant, 1988) of ICH may occur *in utero* from as early as 19 weeks' gestation (Giovangrandi *et al.*, 1990; Murphy *et al.*, 1993). The risk of ICH increases the longer the platelet count is depressed and, therefore, the maximum risk is during the last trimester. Fetal ICH may result in death, porencephaly or hydrocephalus; 19% of infants with neonatal ICH suffer permanent neurological sequelae.

Although most reported series relate to AITP involving anti-HPA-1a, a series of 39 cases of AITP caused by anti-HPA-5a has recently been described (Kaplan *et al.*, 1991). This seems milder, comparatively, with a higher proportion of asymptomatic cases with higher platelet counts. This may relate to the far fewer number of HPA-5 epitopes compared with HPA1 epitopes on the platelet surface. At birth, 43% of platelet counts were $<30 \times 10^9/l$, with $<10\%$ at $<10 \times 10^9/l$ compared with 42% for AITP owing to anti-HPA-1a. A lower proportion of first pregnancies seems affected.

In any individual patient, the most reliable method of assessing likely disease severity is by comparison with previous pregnancies. In one series, nine subsequent pregnancies were as severely affected as the previous pregnancy, three more severely and just one less severely affected (Reznikoff-Etievant, 1988). Maternal antibody titres bear little relation to disease severity, especially as maternal anti-HPA-1a cannot always be detected in typically HPA-1a incompatible cases. Furthermore, anti-HPA-1a may be detected without fetal TP in the presence of incompatibility, or antibody from a previous pregnancy may be detectable in a compatible pregnancy. Throughout pregnancy, maternal antibody levels may

fall, rise or remain stable (Kaplan *et al.*, 1988), again with no apparent relationship to the fetal platelet count.

Management of FAITP

The timing of ICH is important in deciding management strategies with maximum risk after 30 weeks' gestation. Previous pregnancies are a guide as to the risk of ICH, but since haemorrhage is related to the degree of TP, management of an affected pregnancy should aim to improve the fetal platelet count as soon as TP occurs. This means that treatment may have to start as early as 18 weeks or even earlier. Delivery is a time of very high risk for haemorrhage and management should also aim to reduce the risk of delivery, either by raising the platelet count or by the method of delivery.

Diagnosis of a suspected case

AITP should be suspected in any infant found to be thrombocytopenic, particularly when there is no other apparent cause for fetal or neonatal TP. A threshold platelet count of $<150 \times 10^9/l$ should be considered as this ensures that milder cases, especially those caused by anti-HPA-5 antibodies' are not missed. Other causes of TP such as sepsis, hypoxia, disseminated intravascular coagulation (DIC) and congenital infections are absent. The mother is healthy and in particular has a normal platelet count. The diagnosis is usually made initially on clinical grounds, but with the advent of rapid tests (especially DNA based) for platelet phenotype and antibody screening, laboratory diagnosis can be made within 24 hours (Metcalfe & Waters, 1993; Williamson *et al.*, 1992).

Serological diagnosis need not necessarily involve neonatal samples, since the diagnosis can be made by the demonstration of materno--paternal incompatibility for a platelet antigen and the demonstration of maternal antibodies against the antigen concerned (Bussel *et al.*, 1991a). In the Caucasian population, the demonstration that the mother is HPA-1a negative is sufficient circumstantial evidence for a provisional diagnosis of NAITP, especially if supported by a response to a transfusion of HPA-1a-negative platelets. Subsequent demonstration that the neonate is incompatible for the platelet antigen concerned confirms the diagnosis. Negative antibody testing does not exclude NAITP, as discussed above.

Diagnosis of an affected pregnancy

A pregnancy should be considered at risk of AITP in the following cases (Bussel *et al.*, 1991a): (i) confirmed NAITP in a previous pregnancy; (ii) previous birth of a neonate with unexplained TP ($<100 \times 10^9$/l); (iii) an affected pregnancy in a close blood relative (e.g. sister); (iv) in a woman already known to lack a platelet-specific antigen; (v) in unexplained fetal hydrocephalus.

Percutaneous fetal blood sampling (FBS) and estimation of the platelet count is the only sure way to determine whether a fetus is affected (Daffos et al., 1988; Gruel *et al.*, 1986; Nicolini & Rodeck, 1992). However, preliminary tests will enable an assessment of the risk of TP and selection of the women who should undergo FBS. If the father is homozygous for the incompatible antigen, then all subsequent pregnancies will be incompatible and likely to be affected. If, however, he is heterozygous, then there is only a 50% risk of subsequent pregnancies being incompatible and, therefore, affected. In this situation, the fetal phenotype can now simply be determined by PCR on fluid obtained at amniocentesis (Bennett *et al.*, 1994). Should the fetus be negative for the antigen of interest, no further investigation will be needed.

Detection of a maternal antiplatelet antibody, especially in a nullipara, must also raise suspicion of an affected fetus. The condition may be so severe as to present in a first pregnancy with fetal hydrocephalus caused by ICH. We have recently seen two such patients, one as early as 20 weeks (Montemagno *et al.*, 1994) (Fig. 11.2). Investigations should include fetal platelet count, maternal and fetal phenotyping/genotyping and maternal antibody screening. In HPA-1a-negative women without a history of AIT, HLA phenotyping, particularly with reference to the HLA-DRw52 or, particularly, DRw52a phenotype, aids in assessing risk of alloimmunization and TP (Burrows & Kelton, 1993), since this antigen is associated with an immune response to HPA-1a and HPA-5b. Those negative for HLA-DRw52 appear to have a very low risk of alloimmunization and fetal TP (Anon., 1993).

In the hands of an experienced operator, FBS

Fig. 11.2 *Ultrasound picture of fetal hydrocephalus caused by cerebral haemorrhage in a case of alloimmune TP caused by anti-HPA-1a. (From Montemagno et al., 1994.)*

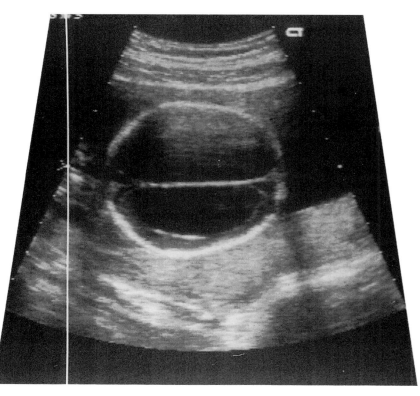

(Chapter 2) can be safely undertaken in the fetus with a bleeding disorder (Daffos *et al.*, 1988; Nicolini & Rodeck, 1992). It is, however, prudent to transfuse compatible platelets after sampling to reduce the risk of haemorrhage and cord tamponade (Anon., 1993) as several fetuses have died of these complications. A fetal platelet count $<100 \times 10^9/l$ in an at-risk pregnancy is strongly suggestive of AITP. Care must be taken to exclude causes of spurious TP, particularly contamination of the sample by amniotic fluid, which, apart from dilutional effects, in smaller amounts can activate the coagulation cascade and cause platelets to be consumed in a clot. In cases of doubt, examination of a blood film will help to validate the platelet count, and assay of clotting factors, particularly factor VIII, will serve to eliminate clotting as a cause of TP. The film will also exclude pseudo-TP, an *in vitro* phenomenon resulting from clumping of the platelets caused by the anticoagulant EDTA (Daffos *et al.*, 1988; Gruel *et al.*, 1986).

FBS should be performed in patients considered at a high risk of TP. Since the fetus is often thrombocytopenic from early in the second trimester, diagnostic FBS is probably best carried out at 21 to 22 weeks' gestation (Anon., 1993; Bussel *et al.*, 1988a; 1990; Kaplan *et al.*, 1988; Kelsey *et al.*, 1991). This allows for early diagnosis and management to be instituted with the aim of improving the fetal platelet count and preventing ICH. An alternative school of thought advocates FBS at 35 to 36 weeks' gestation, to detect the thrombocytopenic fetus, so that an intrauterine platelet transfusion can be given, and the baby delivered within 24 hours of the transfusion (Daffos *et al.*, 1984). This strategy, however, ignores the risk of bleeding earlier in pregnancy, unless maternally administered treatment is given without an initial evaluation of the fetal platelet count. In any individual patient, the course of previous pregnancies can be used as a guide to the degree of intervention necessary. A previous history of an ICH is a strong risk factor for ICH in the current pregnancy and intervention should be early. However, it should be borne in mind that subsequent pregnancies may be more severely affected. This may be particularly the case for alloimmunization to HPA-5.

The finding of a normal platelet count at 20 to 22 weeks' gestation does not preclude an affected fetus, since the platelet count can fall later in pregnancy. FBS should then be repeated at 28 to 32 weeks. The fetal phenotype can be determined by serological or molecular methods, if not already done at amniocentesis, since the finding of a compatible fetus allows exclusion of AITP (Anon., 1993).

Management of the fetus

Management of the affected fetus is aimed at preventing devastating ICH and its sequelae. Treatment aimed at raising the fetal platelet count should ideally start early in the second trimester (Anon., 1993). Three treatment modalities have been described, including maternal steroids, maternal or fetal administration of immunoglobulin and fetal platelet transfusions.

Fetal platelet transfusions (FPTs)

FPTs can be used: (i) to prevent bleeding at the time of FBS; (ii) in a prophylactic fashion at regular intervals through the second and third trimesters; (iii) just before delivery.

The platelets must be compatible with the maternal antibody, i.e. negative for the antigen concerned. The most obvious donor is the mother so that in addition to being negative for the antigen concerned, the risk of transfusion-transmitted infection (CMV, hepatitis, HIV) is reduced. However, maternal plasma contains the pathological antibody and transfusion to the fetus may increase the duration and severity of TP. In addition, maternal HLA antibodies may complicate FPT therapy and direct transfusion into the fetal circulation will increase this effect (Murphy *et al.*, 1993). Maternal platelets should be washed to remove maternal antibody and resuspended in AB plasma (Anon., 1993), but manipulation of platelets in this fashion can lead to activation and loss of function, as well as reduced survival once transfused. Typed platelets are available from unrelated donors obtained from transfusion centres. Platelets are harvested by plateletpheresis and concentrated to give a final count of $\geq 2 \times 10^{12}/l$. This ensures that an adequate platelet increment can be obtained with transfusion of the small volumes required by the second trimester fetus. The donor should be ABO compatible, and CMV antibody negative. Platelet concentrates should be irradiated to prevent graft-versus-host disease and leucodepleted to reduce white cell contamination and possible CMV infection. They should be used as soon as possible after harvesting (preferably within 24 hours) to maximize platelet lifespan after transfusion. The volume of any given concentrate required can be calculated using the formula:

$$V = \frac{\text{FPV} \times F \times \text{Desired increment}}{\text{Concentrate platelet count}}$$

where the fetoplacental blood volume (FPV) for gestational age is derived from previously constructed charts (Murphy *et al.*, 1990; Nicolaides, Clewell & Rodeck, 1987) and a recovery factor (*F*) of 2 used since the immediate platelet increment has been found to be approximately 50% of that expected (Anon., 1993). It is vital to have the facility to perform platelet counts during the FPT, by means of an automated cell counter adjacent to the procedure room. This allows the operator to ensure that an adequate level has been achieved before the transfusion is terminated. A post-transfusion level of $(400–500) \times 10^9/l$ should be aimed for, especially if a programme of repeated FPTs is planned (Nicolini *et al.*, 1988).

Donor platelets survive approximately 4–5 days once transfused into the fetal circulation. To maintain the fetal platelet count at safe levels with repeated platelet transfusions these have to be given at approximately 7–10 day intervals. With a longer interval between transfusions, the platelet count may fall to dangerously low levels and ICH may occur in the interval between FPTs. A regular prophylactic transfusion programme has been successfully used (Fig. 11.3) but is arduous for the mother. In practice, regular transfusions may be started at 26 to 28 weeks (Kelsey *et al.*, 1991; Nicolini *et al.*, 1988). This covers the time of maximum risk for ICH, i.e. the last trimester. However weekly transfusions have been successfully given from 18 weeks onwards (Murphy *et al.*, 1993). If regular prophylactic platelet transfusions are not employed, a platelet transfusion should be given at the time of FBS to prevent procedure-related cord haemorrhage and/or tamponade (Anon., 1993). An FPT immediately before delivery is an effective method for increasing the fetal platelet count to allow for safe vaginal delivery (Daffos *et al.*, 1984).

Apart from the risk of haemorrhage, immediate adverse effects of FPT may result from the acute volume expansion that results when the fetal intravascular volume is increased acutely by the transfusion of platelet concentrate. Fetal bradycardia and occasionally cardiac arrest have occurred. We have observed this in one patient whose fetus had asystole after an uncomplicated transfusion had raised the platelet count to $800 \times 10^9/l$. An increase in viscosity of the blood may have contributed because the fetus was successfully resuscitated by a partial exchange infusion of normal saline into the fetal left ventricle (Rodeck & Roberts, 1994). The risk may be minimized by using as high a platelet concentration as possible. The volume of concentrate may also cause acute dilutional anaemia, which may also contribute to the fetal bradycardia. Up to 60 ml may be given at a rate of 10 ml/min, although this should be slowed if bradycardias occur.

Intravenous gammaglobulin

Maternally administered treatment is simpler and less invasive than direct fetal treatment (e.g. FPTs) but is potentially less effective if one is relying on transplacental transport to gain access to the fetal circulation, e.g. of maternally administered intravenous immunoglobulin (IVIG).

The effectiveness of IVIG in raising the platelet count in childhood AITP, and reports of its effectiveness in neonatal autoimmune TP when administered both to the neonate (Derycke *et al.*, 1985) and to the mother before delivery, has led to its use in NAITP. Antenatal maternal treatment of FAITP with high-dose IVIG has variably been reported to be successful in raising the fetal platelet count and preventing ICH. There are reports of both success and of failure of IVIG (Bussel *et al.*, 1988a; 1990; Kelsey *et al.*, 1991; Nicolini *et al.*, 1990; Shwe *et al.*, 1991) and its role remains unclear.

Maternal IgG starts to cross the placenta into the fetal circulation as early as 14 to 16 weeks' gestation. Studies have suggested that transplacental transfer of gammaglobulin becomes more efficient as gestation progresses, particularly after 30 weeks, implying that relatively higher doses of IVIG would have to be administered to the mother to achieve fetal hypergammaglobulinaemia (Bussel *et al.*, 1988a; Nicolini *et al.*, 1990) early in pregnancy. Maternally administered IVIG may act within the fetal circulation, reducing the rate of platelet destruction, either by reticuloendothelial blockade or by reduction in sensitization of fetal platelets by competi-

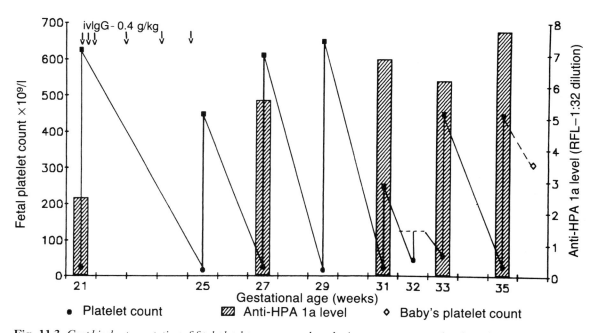

Fig. 11.3 *Graphical representation of fetal platelet counts and maternal antibody levels in a pregnancy complicated by FAITP caused by anti-HPA-1a. The fetus received an initial platelet transfusion at the diagnostic fetal blood sampling at 21 weeks' gestation. Maternal intravenous IgG was given between weeks 21 and 26. FBS at 26 weeks showed no effect of maternal treatment and FPTs were started. These were given at 1–2 week intervals and pre- and post-transfusion platelet counts are shown except for that at 32 weeks (sample clotted – dotted lines). Maternal antibody levels are expressed comparatively as relative fluorescence intensity by a fluorimetric method. The baby was delivered vaginally after a final intrauterine fetal platelet transfusion at 35 weeks. There was no sign of haemorrhage.*

tion. Differences in the timing of maternally administered IVIG, the frequency of administration and the dose administered might account in part for the variable reported success rate in studies of maternal IVIG in FAITP. However, despite the attainment of fetal hypergammaglobulinaemia (Bussel *et al.*, 1988a; Nicolini *et al.*, 1990), treatment failures have been reported. In the mother, hypergammaglobulinaemia may reduce the rate of transplacental transfer of pathological antibody by competition and there is evidence that IVIG may modu-

late the immune system and reduce the rate of maternal antibody production. An issue that has not been explored is the preparation of immunoglobulin employed. Variations in production methods may lead to variation between preparations in effectiveness in ameliorating AITP.

Direct administration of IgG to the fetus early in the second trimester has been tried in several fetuses and has been found to have no effect on severe AITP (Murphy *et al.*, 1993; Weiner *et al.*, 1994), but the fetal reticuloendothelial system may be relatively immature at this stage. Fetal hypergammaglobulinaemia achieved later in pregnancy may be more effective than earlier in pregnancy. However, direct weekly IVIG injections to the fetus produced no effect on the fetal platelet count in one third-trimester case (Weiner *et al.*, 1994).

Bussel *et al.* have reported the successful treatment of 50 patients with previous AITP (Bussel *et al.*, 1988a, 1990; Lynch *et al.*, 1992). After an initial FBS at 20 to 22 weeks, mothers were treated with IVIG 1.0 g/kg weekly if a fetal platelet count of $<100 \times 10^9/l$ was found. FBS was repeated 4–6 weeks later and then prior to delivery. The mean increase in platelet count between first and second sampling was $28 \times 10^9/l$. None of the 50 neonates had ICH compared with 12 of their siblings, and a mean increase in platelet count in the group as a whole was 70 × 10⁹/l higher than their siblings. Nine women also received low-dose steroid therapy and this appeared to have no additional effect on the outcome There were 39 responses out of 50 pregnancies.

The timing of treatment may be important in order to achieve maximal transplacental transfer and thus fetal hypergammaglobulinaemia. Maternal IVIG should be administered during the last trimester, as IVIG given between 21 and 27 weeks' gestation was consistently found to be ineffective (Kelsey *et al.*, 1991). An adequate dose, at least 1.0g /kg weekly, is also important. High-dose IVIG is very expensive and in many cases does not produce a platelet response. Fetal platelet transfusions are required although the risks of this are higher.

Maternal steroid treatment
An isolated case of response to low-dose prednisolone led to the use of steroids in AITP (Murphy *et al.*, 1990). Steroids are thought to act via maternal immuno-suppression, reducing maternal antibody production. Bussel *et al.* found no additional benefit in the use of low-dose dexamethasone in five patients in terms of increase in fetal platelet count and occurrence of fetal ICH, compared with IVIG alone (Bussel *et al.*, 1988b; 1990; Lynch *et al.*, 1992). The role of maternal steroid treatment needs to be explored further (Anon., 1993). An undesirable side effect of long-term dexamethasone treatment in pregnancy is oligohydramnios and possibly fetal growth retardation (Bussel *et al.*, 1988a).

Antenatal management options
Three separate strategies have been described. The first is conservative with maternal rest and frequent ultrasound examinations until delivery once fetal lung maturity is reached. One to two days before delivery, the fetal platelet count is determined and, if reduced, an intrauterine platelet transfusion is administered prior to delivery (Kaplan *et al.*, 1988) and labour then induced. Alternatively, the patient can be delivered by elective caesarean section without the need for FBS. The second involves maternally directed treatment with high-dose IVIG either alone or in conjunction with steroids. This aims at raising the fetal platelet count, with repeat FBS to assess response, either at 26 to 28 weeks' gestation, and/or just before delivery as above. In the event of

nonresponse, fetal platelet transfusions may be administered. The third involves repeated fetal platelet transfusions until fetal maturity is reached, which may be combined with maternally directed treatment (Kelsey *et al.*, 1991). All these mothers should be advised to rest and to avoid antiplatelet drugs like aspirin.

There is no clear evidence to demonstrate one strategy as being superior to the other. Most centres use either maternally directed therapy or serial platelet transfusions, the former being popular in the USA and the latter in Europe. Although serial platelet transfusions seem more efficacious, their cumulative loss rate with repeated procedures may be as great as, and even exceed, the morbidity rate associated with untreated disease (Weiner *et al.*, 1994).

In future, the option of pre-implantation selection of a HPA-compatible embryo may also become a practical possibility (Van den Veyver *et al.*, 1994) to ensure an unaffected pregnancy where the father is heterozygous. The risk of diagnostic error and failure of implantation will need to be weighed against the efficacy and risks of fetal treatment.

Delivery
Delivery is a period of high risk for ICH in the thrombocytopenic fetus. The best method of delivery is controversial: caesarean section has been associated with ICH, and thrombocytopenic fetuses have been delivered vaginally with no adverse effects. One of the aims of antenatal management in FAITP is to raise the platelet count to allow for safe delivery as close to term as possible, according to obstetric indications. FBS close to delivery is recommended, and if antenatal treatment has failed to raise the fetal platelet count >50 × 10⁹/l to allow safe vaginal delivery, then either caesarean section should be performed or labour induced after an intrauterine FPT. Providing delivery occurs within 24 hours of FPT, then the cord platelet count correlates well with the final post-transfusion platelet count (Kelsey *et al.*, 1991).

Post-natal management
Once delivered, the neonate is cut off from the maternal supply of alloantibody and the duration of TP is limited to the survival of maternal antibody within the neonatal circulation. Maternal antiplatelet antibodies have not

been detected in cord serum and it seems in many cases that maternal antibody is rapidly cleared from the neonatal circulation by interaction with neonatal platelets. The platelet count may continue to fall after delivery, and the nadir neonatal platelet count generally occurs between 2 and 5 days post-natally (Mueller-Eckhardt *et al.*, 1989a). In many cases, the platelet count reaches normal levels by day 10.

The true incidence of ICH in infants with AITP is unknown since cranial ultrasound is often only performed in selected cases. ICH should be sought at birth, both to document its incidence and to differentiate ICH that occurred antenatally from those that occurred perinatally. Documentation of ICH by ultrasound allows for appropriate post-natal follow-up. Some experts also recommend long-term immunological follow-up of cases where maternal IVIG has been given as the long-term sequelae of this treatment is unknown (Anon., 1993).

Autoimmune thrombocytopenia

In contrast to AITP, the pathogenic antibodies in immune TP (ITP) have the potential to cause TP in the mother as well as the fetus. TP is a relatively frequent occurrence among pregnant women, but not all cases are immune in origin. The risk of fetal TP in immune and nonimmune maternal TP has been the subject of debate, and recent studies have attempted to determine both the frequency of maternal TP and the risk of associated fetal TP (Burrows & Kelton, 1988; 1990b; 1993; Bussel *et al.*, 1991b; von dem Borne *et al.*, 1986). In general, the severity of fetal and neonatal TP caused by maternal autoantibodies appears to be less than that alloantibodies. AITP is the most common cause of severe neonatal immune TP and accounts for the majority of reported cases of severe haemorrhage (Burrows & Kelton, 1993).

Pathogenesis and serology

Harrington first demonstrated that plasma contained a thrombocytopenic factor in patients with idiopathic TP, through cross transfusion studies (Harrington *et al.*, 1953). The demonstration of increased platelet surface

immunoglobulin in 92–100% of cases and the presence of free platelet-reacting immunoglobulin in 62% of patients with idiopathic TP confirmed the immune nature of platelet destruction (von dem Borne *et al.*, 1986). Platelets become coated with antibody and are destroyed in the reticuloendothelial system, particularly the spleen, through the interaction of the bound antibody with Fc receptors on the surface of macrophage cells. The amount of antibody on the platelet surface is related to the rate of platelet destruction and hence TP in any individual case, but free platelet antibody can persist despite a normal platelet count either owing to treatment or to removal of the major site of destruction (i.e. splenectomy). This is obviously of importance in the pregnant woman where free antibody will be available to cross into the fetal circulation with the potential to cause fetal TP despite a normal maternal platelet count.

Platelet surface antibody is of the IgG class in 82–100% of cases (von dem Borne *et al.*, 1986). Complement is rarely detected on the platelet surface. As well as binding to the platelet surface via the specific antibody activity of the Ig molecule, immune complexes may bind via platelet surface Fc receptors. This nonspecific binding may result in accelerated platelet destruction; however, immune complexes do not cross the placenta and, therefore, cannot cause fetal TP.

In true ITP, the antibodies have specificity for platelet surface antigens. These include platelet glycoproteins, sphingolipids, phospholipids and other platelet surface components such as cardiolipin and proteins. The major platelet GPs are frequently the target of platelet autoantibodies (McMillan *et al.*, 1987), directed against GP IIb/IIIa in up to 62% and against GP Ib in 32 to 38% of cases. Antibodies against GP V have also been described. Anticardiolipin antibodies are found in association with TP in systemic lupus erythematosus (SLE) and occasionally interfere with GP function.

Clinical features

In adults, ITP is often chronic, with persistent and fluctuating TP. The male:female ratio is 1:2 with a peak incidence at 20–60 years. It frequently coincides with pregnancy, estimated to occur in 1 in 300–600 pregnancies (Burrows & Kelton, 1990b).

Clinically, the findings in the mother reflect the

degree of TP, with petechiae, purpura, epistaxis and mucosal membrane bleeding. Platelet size, expressed as mean platelet volume, is raised, reflecting increased platelet turnover with production of young, immature forms. The rest of the blood count is normal unless haemorrhage has led to anaemia and iron deficiency. Clotting studies are normal. In some patients, the haemorrhagic manifestations are less than expected for the degree of TP because of the circulation of large relatively young platelets that are fully functional. An occasional case has been described in which the antibody binds to a vital functional epitope on the platelet surface and interferes with platelet function as well as increasing the rate of destruction. In this case bleeding may be prominent.

Diagnosis is by the exclusion of other causes of TP and by the demonstration of normal or increased numbers of megakaryocytes in the bone marrow, thus excluding marrow failure. The demonstration of increased platelet surface immunoglobulin has a sensitivity of 82–100% and a specificity of 30% for immune destruction of platelets (von dem Borne & Ouwehand, 1989).

Treatment is aimed at raising the platelet count and is usually in the form of immunosupression, particularly with glucocorticoids. This raises the platelet count initially by causing reticuloendothelial blockade and then possibly by modulating antibody production. An initial course of steroids will induce remission in 60% of patients. However, there is a relatively high treatment failure and relapse rate. Splenectomy, by removing the major site of destruction of platelets and a possible site of antibody production will induce remission in 60–70% of patients, including those who have failed first-line steroid therapy. It may induce a clinical but not serological remission and antibody production may persist. This is of relevance in the pregnant woman who may have a normal platelet count, but whose fetus is still at risk of TP. IVIG frequently produces a reliable response in the platelet count but this is rarely maintained, relapse occurring within 3–4 weeks. Its main use is in preparation for surgery, e.g. splenectomy or delivery, in a woman with steroid-unresponsive disease.

Pregnancy associated TP

With the advent of automated blood counters and the routine assessment of the maternal full blood count, it has become recognised that up to 7–9% of women will become mildly or moderately thrombocytopenic during pregnancy. The platelet count is $<150 \times 10^9/l$, but rarely $<50 \times 10^9/l$ (Burrows & Kelton, 1990b; 1993). The mean platelet volume is raised and clotting studies and biochemistry are normal. This is thought to represent an exaggeration of the normal increase in platelet consumption seen in pregnancy and is termed asymptomatic TP or gestational TP (GTP) of pregnancy (Burrows & Kelton, 1993; Christiaens & Helmerhorst, 1987; Kaplan *et al.*, 1990). However, a proportion of cases may represent previously undiagnosed ITP, particularly those with a more profound TP and this carries a higher risk of fetal TP than GTP. It is important, therefore, to try to distinguish ITP from GTP since the latter seems to carry little increased risk of fetal TP or maternal bleeding.

Measurement of platelet surface immunoglobulin is of little use since raised values have been found in GTP (Hart *et al.*, 1986). The only true diagnostic test is to observe recovery after delivery, which is of little use in the current pregnancy. Documentation of a normal platelet count earlier in the index pregnancy is supportive of GTP, whereas an initially depressed count may be more suggestive of ITP. The degree of TP may be useful, GTP rarely falls below $<50 \times 10^9/l$.

Risk of fetal thrombocytopenia

ITP

Several recent studies have attempted to address the true incidence of fetal TP in maternal ITP. Older studies have often been retrospective, and reported incidences of 15 to 65% for fetal TP were probably a result of case selection. These studies also varied in the degree of TP reported. In general, mild TP is taken as 101 to 150, moderate as 51 to 100 and severe as $<50 \times 10^9/l$. More recent prospective or carefully controlled retrospective studies have found an incidence of TP varying between 15% and 52%, with that of severe P between 5% and 20% (Table 11.2). Maternal platelet count has not been found to correlate with severity of

Table 11.2 *Incidence of neonatal TP in maternal autoimmone TP*

	No. of patients	Infants with platelet count[a]	
		<150(%)	<50(%)
Burrows & Kelton, 1988	5	20	NS
Kaplan et al., 1990	33	33	12
Samuels et al., 1990	88	52	20
Burrows & Kelton, 1990	61	15	5
Bussell et al., 1991	24	46	NS
Burrows & Kelton, 1993	46	NS	9

NS, not stated.
[a] Platelet count $\times$ 10^9/l.

fetal TP. Maternal disease may be in remission, usually as a result of treatment and yet the neonate found to be thrombocytopenic. The level of platelet-associated antibody does not correlate with the severity of fetal disease, but the presence of free antiplatelet antibody has been found to be a significant risk factor for fetal TP (Burrows & Kelton, 1990a; Cines *at al.*, 1982; Samuels *et al.*, 1990). In particular, the absence of circulating antibody in one study was associated with a negative predictive value of 100% despite a previous history of ITP (Cines *et al.*, 1982). A history of ITP prior to pregnancy is the most significant risk factor for fetal TP (Cines *et al.*, 1982; Samuels *et al.*, 1990). The presence of free antibody has an additional positive predictive value of 26% (Samuels *et al.*, 1990).

Gestational TP
The risk of fetal TP in carefully selected cases of GTP seems no more than that of a normal pregnancy (4.3% vs 1.9%) (Burrows & Kelton, 1988; Samuels *et al.*, 1990). Burrows and Kelton (1988) found that the TP was moderate, with no counts below <50 $\times$ 10^9/l. This is in contrast to Kaplan *et al.* (1990) who found severe TP in 3% of neonates born to women with incidental TP of pregnancy. However, their series included a greater proportion of women with very low platelet counts (<50 $\times$ 10^9/l) at delivery, suggesting that this series included cases other than GTP, possibly cases of previously undiagnosed ITP. Using the criteria of a platelet count falling from normal during the first trimester, a

count >75 $\times$ 10^9/l and the absence of a previous history of ITP, the risk of severe neonatal TP in GTP appears very low (Table 11.3).

Management of an affected pregnancy

Opinions regarding the optimum management of a pregnancy complicated by maternal ITP are divided. A major area of dispute is the optimum mode of delivery of a potentially thrombocytopenic fetus, and whether assessment of the fetal platelet count, either by fetal blood sampling before or scalp sampling after the onset of labour, should be attempted. In contrast to AITP, the incidence of fetal TP is less predictable (Burrows & Kelton, 1990a), although the problem of autoimmune TP in pregnancy is more common. Furthermore, the severity of TP is generally less. A management strategy must, therefore, take into account the fact that the majority of infants will be unaffected, and that of those affected, only a minority will have a platelet count at birth to cause concern. The risk of severe fetal TP in a woman presenting with a documented fall in platelet count from normal in pregnancy, and no history to suggest ITP, is very low (Burrows & Kelton, 1988; 1990b; Kaplan *et al.*, 1990; Bussel *et al.*, 1991b) and probably not sufficient to justify intervention such as FBS to determine the fetal platelet count, given the inherent, albeit low, risk of the procedure. The pregnancy should be managed according to obstetric indications.

A history of maternal ITP prior to the pregnancy

Table 11.3 *Incidence of neonatal TP in GTP of pregnancy*

	No. of patients	Infants with platelet count[a]		
		>150(%)	>100(%)	<50(%)
Burrows & Kelton, 1988	122	4	NS	None
Burrows & Kelton, 1990	334	4	NS	None
Kaplan *et al.*, 1990	31	13	10	3
Samuels *et al.*, 1990	74	15	4	None
Burrows & Kelton, 1993	761	NS	NS	0.001

NS, not stated.

[a] Platelet count × 10⁹/l.

requires careful consideration of fetal risk, whether the mother is in remission or not. Regarding the mother, treatment should be aimed at raising the platelet count to a safe level for delivery (generally accepted to be >50 × 10⁹/l). This may be achieved with an infusion of IVIG a week to 10 days prior to delivery. If treatment is required earlier in pregnancy a course of 0.5–1.0 mg/kg per day oral prednisolone should be tried. However side effects have to be borne in mind, such as induction of maternal diabetes, hypertension and oligohydramnios.

The risk of severe TP (<50 × 10⁹/l) is between 5 and 20% in neonates of mothers with ITP. While vaginal delivery is thought safe in fetuses with a platelet count >50 × 10⁹/l, the best route of delivery at platelet counts less than this is contentious. In one study, vaginal delivery was associated with ICH in 2/17 patients compared with 0/76 neonates of mothers with ITP who were delivered by caesarean section (Samuels *et al.*, 1990). However, the timing of ICH relative to delivery and the occurrence of TP were not made clear. At least one bleed occurred in the post-partum period. In contrast, in another study (Burrows & Kelton, 1990a) there were no adverse consequences in two infants with nadir platelets <50 × 10⁹/l allowed to deliver vaginally. It is worth bearing in mind that the nadir neonatal platelet count usually occurs 2 to 3 days post-delivery and that, despite counts falling to below 50 × 10⁹/l, the platelet count at delivery may well have been safe for vaginal delivery. Tests for free circulating antiplatelet antibody may be of use in identifying patients with a low risk of fetal TP (Bussel *et al.*, 1991b). A negative result is found in approximately 26% of patients, leaving 74% of patients

for whom the risk of severe fetal TP is in the order of 26%. However, there are no tests to help distinguish those fetuses at risk from those not at risk. A policy of elective caesarean section in all these patients would mean approximately two out of three operative deliveries being unnecessary.

Fetal scalp sampling has been used to assess the platelet count at the onset of labour. In contrast to cord puncture, this technique is universally available. However, some cervical dilatation, descent of the fetal head and rupture of the membranes are required to obtain the blood sample. Labour is well established by this stage and a degree of cranial compression will already have occurred. Fetal scalp blood samples are associated with a high rate of falsely low platelet counts because of amniotic fluid contamination. The finding of a normal platelet count in general gives a true impression of the neonatal platelet count, but the finding of a low platelet count was found to be erroneous in 4/18 patients and in a further 8/18 patients sampling was unsatisfactory because of amniotic fluid contamination and an inadequate sample (Burrows & Kelton, 1990b; Christiaens & Helmerhorst, 1987).

Some authors recommend cord puncture in all cases of maternal ITP and in cases of severe maternal TP of unknown origin (Kaplan *et al.*, 1990; Christiaens & Helmerhorst, 1987) in order to detect profound fetal TP and allow for delivery by caesarean section. However, this procedure is not without some fetal morbidity and mortality, especially in the thrombocytopenic fetus. Given the rarity of severe TP in GTP, FBS is not indicated unless there is sufficient doubt about the diagnosis, for instance early maternal TP. In ITP, the previous obstetric history, if available, is of use in judging whether subsequent pregnancies will be affected. It is not clear whether caesarean section protects against fetal haemorrhage and opinion has recently swung away from fetal intervention, except for very unusual circumstances of a previously affected child in a patient with severe TP.

All neonates should have their platelet counts monitored on a daily basis until the nadir count has been reached. Treatment should be instituted if the infant develops haemorrhagic symptoms or if the platelet count falls below $50 \times 10^9/l$. Because of the autoimmune nature of the antibody, platelet transfusions usually have a short duration of action and should be reserved for urgent control of bleeding and then combined with other treatment modes. IVIG 0.4 g/kg daily for 3 to 5 days is the treatment of choice in passive neonatal ITP. As with AITP, it is good practice to check for ICH with cranial ultrasound in all infants with platelet counts of $<100 \times 10^9/l$.

Conclusions

Both AITP and ITP present diagnostic challenges as far as the fetal condition is concerned. The progress and management of the two diseases is markedly different. In ITP, the outlook is good and nonintervention during pregnancy is appropriate. In AITP, however, the fetus is at grave risk and antenatal treatment is required. In the USA, maternal treatment with IVIG is widespread, while in Europe the usual approach has involved repeated intrauterine platelet transfusion. What the best method is remains to be established.

References

Anon. (1993). Prenatal management of fetal alloimmune thrombocytopenia. *Vox Sanguinis*, 65, 180–9.

Bennett, P. R., Warwick, R., Letsky, E. & Fisk, N. M. (1994). Determination of fetal Rh D type amplification from fetal skin following massive fetomaternal haemorrhage and fetal death *in utero*. *British Journal of Obstetrics and Gynaecology*, 101, 636–7.

Berndt, M. C., Fournier, D. J. & Castaldi, P. A. (1989). Bernard–Soulier syndrome. In *Ballière's Clinical Haematology* 2:3, pp. 585–608. London: Ballière Tindall.

Bettaieb, A., Rodet, M., Fromont, P., Godeau, B., Duedari, N. & Bierling, P. (1991). Br^b, a platelet alloantigen involved in neonatal alloimmune thrombocytopenia. *Vox Sanguinis*, 60, 230–4.

Blanchette, V. S., Chen, L., Salomon de Freidberg, S., Hoghan, V. A., Trudel, E. & Decary, F. (1990). Immunization to the Pl^A1 antigen: results of a prospective study. *British Journal of Haematology*, 74, 209–15.

Burrows, R. F. & Kelton, J. G. (1988). Incidentally detected thrombocytopenia in healthy mothers and their infants. *New England Journal of Medicine*, 319, 142–5.

Burrows, R. F. & Kelton, J. G. (1990a). Low fetal risks in pregnancies associated with idiopathic thrombocytopenic purpura. *American Journal of Obstetrics and Gynecology*, 163, 1147–50.

Burrows, R. F. & Kelton, J. G. (1990b). Thrombocytopenia at delivery: a prospective survey of 6715 deliveries. *American Journal of Obstetrics and Gynecology*, 163, 731–4.

Burrows, R. F. & Kelton, J. G. (1993). Fetal thrombocytopenia and its relation to maternal thrombocytopenia. *New England Journal of Medicine*, 329, 1463–6.

Bussel, J. B., Berkowitz, R. L., McFarland, J. G., Lynch, L. & Chitkara, U. (1988a). Antenatal treatment of neonatal alloimmune thrombocytopenia. *New England Journal of Medicine*, 319, 1372–8.

Bussel, J. B., Druzin, M. L., Cines, D. B. & Samuels, P. (1991a). Thrombocytopenia in pregnancy. *Lancet*, 337, 251.

Bussel, J. B., McFarland, J. G. & Berkowitz, R. L. (1990). Antenatal management of fetal alloimmune and autoimmune thrombocytopenia. *Transfusion Medicine* Reviews, IV, 149–62.

Bussel, J. B., McFarland, J. G., Kaplan, C. and the Working Party on Neonatal Thrombocytopenia of the Neonatal Haemostasis Subcommittee of the Scientific and Standardisation Committee of the ISTH (1991b). Recommendations for the evaluation and treatment of neonatal autoimmune and alloimmune thrombocytopenia. *Thrombosis and Haemostasis*, 65, 631–4.

Bussel, J. B. and the Neonatal Immune Thrombocytopenia Study Group (1988b). Neonatal alloimmune thrombocytopenia (NAIT): information derived from a prospective international registry. (Abstract) *Paediatric Research*, 23, 337A.

Caen, J. P. (1989). Glanzmann's thrombasthenia. In *Ballière's Clinical Haematology*, 2:3, 609–26. London: Ballière Tindall.

Christiaens, G. C. M. L. & Helmerhorst, F. M. (1987). Validity of intrapartum diagnosis of fetal thrombocytopenia. *American Journal of Obstetrics and Gynecology*, 157, 864–5.

Cines, D. B., Dusak, B., Tomaski, A., Mennuti, M. & Schreiber, A. (1982). Immune thrombocytopenic purpura and pregnancy. *New England Journal of Medicine*, 306, 826–31.

Daffos, F., Forestier, F., Kaplan, C. & Cox, W. (1988). Prenatal diagnosis and management of bleeding disorders with fetal blood sampling. *American Journal of Obstetrics and Gynecology*, 158, 939–46.

Daffos, F., Forestier, F., Muller, J. Y., Reznikoff-Etievant, M. H., Habibi, B., Capella-Pavlova, M., Maigret, P. & Kaplan, C. (1984). Prenatal treatment of alloimmune thrombocytopenia. *Lancet*, ii, 632.

Decary, F., L'Abbe, D., Tremblay, L. & Chartrand, P. (1991). The immune response to the HPA-1a antigen: association with HLA-DRw52a. *Transfusion Medicine*, 1, 55–62.

Derycke, M., Dreyfus, M., Ropert, J. C. & Tchernia, G. (1985). Intravenous immunoglobulin for neonatal isoimmune thrombocytopenia. *Archives of Disease in Childhood*, 60, 667–9.

de Waal., L. P., van Dalen, C. M., Engelfreit, C. D. & von dem Borne, A. E. G. (1986). Alloimmunization against the platelet-specific antigen resulting in neonatal alloimmune thrombocytopenia and post transfusion purpura is associated with the supertypic DRw52 antigen including DR3 and DRw6. *Human Immunology*, 17, 45–53.

de Vries, L. S., Counell, J., Bydder, G. M., Dubowitz, L. M. S., Rodeck, C. H., Mibashan, R. S. & Waters, A. H. (1988). Recurrent intracranial haemorrhage *in utero* in an infant with alloimmune thrombocytopenia. *British Journal of Obstetrics and Gynaecology*, 95, 299–302.

Dunstan, R. A. & Simpson, M. B. (1985). Heterogeneous distribution of antigens on human platelets demonstrated by flow cytometry. *British Journal of Haematology*, 61, 603–9.

Flug, F., Karpatkin, M. & Karpatkin, S. (1994). Should all pregnant women be tested for their PLA phenotype? *British Journal of Haematology*, 86, 1–5.

Friedman, J. M. & Aster, R. H. (1985). Neonatal alloimmune thrombocytopenic purpura and congenital porencephaly in two siblings associated with a new maternal anti-platelet antibody. *Blood*, 65, 1412–15.

Giovangrandi, Y., Daffos, F., Kaplan, C., Forestier, F., MacAleese, J. & Moirot, M. (1990). Very early intracranial haemorrhage in alloimmune thrombocytopenia. *Lancet*, 336, 310.

Gruel, Y., Boizard, B., Daffos, F., Forestier, F., Caen, J. & Wautier, J. L. (1986). Determination of platelet antigens and platelet glycoproteins in the human fetus. *Blood*, 68, 488–92.

Harrington, W. J., Sprague, C. C., Minnich, V., Moore, C. V., Aulvin, R. C. & Dubach, R. (1953). Immunologic mechanisms in idiopathic thrombocytopenic purpura. *Annals of Internal Medicine*, 38, 433–69.

Hart, D., Dunetz, C., Nardi, M., Porges, R. F., Weiss, A. & Karpatkin, M. (1986). An epidemic of maternal thrombocytopenia associated with elevated anti-platelet antibody. *American Journal of Obstetrics and Gynecology*, 154, 878–83.

Herman, J. H., Jumbelic, M. I., Ancona, R. J. & Kickler, T. S. (1986). *In utero* cerebral haemorrhage in alloimmune thrombocytopenia. *American Journal of Pediatric Haematology and Oncology*, 8, 312–17.

Johnson, J. M., McFarland, J. G., Blanchette, V. S., Freedman, J. & Siegel-Bartelt, S. (1993). Prenatal diagnosis of neonatal alloimmune thrombocytopenia using an allele specific oligonucleotide. *Prenatal Diagnosis*, 134, 1037–42.

Kaplan, C., Daffos, F., Forestier, F., Cox, W. L., Lyon-Caen, D., Dupuy-Montbrun, M. C. & Salmon, C. (1988). Management of alloimmune thrombocytopenia: antenatal diagnosis and *in utero* transfusion of maternal platelets. *Blood*, 72, 340–3.

Kaplan, C., Daffos, F., Forestier, F., Tertian, G., Catherine, N., Pons, J. C. & Tchernia, G. (1990). Fetal platelet counts in thrombocytopenic pregnancy. *Lancet*, 336, 979–82.

Kaplan, C., Dehan, M. & Tchernia, G. (1992). Fetal and neonatal thrombocytopenia. *Platelets*, 3, 61–7.

Kaplan, C., Morel-Kopp, M. C., Kroll, H., Kiefel, V., Schlegel, N., Chesnel, N. & Mueller-Eckhardt, C. (1991). HPA-5b (Br^a) neonatal alloimmune thrombocytopenia: clinical and immunological analysis of 39 cases. *British Journal of Haematology*, 78, 425–9.

Kelsey, H., Christopoulos, C., Machin, S. J., Huehns, E. R. & Rodeck, C. H. (1991). Antenatal management of fetal alloimmune thrombocytopenia with early fetal blood sampling, maternal intravenous gammaglobulin and repeated prophylactic fetal platelet transfusions. (Abstract) *British Journal of Haematology*, 79, 675.

Kekomaki, B., Jouhikainen, T., Ollikainen, J., Westman, P. & Laes, M. (1993). A new platelet alloantigen, Tu^a, on glycoprotein IIb/IIIa associated with neonatal alloimmune thrombocytopenia in two families. *British Journal of Haematology*, 83, 306–10.

Kekomaki, R., Raivio, P. & Kero, P. (1992). A new low frequency platelet alloantigen, Va^a, on glycoprotein IIb/IIIa associated with neonatal alloimmune thrombocytopenia. *Transfusion Medicine*, 2, 27–33.

Kiefel, V., Santoso, S., Katzmann, B. & Mueller-Eckhardt, C. (1988). A new platelet-specific alloantigen Br^a. Report of 4 cases with neonatal alloimmune thrombocytopenia. *Vox Sanguinis*, 34, 101–6.

Kuijpers, R. W. A. M., Faber, N. M., Kanhai, H. H. & von dem Borne, A. E. G. (1991). Typing of fetal platelet alloantigens when platelets are not available. *Lancet*, 336, 1319.

Kuijpers, R. W. A. M, Simsek, S., Faber, N. M., Goldschmeding, R., van Wermerkerken, R. K. V. & von dem Borne, A. E. G. (1993). Single point mutation in human glycoprotein IIIa is associated with a new platelet-specific alloantigen (Mo) involved in neonatal alloimmune thrombocytopenia. *Blood*, 81, 70–6.

Liebert, M., Aster, R. H. & Izatkowski, N. S. (1977). Expression of HLA B12 on platelets, lymphocytes and in serum. *Tissue Antigens*, 9, 199–208.

Lipitz, S., Ryan, G., Murphy, M. F., Robson, C., Haeusler, M. C. H., Metcalfe, P., Kelsey, H. & Rodeck, C. H. (1992). Neonatal alloimmune thrombocytopenia due to anti-Pl^A1 (anti-HPA-1a): importance of paternal and fetal platelet typing for assessment of fetal risk. *Prenatal Diagnosis*, 12, 955–8.

Lynch, L., Bussel, J. B., McFarland, J. G., Chitkara, U. & Berkowitz, R. L. (1992). Antenatal treatment of alloimmune thrombocytopenia. *Obstetrics and Gynecology*, 62, 67–71.

McFarland, J. G., Aster, R. H., Bussel, J. B., Gianopoulos, J. G., Derbes, R. S. & Newman, P. J. (1991). Prenatal diagnosis of neonatal alloimmune thrombocytopenia using allele specific oligonucleotide probes. *Blood*, 78, 2276–82.

McFarland, J. G., Blanchette, V., Collins, J., Newman, P. J., Wang, R. & Aster, R. H. (1993). Neonatal alloimmune thrombocytopenia due to a new platelet-specific alloantibody. *Blood*, 81, 3318–23.

McMillan, R., Tani, P., Milland F., Berchtold, P., Renshaw, L. & Woods, V. L. (1987). Platelet associated and plasma anti-glycoprotein autoantibodies in chronic ITP. *Blood*, 70, 1040–5.

Metcalfe, P. & Waters, A. H. (1993). HPA-1 typing by PCR amplification with sequence specific primers (PCR-SSP): a rapid and simple technique. *British Journal of Haematology*, 85, 227–9.

Millar, D., Davis, D. L., Rodeck, C. H., Nicolaides, K. H. & Mibasham, R. S. (1985). Normal blood cell values in the early mid trimester fetus. *Prenatal Diagnosis*, 5, 367–73.

Montemagno, R., Soothill, P. W., Scarcelli, M., O'Brien, P. & Rodeck, C. H. (1994). Detection of alloimmune thrombocytopenia as a cause of isolated hydrocephalus by fetal blood sampling. *Lancet*, 343, 1300–1.

Mueller-Eckhardt, G., Hanck, M., Kayser, W. & Mueller-Eckhardt, C. (1980). HLA C antigens on platelets. *Tissue Antigens*, 16, 91–4.

Mueller-Eckhardt, C., Kiefel, V., Grubert, A., Kroll, H., Weisheit, M., Schmidt, S., Mueller-Eckhardt, G. & Santoso, S. (1989a). 348 cases of suspected neonatal alloimmune thrombocytopenia. *Lancet*, i, 363–6.

Mueller-Eckhardt, C., Kiefel, V., Kroll, H. & Mueller-Eckhardt, G. (1989b). HLA-DRw6, a new immune response marker for immunization against the platelet alloantigen Br[a]. *Vox Sanguinis*, 57, 90–1.

Murphy, M. F., Metcalfe, P., Waters, A. H., Ord, J., Hambley, H. & Nicolaides, K. (1993). Antenatal management of severe feto-maternal alloimmune thrombocytopenia: HLA incompatibility may affect responses to fetal platelet transfusions. *Blood*, 81, 2174–9.

Murphy, M. F., Pullon, H. W. H., Metcalfe, P., Jenkins, E., Waters, A. H., Nicolaides, K. H. & Mibashan, R. S. (1990). Management of fetal alloimmune thrombocytopenia by weekly *in utero* platelet transfusions. *Vox Sanguinis*, 58, 45.

Nicolaides, K. H., Clewell, W. & Rodeck, C. H. (1987). Measurement of human fetoplacental blood volume in erythroblastosis fetalis. *American Journal of Obstetrics and Gynecology*, 157, 50–3.

Nicolini, U. & Rodeck, C. H. (1992). Fetal blood and tissue sampling. In *Prenatal Diagnosis and Screening*, ed. D. J. H. Brock, C. H. Rodeck & M. A. Ferguson-Smith, pp. 39–51. London: Churchill Livingstone.

Nicolini, U., Rodeck, C. H., Kochenur, N. K., Greco, P., Fisk, N. M. & Letsky, E. (1988). *In utero* platelet transfusion for alloimmune thrombocytopenia. *Lancet*, ii, 506.

Nicolini, U., Tannirandorn, Y., Gonzalez, P., Fisk, N. M., Beecham, J., Letsky, E. A. & Rodeck, C. H. (1990). Continuing controversy in alloimmune thrombocytopenia: fetal hyperimmunoglobulinemia fails to prevent thrombocytopenia. *American Journal of Obstetrics and Gynecology*, 163, 1144–6.

Omshi, S., Okubo, S., Matsuzaki, T., Ishidia, T. & Yasunagak, K. (1992). Report of two cases of neonatal alloimmune thrombocytopenia caused by anti-HLA antibodies and their screening using umbilical cord blood. *Japanese Journal of Clinical Haematology*, 33, 42–7.

Pearson, H. A., Shulman, N. R., Marder, V. J. & Cone, T. E. (1964). Isoimmune neonatal thrombocytopenic purpura – clinical and therapeutic considerations. *Blood*, 23, 154–77.

Reznikoff-Etievant, M. E. (1988). Management of alloimmune neonatal thrombocytopenia and antenatal thrombocytopenia. *Vox Sanguinis*, 55, 193–201.

Reznikoff-Etievant, M. F., Muller, J. Y., Julien, F. & Patereau, C. (1983). An immune response gene linked to HLA in man. *Tissue Antigens*, 22, 312–14.

Rodeck, C. H. & Roberts, L. (1994). Successful treatment of fetal cardiac arrest by left ventricular exchange transfusion. *Fetal Diagnosis and Therapy*, 9, 213–17.

Samuels, P., Bussel, J. B., Braitman, L. E., Tomaski, A., Druzin, M. L., Mennuti, M. T. & Cines, D. B. (1990). Estimation of the risk of thrombocytopenia in the offspring of pregnant women with presumed immune thrombocytopenic purpura. *New England Journal of Medicine*, 323, 229–35.

Shibata, Y., Matsuda, I., Miyaji, T. & Ichikawa, Y. (1986). Yuk^a, a new platelet antigen involved in two cases of neonatal alloimmune thrombocytopenia. *Vox Sanguinis*, 50, 177–80.

Shwe, K. H., Love, E. M., Lieberman, B. A. & Newland, A. C. (1991). High dose intravenous immunoglobulin in the prenatal management of neonatal alloimmune thrombocytopenia. *Clinical and Laboratory Haematology*, 13, 75–9.

Van den Hof, M. C. & Nicolaides, K. H. (1990). Platelet count in normal, small, and anemic fetuses. *American Journal of Obstetrics and Gynecology*, 162, 735–9.

Van den Veyver, I. B., Chong, S. S., Kristjansson, K., Snabes, M. C., Moise, K. J. Jr & Hughes, M. R. (1994). Molecular analysis of human platelet antigen system 1 antigen on single cells can be applied to preimplantation genetic diagnosis for prevention of alloimmune thrombocytopenia. *American Journal of Obstetrics and Gynecology*, 170, 801–12.

von dem Borne, A. E. G. & Decary, F. (1990). Nomenclature of platelet-specific antigens. *Human Immunology*, 29, 1–2.

von dem Borne, A. E. G. & Ouwehand, W. H. (1989). Immunology of platelet disorders. In *Ballière's Clinical Haematology*, 2:3, pp. 749–781. London: Ballière Tindall.

von dem Borne, A. E. G., Vos, J. J., van der Lelie, E., Bossers, B. & van Dalen, C. M. (1986). Clinical significance of a positive platelet immuno-fluorescence test in thrombocytopenia. *British Journal of Haematology*, 64, 767–76.

Weiner, E., Zosmer, N., Bajoria, R., Sepulveda, W., Vaughan, J. I., Letsky, E. A., Fisk, N. M. (1994). Direct fetal administration of immunoglobulins: another disappointing therapy in alloimmune thrombocytopenia. *Fetal Diagnosis and Therapy*, 9, 159–64.

Williamson, L. M., Bruce, D., Lubenko, A., Chana, H. J. & Ouwehand, W. H. (1992). Molecular biology for platelet alloantigen typing. *Transfusion Medicine*, 2, 225–64.

12 Fetal arrhythmias

JOSHUA A. COPEL AND CHARLES S. KLEINMAN

Introduction

With recent greater attention to fetal cardiac imaging and fetal heart rate monitoring, there has been a heightened awareness of the diagnosis and management of fetal cardiac arrhythmias. In this chapter, we shall review the major categories of fetal arrhythmias, their pathophysiology and clinical consequences, and consider the potential areas in which fetal treatment may be helpful. Throughout such discussions the overriding consideration must be the safety of both mother and fetus. For that reason any therapy must be based on an understanding of the underlying electrophysiology of the arrhythmia and on knowledge of the fetomaternal pharmacology and the pharmacokinetics of antiarrhythmic agents. A rational risk–benefit analysis must take place, since every available antiarrhythmic agent carries the potential for significant toxicity. In reviewing fetal arrhythmias and their treatment, we will discuss selected treatment approaches and drugs in this context, although the details of the biochemistry of the drugs will not be discussed in detail. An extensive review of the electrophysiology of fetal tachyarrhythmias and the drugs in common use for their treatment can be found in a number of recent publications (Kleinman & Copel, 1991; 1996). A review of our experience is illustrated in Table 12.1.

Fetal rhythm analysis

While the ideal clinical tool for the analysis of arrhythmias is the electrocardiogram, this is a technique that is currently unavailable for use in the fetus without placing electrodes directly on the fetal body. This would require the use of electrodes placed on a surgically exposed fetus or, alternatively, the application of internal leads applied intrapartum to a fetal presenting part. Since most fetal arrhythmias require diagnosis before the onset of labour, other noninvasive approaches must be utilized. The ultrasonographic techniques that have been used for fetal cardiac rhythm analysis include M-mode echocardiography, pulsed Doppler, and Doppler colour flow-encoded M-mode echocardiography, M/Q tracings.

In the absence of a high-fidelity electrocardiographic tracing offering visualization of electrical depolarization and repolarization of the atria (P waves) and ventricles (QRS complexes and T waves), cardiac ultrasound is used to detect mechanical events in the cardiac cycle by M-mode echocardiography that represent the mechanical responses to the preceding electrical stimulation. These are recorded in hard copy against time. Reasoning backward from the mechanical undulation of the atrial or ventricular walls, and undulations of the atrioventricular and/or semilunar valves to the preceding electrical event allows an indirect analysis of the electrophysiology of the underlying rhythm (Kleinman et al., 1980; 1983; DeVore, Siassi & Platt, 1983; Silverman et al., 1985). Because the sampling rate of M-mode echocardiography is quite rapid (1000/second) the tracings obtained by this technique represent virtually continuous tracings of wall and valve movement against time. Many of the changes in wall or valve motion cannot be detected through the use of techniques involving a significantly slower sampling rate such as real-time two-dimensional imaging. In the fetus, atrial flutter rates, for example, may approach 500 beats/min (8/second), making two-dimensional recordings of wall motion

Table 12.1 *Fetal cardiac arrhythmias: the Yale experience*

Arrhythmia type	No. of fetuses
Isolated extrasystoles	1026
Supraventricular tachycardia	58
Atrial flutter	17
Atrial fibrillation	2
Sinus tachycardia	6
Junctional tachycardia	1
Ventricular tachycardia	6
Complete heart block	29
Second degree AV block	8
Sinus bradycardia	6
Total	1159

atrial and ventricular activity simultaneously, allowing the rate and atrioventricular contraction sequence to be discerned (Fig. 12.1). Such alignment is not always simple to obtain and is, to a large extent, dependent upon fetal position. Fetal movement and fetal breathing may complicate the process.

Pulsed Doppler analysis may be a useful tool for fetal cardiac rhythm analysis in selected situations (Kleinman, 1986; Strasburger, 1986; Steinfeld, 1986; Reed, 1987; Lingman, 1987). This records intravascular or intracardiac blood flow events in hard copy against time. Just as M-mode tracings are analysed to relate mechanical events to the preceding electrical stimulation, the pulsed Doppler evaluation relates the flow patterns within the cardiovascular system to the immediately preceding mechanical and electrical events. Typically, signals representing flow across the atrioventricular junction in the fetus differ significantly from those seen postnatally (Kleinman, Weinstein & Copel, 1986). Because the fetal ventricular myocardium is less compliant than that of the neonate or older children, the fetal heart is more dependent upon active atrial contraction for adequate ventricular filling (Romero, Covell & Friedman, 1972). The biphasic

inadequate for detailed analysis of atrioventricular contraction sequences.

Obtaining diagnostic tracings may be a time consuming process, since the M-mode sampling line must be oriented in a fashion that allows identification of the structures being examined. It is crucial to align the M-mode cursor to transect structures that represent

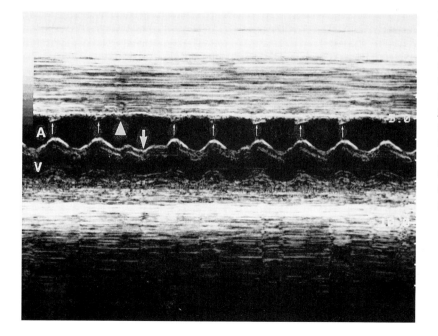

Fig. 12.1 *M-mode echocardiogram through the atrium (A) and ventricle (V), showing normal, regular atrial contractions (small arrows), with a premature atrial beat (arrowhead) that is followed by a ventricular response reflected by downward movement of the atrioventricular valve (large arrow).*

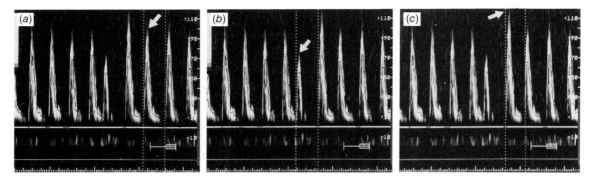

Fig. 12.2 *Pulsed Doppler waveforms from the aortic arch in a fetus with premature atrial beats. The flow velocity integral is measured from the waveform as indicated between the white vertical markers. (a) A normal beat, with a flow-velocity integral of 20.4 cm/s (white arrow); (b) a premature atrial beat, with a diminished flow–velocity integral, 18.0 cm/s (white arrow); (c) post-extrasystolic beat with enhanced flow–velocity integral, 26.4 cm/s (white arrow).*

Doppler flow waveform of transmitral or transtricuspid valve flow, therefore, shows less flow in the early passive filling phase (E wave) than in the active filling phase of diastole (A wave).

If pulsed Doppler flow analysis is used for fetal cardiac rhythm analysis, a particularly useful location for the placement of the sample volume is in the left ventricle, at the junction of the ventricular inflow tract and the left ventricular outflow tract to the aorta. In this location, both ventricular filling and emptying patterns can be seen with inflow and outflow represented on opposite sides of the Doppler baseline, since flow directions are opposite to one another. A similar strategy has been recently described in which the Doppler sample volume is placed in a position overlapping pulmonary venous flow with pulmonary arterial outflow from the heart (Devore & Horenstein, 1993). Visualization of an abnormal early A wave during diastole can identify early electrical stimulation of the fetal atrium, as shown in Fig. 12.1. While we find the M-mode echocardiogram much more helpful and understandable than pulsed Doppler tracings for rhythm analysis, Doppler evaluation has been particularly helpful in providing information regarding the physiological impact of fetal arrhythmias on

the fetal cardiovascular system (Reed *et al.*, 1987) (Fig. 12.2).

The advent of Doppler colour flow mapping has allowed superimposition of flow information onto the two-dimensional image, thus providing the equivalent of a noninvasive angiocardiogram. When used for postnatal echocardiographic study, the colour flow map may provide invaluable physiological information that is superimposed on the two-dimensional image (Ortiz *et al.*, 1985; Chiba *et al.*, 1990; Copel *et al.*, 1991). The colour flow information has no intrinsic temporal resolution, making simultaneous recording of an electrocardiogram a requisite part of the colour flow analysis postnatally.

The lack of availability of a fetal electrocardiogram is the reason that echocardiographic techniques are employed for fetal rhythm analysis. The simultaneous inscription of colour flow information upon a background of timed mechanical events represented by the M-mode echocardiogram enables the fetal cardiologist to obtain colour flow data that have temporal resolution imparted by the M-mode trace. For this reason, the colour flow encoded M-mode echocardiogram has been termed 'M/Q Doppler' (Eyer *et al.*, 1981). As previously described with pulsed Doppler, the most effective strategy for the use of this modality has been to orient the M-mode cursor across the junction of ventricular inflow and outflow streams, making flow into the ventricle 180° different from the outflow. Typically in normal sinus rhythm, ventricular filling will appear as a biphasic blush of one colour, while ventricular outflow will appear as a uniphasic signal in the opposite colour (Fig. 12.3). The outflow pattern will often alias because of relatively high physiological velocities exceeding the Nyquist limit of the colour flow systems.

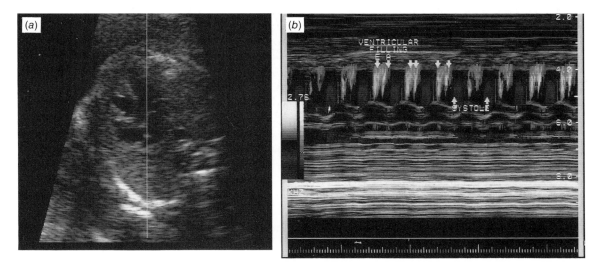

Fig. 12.3 (a) *Four chamber view of the fetal heart with M-mode cursor through the left ventricle and aortic outflow tract.* (b) *Colour Doppler M-mode study showing normal biphasic ventricular filling (E, A), and ventricular systole as indicated. Fetus is in normal sinus rhythm.*

The irregular fetal heart rhythm

Assessment

The most common indication for fetal rhythm analysis is an irregular fetal cardiac rhythm. Because physiological variable decelerations are commonly encountered in the second trimester, especially while the patient lies supine (Sorokin *et al.*, 1982), it is important to distinguish a transient slowing of the fetal heart from a true irregularity of rhythm. The former is benign and does not require further investigation, while the latter, most often also benign, may warrant further investigation.

The most common irregularity of fetal cardiac rhythm occurs with variable frequency against a background normal rate. The pattern that is detected may suggest either a pause or an extra beat. The difference between these two manifestations lies in the timing of the extrasystoles. If a supraventricular extrasystole occurs very early in diastole it may occur during the refractory period of the atrioventricular conduction system. Such beats will not be conducted into the ventricle and will not be associated with ventricular ejection. The atrial pace-

maker will be reset, and there will be a longer pause between ventricular ejections than normal. Since most fetal cardiac auscultation involves the use of Doppler devices, the absence of ejection into the fetal arteries will result in the perception of a skipped beat, even when the underlying electrophysiology actually is that of an early or extra beat. M-mode or Doppler flow analysis will demonstrate passive E wave filling of the ventricle after ventricular systole, with the early A wave appearing closer to, or even superimposed upon, the E wave. If the premature A wave is not obscured in the passive filling phase, the time to the next A wave can be demonstrated to be the same as that between normal beats.

If a supraventricular extrasystole occurs slightly later in diastole, it may encounter the atrioventricular conduction system at a time allowing conduction into the ventricle. Even then diastolic filling of the ventricle may be inadequate to permit significant ejection of blood into the fetal arterial system secondary to an inadequate stroke volume. In such cases, the Doppler flow detectors may note a weak pulse or no pulse at all, again leading to the perception of a pause rather than an extra beat. Typically the postextrasystolic beat is more forceful than usual (Reed *et al.*, 1987). This relates to enhanced diastolic filling of the ventricle during the prolonged diastolic filling period of the postextrasystolic pause. This increased diastolic volume enhances ventricular ejection in the intact fetal ventricle via the Frank–Starling mechanism, which is limited but extant in the human fetus (Romero *et al.*, 1972; Rudolph, 1974). In addition, there is a longer period for diastolic runoff during the prolonged postextrasystolic period, which leads to lower arterial diastolic pressures. The first postextrasystolic beat, therefore, occurs in a setting of enhanced fetal ventricular preload and decreased arterial afterload. The absence of a potentiated post-extrasystolic beat may be a means of detecting intrinsic impairment of fetal ventricular myocardium.

The distinction of extrasystoles arising from atrial, junctional, or ventricular sites is quite time-consuming and difficult even postnatally. The distinction of ventricular from junctional and, occasionally, atrial from junctional extrasystoles may be demanding, if not impossible. Such exercises, while helpful in developing experience in the analysis of fetal cardiac M-mode and Doppler tracings, have little pragmatic significance, since the isolated extrasystole is of importance only as a potential harbinger of sustained tachyarrhythmias in the future (Kleinman & Copel, 1994). In such cases, the usual underlying mechanism involves reentry circuits, either within areas of diseased atrial or ventricular myocardium or, more frequently, involving accessory conduction pathways at the level of the atrioventricular junction (Kleinman & Copel, 1991). At this stage of our experience, we have noted the onset of sustained fetal or neonatal supraventricular tachycardia in five fetuses out of almost 1200 who were discerned to have isolated extrasystoles during fetal life, a risk of approximately 0.5%. Four of these occurred prenatally, the fifth occurred on the third day of life in a neonate who was diagnosed to have blocked atrial bigeminy *in utero* that had been incorrectly diagnosed as complete heart block in another hospital. This neonate had Wolff–Parkinson–White syndrome on the neonatal electrocardiogram and developed sustained supraventricular tachycardia on the third day of life. An additional fetus referred for only isolated extrasystoles identified during a routine prenatal visit was found to have brief runs of supraventricular tachycardia when the fetal echocardiogram was performed the next day.

Management

We generally recommend that fetuses with extrasystoles have fetal heart rate checks at least weekly until several visits fail to demonstrate remaining irregularities. By not allowing more than a week between heart rate evaluations, the potential for the development of nonimmune hydrops caused by sustained supraventricular tachycardia between visits is minimized. These heart rate checks can be undertaken using Doppler stethoscope auscultation rather than continuous electronic fetal heart rate monitoring. In selected situations, the pregnant woman or another family member may be trained to perform such auscultation. We approach the fetus with frequent premature beats or even atrial bigeminy in exactly the same fashion. If premature couplets or triplets are noted, the potential for sustained tachycardia is greater. We have been quite pleased to find that the same management strategy has been quite effective for the management of 99.5% of fetuses with isolated extrasystoles, or even short nonsustained episodes of tachycardia.

We also recommend that the mother avoids stimulants such as caffeine or medications with sympathomimetic effects. Management of the patient with fetal extrasystoles who also has preterm labour is problematic, as β-adrenergic agents may also provoke atrial or ventricular ectopy. The potential for the precipitation of clinically significant sustained tachycardia certainly exists in such cases. Alternative tocolytics such as intravenous magnesium or oral nifedipine may be preferable in these patients.

The major complication we have encountered with extrasystoles *per se* has been in the patient with persistent fetal premature beats who presents in labour. If the extrasystoles are very frequent, they may render electronic fetal heart rate monitoring in labour difficult. This can usually be overcome with sufficient patience and an attempt to look at the long-term fetal heart rate pattern, rather than small portions of the tracing. The small but finite possibility that structural abnormalities or cardiomyopathies might underlie the presentation with isolated extrasystoles, and the rare fetus with atrial flutter and variable block or brief episodes of reentrant tachycardia who may sound similar to the fetus with extrasystoles, make us continue to recommend full fetal echocardiographic evaluation for all fetuses presenting with irregular fetal heart rates. The rarity with which complications occur in the fetus with isolated extrasystoles and the benign course that is anticipated when isolated extrasystoles occur in the neonate or child argue strongly against any attempt to suppress these extrasystoles with maternal medications (Blandon & Leandro, 1985).

Tachycardias

Fetal tachycardia can be defined as a heart rate of 180 beats/min. This arrhythmia occurs less frequently than the irregular fetal heart rhythm; however, tachycardias are more common than fetal bradycardia. Fetal tachycardias can be generally divided into supraventricular tachycardia, atrial flutter, atrial fibrillation, ventricular tachycardia and sinus tachycardia.

Supraventricular tachycardia

Pathophysiology

The most common type of pathologic tachycardia we have encountered has been supraventricular tachycardia (SVT). This is most often reciprocating or atrioventricular reentrant tachycardia. In this situation, a circular movement of electrical impulses is initiated by an extrasystole that is conducted slowly through the atrioventricular node to the ventricle and then reenters the atrial tissue by way of an accessory conduction pathway that bypasses the atrioventricular node (Kleinman & Copel, 1991). In many neonates presenting with SVT, the electrocardiogram demonstrates a narrow QRS complex during tachycardia with retrograde P waves, suggesting atrial depolarization by way of an impulse reentering the atrium from the region of the atrioventricular junction. When these neonates are converted electrically or pharmacologically to normal sinus rhythm, many will demonstrate antegrade conduction through an accessory conduction pathway that results in a short PR interval with a slurred initial ventricular depolarization demonstrated as a delta wave and a broadened QRS complex. This is the pattern typical of the Wolff–Parkinson–White syndrome.

Most patients are found to have a normal electrocardiogram during sinus rhythm because the accessory conduction pathway does not conduct in an antegrade direction from the atrium to the ventricle. In these patients, the accessory pathway is only available to conduct in the retrograde direction if unmasked by an extrasystole. This extrasystole must occur with just the right timing to allow the spreading electrical impulse in the ventricular muscle to encounter the ventricular terminus of the accessory connection when it is ready to conduct retrograde into the atrial muscle. This establishes a circular, reentrant or reciprocating circuit that depolarizes the atrium and the ventricle at a rate that exceeds and is independent of the rate of depolarization of the normal sinus node. While the potential exists to recognize a characteristic undulation of the ventricular septum on the M-mode echocardiogram of some patients with right-sided accessory atrioventricular connections, this is quite rare and often not reproducible. To date, we have suspected the presence of a right-sided bypass tract in only one fetus with SVT and an early or presystolic notch in ventricular septal motion.

Reciprocating atrioventricular reentrant tachycardia depends upon the presence of an accessory pathway with a different conduction velocity and effective refractory period to that of the atrioventricular node for the initiation and maintenance of this arrthymia. The rationale of therapy is usually directed at altering the conduction velocities and/or refractory periods of the atrioventricular nodal tissue, while less frequently the accessory conduction tissue is targeted (Kleinman & Copel, 1991). In addition, the intrinsic properties of the atrioventricular nodal and accessory conduction tissue constituting the electrical circuit appear to impart relatively distinct characteristics to this type of tachycardia. The rate is virtually always 240–260 beats/min. While we are reluctant to use absolute terms, the experience that we have had suggests that any sustained tachycardia outside of this range should be viewed as being something other than atrioventricular reciprocating tachycardia unless proved otherwise. This does not mean that any tachycardia in the 240–260 beats/min range must be atrioventricular reciprocating tachycardia, but if the rate is not in this range one should have serious doubts about the underlying aetiology of the arrhythmia.

Assessment

The initial determination of the need for antiarrhythmic therapy must be based upon a logical analysis of a number of factors. These include gestational age, the presence or absence of fetal hydrops and the relative amount of time spent in the tachycardia. As an example, a nonhydropic fetus presenting with occasional nonsustained episodes of tachycardia at term is best managed by delivery and postnatal evaluation and possible treatment. However, a hydropic fetus in the midtrimester with an incessant tachycardia merits a completely different approach. Most patients, however, fail to fall into either of these extremes, and the approach to each patient must be individualized according to local experience with postnatal management of premature neonates with sustained cardiac arrhythmias. The dismal prognosis expected for severely hydropic premature infants suggests that many of these fetuses are better candidates for *in utero* rather than postnatal therapy.

In the absence of fetal hydrops, it has become our practice to employ continous fetal heart rate monitoring for a prolonged period, generally at least overnight, in order to establish the pattern of time spent in the tachycardia. Such monitoring allows us to determine whether fetal therapy is indicated and may allow us to detect whether initial doses of medication are having an influence on the frequency and duration of the arrhythmia.

Whether or not a fetus with intermittent tachycardia will develop hydrops is a central question in determining the need for fetal therapy. It is not clear why some fetuses take a longer period of time to develop oedema while others seem to develop severe hydrops in a short period of time. Critical factors may include venous hydrostatic pressure and serum oncotic pressure. Doppler studies of flow in the fetal inferior vena cava during atrial ectopy and during sustained SVT demonstrate prominent retrograde flow into the hepatic circulation. Previous experiences in our laboratory have demonstrated that fetuses who remain hydropic for many days after conversion of fetal tachycardia to sinus rhythm also have marked fetal hypoalbuminaemia with consequent hypoosmolality. The fetal hypoalbuminaemia may be related to passive hepatic congestion and secondary impairment of hepatic synthetic function. We believe that the hypoosmolality and associated low serum oncotic pressure explain why agents such as frusemide do not appear to be beneficial in the treatment of such fetuses.

Another potentially important factor is the site of initial atrial depolarization, which might affect atrial emptying. Initial depolarization of the left atrium, by transiently increasing left atrial pressure above right, could partially close the atrial foramen ovale. This would trap more blood than usual returning from the inferior vena cava in the right heart (Buis-Liem *et al.*, 1987). A higher systemic venous pressure would occur and render the fetus more prone to the development of hydrops. Two human fetuses recently encountered in our laboratory appear to support this mechanism. Similarly, atrial pacing studies in lamb fetuses have demonstrated that altering the location of atrial pacing significantly alters ventricular outputs and flow distribution (Nimrod *et al.*, 1987).

Therapeutic modalities

The postnatal approach to reciprocating atrioventricular tachycardia involves the use of rapidly acting pharmacologic agents such as adenosine to cause transient atrioventricular block to break the reentry circuit, leading to an immediate resolution of the tachycardia (Camm & Garratt, 1991). Alternatively, oesophageal or intracardiac overdrive pacing and/or electrical cardioversion can be utilized. Such treatments have a limited role in fetal therapy. Postnatally, the application of physical techniques to increase vagal tone, such as eliciting the diving seal reflex through ice application to the neonate's face or the use of carotid massage, can be used to break runs of tachycardia. Prenatal manoeuvres such as external compression of the umbilical cord may also result in transient breaks in tachycardia (Martin Nijhuis & Weijer, 1984; Fernandez *et al.*, 1988). Such treatments may be useful as diagnostic tests to determine whether the underlying electrophysiological mechanism of the tachycardia is reentrant, involving the atrioventricular node as one limb of the reentrant circuit. However, one would not expect more than a transient reversion to sinus rhythm with these manoeuvres. The preexisting extrasystoles which are almost always present quickly result in recurrent tachycardia. While the temptation may exist to reapply such therapies, we believe them not worthwhile, since prophylaxis against recurrent tachycardia is the most important objective once the tachycardia has been established to have a reciprocating atrioventricular reentry mechanism.

Typical agents used in the treatment of reentrant tachycardia depress conduction and prolong the effective refractory period of the atrioventricular node

(Kleinman & Copel, 1991). The cardiac glycoside digoxin (Kleinman *et al.*, 1985), β-blockers propranolol and labetalol, calcium channel blockers verapamil and diltiazem, and adenosine are included in this group. Agents that have their primary impact on the accessory conduction pathways include the type IA antiarrhythmic agents such as quinidine, procainamide and disopyramide (Gunteroth *et al.*, 1985), and 1C agents such as flecainide and sotalol (Wren & Hunter, 1988; Allan *et al.*, 1991; Kofinas *et al.*, 1991; Perry, Ayres & Carpenter, 1991). Amiodarone, a type III agent, has been reported to be useful in some fetuses after oral administration to the mother or direct intravenous administration to the fetus (Arnoux *et al.*, 1987; Gembruch *et al.*, 1989). However, the extremely protracted half life and potential danger of associated side effects, including interference with normal fetal thyroid function (Laurent *et al.*, 1987; Rovet, 1987) and myocardial development (Nag, 1990), have led us to consider this as a medication of last resort.

Protocols for the treatment of paediatric arrhythmias vary from institution to institution. There should be little wonder, therefore, that there is no unanimity of opinion regarding the best protocol for *in utero* antiarrhythmic therapy. Any approach seeking a magic bullet that will treat all arrhythmias is quite naive, since the variability of response of accurately diagnosed arrhythmias postnatally has led to a large number of therapies, including radio frequency ablation in refractory cases (Kugler *et al.*, 1994). Yet the literature concerning antenatal antiarrhythmic therapy seems to suggest a simplistic approach that is based only on the transplacental passage of these medications. The complex interactions between drug disposition in the mother, fetus and placenta make it likely that most of these agents will vary in bioavailability from patient to patient and, potentially, even within the same patient. Such factors as regional blood flow, serum protein levels and pH shift with changing degrees of haemodynamic stability affect the pharmacokinetics of these agents. Even the most widely used agent, digoxin, is known to have variable penetration to the fetus, particularly in the presence of placental oedema secondary to nonimmune hydrops (Weiner, Landas & Persoon, 1987, Weiner & Thompson, 1988; Younis & Granat, 1987). To avoid this problem, direct fetal administration of digoxin has been advocated. Digoxin has been administered either intravenously

(Schlebusch, 1991) or intramuscularly (Weiner & Thompson, 1988).

The desire to provide a simple treatment algorithm for fetal arrhythmias is very strong. Perhaps a brief historical review of the evolution of such algorithms at our centre is in order. Years ago, we arrived at the conclusion that digoxin was a logical drug to offer mothers for therapy of fetal SVT: (i) it has been in use in one or another form for over two centuries; (ii) its safety in pregnancy has been well documented over many decades; (iii) it is widely available and is relative inexpensive; (iv) unique among antiarrhythmic agents, it is a positive rather than a negative inotropic agent; and (v) serum assays are readily available. Empirical use of this agent demonstrated its utility for use in postnatal SVT and it proved to be quite effective in the therapy of fetal SVT. Not surprisingly, based on its efficacy in conversion of approximately 60% of neonatal SVTs, this agent did not result in control of all cases of SVT. It remains the first-line drug in our protocol for therapy of fetal SVT, but in about 40% of cases a second agent is required. We quickly became disenchanted with the use of propranolol, as this agent did not seem to be efficacious in our experience, despite the use of very high oral doses.

Verapamil was introduced as an alternative for the treatment of neonatal reentrant SVT. We administered it to several mothers, using oral dosages that were gradually increased to levels as high as 160 mg four times daily in one patient, and 200 mg four times daily in a second. The worst side effect that we encountered in eight patients was maternal constipation. We administered the verapamil intravenously to the first mother we treated, but in the subsequent seven mothers used only oral administration. This agent was effective and we were satisfied that it should be administered as the drug of second choice in our emerging algorithm. In 1987, we were alarmed to read a report associating the use of verapamil for control of neonatal SVT with congestive heart failure and the potential for haemodynamic collapse in 10–20% of neonates receiving it by intravenous injection (Garson, 1987). While we were not administering the agent intravenously, we certainly were administering it to immature patients with an immature, presumably calcium flux-dependent, myocardium. This led us to discontinue the use of verapamil. The speed at which agents such as verapamil are viewed as first beneficial and later potentially harmful is alarming but points out the need to remain abreast of changes in therapy. This further emphasizes the importance of a multidisciplinary approach to such patients.

Another agent with a similar record is flecainide, a type 1C agent introduced as a potential remedy for all forms of supraventricular and ventricular tachycardia. An agent with a spectrum of antiarrhythmic activity so broad that the accuracy of the electrophysiologic diagnosis of the fetal arrhythmia becomes much less important would be attractive. Flecainide appeared to be such an agent as it has been found useful for the treatment of a wide variety of paediatric arrhythmias. Its use in the treatment of fetal arrhythmias has also been described (Wren & Hunter, 1988; Allan *et al.*, 1991; Kofinas et al,, 1991; Perry *et al.*, 1991). Unfortunately, agents in this class have been reported to cause proarrhythmic deaths with alarming frequency in a group of adult patients treated prophylactically for ventricular arrhythmias following myocardial infarction (CAST Investigators, 1989). This study led to a reconsideration of the use of 1C agents. Subsequent experience, especially in the paediatric population (Fish, Gillette & Benson, 1991), has suggested that Class 1C drugs may be quite useful. The cardiovascular status of the older men surviving myocardial infarctions who comprised the population of the CAST study is quite different from the fetus and the pregnant mother. Nonetheless the potential for a ventricular proarrhythmic effect of this agent clearly exists. A recent preliminary report of a multicentre trial of propafenone, another type of 1C agent, suggests its usefulness for supraventricular and ventricular arrhythmias. Sudden death occurred in 1 of 58 patients studied (Reimer, Paul, & Kallfelz, 1991).

Even our most fundamental antiarrhythmic agent, digoxin, has been reexamined in the light of potential problems. The role of digoxin has been placed in doubt by the reports of a 1% incidence of sudden death among children receiving it for long-term treatment of SVT in the presence of Wolff–Parkinson–White syndrome (Deal *et al.*, 1985). Certainly, adults and older children with the Wolff–Parkinson–White syndrome receiving digoxin are at risk of a shortened antegrade effective refractory period in the accessory pathway, which may cause rapid conduction of intercurrent atrial fibrillation and be fatal (Wellens & Durrer, 1973). Some have

suggested that digoxin should not be used at all in cases of Wolff–Parkinson–White syndrome at any age (Duvernoy, 1977). Gillette has suggested that if the effective refractory period is above 220 ms during treatment, infants may be safely treated with digoxin, even in the presence of Wolff–Parkinson–White syndrome (Gillette, Blair & Crawford, 1990). In addition, this agent has been used for years for neonatal SVT and empirical experience has shown that it is effective. We still consider digoxin our drug of first choice when reciprocating atrioventricular tachycardia requires treatment in the fetus.

It has been demonstrated that a digoxin-like immunoreactive substance can be found in the serum of pregnant women, especially in the presence of polyhydramnios and hydrops fetalis. This same substance can been found in the fetal circulation as well (González *et al.*, 1987; Weiner *et al.*, 1987). This has been identified to be ouabain-like, with Na^+K^+-ATPase blocking activity (Ebara *et al.*, 1988; Morris *et al.*, 1988). It has been suggested that digoxin administered to the pregnant patient does not reach the hydropic fetus across the hydropic placenta, and that serum assays suggesting otherwise are confounded by the digoxin-like immunoreactive substance (Younis & Granat, 1987; Weiner *et al.*, 1987; Weiner & Thompson, 1988). However, the use of digoxin has resulted in the resolution of fetal SVT in approximately 60% of patients. It is unclear whether the potential for inducing maternal and/or fetal digoxin toxicity exists, since exogenous drug is being added to a system that is producing endogenous ouabain. We are unaware of any cases in which such toxicity has been suggested.

Recommended management protocol

We believe that it is important for obstetric and paediatric cardiology consultants to collaborate to develop a local protocol for the treatment of sustained fetal arrhythmias. Such protocols should include indications for therapy and should be logically based on an understanding of the electrophysiology of the arrhythmia and the pharmacology and pharmacokinetics of the agents employed. The sequential administration of antiarrhythmic agents should be logically based on an understanding of the mechanism of action of the drug. The use of redundant agents that act through the same molecular mechanism may increase the potential for disastrous proarrhythmic side effects with no likelihood of added therapeutic efficacy. A case in point is an algorithm that has been suggested for therapy of hydropic fetuses who are unresponsive to digoxin therapy for sustained SVT. This algorithm suggests that the second line of therapy should include the simultaneous maternal administration of procainamide and quinidine (DeVore, Siassi & Platt, 1990). Both these agents are class IA and are associated with the potential for proarrhythmic effects that may result in fatal torsades de pointe secondary to pathologic prolongation of the QT interval. The concomitant use of these agents represents a rarely used and very controversial combination of drugs that most electrophysiologists would consider potentially lethal to both mother and fetus.

The typical presentation of fetal SVT with hydrops is so dramatic as to appear to be a dire emergency that must be immediately controlled. It is clear that some fetuses may die soon after diagnosis. One of our patients had a fetal demise within one hour of arrival at our hospital, before therapy could be instituted. In general, however, these fetuses are not moribund and may be safely observed and treated in a logical fashion, without a high likelihood of immediate demise. Antiarrhythmic agents may require hours or days to reach therapeutic levels. Equally important, many of these agents, such as flecainide and amiodarone, have significantly long half lives and may remain in the maternal or fetal bloodstream or tissue for many days after discontinuation of medication. There should be a logical sequence followed if medications are to be changed in order to avoid the potential toxicity of having multiple antiarrhythmic agents present simultaneously.

We currently employ digoxin as our agent of first choice in the treatment of reciprocating SVT in the preterm hydropic fetus. We use an intravenous loading dose of 1.0 mg divided over 12 hours. A loading dose of 0.5 mg is followed by two 0.25 mg doses at six hour intervals. We monitor the maternal response with continuous cardiac monitoring after ascertaining that the maternal electrolytes and EKG are normal. The fetus is observed by continuous external electronic monitoring and fetal ultrasound is performed at least daily.

We believe that all antiarrhythmic therapy should be initiated on an in-patient basis, even in this day of streamlining medical care to reduce medical costs. Incremental intravenous doses of digoxin are frequently required, and the total loading dose over the first 24 to 36 hours of treatment may be as high as 2.0 mg. Thereafter, oral maintenance therapy is instituted, again monitoring for EKG or subjective evidence of maternal digoxin toxicity. Maternal serum digoxin levels of 1.5 to 2.0 ng/ml are sought, as long as there is no EKG or subjective evidence of digoxin toxicity. Achieving therapeutic maternal serum levels often requires surprisingly high doses of digoxin (0.50–1.0 mg/day). If any other medications are ultimately needed, it is essential to remember that some antiarrhythmic agents, including quinidine, verapamil and amiodarone, increase digoxin serum levels and bioavailability even if digoxin has been in steady-state for long periods. Digoxin serum levels should be monitored, and digoxin doses should be empirically reduced by 50% or more to prevent inadvertent digoxin toxicity.

The absence of the desired therapeutic response may relate to inadequate delivery of drug to the fetus. It is also possible that the arrhythmia has been incorrectly diagnosed. The differential diagnosis of fetal atrial tachycardia includes ectopic focus tachycardia. In this syndrome, the heart rate arises from an irritable focus of atrial tissue, which serves as an inappropriate and rapid pacemaker and usurps the normal sinus pacemaker, resulting in an incessant tachycardia (Knudson et al., 1994). This is the mechanism of approximately 10% of fetal and neonatal tachycardia. This condition is extremely difficult to treat and may fail to respond to any of the medications described previously. Digoxin may induce atrioventricular block, but blocking the atrioventricular node does not break such tachycardia. Likewise, agents such as adenosine, verapamil, pacing and electrical cardioversion are ineffective for such arrhythmias. Type IA or 1C agents may have some efficacy for ectopic focus tachycardia.

We currently consider flecainide our drug of second choice but undertake extensive risk–benefit discussions with the parents beforehand and are very concerned about the potential for fetal or maternal proarrhythmic effects.

We view the presence of hydrops as evidence of a very poor prognosis that justifies the uncertainties and risks of transplacental antiarrhythmic therapy. Short of such

Table 12.2 *Perinatal outcome in fetal tachycardias*

Fetal tachycardias	
Supraventricular (reentrant) tachycardia (n = 58)	
Gestational age (weeks)	19–39
Hydrops fetalis	32 (55%)
Congenital heart disease	1 (0.02%)
Deaths	3 (0.05%)
*Atrial flutter (*n = 17)	
Gestational age (weeks)	24–38
Hydrops fetalis	9 (0.53%)
Congenital heart disease	5 (0.29%)
Deaths	4 (0.24%)
*Atrial fibrillation (*n = 2)	
Gestational age (weeks)	19–38
Hydrops fetalis	0
Congenital heart disease	0
Deaths	0

an overwhelming risk–benefit analysis, we believe that close fetal monitoring should be considered for patients who are not hydropic, and we are reluctant to be more aggressive than treatment with digoxin alone.

Outcome

Table 12.2 describes the perinatal outcome of fetuses with SVT. Only one patient in our series of 58 cases of fetal reciprocating SVT had a congenital cardiac malformation, a prematurely closed foramen ovale. This fetus represented one of the three fetuses who died despite restoration of normal sinus rhythm for several days prior to delivery. We postulate that premature closure of the ovale foramen may have resulted from early left atrial depolarization via a left-sided accessory connection. Premature depolarization of the left atrium would then result in an 'a' wave gradient, with left atrial pressure prematurely exceeding right, closing the flap of the foramen ovale over the normally patent interatrial communication (Buis-Liem *et al.*, 1987).

Atrial flutter/fibrillation

The frequency of atrial flutter and fibrillation in our patients suggests that these arrhythmias are more rare

than SVT in the fetus. This comes as no surprise, based on the relative rarity of these arrhythmias in newborns. Our series demonstrates a high incidence of nonimmune hydrops fetalis in this group. The relatively high mortality rate noted in Table 12.2 reflects both the difficulty encountered in controlling these rhythms prenatally and their common association with major structural heart disease.

Assessment

Atrial flutter results from a circular reentrant movement of electrical energy occurring totally within the atrial musculature. Postnatal atrial flutter rates are usually in the range of 300 to 400 beats/min, whereas in the fetus monotonous atrial flutter rates of 400 to 480 are common. Varying degrees of atrioventricular block may be seen in association with fetal atrial flutter, resulting in varying ventricular response rates. These may be fixed and unresponsive to fetal activity, as in the case of a fixed 2:1 atrioventricular block, or quite irregular, as in cases with variable atrioventricular block. The frequent association of atrial flutter with atrioventricular block is further evidence that this arrhythmia does not involve atrioventricular reentry via the atrioventricular node as the underlying electrophysiological mechanism.

Management

Postnatal therapy for atrial flutter is based upon the principle of decreasing the ventricular response rate in an effort to decrease the degree of heart failure. By contrast, prenatal control of the ventricular response rate alone in hydropic fetuses with atrial flutter has proved disappointing in our experience. We believe that this is because of the unique haemodynamics of the fetus with its restrictive ventricular myocardium and relatively volume loaded right heart (Romero *et al.*, 1972; Rudolph, 1974). The fetal cardiovascular decompensation accompanying sustained supraventricular tachyarrhythmias may, therefore, reflect diastolic, rather than systolic, pump dysfunction. The normal function of the fetal ventricle is dependent upon an active and effective atrial pump. Therefore, unless the atrial flutter is controlled, atrial contractions will continue to occur against a closed or partially closed atrioventricular valve. This results in elevated atrial pressures and dilatation of the failing atrial pump. The resultant rise in systemic venous pressure retards the resolution of fetal oedema and effusions. The goal of antiarrhythmic therapy for fetal atrial flutter must, therefore, be restoration of normal sinus rhythm, with resumption of a 1:1 atrioventricular contraction sequence. The usual approach taken is to initiate treatment with digoxin to control the ventricular response rate by slowing conduction at the level of the atrioventricular node, followed by the addition of a type I agent such as procainamide or flecainide. Careful attention to the maternal digoxin level is important. The corrected QT interval of the maternal EKG must be monitored carefully until stable doses and drug levels are reached.

Atrial fibrillation appears to be even less common in the fetus than atrial flutter. Our two patients responded to digoxin therapy alone. However, had the arrhythmia persisted despite control of the ventricular response rate, we would have added a type I antiarrhythmic agent for the same reasons described for the treatment of atrial flutter.

Outcome

The high mortality rate of 31% in our series of fetuses with atrial flutter/fibrillation reflects the association with congenital heart disease in an equal percentage of fetuses. Structural defects included two with critical pulmonary outflow obstruction and tricuspid insufficiency, one with Ebstein malformation of the tricuspid valve with severe tricuspid insufficiency and one with left atrial isomerism, AV valve insufficiency and complete heart block. In these four fetuses, marked atrial dilatation was associated with the development of atrial flutter. The four deaths in our series included three of these patients with associated congenital heart disease.

Ventricular tachycardia

We have only diagnosed ventricular tachycardia in seven fetuses. In each, the heart rate during the tachycardia did not fall into the usual range of 240 to 260 beats/min seen in fetuses with AV reciprocating SVT. Although this was likely to be a coincidence, it was quite helpful in alerting us to the likelihood that this was not reciprocating atrioventricular tachycardia. When there is a tachycardia with a rate outside this range, we have a strong suspicion that we are dealing with an unusual tachycardia. Atrio-

ventricular dissociation was present in each of the fetuses in our series, although it is possible for fetuses with ventricular tachycardia to have a 1:1 atrioventricular relationship based on retrograde atrial activation. Therefore, one cannot rely solely on atrioventricular dissociation to establish the diagnosis of fetal ventricular tachycardia.

Not all neonates with ventricular tachycardia are ill, and many do not require treatment. Five of our fetal patients were non-hydropic, had structurally normal hearts and were not treated *in utero*. None of these required antiarrhythmic therapy as neonates. In light of the infrequency of episodes of postnatal tachycardia, the lack of symptoms during tachycardia and the rarity of associated structural heart disease, it has been our impression that conservative management of fetal ventricular tachycardia is often preferable to aggressive therapy.

A sixth fetal patient presented during labour with ventricular tachycardia associated with marked right ventricular and right atrial dilatation. No therapy was administered until after delivery. The neonate had significant right ventricular dilatation and congestive heart failure with prolonged episodes of ventricular tachycardia. A diagnosis of arrhythmogenic right ventricular dysplasia was established and the neonate was successfully treated with intravenous lidocaine, followed by oral mexiletine.

Our final case of fetal ventricular tachycardia occurred in a labouring patient who received intravenous ephedrine for maternal hypotension after insertion of an epidural. The episode lasted less than one hour and spontaneously resolved prior to delivery without sequelae.

If ventricular tachycardia is diagnosed in a previable fetus with evidence of congestive cardiac failure, antiarrhythmic therapy should be considered. Digoxin should be avoided. Instead strategies such as the direct umbilical venous infusion of lidocaine or procainamide followed by maternal oral therapy with procainamide, flecainide or propranolol should be considered.

Sinus tachycardia

Fetuses with mild degrees of tachycardia in the range of 180 to 210 beats/min need not have a cardiac arrhythmia as the underlying cause. The traditional obstetrical differential diagnoses must be considered for fetuses with apparent sinus tachycardia, bearing in mind that a ventricular tachycardia with 1:1 retrograde conduction may also present in this manner. It is particularly important to consider maternal fever or bacterial intrauterine infection as causes of fetal sinus tachycardia. In addition, fetal distress may cause a baseline tachycardia with loss of beat-to-beat variability. Maternal or fetal hyperthyroidism can also cause fetal tachycardia; a fetal goitre can be excluded with ultrasound. Finally, the use of such medications as β-mimetics that are known to cause fetal tachycardia should be excluded. For these causes of tachycardia, treatment of the underlying cause is important, rather than treatment of the tachycardia *per se*.

Bradycardias

We consider a significant bradycardia to be a fetal heart rate that is persistently below 100 beats/min. Fetal sinus bradycardia is uncommon. We have seen only six cases, nine with a rate lower than 90 beats/min. To establish this diagnosis, 1:1 atrioventricular concordance must be present, and some heart rate variability should be sought, depending on the gestational age of the fetus. Fetuses having intermittent slowing of the fetal heart should be evaluated using traditional obstetric criteria for significant decelerations that may require prompt intervention, rather than engendering delay by waiting for a fetal echocardiogram. However, a rapid screening ultrasound of the fetus with a persistent bradycardia may demonstrate good fetal movements and obvious atrioventricular discordance. In these cases, an emergency caesarean delivery can be avoided and appropriate cardiac evaluation initiated. The patient having apparent episodes of fetal bradycardia in the setting of an irregular fetal heart rate can usually be demonstrated to have atrial premature beats. During periods of fetal atrial bigeminy, every other beat will be premature and be blocked at the atrioventricular node. This can be distinguished from simple Mobitz type II second-degree atrioventricular block or from complete heart block by noting the regular irregularity of the atrial contractions when every second beat is premature. In contrast, fetuses with Mobitz type

II second-degree block or complete heart block will be noted to have a regular atrial rate.

Complete heart block

Fetuses with complete heart block are of intense interest to most fetal cardiologists. Approximately half of these fetuses have complex structural cardiac anomalies as the underlying cause, most involving the atrioventricular junction. Often left atrial isomerism is present, while in those patients without visceral heterotaxia, atrioventricular discordance can usually be demonstrated. These 'heterotaxy' syndromes are also described in relation to the abdominal abnormalities that accompany them. In left atrial isomerism, multiple small spleens are frequently present, a condition referred to as polysplenia. In right atrial isomerism, the spleen may be absent, a condition known as asplenia syndrome. The combination of complete heart block and severe structural heart disease is usually poorly tolerated by the fetus, especially when atrioventricular valve regurgitation is present, because of the propensity of these fetuses to develop nonimmune hydrops. The association of fetal hydrops with structural heart disease and complete heart block carries a poor prognosis, with survival being extremely unlikely (Kleinman, Copel & Hobbins, 1987; Machado *et al.*, 1988; Wladimiroff, Stewart & Tonge, 1988; Schmidt *et al.*, 1991).

Pathophysiology

The remaining fetuses with complete heart block are affected by an immune process initiated by maternal autoantibodies (Chamiedes *et al.*, 1977; Esscher & Scott, 1979; Scott *et al.*, 1983; Litsey *et al.*, 1985; Taylor *et al.*, 1986; Lee *et al.*, 1987). These antibodies, typically found in Sjögren syndrome and systemic lupus erythematosus, are called anti-SSA/Ro and anti-SSB/La. They have a particular affinity for the fetal cardiac conduction system and provoke an intense inflammatory response. Fetal myocarditis can also be demonstrated (Horsfall *et al.*, 1991). The frequent development of nonimmune hydrops in fetuses with immune heart block may be the result of a number of significant factors. The combination of a sudden drop in fetal ventricular rate and a lack of coordination between the fetal atria and ventricles is difficult for the fetus to tolerate because of the reliance of the fetal heart on active atrial contraction for normal ventricular filling. The addition of myocarditis would be expected to reduce ventricular compliance, increasing the reliance of the heart on coordinated atrial contraction for adequate ventricular filling, and to reduce ventricular contractility. These factors may well contribute to the development of hydrops in these fetuses.

Management

Several treatment approaches have been advocated for the fetus with heart block. A surgical approach has been suggested to place a pacemaker in the fetus. One report has shown the feasibility of percutaneous pacemaker lead placement and transient ventricular capture, although the fetus was moribund when the procedure was undertaken, with little fetal response (Carpenter *et al.*, 1986). A further attempt at transvenous pacing has been reported. Although a sinus rhythm was achieved, the fetus died (Walkinshaw *et al.*, 1994). Another attempt by the UCSF group utilizing open fetal surgery was similarly unsuccessful (M. Harrison, personal communication). Whether direct fetal pacing will be successful will await the development of better fetal surgical techniques. It is uncertain whether ventricular pacing alone will suffice or whether sequential atrioventricular pacing will be necessary to eliminate the cannon waves of reflected 'a' waves from atrial contractions against closed atrioventricular valves that elevate mean atrial pressures, impeding resorption of fetal oedema. The pacemaker itself must be placed in such a way as to avoid having wires floating freely in the amniotic fluid, as would be the case if the generator is outside the uterus. Such wires could represent a hazard to the fetus should the umbilical cord become intertwined with them, a situation analogous to the umbilical cord entanglement seen in monoamniotic twins. The ideal surgical solution would be a sequential atrioventricular pacemaker placed subcutaneously in the fetus or threaded through the umbilical cord from the placental insertion, a formidable challenge.

We have observed the progression of a second-degree heart block to complete heart block in an occasional fetus. This suggests the possibility of a need for medical therapy in these fetuses. Treatments suggested in the past have included plasmapheresis and corticosteroids

(Buyon *et al.*, 1986; Bierman *et al.*, 1988; Watson & Katz, 1991), although the agent used most often in the past was prednisone, which crosses the placenta poorly. We reasoned that selecting a steroid that would cross the placenta efficiently coupled with the initiation of treatment early in the course of the disease might ameliorate the myocarditis and alter the rhythm. It was also notable to us that the onset of immune fetal heart block was usually reported at approximately 20 to 24 weeks' gestation. In addition, this arrhythmia had not been reported prior to 17 to 18 weeks' gestation, when the fetal immune system is considered immature. The analogy to fetal syphilis and viral infections, which may cross the placenta but do not provoke a fetal response until immunocompetence develops, further suggested that immune suppression to reduce the inflammatory response might be an appropriate approach.

We have treated five fetuses to date with maternal dexamethasone in a dose of 4 mg orally each day and have seen evidence of fetal response in four (Copel, Buyon & Kleinman, 1994). The nonimmune hydrops completely resolved in two fetuses and one of these transiently reverted to second-degree atrioventricular block. One additional fetus presenting with second-degree block accompanied by high maternal anti-SSA/Ro and anti-SSB/La titres reverted to first-degree block. A second fetus presenting with mixed second- and third-degree block is stable postnatally in second-degree block. While these results are encouraging, clearly the resolution of fetal hydrops may have been coincidental to the initiation of treatment as the fetal myocardium adjusted to the atrioventricular dissociation. However, we have never observed spontaneous improvement in the heart rate in cases of immune-mediated block, suggesting that some real effects are present. A randomized trial will be necessary to confirm the benefits of this treatment.

The risk for fetal demise has justified the use of agents such as amiodarone and flecainide in the treatment of fetal arrhythmias. It should be emphasized, however, that maternal administration of these agents causes significant blood levels in the mother and exposes her to the life-threatening risks of proarrhythmic effects from these agents (Morganroth, 1987). The loss of a fetal patient is a tragedy for the parents and for the treating physician. This tragedy would be dwarfed, however, by that of an iatrogenic maternal death. For this reason, we urge that agents with significant proarrhythmic potential be used only in the presence of dire risk to the fetus, and only after informed consent is obtained from the parents. It is also incumbent upon the treating physician to recognize that families faced with this desperate situation will often accept fetal therapy. In this circumstance, the physician's desire to intervene in the fetal condition may result in poorly conceived treatment protocols. For this reason, it is essential that a team approach be employed and appropriate counselling be given for the needs of both maternal and fetal risks.

Conclusions

The majority of fetal arrhythmias are benign extrasystole and do not require treatment. SVT should be treated when sustained or associated with hydrops fetalis. Maternal administration of digoxin achieves fetal sinus rhythm in 60% of patients, while in the remainder second-line therapy with flecainide is required. Steroid therapy may have a role in complete heart block secondary to maternal autoimmune disease.

Management of the fetus with an arrhythmia requires a team approach by perinatologists and paediatric cardiologists with due consideration to the risk–benefit ratio of the mother and fetus.

References

Allan, L. D., Chita, S. K., Sharland, G. K., Maxwell, D. & Priestley, K. (1991). Flecainide in the treatment of fetal tachycardias. *British Heart Journal*, 65, 46–8.

Arnoux, P., Seyral, P., Llurens, M., Djiane, P., Potier, A., Unal, D., Cano, J. P., Serradimigni, A. & Rouault, F. (1987). Amiodarone and digoxin for refractory fetal tachycardia. *American Journal of Cardiology*, 59, 166–7.

Bierman, F. Z., Baxi, L., Jaffe, I. & Driscoll, J. (1988). Fetal hydrops and congenital complete heart block, response to maternal steroid therapy. *Journal of Pediatrics*, 112, 646–8.

Blandon, R. & Leandro, I. (1984). Fetal heart arrhythmia, Clinical experience with antiarrhythmic drugs. In *Pediatric Cardiology, Proceedings of the Second World Congress*, ed. E. F. Doyle, M. A. Engle, W. M. Gersony, W. J. Rashkind, N. S. Talner, pp. 483–4. New York: Springer-Verlag.

Buis-Liem, T. N., Ottenkamp, J., Meerman, R. H. & Verwey, R. (1987). The concurrence of fetal supraventricular tachycardia and obstruction of the foramen ovale. *Prenatal Diagnosis*, 7, 425–31.

Buyon, J. P., Swersky, S. H., Fox, H. E., Bierman, F. Z. & Winchester, R. J. (1986). Intrauterine therapy for presumptive fetal myocarditis with acquired heart block due to systemic lupus erythematosus. Experience in a mother with a predominance of SS-B (La) antibodies. *Arthritis and Rheumatism*, 30, 44–9.

Camm, A. J. & Garratt, C. J. (1991). Adenosine and supraventricular tachycardia. *New England Journal of Medicine*, 325, 1621–9.

CAST (The Cardiac Arrhythmia Suppression Trial Investigators) (1989). Preliminary report. Effect of encainide and flecainide on mortality in a randomized trial of arrhythmia suppression after myocardial infarction. *New England Journal of Medicine*, 321, 406–12.

Carpenter, R. J., Jr, Strasburger, J. F., Garson, A., Jr, Smith, R. T., Deter, R. L. & Engelhardt, H. T., Jr (1986) Fetal ventricular pacing for hydrops secondary to complete atrioventricular block. *Journal of American College of Cardiology*, 8, 1434–6.

Chameides, L., Truex, R. C., Vetter, V., Rashkind, W. J., Galioto, F. M., Jr & Noonan, J. A. (1977). Association of maternal systemic lupus erythematosus with congenital complete heart block. *New England Journal of Medicine*, 297, 1204–7.

Chiba, Y., Kanzaki, T., Kobayashi, H., Murakami, M. & Yutani, C. (1990). Evaluation of fetal structural heart disease using color flow mapping. *Ultrasound in Medicine and Biology*, 16, 221.

Copel, J. A., Buyon, J. P. & Kleinman, C. S. (1994). Successful *in utero* treatment of fetal heart block. *American Journal of Obstetrics and Gynecology*, 170, 280.

Copel, J. A., Morotti, R., Hobbins, J. C. & Kleinman, C. S. (1991). The antenatal diagnosis of congenital heart disease using fetal echocardiography, Is color flow mapping necessary? *Obstetrics and Gynecology*, 78, 1–8.

Deal, B. J., Keane, J. F., Gillette, P. C. & Garson, A., Jr (1985). Wolff–Parkinson–White syndrome and supraventricular tachycardia during infancy, management and follow-up. *Journal of the American College of Cardiology*, 5, 130–5.

DeVore, G. R. & Horenstein, J. (1993). Simultaneous Doppler recording of the pulmonary artery and vein, a new technique for the evaluation of a fetal arrhythmia. *Journal of Ultrasound in Medicine*, 12, 669–71.

DeVore, G. R., Siassi, B. & Platt, L. D. (1983). Fetal echocardiography III. The diagnosis of cardiac arrhythmias using real-time-directed M-mode ultrasound. *American Journal of Obstetrics and Gynecology*, 146, 792–9.

DeVore, G. R., Siassi, B. & Platt, L. D. (1990). The fetus with cardiac arrhythmias. In *The Unborn Patient, Prenatal Diagnosis and Treatment*, 2nd edn, ed. M. R. Harrison, M. S. Golbus & R. A. Filly, pp. 249–63. Philadelphia, PA: W. B. Saunders.

Duvernoy, W. F. C. (1977). Sudden death in Wolff–Parkinson–White syndrome. *American Journal of Cardiology*, 39, 472–8.

Ebara, H., Suzuki, S., Nagashima, K. & Kuroume, Y. (1988). Natriuretic activity of digoxin-like immunoreactive substance extracted from cord blood. *Life Sciences*, 42, 303–9.

Esscher, E. & Scott, J. S. (1979). Congenital heart block and maternal systemic lupus erythematosus. *British Medical Journal*, i, 1235–8.

Eyer, M. K., Brandestini, M. A., Phillips, D. J. & Baker, D. W. (1981). Color digital echo/Doppler image presentation. *Ultrasound in Medicine and Biology*, 7, 21–31.

Fernandez, C., De Rosa, G. E., Guevara, E., Velazquez, H., Pueyrrdon, H. R., Casavilla, F. & Suarez, L. D. (1988). Reversion by vagal reflex of a fetal paroxysmal atrial tachycardia detected by echocardiography. *American Journal of Obstetrics and Gynecology*, 159, 860–1.

Fish, F. A., Gillette, P. C. & Benson, D. W., Jr (1991). Proarrhythmia, cardiac arrest and death in young patients receiving encainide and flecainide. The Pediatric Electrophysiology Group. *Journal of American College of Cardiology*, 18, 356–65.

Garson, A., Jr (1987). Medicolegal problems in the management of cardiac arrhythmias in children. *Pediatrics*, 79, 84–8.

Gembruch, U., Manz, M., Bald, R., Ruddel, H., Redel, D. A., Schlebusch, H., Nitsch, J. & Hansmann, M. (1989). Repeated intravascular treatment with amiodarone in a fetus with refractory supraventricular tachycardia and hydrops fetalis. *American Heart Journal*, 118, 1335–8.

Gillette, P. C., Blair, H. L. & Crawford, F. A. (1990). Preexcitation syndromes. In *Pediatric Arrhythmias, Electrophysiology and Pacing*, ed. P. C. Gillette & A. Garson, Jr, pp. 376–7. Philadelphia: W. B. Saunders.

González, A. R., Phelps, S. J., Cochran, E. B. & Sibai, B. M. (1987). Digoxin-like immunoreactive substance in pregnancy. *American Journal of Obstetrics and Gynecology*, 157, 660–4.

Guntheroth, W. G., Cyr, D. R., Mack, L. A., Benedetti, T., Lenke, R. R. & Petty, C. N. (1985). Hydrops from reciprocating atrioventricular tachycardia in a 27-

week fetus requiring quinidine for conversion. *Obstetrics and Gynecology*, 66, 29S–33S.

Horsfall, A. C., Venables, P. J., Taylor, P. V. & Maini, R. N. (1991). Ro and La antigens and maternal anti-La idiotype on the surface of myocardial fibres in congenital heart block. *Journal of Autoimmunity*, 4, 165–76.

Kleinman, C. S. & Copel, J. A. (1991). Electrophysiologic principles and fetal antiarrhythmic therapy. *Ultrasound in Obstetrics and Gynecology*, 1, 286–97.

Kleinman, C. S. & Copel, J. A. (1994). Fetal cardiac arrhythmias, Diagnosis and therapy. In *Maternal–Fetal Medicine, Principles and Practice*, 3rd edn, ed. R. K. Creasy & R. Resnick, pp. 326–41. Philadelphia, Pa: W. B. Saunders.

Kleinman, C. S. & Copel, J. A. (1996). Diagnosis and treatment of fetal supraventricular tachycardia. *Progressive Pediatric Cardiology*, in press.

Kleinman, C. S., Copel, J. A. & Hobbins, J. C. (1987). Combined echocardiographic and Doppler assessment of fetal congenital atrioventricular block. *British Journal of Obstetrics and Gynecology*, 94, 967–74.

Kleinman, C. S., Copel, J. A., Weinstein, E. M., Santulli, T. V., Jr & Hobbins, J. C. (1985). Treatment of fetal supraventricular tachyarrhythmias. *Journal of Clinical Ultrasound*, 13, 265–73.

Kleinman, C. S., Donnerstein, R. L., Jaffe, C. C., DeVore, G. R., Weinstein, E. M., Lynch, D. C., Talner, N. S., Berkowitz, R. L. & Hobbins, J. C. (1983). Fetal echocardiography. A tool for evaluation of *in utero* cardiac arrhythmias and monitoring of *in utero* therapy, analysis of 71 patients. *American Journal of Cardiology*, 51, 237–43.

Kleinman, C. S., Hobbins, J. C., Jaffe, C. C., Lynch, D. C. & Talner, N. S. (1980). Echocardiographic studies of the human fetus, prenatal diagnosis of congenital heart disease and cardiac dysrhythmias. *Pediatrics*, 65, 1059–67.

Kleinman, C. S., Weinstein, E. M. & Copel, J. A. (1986). Pulsed Doppler analysis of human fetal blood flow. *Clinical Diagnostic Ultrasound*, 17, 173–85.

Knudson, J. M., Kleinman, Copel, J. A., Rosenfeld, L. E. (1994). Ectopic atrial tachycardia *in utero*. *Obstetrics and Gynecology*, 84, 686–9.

Kofinas, A. D., Simon, N. V., Sagel, H., Lyttle, E., Smith, N. & King, K. (1991). Treatment of fetal supraventricular tachycardia with flecainide acetate after digoxin failure. *American Journal of Obstetrics and Gynecology*, 165, 630–1.

Kugler, J. D., Danford, D. A., Deal, B. J., Gillette, P. C., Perry, J. C., Silka, M. J., Van Hare, G. F. & Walsh, E. P. (1994). Radiofrequency catheter ablation for tachyarrhythmias in children and adolescents. The Pediatric Electrophysiology Society. *New England Journal of Medicine*, 330, 1481–7.

Laurent, M., Betremieux, P., Biron, Y. & LeHelloco, A. (1987). Neonatal hypothyroidism after treatment by amiodarone during pregnancy. *American Journal of Cardiology*, 60, 942.

Lee, L. A., Coulter, S., Erner, S. & Chu, H. (1987). Cardiac immunoglobulin deposition in congenital heart block associated with maternal anti-Ro autoantibodies. *American Journal of Medicine*, 83, 793–6.

Lingman, G. & Marsál, K. (1987). Fetal cardiac arrhythmias, Doppler assessment. *Seminars in Perinatology*, 11, 357–61.

Litsey, S. E., Noonan, J., O'Connor, W. N., Cottrill, C. M. & Mitchell, B. (1985). Maternal connective tissue disease and congenital heart block. Demonstration of immunoglobulin in cardiac tissue. *New England Journal of Medicine*, 312, 98–100.

Machado, M. V., Tynan, M. J., Curry, P. V. & Allan, L. D. (1988). Fetal complete heart block. *British Heart Journal*, 60, 512–15.

Martin, C. B., Jr, Nijhuis, J. G. & Weijer, A. A. (1984). Correction of fetal supraventricular tachycardia by compression of the umbilical cord, report of a case. *American Journal of Obstetrics and Gynecology*, 150, 324–6.

Morganroth, J. (1987). Risk factors for the development of proarrhythmic events. *American Journal of Cardiology*, 59, 32E–7E.

Morris, J. F., Poston, L., Wolfe, C. D., Hilton, P. J. (1988). A comparison of endogenous digoxin-like immunoreactivity and sodium transport inhibitory activity in umbilical arterial and venous serum. *Clinical Science*, 75, 577–9.

Nag, A. C., Lee, M. L., Shepard, D. (1990). Affect of amiodarone on the expression of myosin isoforms and cellular growth of cardiac muscle cells in culture. *Circulation Research*, 67, 51–60.

Nimrod, C., Davies, D., Harder, J., Iwanicki, S., Kondo, C., Takahashi, Y., Maloney, J., Persaud, D., Nicholson, S. (1987). Ultrasound evaluation of tachycardia-induced hydrops in the fetal lamb. *American Journal of Obstetrics and Gynecology*, 157, 655–9.

Ortiz, E., Robinson, P. J., Deanfield, J. E., Franklin, R., Macartney, F. J. & Wyse, R. K. H. (1985). Localisation of ventricular septal defects by simultaneous display of superimposed colour Doppler and cross sectional echocardiographic images. *British Heart Journal*, 54, 53–60.

Perry, J. C., Ayres, N. A. & Carpenter, R. J., Jr. (1991). Fetal supraventricular tachycardia treated with flecainide acetate. *Journal of Pediatrics*, 118, 303–5.

Reed, K. L., Sahn, D. J., Marx, G. R., Anderson, C. F. & Shenker, L. (1987). Cardiac Doppler flows during fetal arrhythmias, physiologic consequences. *Obstetrics and Gynecology*, 70, 1–6.

Reimer, A., Paul, T. & Kallfelz, H. C. (1991). Efficacy and safety of intravenous and oral propafenone in pediatric cardiac dysrhythmias. *American Journal of Cardiology*, 68, 741–4.

Romero, T., Covell, J. W. & Friedman, W. F. (1972). A comparison of pressure–volume relations of the fetal, newborn and adult heart. *American Journal of Physiology*, 222, 1285–90.

Rovet, J., Ehrlich, R. & Sorbara, D. (1987). Intellectual ourcome in children with fetal hypothyroidism. *Journal of Pediatrics*, 110, 700–4.

Rudolph, A. M. (1974). *Congenital Diseases of the Heart*. Chicago: Yearbook.

Schlebusch, H., von Mende, S., Grunn, U., Gembruch, U., Bald, R. & Hannsmann, M. (1991). Determination of digoxin in the blood of pregnant women, fetuses and neonates before and during anti-arrhythmic therapy, using four immunochemical methods. *European Journal of Clinical Chemistry and Clinical Biochemistry*, 29, 57–5.

Schmidt, K. G., Ulmer, H. E., Silverman, N. H., Kleinman, C. S. & Copel, J. A. (1991). Perinatal outcome of fetal complete atrioventricular block, a multicenter experience. *Journal of the American College of Cardiology*, 17, 1360–6.

Scott, J. S., Maddison, P. J., Taylor, P. V., Esscher, E., Scott, O. & Skinner, R. P. (1983). Connective-tissue disease, antibodies to ribonucleoprotein, and congenital heart block. *New England Journal of Medicine*, 309, 209–12.

Silverman, N. H., Enderlein, M. A., Stanger, P., Teitel, D. F., Heymann, M. A. & Golbus, M. S. (1985). Recognition of fetal arrhythmias by echocardiography. *Journal of Clinical Ultrasound*, 13, 255–63.

Sorokin, Y., Bottoms, S. F., Dierker, L. J., Jr. & Rosen, M. G. (1982). The clustering of fetal heart rate changes and fetal movements in pregnancies between 20 and 30 weeks of gestation. *American Journal of Obstetrics and Gynecology*, 143, 952–7.

Steinfeld, L., Rappaport, H. L., Rossbach, H. C. & Martinez, E. (1986). Diagnosis of fetal arrhythmias using echocardiographic and Doppler techniques. *Journal of the American College of Cardiology*, 1986, 1425–33.

Strasburger, J. F., Huhta, J. C., Carpenter, R. J., Garson, A., Jr & McNamara, D. G. (1986). Doppler echocardiography in the diagnosis and management of persistent fetal arrhythmias. *Journal of the American College of Cardiology*, 7, 1386–91.

Taylor, P. V., Scott, J. S., Gerlis, L. M., Esscher, E. & Scott, O. (1986). Maternal antibodies against fetal cardiac antigens in congenital complete heart block. *New England Journal of Medicine*, 315, 667–72.

Walkinshaw, S. A., Welch, C. R., McCormack, J. & Walsh, K. (1994). *In utero* pacing for fetal congenital heart block. *Fetal Diagnostic Therapy*, 9, 183–5.

Watson, W. J. & Katz, V. L. (1991). Steroid therapy for hydrops associated with antibody-mediated congenital heart block. *American Journal of Obstetrics and Gynecology*, 165, 553–4.

Weiner, C. P., Landas, S. & Persoon, T. J. (1987). Digoxin-like immunoreactive substance in fetuses with and without cardiac pathology. *American Journal of Obstetrics and Gynecology*, 157, 368–71.

Weiner, C. P. & Thompson, M. I. (1988). Direct treatment of fetal supraventricular tachycardia after failed transplacental therapy. *American Journal of Obstetrics and Gynecology*, 158, 570–3.

Wellens, H. J. & Durrer, D. (1973). Effect of digitalis on atrioventricular conduction and circus–movement tachycardias in patients with Wolff–Parkinson–White syndrome. *Circulation*, 47, 1229–33.

Wladimiroff, J. W., Stewart, J. W. & Tonge, H. M. (1988). Fetal bradyarrhythmia, diagnosis and outcome. *Prenatal Diagnosis*, 8, 53–7.

Wren, C. & Hunter, S. (1988). Maternal administration of flecainide to terminate and suppress fetal tachycardia. *British Medical Journal*, 296, 249.

Younis, J. S. & Granat, M. (1987). Insufficient transplacental digoxin transfer in severe hydrops fetalis. *American Journal of Obstetrics and Gynecology*, 157, 1268–9.

13 Oligohydramnios and polyhydramnios
PHILLIPA M. KYLE AND NICHOLAS M. FISK

Introduction

Amniotic fluid surrounds the fetus in intrauterine life, providing a protected, low-resistance space suitable for growth and development. It arises from secondary partitioning of water within the fetoplacental extracellular space and reflects fetal fluid balance. The relative constancy of amniotic fluid volume (AFV) in the presence of a high turnover rate and several pathways of exchange indicates a remarkable coordination in its control. Breakdown of this leads to oligo- and polyhydramnios, each of which is associated with increased perinatal mortality and morbidity, in relation to the degree of aberrant fluid volume (Chamberlain et al., 1984a,b). Management of both conditions is based on determining the underlying aetiology and then, if appropriate, instituting therapy to restore the normal level of AFV. There are two approaches to therapy. The first and preferable one is to correct the underlying cause. However, when this option is not available, non-specific drainage and infusion techniques can be used. This chapter reviews the place of current and potential future therapies in the management of oligo- and polyhydramnios.

Determinants of AFV

Source and control

The factors determining AFV regulation remain poorly understood. In early pregnancy, amniotic fluid is considered initially a maternal dialysate and then a fetal transudate, since its composition resembles that of maternal and then fetal serum (Lind, Kendall & Hytten, 1972). After 20 to 25 weeks, with progressive impermeability of fetal skin, amniotic fluid becomes increasingly hypotonic with greater concentrations of urea and creatinine, implicating fetal urine as the major contributor (Lind, Billewicz & Cheyne, 1971). A net outflow of lung liquid from the fetal trachea also contributes to amniotic fluid, although swallowing may prevent much of this reaching the amniotic cavity (Harding et al., 1984).

Fetal swallowing is a major route of clearance. Human fetuses with lesions preventing swallowing often develop polyhydramnios (Moya et al., 1960), as do sheep after oesophageal occlusion (Fujino et al., 1991). The other major route of clearance is bulk flow across permeable membranes between maternal, fetal and amniotic compartments in response to osmotic (Gilbert & Brace, 1988) and hydrostatic gradients (Ross et al., 1983). Consistent with this is the correlation between maternal plasma and AFV in human pregnancies with both normal and abnormal quantities of amniotic fluid (Goodlin, Anderson & Gallagher, 1983). In sheep, the transmembranous pathway from the amniotic cavity to the maternal circulation is not a major route for fluid flow, whereas the intramembranous route from the amniotic cavity via vascularized membranes into the fetal circulation appears to be (Gilbert & Brace, 1989). However, human placental and membranous anatomy differs from that in sheep, and it is not yet known whether the intramembranous pathway plays a role in AFV control in the human. The fetus is known to be able to alter its urine production by releasing vasoactive peptides such as vasopressin and atrial natriuretic peptide in response to changes in maternal and fetal intravascular volume (Schroder, Gilbert & Power, 1984; Lumbers & Stevens,

1983). This suggests that alterations in AFV in response to changes in maternal fluid balance occur via their effect on fetal fluid balance (Stevens & Lumbers, 1985).

Measurement

AFV has been measured in normal human pregnancy by direct collection (Abramovich, 1968) or indicator dye dilution techniques (Queenan *et al.*, 1972). Pooled data from several studies suggest that mean AFV increases rapidly to 630 ml at 22 weeks, and then more slowly to a peak of 817 ml at 33 weeks, declining thereafter to 715 ml at 40 weeks (Brace & Wolf, 1989). The 95% reference range for volumes at each gestation is wide.

Direct quantification of AFV is not performed in clinical practice because dye dilution requires two invasive procedures with attendant risks and its accuracy has been questioned (Brans *et al.*, 1989). Accordingly, definitions of increased and decreased AFV are based on non-invasive ultrasonographic criteria. These include subjective assessment and measurement of the maximum vertical pocket (MVP) and amniotic fluid index (AFI). The last two methods were derived to provide reproducible, semiquantitative assessments and later were shown to be of prognostic value. The AFI is now preferred to the MVP technique because (i) the latter does not allow for an asymmetrical fetal position within the uterus; (ii) the regression curve between AFI and gestational age is similar in shape to that between AFV and gestational age (Brace & Wolf, 1989) and has been used to derive a reference range for AFI from 16–42 weeks (Moore & Cayle, 1990); and (iii) the AFI appears superior to the MVP in diagnosis and classification of severity of both oligohydramnios and polyhydramnios (Moore, 1990). Nevertheless, both techniques overestimate the incidence of oligohydramnios and underestimate that of polyhydramnios when compared with direct volume measurement (Dildy *et al.*, 1992). Both methods are also influenced by transducer pressure, which may explain the poor reproducibility reported (Flack *et al.*, 1994). These difficulties may be obviated by development of new methods for AFV estimation such as three-dimensional ultrasound.

Using the MVP, mild and severe polyhydramnios have been arbitrarily defined as a deepest pool >8 and 15 cm, respectively (Chamberlain *et al.*, 1984b), while oligohydramnios has been variously defined as a deepest pool ≤3, 2 or 1 cm (Crowley, 1980; Manning, Hill & Platt, 1981; Chamberlain *et al.*, 1984a). The more stringent criteria have been used to indicate moderate to severe oligohydramnios. The AFI definitions for poly- and oligohydramnios are values outside the 97.5th and 2.5th centile for gestation, respectively (Moore & Cayle, 1990).

Oligohydramnios

Oligohydramnios is found in 3 to 5% of pregnancies in the third trimester (Chamberlain *et al.*, 1984a) but only 0.2% in the midtrimester (Barss, Benacerraf & Frigoletto, 1984). Severe oligohydramnios is least common. Much of the literature evaluating diagnosis and prognosis in oligohydramnios was performed before the availability of colour flow Doppler, a tool which distinguishes the umbilical cord from amniotic fluid. The incidence and severity of oligohydramnios may, therefore, have been underestimated in the past. Studies should now be repeated using colour Doppler to determine the true incidence of oligohydramnios.

Aetiology

Oligohydramnios may be caused by renal hypofunction, urinary obstruction, rupture of the membranes or intrauterine growth retardation (IUGR), their relative frequency as causes depending on gestation and severity. In late pregnancy, IUGR and ruptured membranes predominate (Chamberlain *et al.*, 1984a; Mercer *et al.*, 1984) whereas urinary tract anomalies leading to oligohydramnios are usually detected on routine ultrasound in the midtrimester. The aetiology in the remainder of patients is idiopathic with the reduction in AFV being less severe than in other aetiological groups (Moore *et al.*, 1989).

Prelabour rupture of the membranes (PROM) complicates 3 to 17% of pregnancies (Gunn, Mishell & Morton, 1970) and is responsible for a quarter of cases of oligohydramnios (Mercer *et al.*, 1984), the majority occurring near term. Oligohydramnios from PROM is usually short-lived, as the latent period to onset of labour exceeds a week in only 2–5% and 20–40% of those with term and preterm PROM, respectively (Kappy *et al.*, 1979; Moretti & Sibai, 1988).

IUGR leads to oligohydramnios (Philipson, Sokol & Williams, 1983) with significantly lower MVP measurements in small versus appropriate-for-gestational age fetuses. Oligohydramnios in IUGR seems secondary to fetal oliguria, which probably reflects a renovascular response to hypoxia, with reflex redistribution of blood flow away from kidneys and viscera towards the brain (Cohn *et al.*, 1974; Peeters *et al.*, 1979). Support for renal hypoperfusion being the mechanism comes from human studies showing correlations between increased resistance in the renal artery and reduced AFV (Arduini & Rizzo, 1991) and between reduced urine production and fetal hypoxaemia (Nicolaides *et al.*, 1990). Hypoxia-induced release of vasopressin may also contribute (Robillard *et al.*, 1981).

Major congenital abnormalities are found in 4 to 7% of pregnancies with oligohydramnios (Mercer *et al.*, 1984), rising to 26 to 35% in the midtrimester (Moore *et al.*, 1989). This frequency approaches 50% in severe oligohydramnios compared with 14% in mild/moderate cases (Moore *et al.*, 1989). Furthermore, if separation between the amnion and chorion is present together with oligohydramnios, the incidence of congenital abnormalities is even higher (Bronstein & Zimmer, 1995). Bilateral urinary tract pathology such as renal agenesis, multicystic or polycystic disease and lower tract obstruction are most frequent, occurring in 33 to 57% of patients (Mercer & Brown, 1986).

Perinatal complications

These are significantly increased in oligohydramnios, as a result of both the underlying aetiology and related sequelae such as pulmonary hypoplasia (PH). Perinatal mortality is infrequent in mild oligohydramnios in the third trimester, whereas in two series of midtrimester oligohydramnios, 43 and 88% of perinates succumbed (Moore *et al.*, 1989; Mercer *et al.*, 1986). Prognosis is worse when maternal serum alpha-fetoprotein is raised (Dyer, Burton & Nelson, 1987) and is also dependent on the severity of oligohydramnios; the mortality rate being 88% in association with severe reduction in AFV compared with 11% in mild/moderate midtrimester oligohydramnios (Moore *et al.*, 1989).

Poor outcome in PROM is largely confined to pregnancies with rupture prior to 29 weeks; in this group mortality rates of 37 to 76% have been reported. Gestational age at delivery is the most important variable, with infrequent survival before 24 to 25 weeks (Beydoun & Yasin, 1986; Morettii & Sibai, 1988). Perinatal death and PH in preterm PROM are independently associated with early gestational age at rupture and persistent oligohydramnios (i.e. MVP <2 cm) (Vintzileos *et al.*, 1985a; Hadi, Hodson & Strickland, 1994; Vergani *et al.*, 1994).

Some of the fetal complications such as PH and soft tissue deformities may be attributed to reduced AFV, whereas others such as infection result from the underlying condition. In PROM, proven neonatal sepsis occurs in only 17 to 29%, confirming that prematurity rather than infection is the greater cause of perinatal morbidity and mortality (Moretti & Sibai, 1988). PROM with oligohydramnios leads to a higher frequency of chorioamnionitis and neonatal sepsis than PROM with normal AFV (Hadi *et al.*, 1994).

PH is a disorder of impaired lung growth and is found in 13 to 21% of perinatal autopsies, of which the most common aetiology is oligohydramnios (Wigglesworth & Desai, 1982; Knox & Barson, 1986). The most vulnerable period of lung development to lack of amniotic fluid is the canalicular phase, which in humans extends from 17 to 26 weeks (Burri, 1984). The likelihood of PH after oligohydramnios depends on the gestational age at onset and the duration and the severity of oligohydramnios (Hadi *et al.*, 1994; Vergani *et al.*, 1994; Moore *et al.*, 1989) (Fig. 13.1). Although a causal relationship between lung hypoplasia and oligohydramnios has been well established, its underlying mechanism remains controversial (Fisk, 1992a). Older theories of oligohydramnios causing chest compression (Gruenwald, 1957; Nakayama *et al.*, 1983) have been challenged by the finding of low pressure within the uterine cavity in oligohydramnios (Fisk *et al.*, 1990) and by the lack of change with restoration of AFV in biophysical variables considered indicative of compression (Fisk *et al.*, 1992a,b). Cessation of fetal breathing movements is not the mechanism, as these remain present throughout oligohydramnios in both human (Moessinger *et al.*, 1987) and animal (Harding, Hooper & Dickson, 1990) studies. Oligohydramnios-related PH is known to in

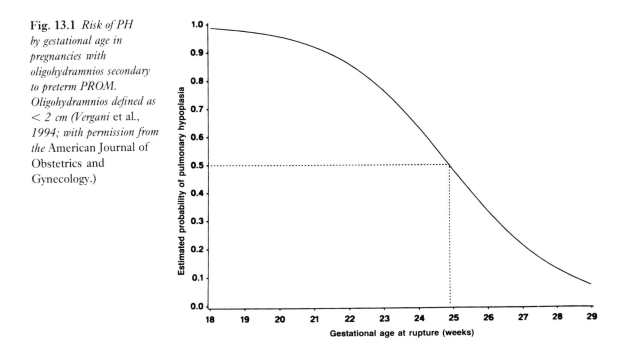

Fig. 13.1 *Risk of PH by gestational age in pregnancies with oligohydramnios secondary to preterm PROM. Oligohydramnios defined as < 2 cm (Vergani et al., 1994; with permission from* the *American Journal of Obstetrics and Gynecology.)*

volve chronic loss of lung liquid (Adzick *et al.*, 1984; Harding *et al.*, 1990), most likely by altering the tracheo-amniotic pressure gradient. Recent studies in fetal sheep indicate that pressure gradients in the upper airways are not affected by low amniotic pressure (Fisk *et al.*, 1992c); instead these gradients increase during non-labour uterine contractions (Harding *et al.*, 1990), suggesting that intermittent chest compression may impair lung development by increasing lung liquid loss.

Other sequelae related to oligohydramnios are soft tissue and skeletal deformities comprising flattened facies, flexion contractures and talipes. Their relationship to oligohydramnios seems different from that of PH, in that the severity and duration are more important than gestational age at onset (Rotschild *et al.*, 1990). Because amniotic pressure is low in oligohydramnios (Fisk *et al.*, 1990), they most likely result from fetal immobilization rather than compression. Nevertheless, severe soft-tissue deformities are seldom found in the absence of PH.

Oligohydramnios is also associated with an increased risk of fetal distress and birth asphyxia (Mercer *et al.*, 1984). These may reflect the underlying condition, such as IUGR and postmaturity, but the high frequency of fetal heart rate decelerations in labouring patients with ruptured membranes (Vintzileos *et al.*, 1985a) suggests that oligohydramnios *per se* may adversely affect fetal well being. Oligohydramnios in the absence of labour does not appear to affect fetal well being, in as much as fetal Doppler waveforms are normal in the absence of IUGR (Hackett, Nicolaides & Campbell, 1987) and are unaltered by restoration of AFV (Fisk, 1992a).

Diagnostic approach

The aim is to determine the underlying aetiology, the presence of associated anomalies and the severity of oligohydramnios. History and physical examination reveal most cases of PROM, except for a few very early in gestation in whom the small quantities of vaginal fluid are lost unnoticed (Fisk *et al.*, 1991a). Detailed examination of fetal anatomy is also crucial for diagnosis, but just when optimal ultrasonographic views are required, they are limited in severe oligohydramnios by lack of an acoustic window and pronounced fetal flexion.

Ultrasound

In the absence of amniotic fluid, renal agenesis is a notoriously difficult diagnosis which rests on demonstration of vacant renal fossae (Romero *et al.*, 1985). If the fetal abdomen is within the lower half of the uterus, transvaginal ultrasound may facilitate views of the fetal renal fossae (Benacerraf, 1990). Maternal administration of furosemide to provoke fetal diuresis (Wladimiroff, 1975) is no longer recommended as it produced numerous false-negative diagnoses (Harman, 1984; Romero *et al.*, 1985). In addition, furosemide administered to the pregnant ewe is now known not to produce a fetal diuresis nor indeed to cross the placenta (Chamberlain *et al.*, 1985). In contrast, lower urinary tract obstruction is relatively easy to diagnose because of the enlarged bladder. Nevertheless, visualization of other urinary structures of prognostic value, such as the renal cortex and upper urethra, and of extra-renal anatomy for associated anomalies remains suboptimal.

Diagnostic amnioinfusion (Gembruch & Hansmann, 1988; Fisk *et al.*, 1991a) has been recommended to facilitate ultrasonographic resolution in cases of moderate to severe oligohydramnios in which the underlying aetiology is uncertain and the ultrasound view is suboptimal. The procedure is described in detail in Chapter 2.

Ultrasonographic resolution after infusion is superior to that beforehand, providing that vaginal leakage does not prevent retention of infused fluid. In many cases, fetal abnormalities suspected before amnioinfusion can then be confirmed, an important issue if pregnancy termination is to be offered. In other cases, suspected anomalies will not be confirmed. Amnioinfusion was considered necessary in one series for definitive diagnosis of renal agenesis in 5 of 16 cases (Reuss *et al.*, 1987). In another series, bilateral renal agenesis was suspected in three fetuses on the initial scan, but following amnioinfusion kidneys were clearly demonstrated (Fisk *et al.*, 1991a). Alternatively, fetal intraperitoneal infusion has been used to facilitate diagnosis of renal agenesis (Nicolini *et al.*, 1989). Up to 100 ml saline has been infused without sequelae, although in our experience much smaller volumes are usually sufficient. As with diagnostic amnioinfusion, therefore, we recommend instilling the minimum volume to improve the ultrasonographic view. A potential advantage of this procedure over amnioinfusion is that a smaller volume of fluid is required, which may reduce the risk of ruptured membranes. Amnioinfusion, however, also improves ultrasonographic demonstration of other fetal structures, revealing unsuspected anomalies in 9 to 18% of fetuses (Gembruch & Hansmann, 1988; Fisk *et al.*, 1991a; Quetel *et al.*, 1992). Other advantages of amnioinfusion include diagnosis of ruptured membranes by demonstration of liquor leakage and/or membranous detachment on ultrasound (Fisk *et al.*, 1991a) and an opportunity to obtain 'amniotic fluid' for karyotyping (Gembruch & Hansmann, 1988), an important manoeuvre if fetal blood sampling is not possible.

Colour Doppler

More recently, colour Doppler has been used to visualize the renal arteries. In a series of 33 patients, absence of flow signals accurately predicted all cases of renal agenesis, and the only false-positive diagnoses were with severely dysplastic kidneys, functionally similar to agenesis (Sepulveda *et al.*, 1995).

The severity of oligohydramnios is also assessed, not only for clues to aetiology, but also for prognosis. Colour flow mapping improves the differentiation of residual pockets of amniotic fluid from loops of umbilical cord.

Karyotyping

Since it may be impossible to inspect minor structures such as the face and limbs for features of aneuploidy, rapid karyotyping is recommended in midtrimester oligohydramnios. Chromosomal abnormalities will be found in 5 to 10% of fetuses (Hackett *et al.*, 1987).

Therapy

The aim of therapy in oligohydramnios is chiefly to restore AFV to allow continued lung development during the canalicular phase. The experimental basis for restitution of amniotic volume to prevent PH has been well established in animal models (Harrison *et al.*, 1982a; Nakayama *et al.*, 1983). PH induced by urethral obstruction in fetal lamb was ameliorated by *in utero* suprapubic cystostomy 20 days later, with restoration of AFV and greater survival in lambs that underwent decompression of their urinary tract compared with those that did not (Harrison *et al.*, 1982). In another study,

oligohydramnios and PH induced in fetal rabbits by
bladder neck obstruction was reversed by continuous
infusion of normal saline into the amniotic cavity
(Nakayama *et al.*, 1983). Therefore, in fetuses with
experimental bladder outlet obstruction, restoration of
AFV by either diversion of urine or infusion of saline into
the amniotic cavity has significant beneficial effects on
lung development and allows survival at birth. In human
oligohydramnios, several approaches have been tried,
but no controlled data yet exist to confirm any benefit .

Vesico-amniotic shunting

In fetuses with lower obstructive uropathy, urinary decompression (Harrison *et al.*, 1982b; Manning *et al.*,
1986) aims not only to relieve obstruction to prevent
renal dysplasia (Chapter 17) but also to restore AFV to
facilitate lung development. However, PH was the cause
of death in almost all of the shunted fetuses that died in
the International Fetal Surgery Registry (Manning *et al.*,
1986). There is, therefore, considerable scepticism
about this procedure (Elder, Duckett & Snyder, 1987;
Reuss *et al.*, 1988) in particular whether it can restore
AFV long term in fetuses with severe oligohydramnios.

Cervical occlusion

In patients with preterm PROM, attempts have been
made to restore AFV either by preventing leakage with a
cervical plug (Ogita *et al.*, 1984) or occluding the cervix
with fibrin gel (Baumgarten & Moser, 1986). Although
sometimes initially effective, neither of these methods
prevented amniotic fluid drainage long term. We have
used fibrin gel in three pregnancies with severe mid-
trimester oligohydramnios, all of which miscarried and/
or developed intrauterine infection despite prophylactic
antibiotics. An alternative use of the double balloon
catheter has been to infuse normal saline into the amniotic cavity to maintain the deepest pool >5 cm (Imanaka,
Ogita & Sugawa, 1989). This device has been mainly
used to prevent infective complications of PROM in the
late second and early third trimester (Ogita *et al.*, 1988;
Shalev *et al.*, 1994) rather than in the second trimester to
prevent PH. Antibiotics can be directly infused, leading
to levels in amniotic fluid which are higher than after
maternal oral or intravenous administration. Any effect
on outcome is difficult to determine from the available
studies because of the absence of controls.

Serial amnioinfusions

Another option to prevent PH is to maintain AFV by
repeated amnioinfusions (Gembruch & Hansmann,
1988; Fisk *et al.*, 1991a; Hansmann *et al.*, 1991).
Gembruch & Hansmann (1988) performed two to four
amnioinfusions between 17 and 36 weeks in each of 15
pregnancies, with only two neonatal survivors. At least
half their fetuses, however, had bilateral lethal renal
pathology with the indication for the procedure being to
gain sufficient fluid for karyotyping rather than to promote lung development.

Our group conducted a pilot study of serial therapeutic infusions to prevent oligohydramnios sequelae in
nine women with appropriately grown euploid singleton
fetuses in whom severe oligohydramnios had been documented before 22 weeks (Fisk *et al.*, 1991a). Two of the
fetuses had lower urinary tract obstruction, three had no
apparent cause for the oligohydramnios and the remainder had evidence suggesting a 'high leak' membrane rupture. Forty infusions were performed with
sufficient normal saline to restore qualitatively normal
AFV at approximately weekly intervals until the end of
the canalicular phase. In 27/31 subsequent infusions,
the MVP was ⩽2 cm before each procedure. Therefore,
in the majority of patients the fluid was not retained in
the amniotic cavity for longer than seven days, and in fact
vaginal leakage within 24 hours occurred after 10 of 18
infusions in those with ruptured membranes. Preterm
labour occurred in four patients 3 to 12 weeks after the
final infusion; another developed clinical amnionitis two
days after her sixth and final infusion. Three infants
survived of the six born alive; one of the six perinatal
deaths had a reduced lung:body weight ratio and another
with a borderline ratio had clinical evidence of PH (Fig.
13.2). Lung hypoplasia was, therefore, found in two of
nine pregnancies (22%) complicated by severe
oligohydramnios diagnosed ⩽22 weeks, which
compares favourably with 60% reported in severe
oligohydramnios diagnosed ⩽28 weeks (Moore *et al.*,
1989). None of the fetuses had evidence of skeletal
deformities. This study concluded that serial amnioinfusion may be associated with a low incidence of
oligohydramnios sequelae. Furthermore, there were no
specific complications attributed to serial as opposed to
single infusions. Four of seven patients undergoing
serial infusions who reached viability had preterm

labour, which compares favourably with a frequency of 75% reported in midtrimester oligohydramnios (Mercer & Brown 1986).

In another study of multiple amnioinfusions in nine pregnancies with no fetal malformations or infection, seven of nine neonates survived and none demonstrated compression abnormalities (Hansmann et al., 1991). However, in only five of these were infusions commenced before 26 weeks, and only three of these fetuses survived. Furthermore, the definition of oligohydramnios used for patient selection was not described, rendering interpretation of these data less clear.

Identifying patients with oligohydramnios who might benefit from serial amnioinfusion is difficult and currently based on clinical risk factors. However, selection could alternatively be based on various ultrasonographic measurements of lung size considered predictive of PH, including fetal lung length (Roberts & Mitchell, 1990), fetal chest circumference (Nimrod et al., 1986) and/or its ratio to parameters independent of gestational age such as head circumference, abdominal circumference or femur length (De Vore, Horenstein & Platt, 1986; Vintzileos et al., 1989). These parameters, however, have not been widely adopted in practice because of concerns about their reproducibility in the presence of severe

oligohydramnios. A newer approach involves Doppler interrogation of the fetal pulmonary circulation (van Eyck, van der Mooren & Wladimiroff, 1990), with reduced ductal velocity modulation during fetal breathing predicting PH. However, longitudinal studies suggest that in PH progressive lag in all these biophysical parameters does not occur until at least 24 weeks (Roberts & Mitchell, 1990; van Eyck et al., 1990). As the critical canalicular phase is virtually completed by then, it is most likely that ultrasonographic measurement of fetal pulmonary parameters is of value only in indicating the presence of PH and not in selecting patients for preventative or therapeutic interventions.

The optimal infusate for therapeutic amnioinfusion has not been determined. Most groups use isotonic solutions such as 0.9% saline, 5% glucose or Ringer's lactate although Gembruch & Hansmann (1988) chose a hyperosmolar solution, presumably in an attempt to promote fluid influx into the amniotic cavity along an osmotic gradient. They also considered the pentoses in their solution, sorbite and xylite, produced a sugary taste which might encourage fetal swallowing. Animal studies, however, suggest that the primary determinant of fetal swallowing is the state of fetal hydration (Ross et al., 1989). In this regard, rapid filling of the human fetal

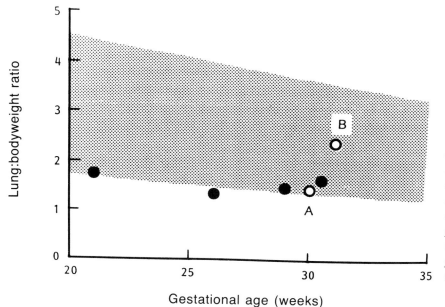

Fig. 13.2 *Lung:body weight ratios in six fetal and neonatal deaths among nine pregnancies with severe oligohydramnios that underwent serial amnioinfusions plotted against the 95% reference range. As ventilation may artefactually elevate lung:body weight ratios, the two ventilated neonates are indicated (O); one of these (A) had clinical evidence of pulmonary hypoplasia (Fisk, 1992a; with permission from Obstetrics and Gynecology.)*

stomach has been observed on ultrasound following amnioinfusion of 0.9% saline (Fisk *et al.*, 1991a). There has been some concern, both theoretical and based on animal studies, that 0.9% saline may be associated with fetal acidosis (Shields & Brace, 1993). Little clinical information is available, although a recent non-randomized study of 53 patients in which either normal saline or Ringer's lactate was infused during labour showed no differences in neonatal electrolytes, outcome or cord blood gas variables (Puder *et al.*, 1994). Use of any of the commonly available isotonic infusates seems appropriate at this time.

The main disadvantage of serial amnioinfusion, even if confirmed to be beneficial, is that only a very small proportion of patients will be eligible for treatment. Idiopathic oligohydramnios is rare and the therapy is impractical for many cases of ruptured membranes. It is unlikely to be beneficial in cases of oligohydramnios secondary to IUGR and major malformations associated with oligohydramnios, primarily because the underlying pathology will result in fetal demise. An example is a case report of renal agenesis in which ten amnioinfusions were performed between 17 and 33 weeks' gestation (Cameron *et al.*, 1994). At birth, the neonate was placed on immediate peritoneal dialysis and although the infant did not exhibit clinical evidence of PH or compression deformities, he died three weeks later from unsuccessful dialysis. Therefore, although this case indicates that therapeutic amnioinfusions can prevent oligohydramnios sequelae, it does remind us that until primary therapy is available for the underlying malformation at birth, repeated amnioinfusions to permit neonatal survival should be considered ethically questionable.

Maternal hydration

A potential option for the treatment of oligohydramnios would be to manipulate maternal fluid balance, since changes in the state of maternal hydration are known to result in similar changes in fetal hydration. Iatrogenic water intoxication in the mother induces marked hypotonicity in fetal serum (Battaglia *et al.*, 1960) while in the ovine fetus maternal dehydration decreases urine production (Bell *et al.*, 1984; Ross *et al.*, 1983). Reports of correction of AFV by maternal intravenous hydration in a severely hypovolaemic woman (Sherer *et al.*, 1990) and of changes in AFI secondary to subtotal immersion, in

which pregnant women are immersed in shoulder-deep water to reduce dependent oedema (Strong, 1993), further suggest that AFV is dependent on maternal intravascular volume.

Two studies have reported that acute maternal oral hydration increases the AFI in women with third-trimester oligohydramnios compared with controls (Kilpatrick *et al.*, 1991; Flack *et al.*, 1995). However, the mechanism of this effect is unclear because in the latter study, although there was an improvement *in utero* placental function, fetal urine production did not change (Flack *et al.*, 1995). Transmembranous passage of fluid may account for some of this increase in AFV. These studies were of acute maternal hydration and it seems likely that the additional fluid load may be cleared rapidly from the maternal circulation. Nevertheless, chronic maternal hydration warrants investigation as a possible therapy.

Intrapartum amnioinfusion

Oligohydramnios in labour is associated with umbilical cord compression leading to variable decelerations, fetal acidosis, meconium staining and increased rates of operative delivery (Robson *et al.*, 1992). A rational approach to the prevention and treatment of such problems in labour is amnioinfusion, either transcervically (Miyazaki & Nevarez, 1985; Nageotte *et al.*, 1985) or transabdominally (Mandelbrot, Dommergues & Dumez, 1992; Mandelbrot *et al.*, 1993). A meta-analysis of the controlled studies of transcervical amnioinfusion has shown that although variable decelerations and operative delivery rates were decreased in the study compared with the control groups the fetal outcome was similar (Hofmeyer, 1993a). In these studies, fetal scalp pH testing was not used to interpret decelerative cardiotocograph changes and, therefore, this limits the value and application of these results in countries such as the UK where scalp sampling is used. Alternatively, in countries such as the USA, in which the practice is solely based on cardiotocographic changes, amnioinfusion for variable decelerations is widely used and beneficial in reducing rates of operative intervention.

Maternal endometritis was actually decreased in the study group, presumably the result of fewer caesarean sections. Transabdominal infusions in women entering labour with an unfavourable cervix and oligohydramnios may be more useful than transcervical infusions (Mandelbrot *et al.*, 1992; 1993) and there may be less risk of cord prolapse. Prophylactic versus therapeutic amnioinfusion does not appear to confer any benefit in cases of term intrapartum oligohydramnios (Ogundipe, Spong & Ross, 1993). However, in the one randomized trial reported to date, cases of preterm PROM treated in early labour with prophylactic amnioinfusion appeared promising and showed a reduced incidence of decelerations and a higher mean cord arterial pH than in controls (Nageotte *et al.*, 1985).

A more convincing benefit of intrapartum amnioinfusion is its ability to decrease morbidity and mortality from meconium aspiration (Hofmeyer, 1993b) (Fig. 13.3). In all published studies, intrapartum amnioinfusion for thick meconium reduced the incidence of meconium below the cords and the meconium aspiration syndrome (Sadovsky *et al.*, 1989; Wenstrom & Parsons, 1989). However, because meconium staining usually only appears thick in the presence of oligohydramnios, the reduction in incidence of meconium aspiration syndrome may possibly be the result of correction of oligohydramnios. The mechanism may be either direct dilution of meconium or improvement in uterine and fetal blood flow, the latter leading to improved fetal condition and thus prevention of intrauterine gasping.

An intrauterine pressure catheter is introduced into the amniotic cavity. Approximately 800 ml of normal saline or Ringer's lactate is infused at 15 to 25 ml/min through the catheter. If a slower infusion rate of approximately 10 to 15 ml/min is used, it is unnecessary to warm the solution. A continuous infusion of 3 ml/min may then be used, or repeat bolus infusions at approximately six hourly intervals, up until delivery. The single or continuous infusion is monitored by both the AFI, which should be in the normal range (7–24 cm), and the fetal heart rate trace. Furthermore, it seems prudent to insert a second intrauterine pressure catheter to allow simultaneous intrauterine pressure readings to prevent uterine hypertonus.

There are a number of potential risks associated with intrapartum amnioinfusion including uterine overdistension or elevated intrauterine pressure (Posner, Ballagh & Paul, 1990) and amniotic fluid embolism (Maher *et al.*, 1994). Nevertheless, limiting infusion rates combined with simultaneous uterine pressure monitoring and ultrasonographic AFV estimation should minimize such complications.

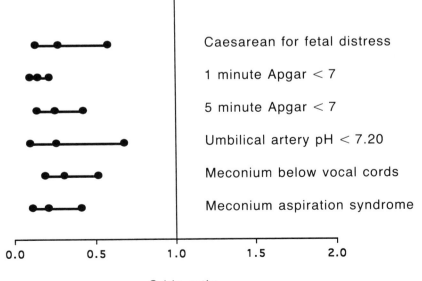

Caesarean for fetal distress

1 minute Apgar < 7

5 minute Apgar < 7

Umbilical artery pH < 7.20

Meconium below vocal cords

Meconium aspiration syndrome

Fig. 13.3 *Meta-analysis of amnioinfusion in meconium liquor (adapted from Hofmeyer, 1993b).*

Odds ratio

Therefore, amnioinfusion appears advantageous in labours with oligohydramnios and variable decelerations when labour management does not include fetal scalp pH testing, in patients with preterm PROM as prophylaxis in early labour, and finally in cases of thick meconium (i.e. and oligohydramnios).

Polyhydramnios

Ultrasound studies have shown a prevalence of polyhydramnios of 1.0 to 3.2% using the 8 cm MVP definition (Chamberlain *et al.*, 1984b; Hill *et al.*, 1987). Polyhydramnios is defined as mild (MVP 8 to 12 cm), moderate (MVP 12 to 15 cm) and severe (MVP ≥15 cm). Severe polyhydramnios occurs less frequently, in only 5% of these cases (Hill *et al.*, 1987).

Aetiology

Various maternal and fetal conditions are associated with polyhydramnios. In two series, 60% of cases were classified as idiopathic, 12 to 19% related to fetal anomalies, 5 to 19% to maternal diabetes, 8 to 13% to multiple pregnancy and the remainder idiopathic (Landy, Isada & Larsen, 1987; Ben-Chetrit *et al.*, 1990). In 7% of cases, polyhydramnios was associated with fetal hydrops.

The more severe the polyhydramnios, the more likely that an underlying cause will be found. In a series of 102 cases, 83% of mild polyhydramnios was idiopathic, whereas only 8% of severe polyhydramnios remained unexplained (Hill *et al.*, 1987).

Central nervous system, gastrointestinal and musculoskeletal disorders are the main fetal anomalies associated with polyhydramnios (Ben-Chetrit *et al.*, 1990; Queenan & Gadow, 1970). Impairment of fetal swallowing seems the predominant mechanism and explains the high frequency of polyhydramnios in fetuses with upper gastrointestinal obstruction, skeletal dystrophies affecting the thorax, neurological deficits such as myotonic dystrophy and intrathoracic space-occupying lesions such as diaphragmatic hernia and pleural effusions. Nevertheless, while almost all anencephalic fetuses do not swallow, only 67% develop polyhydramnios (Nichols & Schrepfer, 1966), which suggests that alternative mechanisms contribute, such as meningeal

transudation or vasopressin deficiency producing fetal polyuria (Naeye, Milic & Blanc, 1970).

Maternal diabetes as a cause for polyhydramnios has recently declined in frequency to 5–13% (Hill *et al.*, 1987) from 22–26% in older series (Queenan & Gadow, 1970; Jacoby & Charles, 1966) probably because of tighter glucose control. Although fetal polyuria secondary to an osmotic diuresis seems the obvious mechanism, normal fetal urine production rates have been reported in diabetic pregnancies with mild polyhydramnios (van Otterlo, Wladimiroff & Wallenburg, 1977). However, the measurement technique used is now known to underestimate fetal urine output considerably (Rabinowitz *et al.*, 1989), although it has been used to demonstrate polyuria in a fetus with diabetes insipidus and polyhydramnios (Kirshon, 1989). Recipient fetuses in feto–fetal transfusion syndrome (FFTS) have been shown to be polyuric *in vivo* (Kirshon, 1989) and histologically have enlarged glomeruli and dilated distal collecting tubules (Achiron, Rosen & Zakut, 1987). Increased cardiac output may underlie polyhydramnios in FFTS and in some cases of hydrops and Rh alloimmunization, although investigations in sheep have suggested that this may be an oversimplification of the mechanism (Anderson & Faber, 1989; Powell & Brace, 1991). Recent work has shown infusion of angiotensin I into fetal sheep with functional kidneys leads to polyhydramnios (Anderson *et al.*, 1989; Faber & Anderson, 1994), although this mechanism is poorly understood.

The term 'acute polyhydramnios' essentially means severe polyhydramnios. Most cases occur before 24 to 26 weeks in one sac of monochorial multiple pregnancies as a manifestation of FFTS (Chapter 14).

Complications

Severe polyhydramnios may produce maternal abdominal discomfort, respiratory embarrassment, renal failure and uterine irritability (Vintzileos *et al.*, 1985b; Cardwell, 1987). It is associated with preterm delivery; although the high incidence of anomalies and multiple pregnancy makes derivation of an exact risk for spontaneous preterm labour difficult, a rate corrected for congenital anomalies of 22% has been reported (Hill *et al.*, 1987). In many cases, PROM precedes the onset of preterm labour (Cardwell, 1987). Because amniotic pressure is raised in polyhydramnios (Fisk et al., 1990), these complications have all been attributed to uterine overdistension.

Perinatal mortality rates are high at 13 to 29% (Queenan & Gadow, 1970; Hill et al., 1987), reflecting the increased incidence of congenital malformations, preterm labour and asphyxial complications such as abruption, cord prolapse and placental insufficiency. Three main variables influence perinatal survival in polyhydramnios: the presence of congenital anomalies, gestational age at delivery and severity of polyhydramnios. In a series of 537 singletons with polyhydramnios, perinatal mortality was 61% in the presence of fetal or placental malformations, 10% with maternal diabetes and only 2.4% in their absence (Desmedt, Henry & Beischer, 1990). Perinatal mortality exceeds 50% in FFTS associated with polyhydramnios and, when detected before 28 weeks, mortality rates of 80–100% have been reported (Gonsoulin et al., 1990; Urig, Clewell & Elliott, 1990).

Although this excess perinatal morbidity and mortality has been attributed to preterm delivery and congenital malformations, these associations do not entirely account for the adverse outcome attributed to polyhydramnios, in particular an excess of unexplained stillbirths with normal anatomy. It has been suggested that raised amniotic pressure in polyhydramnios impairs uteroplacental perfusion (Tabor & Maier, 1987); this is based on observations of changes in fetal condition during iatrogenic polyhydramnios from intrapartum amnioinfusion. Indeed, in a study of fetuses with polyhydramnios investigated by blood sampling, fetal pH and pO_2 were inversely correlated with amniotic pressure (Fisk, Vaughan & Talbert, 1994) and severity (Fisk et al., 1990). In contrast, fetal blood gas status in the sheep model does not change during experimental polyhydramnios, although the differences in response may be explained by only a modest rise in amniotic pressure in the ovine uterus, which is more compliant than that of the human (Fisk et al., 1991b).

Diagnostic approach

The aim is to determine the underlying aetiology, the presence of associated anomalies and the severity of the polyhydramnios.

Ultrasound

A detailed ultrasound is performed for structural malformations, with particular emphasis on the upper gastrointestinal tract and its associated structures. Neurological function is assessed by observing fetal movements, and in twin pregnancies chorionicity is determined if not previously done. Repeated sonographic measurements of bladder size (Rabinowitz et al., 1989) may be used to calculate the hourly fetal urine production rate to distinguish polyhydramnios caused by fetal polyuria from other causes (Kirshon, 1989). In our experience, however, this is unnecessary as frequent and incomplete emptying gives the polyuric bladder the appearance of being chronically full; this can be simply determined from three to four observations during a 15 to 20 minute ultrasound.

The severity of polyhydramnios is quantified, both as a baseline and for prognosis.

Karyotyping

In view of a 5% chance of chromosomal abnormality, rapid karyotyping is recommended, especially in moderate/severe polyhydramnios associated with structural anomalies (Landy et al., 1987).

Others

Maternal diabetes should be excluded by testing carbohydrate tolerance and alloimmunization by maternal blood serology. With fetal hydrops unassociated with a congenital malformation, viral titres are performed on mother and fetus and fetal anaemia is excluded by fetal blood sampling.

Therapy

The aim of therapy for polyhydramnios is to relieve maternal symptoms and prolong gestation. However, as many cases are not at risk of either complication, treatment is usually only warranted in moderate to severe polyhydramnios in the mid or early third trimester. The criteria we use for intervention are either excessive maternal symptoms or an AFI >40 cm and/or MVP >12 cm, above which intra-amniotic pressure is known to be increased (Fig. 13.4). Ideally, treatment should be directed at the underlying aetiology, but this is only possible in a limited number of cases such as correction

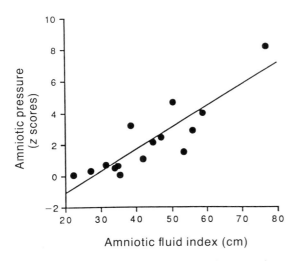

Fig. 13.4 *The relationship between amniotic pressure in z scores (standard observations from the mean for gestational age) and AFI.* y = −3.9 + 0.13 x, *when* y = *AP z score and* x = *AFI in com,* r = 0.88l, p <0.001. (Fisk, 1992b.)

of fetal anaemia by transfusion and drainage of pleural effusions by pleuro-amniotic shunts. Polyhydramnios secondary to FFTS is the most frequent indication for treatment.

Prostaglandin synthetase inhibitors

Indomethacin has mainly been used as a tocolyte. However, following recognition of decreased urinary flow rates in neonates given indomethacin (Cifuentes *et al.*, 1979), indomethacin was shown to reduce hourly fetal urine production (Kirshon *et al.*, 1988) and AFV (Kirshon, Mari & Moise, 1990). This group showed that eight patients receiving indomethacin for preterm labour had a marked decline in fetal urine output five hours after starting treatment (Kirshon *et al.*, 1988). In a study of eight singleton pregnancies with symptomatic poly-hydramnios between 21 and 34 weeks, indomethacin reduced fundal height, umbilical perimeter and qualita-tive AFV, all of which increased after cessation of therapy (Cabrol *et al.*, 1987). Similarly, a significant fall in qualitative AFV has been reported following treat-ment in both singleton (Mamopoulos *et al.*, 1990) and twin pregnancies (Lange *et al.*, 1989). Indomethacin appears effective in treating symptomatic polyhydram-nios when the underlying aetiology is associated with

increased urine output. The response is limited when polyhydramnios is secondary to poor fetal swallowing, such as in neuromuscular disorders or gastrointestinal obstruction (Kirshon *et al.*, 1990).

Indomethacin crosses the placenta freely (Moise *et al.*, 1990). Although indomethacin has been considered to reduce urine output by a renovascular mechanism (Millard, Baig & Vatner, 1979), Doppler studies of the renal artery have shown no change from baseline values during treatment (Mari *et al.*, 1990). A study in fetal sheep exposed to indomethacin has shown that, while renal blood flow is unchanged, the blood flow distributed to the inner cortex is reduced (Stevenson & Lumbers, 1992). Therefore, with blood flow directed away from the inner and more mature nephrons, urine production may be altered. Another proposed mechanism is re-duced inhibition of arginine vasopressin by prosta-glandin E in the renal collecting duct (Seyberth *et al.*, 1983). Concomitant administration of an arginine vas-opressin V2-receptor antagonist with indomethacin in sheep blocks the oliguric and free water clearance effect of indomethacin alone (Walker *et al.*, 1994).

Although indomethacin appears to be a promising drug for treatment of polyhydramnios, concern has been raised about maternal and particularly fetal side-effects. Reports of maternal side-effects after oral or rectal administration have mainly been limited to the gastro-intestinal tract. Nevertheless, a case of renal insuffi-ciency, another of cholestatic jaundice and two of pulmonary oedema have been reported from one institu-tion (Kramer, van den Veyver & Kirshon, 1994). Pros-taglandin synthetase inhibitors are relatively contraindicated in patients with renal insufficiency, pep-tic ulcer disease or coagulation disorders. Oral admin-istration is preferred because the drug is well absorbed and rectal irritation can be avoided. Although doses up to 50 mg six-hourly have been used, 25 mg every six hours seems adequate to achieve a reduction in urine output (Kirshon *et al.*, 1990a).

Fetal side-effects still remain the predominant con-cern, particularly oligohydramnios (Hendricks *et al.*, 1990), premature closure of the ductus arteriosus (Moise *et al.*, 1988) and cerebral vasoconstriction (Cowan, 1986). Monitoring ductal patency by Doppler has been recommended, particularly when treatment lasts longer than 72 hours, as it is presumed that cases of neonatal pulmonary hypertension and persistent fetal circulation occur in fetuses with prolonged ductal constriction *in utero* (Moise *et al.*, 1988). Neonatal complications from premature closure of the ductus *in utero* appear rare, and overall only 26% of exposed fetuses develop abnormal ductal waveforms (Respondek, Weil & Huhta, 1995). However, 50% of fetuses will demonstrate ductal constriction and/or tricuspid regurgitation by 32 weeks' gestation (Moise, 1993) and, therefore, therapy is not recommended beyond this gestation. Fetal echocardiography in patients on long-term indomethacin is recommended 24 hours after initiation of medication and weekly thereafter (Moise, 1993). If ductal constriction occurs, the dose should be reduced, but if ductal constriction and/or tricuspid regurgitation persist 24 hours later, therapy is stopped. Using this regimen, ductal and cardiac findings returned to normal in all cases within 24 hours (Kirshon *et al.*, 1990b). Other reported fetal complications of indomethacin therapy include neonatal renal failure (Buderus *et al.*, 1992; van der Heijden *et al.*, 1994), increased incidence of neonatal patent ductus arteriosus, necrotizing enterocolitis (Norton *et al.*, 1993) and fetal pleural effusions (Murray *et al.*, 1993); these, however, are all derived from either one or two case reports (Buderus *et al.*, 1992; Murray *et al.*, 1993) or from a retrospective, poorly controlled study (Norton *et al.*, 1993). Their significance, therefore, remains uncertain.

A further disadvantage to the use of indomethacin is that amelioration in AFV is not rapid; one study reported a median time to achieve normal volume of 12.5 days. Accordingly, one group advocates initial amnioreduction followed by maternal indomethacin (Kirshon *et al.*, 1990a). Indomethacin may also be useful in moderate polyhydramnios to avoid the need for amnioreduction. Indomethacin is not recommended in FFTS (Chapter 14) because of concern about further jeopardizing renal function in the already oliguric donor (Buderus *et al.*, 1992).

Sulindac, an alternative prostaglandin synthetase inhibitor with similar structure to indomethacin, has recently been introduced in obstetric practice. It is administered orally as a prodrug; after absorption it is irreversibly oxidized to the inactive sulphone metabolite or reversibly oxidized to the active sulphide metabolite. Initial evaluation showed sulindac to be as effective a

tocolytic as indomethacin but it appeared to have a much weaker effect on fetal urine output and no effect on the ductus arteriosus (Carlan *et al.*, 1992). In 36 women with refractory preterm labour randomized to either indomethacin or sulindac, the fall in urine flow rate at 24 hours was 56% and 25% with each drug, respectively, and changes in the ductal flow velocities were only observed with indomethacin. The relative lack of fetal effects were initially attributed to poor transplacental passage of the drug or failure of metabolism of the prodrug within the fetus. The active form of sulindac has been recently shown to cross the human placenta (Kramer *et al.*, 1995). The fetal sulphide levels, the active metabolite, were only 50% of that in the mother, whereas maternal and fetal sulindac levels, the inactive forms of the drug, were similar. Therefore, as the active form of sulindac seems reduced in the fetus, this drug is potentially as effective a tocolytic as indomethacin but with a lower risk of fetal side-effects. Not withstanding, fetal effects still occur with sulindac. At the recommended oral dose of 200 mg 12 hourly, we have used sulindac successfully to reduce AFV in two sets of monoamniotic twins in the second trimester to reduce gross fetal movements and avoid further cord entanglement. AFV was reduced from normal to relative oligohydramnios and there was no evidence of ductal constriction during the course of therapy (M. J. Peek *et al.*, submitted for publication). Although further studies are required, sulindac appears to have a role in treating polyhydramnios. In comparison to indomethacin, it may have a less pronounced effect on fetal urine production, but the constrictive effects on the ductus arteriosus may be less likely.

New research into prostaglandin involvement in the onset and mechanism of labour shows that uterine contractions are mediated by cyclooxygenase 2 (COX-2) (Slater *et al.*, 1995) whereas prostaglandins available for fetal renal and ductal function are mediated by cyclooxygenase 1 (COX-1). Indomethacin is known to inhibit both isoenzymes, but the relative effects of sulindac on COX-1 and COX-2 are unknown (P. Bennett, personal communication). If a differential effect on the two enzymes was found to be evident, this could also explain sulindac's relative lack of fetal side-effects. Although not useful for the treatment of polyhydramnios, if a specific COX-2 inhibitor became available, it should theoretically function as a tocolytic free of fetal side-effects.

Amnioreduction

Since the first description of amnioreduction (Rivett, 1933), numerous case reports have claimed the procedure to be successful in reducing maternal symptoms and prolonging gestation in both singleton and twin pregnancies. In contrast, others have found that rapid re-accumulation of fluid rendered amnioreduction to be of little benefit (Fisk & Moessinger, 1994).

Most workers were initially conservative in the selection of the amniotic volume to be removed in view of concerns regarding precipitation of abruption or preterm labour (Feingold *et al.*, 1986; Cabrera-Ramirez & Harris, 1976). Indeed, raised amniotic pressure in severe polyhydramnios is restored to normal by removal of relatively small volumes (Fisk *et al.*, 1990) (Fig. 13.5). However, with rapid reaccumulation of fluid, it seems likely that amniotic pressure soon rises again. Accordingly, one group (Urig *et al.*, 1990) considered restitution of normal AFV the more important goal and drained much larger volumes of up to 5000 ml in 29 procedures. Their promising results using 'aggressive therapeutic amniocentesis' with reversal of hydrops in the recipient

and oligohydramnios in the donor support their claim (Elliot, Urig & Clewell, 1991).

A recent review of 200 'large volume' reduction amniocenteses in single and twin pregnancies suggests that the complication rate is low at 1.5% (Elliot *et al.*, 1994). One patient developed chorioamnionitis, another presented with ruptured membranes 24 hours following the procedure and a further pregnancy was complicated by an abruption following removal of 10 litres of amniotic fluid prior to inducing labour with an anencephalic fetus. It may be prudent to remove no more than an upper limit of 5 to 6 litres of fluid to avoid this complication. Patients having contractions at the time of amnioreduction are known to have a greater risk of preterm delivery following the procedure (Caldeyro-Barcia, Pose & Alvarez, 1957). Therefore, amnioreduction should be ideally performed before the onset of contractions or cervical dilatation.

The patient is wedged in the left lateral position to avoid supine hypotension and should be comfortable as the procedure may take up to one hour. We use sterile technique and prophylactic intravenous antibiotics. A

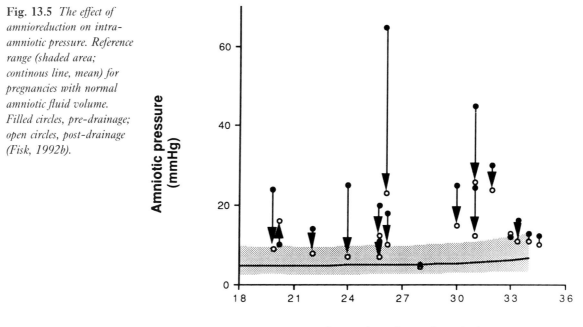

Fig. 13.5 *The effect of amnioreduction on intra-amniotic pressure. Reference range (shaded area; continous line, mean) for pregnancies with normal amniotic fluid volume. Filled circles, pre-drainage; open circles, post-drainage (Fisk, 1992b).*

large amniotic pocket is located by ultrasound which is slightly lateral and midway down the uterus with attention to avoidance of the placenta. This site is chosen to allow maximal flexibility of the needle to minimize maternal discomfort and contractions as the relationship between the overlying skin, uterus and amniotic cavity changes greatly during drainage. Local anaesthetic is instilled and the skin pierced with a scalpel blade. An 18-gauge needle is inserted into the pool under ultrasound guidance. As the trochar is removed, extension tubing is attached to the needle hub, and the intra-amniotic pressure measured. To do this, the three-way tap at the end of the tubing is opened to air and the tubing is raised vertically against a ruler. Once the fluid settles, the meniscus should fluctuate with respiration; the pressure measurement is taken from the meniscus to the top of the uterus in centimetres of H_2O. This represents the intra-amniotic pressure. A 50 ml syringe is then attached to the three-way tap and fluid is aspirated continuously until the AFI is decreased into the low-normal range, usually an MVP <7 cm. We attempt to remove the fluid as rapidly as possible to avoid a lengthy procedure and discomfort to the mother. At the end of the procedure, the intra-amniotic pressure measurement is repeated. Thereafter, the patient is monitored two to three times per week by ultrasound; repeat amnioreductions are indicated in the presence of symptoms or an AFI>40 cm or MVP>12 cm.

The placement of chronic drainage catheters has occasionally been attempted but has often been complicated by a high incidence of infection and blockage. In terms of the latter, the main problem appears to be kinking between the skin and uterine entry sites which move apart as the uterus decreases in volume.

Others

In selected pathologies, correction of the underlying aetiology is preferable to empirical treatment of polyhydramnios. Medical causes of polyhydramnios, with or without hydrops, may respond to transfusion (Chapter 10) or drug therapy (Chapter 15). In fetuses with bilateral hydrothoraces, chronic *in utero* drainage by pleuroamniotic shunting corrects polyhydramnios, providing lung hypoplasia does not prevent lung re-expansion (Chapter 16). Open fetal surgical correction of intrathoracic lesions, such as diaphragmatic hernia or cystic adenomatoid lung malformation (Chapters 18, 19) may also restore transit of amniotic fluid through the upper gastrointestinal tract. In each of the above, the primary aim of treatment is not correction of polyhydramnios but rather prevention of complications from the underlying condition.

Conclusions

Aberrant AFV complicates up to 7% of pregnancies, although many cases will be mild and present in the third trimester with no underlying cause or sequelae. In contrast, severe oligohydramnios and polyhydramnios in the midtrimester are associated with substantial perinatal morbidity and mortality, reflecting both the underlying aetiology and the complications of disordered amniotic volume.

To date, the outcome of therapy for severe oligohydramnios has been disappointing. Preterm PROM and severe IUGR, which comprise the majority of cases of second-trimester oligohydramnios, are presently unamenable to therapy to restore amniotic fluid. Preliminary experience in human oligohydramnios suggests that serial amnioinfusions may facilitate lung growth and improve survival. However, the overriding limitation is that very few cases are suitable.

In some conditions associated with polyhydramnios, the underlying cause is amenable to treatment, but in others, treatment of the polyhydramnios is indicated to prolong gestation and relieve maternal discomfort. Accordingly, FFTS is the most common indication for treatment. Large-volume amnioreduction and, in selected cases, prostaglandin synthetase inhibitors are useful treatment modalities for symptomatic polyhydramnios. Preliminary experience suggests that sulindac has fewer side-effects than indomethacin and may in future become the treatment of choice for polyhydramnios in singletons.

References

Abramovich, D. R. (1968). The volume of amniotic fluid in early pregnancy. *Journal of Obstetrics and Gynaecology of the British Commonwealth*, 75, 728–31.

Achiron, R., Rosen, N. & Zakut, H. (1987). Patho-physiologic mechanism of hydramnios development in twin transfusion syndrome. *Journal of Reproductive Medicine*, 32, 305–8.

Adzick, N. S., Harrison, M. R., Glick, P. L., Villa, R. L. & Finkbeiner, W. (1984). Experimental PH and oligohydramnios: relative contributions of lung fluid and fetal breathing movements. *Journal of Pediatric Surgery*, 19, 658–65.

Anderson, D. F. & Faber, J. J. (1989). Animal model for polyhydramnios. *American Journal of Obstetrics and Gynecology*, 160, 389–90.

Ardiuni, D. & Rizzo, G. (1991). Fetal renal artery velocity waveforms and AFV in growth-retarded and post-term fetuses. *Obstetrics and Gynecology*, 77, 370–3.

Barss, V., Benacerraf, B. & Frigoletto, F. (1984). Second trimester oligohydramnios: a predictor of poor fetal outcome. *Obstetrics and Gynecology*, 64, 608–10.

Battaglia, F., Prystowsky, H., Smisson, C., Hellegers, A. & Bruns, P. (1960). Fetal blood studies. XIII. The effect of the administration of fluids intra-venously to mothers upon the concentrations of water and electrolytes in plasma of human fetuses. *Pediatrics*, 25, 2–10.

Baumgarten, K. & Moser, S. (1986). The technique of fibrin adhesion for premature rupture of the membranes during pregnancy. *Journal of Perinatal Medicine*, 14, 43–9.

Bell, R. J., Congiu, M., Hardy, K. J. & Wintour, E. M. (1984). Gestation-dependent aspects of the response of the ovine fetus to the osmotic stress induced by maternal water deprivation. *Quarterly Journal of Experimental Physiology*, 69, 187–95.

Benacerraf, B. R. (1990). Examination of the severe second trimester fetus with severe oligohydramnios using transvaginal scanning. *Obstetrics and Gynecology*, 75, 491–3.

Ben-Chetrit, A., Hochner-Celnikier, D., Ron, M. & Yagel, S. (1990). Hydramnios in the third trimester of pregnancy: a change in the accompanying fetal anomalies as a result of early ultrasonographic diagnosis. *American Journal of Obstetrics and Gynecology*, 162, 1344–5.

Beydoun, S. N. & Yasin, S. Y. (1986). Premature rupture of the membranes before 28 weeks: conservative management. *American Journal of Obstetrics and Gynecology*, 155, 471–9.

Brace, R. A. (1989). Fetal blood volume, urine flow, swallowing, and AFV responses to long term intravascular infusions of saline. *American Journal of Obstetrics and Gynecology*, 161, 1049–54.

Brace, R. A. & Wolf, E. J. (1989). Normal AFV changes throughout pregnancy. *American Journal of Obstetrics and Gynecology*, 161, 382–8.

Brans, Y., Andrew, D. S., Dutton, E. R., Schwartz, C. A. & Carey, K. D. (1989). Dilution of chemicals used for estimation of water content of body compartments in perinatal medicine. *Pediatric Research*, 25, 377–82.

Bronstein, M. & Zimmer, E. T. (1995). Oligo-hydramnios with amnio-chorionic separation at 15–16 weeks' gestation. *Prenatal Diagnosis*, 15, 161–4.

Buderus S., Thomas B., Fahnenstich H. & Kowalewski, S. (1993). Renal failure in two preterm infants: toxic effect of prenatal maternal indomethacin treatment? *British Journal of Obstetrics and Gynaecology*, 100, 97–8.

Burri, P. H. (1984). Fetal and postnatal development of the lung. *Annual Review of Physiology*, 46, 617–28.

Cabrera-Ramirez, L. & Harris, R. E. (1976). Controlled removal of amniotic fluid in hydramnios. *Southern Medical Journal*, 69, 239–40.

Cabrol, D., Landesman, R., Muller, J., Uzan, M., Sureau, C. & Saxena, B. B. (1987). Treatment of polyhydramnios with prostaglandin synthetase inhibitor (indomethacin). *American Journal of Obstetrics and Gynecology*, 157, 422–6.

Caldeyro-Barcia, R., Pose, S. V. & Alvarez, H. (1957). Uterine contractility in polyhydramnios and the effects of withdrawal of the excess of amniotic fluid. *American Journal of Obstetrics and Gynecology*, 73, 1238–54.

Cameron, D., Lupton, B. A., Farquharson, D. & Hiruki, T. (1994). Amnioinfusions in renal agenesis. *Obstetrics and Gynecology*, 83, 872–6.

Cardwell, M. S. (1987). Polyhydramnios: a review. *Obstetric and Gynecological Survey*, 42, 612–17.

Carlan, S. J., O'Brien, W. F., O'Leary, T. D. & Mastrogiannis, D. (1992). Randomized comparative trial of indomethacin and sulindac for the treatment of refractory preterm labor. *Obstetrics and Gynecology*, 79, 223–8.

Chamberlain, P. F., Cumming, M., Torchia, M. G., Biehl, D. & Manning, F. A. (1985). Ovine fetal urine production following maternal intravenous furosemide administration. *American Journal of Obstetrics and Gynecology*, 151, 815–19.

Chamberlain, P. F., Manning, F. A., Morrison, I., Harman, C. R. & Lange, I. R. (1984a). Ultrasound evaluation of AFV. I. The relationship of marginal and decreased AFVs to perinatal outcome. *American Journal of Obstetrics and Gynecology*, 150, 245–9.

Chamberlain, P. F., Manning, F. A., Morrison, I., Harman, C. R. & Lange, I. R. (1984b). Ultrasound evaluation of AFV. II. The relationship of increased AFV to perinatal outcome. *American Journal of Obstetrics and Gynecology*, 150, 250–4.

Cifuentes, R. F., Olley, P. M., Balfe, J. W., Radde, I. C. & Soldin, S. J. (1979). Indomethacin and renal function in premature infants with persistent patent ductus arteriosus. *Journal of Pediatrics*, 95, 583–7.

Cohn, H. E., Sacks, E., Heyman, M. A. & Rudolph, A. M. (1974). Cardiovascular responses to hypoxemia and acidemia in fetal lambs. *American Journal of Obstetrics and Gynecology*, 120, 817–24.

Cowan, F. (1986). Indomethacin, patent ductus arteriosus, and cerebral blood flow. *Journal of Pediatrics*, 109, 341–4.

Crowley, P. (1980). Non-quantitative measurement of AFV in prolonged pregnancy. *Journal of Perinatal Medicine*, 8, 249–51.

Desmedt, E. J., Henry, O. A. & Beischer N. A. (1990). Polyhydramnios and associated maternal and fetal complications in singleton pregnancies.

British Journal of Obstetrics and Gynaecology, 97, 1115–22.

DeVore, G. R., Horenstein, J. & Platt, L. D. (1986). Fetal echocardiography VI. Assessment of cardiothoracic disproportion – a new technique for the diagnosis of thoracic hypoplasia. *American Journal of Obstetrics and Gynecology*, 155, 1066–71.

Dildy, G. A., Lira, N., Moise, K. J., Riddle, G. D. & Deter, R. L. (1992). AFV assessment: comparison of ultrasonographic estimates versus direct measurements with a dye-dilution technique in human pregnancy. *American Journal of Obstetrics and Gynecology*, 167, 986–94.

Dyer, S. N., Burton, B. K. & Nelson, L. H. (1987). Elevated maternal serum a-fetoprotein levels and oligohydramnios: poor prognosis for pregnancy outcome. American Journal of *Obstetrics and Gynecology*, 157, 336–9.

Elder, J. S., Duckett, J. W. & Snyder, H. M. (1987). Intervention for fetal obstructive uropathy: has it been effective? *Lancet*, ii, 1007–10.

Elliott, J. P., Urig, M. A. & Clewell, W. H. (1991). Aggressive therapeutic amniocentesis for treatment of twin–twin transfusion syndrome. *Obstetrics and Gynecology*, 77, 537–40.

Faber, J. J. & Anderson, D. F. (1994). Hydrops fetalis in nephrectomised fetal lambs infused with angiotensin I. *American Journal of Physiology*, 267, R1522–7.

Feingold, M., Cetrulo, C. L., Newton, E., Weiss, J., Shakr, C. & Shmoys, S. (1986). Serial amnio-centeses in the treatment of twin to twin transfusion complicated with acute polyhydramnios. *Acta Geneticae Medicae et Gemellologiae*, 35, 107–13.

Fisk, N. F. (1992a). Oligohydramnios-related pulmonary hypoplasia. *Contemporary Reviews in Obstetrics and Gynaecology*, 4, 191–201.

Fisk, N. F. (1992b). Amniotic Pressure in Disorders of Amniotic Fluid Volume. PhD Thesis, University of London.

Fisk, N. M., Giussani, D. A., Parkes, M. J., Moore, P. J. & Hanson, M. A. (1991b). Amnioinfusion increases amniotic pressure in pregnant sheep but does not alter fetal acid base status. *American Journal of Obstetrics and Gynecology*, 165, 1459–63.

Fisk, N. M. & Moessinger, A. (1994). Oligohydramnios and polyhydramnios. In *Diseases of the Fetus and Newborn*, 2nd edn, vol. 2, ed. G. B. Reed, A. E. Claireaux, F. Cockburn & M. Connor, pp. 1243–56. London: Chapman Hall.

Fisk, N. M., Parkes, M. J., Moore, P. J., Hanson, M. A., Wigglesworth, J., Rodeck, C. H. (1992c). Mimicking low amniotic pressure by chronic pharyngeal drainage does not impair lung development in fetal sheep. *American Journal of Obstetrics and Gynecology*, 166, 991–6.

Fisk, N. M., Ronderos-Dumit, D., Soliani, A., Nicolini, U., Vaughan, J. I. & Rodeck, C. H. (1991a). Diagnostic and therapeutic transabdominal amnioinfusion in oligohydramnios. *Obstetrics and Gynecology*, 78, 270–8.

Fisk, N. M., Talbert, D. G., Nicolini, U., Vaughan, J. & Rodeck, C. (1992b). Fetal breathing movements in oligohydramnios are not altered by amnioinfusion. *British Journal of Obstetrics and Gynaecology*, 99, 464–8.

Fisk, N. M., Tannirandorn, Y., Nicolini, U., Talbert, D. G. & Rodeck, C. H. (1990). Amniotic pressure in disorders of amniotic fluid volume. *Obstetrics and Gynecology*, 76, 210–14.

Fisk, N. M., Vaughan J. & Talbert D. (1994). Impaired fetal blood gas status in polyhydramnios and its relation to raised amniotic pressure. *Fetal Diagnosis and Therapy*, 9, 7–13.

Fisk, N. M., Welch, C. R., Ronderos-Dumit, D., Vaughan, J. I., Nicolini, U. & Rodeck, C. H. (1992a). Relief of presumed compression in oligohydramnios: amnioinfusion does not affect umbilical Doppler waveforms. *Fetal Diagnosis and Therapy*, 7, 180–5.

Flack, N. J., Doré, C., Southwell, D., Kourtis, P., Sepulveda, W. & Fisk, N. M. (1994). The influence of operator transducer pressure on ultrasonographic measurements of amniotic fluid volume. *American Journal of Obstetrics and Gynecology*, 171, 218–22.

Flack, N. J., Sepulveda, W., Bower, S. & Fisk, N. M. (1995). Acute maternal hydration in third-trimester oligohydramnios: effects on amniotic fluid volume, uteroplacental perfusion, and fetal blood flow and urine output. *American Journal of Obstetrics and Gynecology*, 173, 502–7.

Fujino, Y., Agnew, C. L., Schreyer, P. G., Ervin, M. G., Sherman, D. J. & Ross, M. G. (1991). Amniotic fluid volume response to esophageal occlusion in fetal sheep. *American Journal of Obstetrics and Gynecology*, 165, 1620–6.

Gembruch, U. & Hansmann, M. (1988). Artificial instillation of amniotic fluid as a new technique for the diagnostic evaluation of cases of oligo-hydramnios. *Prenatal Diagnosis*, 8, 33–45.

Gilbert, W. M. & Brace, R. A. (1988). Increase in fetal hydration during long-term intraamniotic saline infusion. *American Journal of Obstetrics and Gynecology*, 159, 1413–17.

Gilbert, W. M. & Brace, R. A. (1989). The missing link in amniotic fluid volume regulation: intramembranous absorption. *Obstetrics and Gynecology*, 74, 748–54.

Gonsoulin, W., Moise, K. J., Kirshon, B., Cotton, D. B., Wheeler, B. & Carpenter, R. J. (1990). Outcome of twin–twin transfusion diagnosed before 28 weeks of gestation. *Obstetrics and Gynecology*, 75, 214–16.

Goodlin, R. C., Anderson, J. C. & Gallagher, T. F. (1983). Relationship between amniotic fluid volume and maternal volume expansion. *American Journal of Obstetrics and Gynecology*, 146, 505–11.

Gruenwald, P. (1957). Hypoplasia of the lungs. *Journal of Mount Sinai Hospital*, 24, 913–19.

Gunn, G. C., Mishell, D. & Morton, D. G. (1970). Premature rupture of the fetal membranes. *American Journal of Obstetrics and Gynecology*, 106, 469–83.

Hackett, G. A., Nicolaides, K. H. & Campbell, S. (1987). Doppler ultrasound assessment of fetal and uteroplacental circulations in severe second trimester oligohydramnios. *British Journal of Obstetrics and Gynaecology*, 94, 1074–7.

Hadi, H. A., Hodson, C. A. & Strickland, D. (1994). Premature rupture of the membranes between 20 and 25 weeks' gestation: role of AFV in perinatal outcome. *American Journal of Obstetrics and Gynecology*, 170, 1139–44.

Hansmann, M., Chatterjee, M. S., Schuh, S., Gembruch, U. & Bald, R. (1991). Multiple antepartum amnioinfusions in selected cases of olighydramnios. *Journal of Reproductive Medicine*, 36, 847–51.

Harding, R., Bocking, A. D., Sigger, J. N. & Wickham, P. J. D. (1984). Composition and volume of fluid swallowed by fetal sheep. *Quarterly Journal of Experimental Physiology*, 69, 487–95.

Harding, R., Hooper, S. B. & Dickson, K. A. (1990). A mechanism leading to reduced lung expansion and lung hypoplasia in fetal sheep during oligo-hydramnios. *American Journal of Obstetrics and Gynecology*, 163, 1904–13.

Harman, C. R. (1984). Maternal furosemide may not provoke urine production in the compromised fetus. *American Journal of Obstetrics and Gynecology*, 150, 322–3.

Harrison, M. R., Golbus, M. S., Filly, R. A., Callen, P. W., Katz, M., de Lorimier, A. A., Rosen, M. & Johsen, A. R. (1982b). Fetal surgery for congenital hydronephrosis. *New England Journal of Medicine*, 306, 591–3.

Harrison, M. R., Nakayama, D. K., Noall, R. & de Lorimier, A. A. (1982a). Correction of congenital hydronephrosis *in utero*. II. Decompression reverses the effects of obstruction on the fetal lung and urinary tract. *Journal of Pediatric Surgery*, 17, 965–74.

Hendricks, S. D., Smith, J. R., Moore, D. E. and Brown, Z. A. (1990). Oligohydramnios associated with prostaglandin synthetase inhibitors in preterm labour. *British Journal of Obstetrics and Gynaecology*, 97, 312–16.

Hill, L. M., Breckle, R., Thomas M. L. & Fries, J. K. (1987). Polyhydramnios: ultrasonographically detected prevalence and neonatal outcome. *Obstetrics and Gynecology*, 69, 21–5.

Hofmeyer, G. J. (1993a). Prophylactic vs. therapeutic amnioinfusion for intrapartum oligohydramnios. In *Pregnancy and Childbirth Module*, ed. M. J. N. C. Keirse, M. J. Renfrew, J. P. Neilson & C. Crowther. London: Cochrane Database of Systematic Reviews, BMJ Publishing Group.

Hofmeyer, G. J. (1993b). Amnioinfusion for meconium-stained liquor in labour. In *Pregnancy and Childbirth Module*, ed. M. J. N. C. Keirse, M. J. Renfrew, J. P. Neilson & C. Crowther. London: Cochrane Database of Systematic Reviews, BMJ Publishing Group.

Imanaka, M., Ogita, S. & Sugawa, T. (1989). Saline solution amnioinfusion for oligohydramnios after premature rupture of the membranes. *American Journal of Obstetrics and Gynecology*, 161, 102–6.

Jacoby, H. E. & Charles, D. (1966). Clinical conditions associated with hydramnios. *American Journal of Obstetrics and Gynecology*, 94, 910–19.

Kappy, K. A., Cetrulo, C. L., Knuppel, R. A., Ingardia, C. J., Sbara, A. J., Scerbo, J. C. & Mitchell, G. W. (1979). Premature rupture of the membranes: a conservative approach. *American Journal of Obstetrics and Gynecology*, 134, 655–61.

Kilpatrick, S. J., Safford, K. L., Pomeroy, T., Hoedt, L., Scheerer, L. & Laros, R. (1991). Maternal hydration increases amniotic fluid index. *Obstetrics and Gynecology*, 78, 1098–1102

Kirshon, B. (1989). Fetal urine output in hydramnios. *Obstetrics and Gynecology*, 73, 240–2.

Kirshon, B., Mari, G. & Moise, K. J. (1990a). Indo-methacin therapy in the treatment of symptomatic polyhydramnios. *Obstetrics and Gynecology*, 75, 202–5.

Kirshon, B., Mari, G., Moise, K. J. & Wasserstrum, N. (1990b). Effect of indomethacin on the fetal ductus arteriosus during treatment of symptomatic polyhydramnios. *Journal of Reproductive Medicine*, 35, 529–32.

Kirshon, B., Moise, K. J., Wasserstrum, N., Ou, C. N. & Huhta, J. C. (1988). Influence of short-term indomethacin therapy on fetal urine output. *Obstetrics and Gynecology*, 72, 51–3.

Knox, W. F. & Barson, A. J. (1986). Effect of induced olighydramnios on fetal lung development. *Early Human Development*, 14, 33–42.

Kramer, W. B., Saade, G., Ou, C., Roguerud, C., Dorman, K., Mayes, M. & Moise, K. J. (1995). Placental transfer of sulindac and its active sulfide metabolite in humans. *American Journal of Obstetrics and Gynecology* , 172, 886–90.

Kramer, W. B., Van den Veyver, I. B. & Kirshon, B. (1994). Treatment of polyhydramnios with indomethacin. *Clinics in Perinatology*, 21, 615–30.

Landy, H. J., Isada, N. B. & Larsen, J. W. (1987) Genetic implications of idiopathic hydramnios. *American Journal of Obstetrics and Gynecology*, 157, 114–17.

Lange, I. R., Harman, C. R., Ash, K. M., Manning, F. A. & Menticoglou, S. (1989). Twins with hydramnios: treating premature labor at source. *American Journal of Obstetrics and Gynecology*, 160, 552–7.

Lind, T., Billewicz, W. Z. & Cheyne, G. A. (1971). Composition of amniotic fluid and maternal blood throughout pregnancy. *Journal of Obstetrics and Gynaecology of the British Commonwealth*, 78, 505–12.

Lind, T., Kendall, A. & Hytten, F. E. (1972). The role of the fetus in the formation of amniotic fluid. *Journal of Obstetrics and Gynaecology of the British Commonwealth*, 79, 289–98.

Lumbers, E. R. & Stevens, A. D. (1983). Changes in fetal renal function in response to infusions of a hyperosmotic solution of mannitol to the ewe. *Journal of Physiology*, 343, 439–46.

Maher, J. E., Wenstrom, K. D., Hauth, J. C. & Meis, P. J. (1994) Amniotic fluid embolism after saline amnioinfusion: two cases and review of the literature. *Obstetrics and Gynecology*, 83, 851–4.

Mamopoulos, M., Assimakopoulos, E., Reece, E. A., Andreou, A., Zheng, X. Z. & Mantalenakis, S. (1990). Maternal indomethacin therapy in the treatment of polyhydramnios. *American Journal of Obstetrics and Gynecology*, 162, 1225–9.

Mandlebrot, L., Dommergues, M. & Dumez Y. (1992). Prepartum transabdominal amnio-infusion for severe oligohydramnios. *Acta Obstetrica et Gynecologica Scandinavica*, 71, 124–5.

Mandlebrot, L., Verspyk, E., Dommergues, M., Bréart, G. & Dumez, Y. (1993). Transabdominal amnioinfusion for the management of nonlaboring postdates with severe oligohydramnios. *Fetal Diagnosis and Therapy*, 8, 412–17.

Manning, F. A., Harrison, M. R., Rodeck, C. H. and members of the International Fetal Medicine and Surgery Society (1986). Catheter shunts for fetal hydronephrosis and hydrocephalus. *New England Journal of Medicine*, 315, 336–40.

Manning, F. A., Hill, L. M. & Platt, L. D. (1981). Qualitative amniotic fluid volume determination by ultrasound: antepartum detection of intrauterine growth retardation. *American Journal of Obstetrics and Gynecology*, 139, 254–8.

Mari, G., Moise, K. J., Deter, R. L., Kirshon, B. & Carpenter, R. J. (1990). Doppler assessment of the renal blood flow velocity waveform during indomethacin therapy for preterm labor and polyhydramnios. *Obstetrics and Gynecology*, 75, 199–201.

Mercer, L. J. & Brown, L. G. (1986). Fetal outcome with oligohydramnios in second trimester. *Obstetrics and Gynecology*, 67, 840–2.

Mercer, L. J., Brown, L. G., Petres, R. E. & Messer R. H. (1984). A survey of pregnancies complicated by decreased amniotic fluid. *American Journal of Obstetrics and Gynecology*, 149, 355–61.

Millard, R. W., Baig, H. & Vatner, S. F. (1979). Prostaglandin control of the renal circulation in response to hypoxemia in the fetal lamb *in utero*. *Circulation Research*, 45, 172–9.

Miyazaki, F. S. & Nevarez, F. (1985). Saline amnioinfusion for relief of repetitive variable decelerations: a prospective randomised study. *American Journal of Obstetrics and Gynecology*, 153, 301–6.

Moessinger, A. C., Fox, H. E., Higgins, A., Rey, H. R. & Al Haidieri, M. (1987). Fetal breathing movements are not a reliable predictor of continued lung development in pregnancies complicated by oligohydramnios. *Lancet*, ii, 1297–1300.

Moise, K. J. (1993) Effect of advancing gestational age on the frequency of fetal ductal constriction in association with maternal indomethacin use. *American Journal of Obstetrics and Gynecology*, 168, 1350–3.

Moise, K. J., Huhta, J. C., Sharif, D. S., Ou, C. N., Kirshon, B., Wasserstrum, N. & Cano, L. (1988). Indomethacin in the treatment of premature labor. Effects on fetal ductus arteriosus. *New England Journal of Medicine*, 319, 327–31.

Moise, K. J., Ou, C. N., Kirshon, B., Cano, L. E., Rognerud, C. & Carpenter, R. J. (1990). Placental transfer of indomethacin in the human pregnancy. *American Journal of Obstetrics and Gynecology*, 162, 549–54.

Moore, T. R. (1990). Superiority of the four-quadrant sum over the single-deepest-pocket technique in ultrasonographic identification of abnormal amniotic fluid volume. *American Journal of Obstetrics and Gynecology*, 163, 762–7.

Moore, T. R. & Cayle, J. E. (1990) The amniotic fluid index in normal human pregnancy. *American Journal of Obstetrics and Gynecology*, 162, 1168–73.

Moore, T. R., Longo, J., Leopold, G. R., Casola, G. & Gosink, B. B. (1989). The reliability and predictive value of an amniotic fluid scoring system in severe second trimester oligohydramnios. *Obstetrics and Gynecology*, 73, 739–42.

Moretti, M. & Sibai, B. M. (1988). Maternal and perinatal outcome of expectant management of premature rupture of membranes in the midtrimester. *American Journal of Obstetrics and Gynecology*, 159, 390–6.

Moya, F., Apgar, V., James, L. S. & Berrien, C. (1960). Hydramnios and congenital anomalies. *Journal of the American Medical Association*, 173, 1552–6.

Murray, H. G., Stone, P. R., Strand, L. & Flower, J. (1993). Fetal pleural effusion following maternal indomethacin therapy. *British Journal of Obstetrics and Gynaecology*, 100, 277–82.

Naeye, R. L., Milic, A. M. B. & Blanc, W. (1970). Fetal endocrine and renal disorders: clues to the origin of hydramnios. *American Journal of Obstetrics and Gynecology*, 108, 1251–6.

Nageotte, M. P., Freeman, R. K., Garite, T. J. & Dorchester, W. (1985). Prophylactic intrapartum amnioinfusion in patients with preterm premature rupture of membranes. *American Journal Obstetrics and Gynecology*, 153, 557–62.

Nakayama, D. K., Glick, P. ll, Harrison, M. R., Villa, R. L. & Noall, R. (1983). Experimental pulmonary hypoplasia due to oligohydramnios and its reversal by relieving thoracic compression. *Journal of Pediatric Surgery*, 18, 347–53.

Nichols, J. & Schrepfer, R. (1966). Polyhydramnios in anencephaly. *Journal of the American Medical Association*, 197, 549–51.

Nicolaides, K. H., Peters, M. T., Vyas, S., Rabinowitz, R., Rosen, D. J. & Campbell, S. (1990). Relation of rate of urine production to oxygen tension in small-for-gestational-age fetuses. *American Journal of Obstetrics and Gynecology*, 162, 387–91.

Nicolini, U., Santolaya, J., Hubinont, C., Fisk, N. M., Maxwell, D. & Rodeck, C. H. (1989). Visualization of fetal intra-abdominal organs in second trimester severe oligohydramnios by intraperitoneal infusion. *Prenatal Diagnosis*, 9, 191–4.

Nimrod, C., Davies, D., Iwanicki, S., Harder, J., Persaud, D. & Nicholson, S. (1986). Ultrasound prediction of pulmonary hypoplasia. *Obstetrics and Gynecology*, 68, 495–7.

Norton, M. E., Merrill, J., Cooper, B. A. B., Kuller, J. A. & Clyman, R. I. (1993). Neonatal complications after the administration of indomethacin for preterm labor. *New England Journal of Medicine*, 329, 1602–7.

Ogita, S., Imanaka, M., Matsumoto, M. & Hatanaka, K. (1984). Premature rupture of the membranes managed with a new cervical catheter. *Lancet*, i, 1330–1.

Ogita, S., Imanaka, M., Matsumoto, M., Oka, T. & Sugawa, T. (1988). Transcervical amnioinfusion of antibiotics: a basic study for managing premature rupture of membranes. *American Journal of Obstetrics and Gynecology*, 158, 23–7.

Ogundipe, O. A., Spong, C. Y. & Ross, M. G. (1994). Prophylactic amnioinfusion for oligohydramnios: a re-evaluation. *Obstetrics and Gynecology*, 84, 544–8.

Peeters, L. L. H., Sheldon, R. E., Jones, M. D., Makowski, E. L. & Meschia, G. (1979). Blood flow to fetal organs as a function of arterial oxygen content. *American Journal of Obstetrics and Gynecology*, 135, 637–46.

Philipson, E. H., Sokol, R. J. & Williams, T. (1983). Oligohydramnios: clinical associations and predictive value for intrauterine growth retardation. *American Journal of Obstetrics and Gynecology*, 146, 271–8.

Posner, M. D., Ballagh, S. A. & Paul, R. H. (1990). The effect of amnioinfusion on uterine pressure and activity: a preliminary report. *American Journal of Obstetrics and Gynecology*, 163, 813–18.

Powell, T. L. & Brace, R. A. (1991). Elevated fetal plasma lactate produces polyhydramnios in the sheep. *American Journal of Obstetrics and Gynecology*, 165, 1595–607.

Puder, K. S., Sorokin,Y., Bottoms, S. F., Hallak, M. & Cotton, D. B. (1994). Amnioinfusion: does the choice of solution adversely affect neonatal electrolyte balance? *Obstetrics and Gynecology*, 84, 956–9.

Queenan, J. T. & Gadow E. C. (1970). Poly-hydramnios, chronic versus acute. *American Journal of Obstetrics and Gynecology*, 108, 349–55.

Queenan, J. T., Thompson, W., Whitfield, C. R. & Shah, S. I. (1972). Amniotic fluid volume in normal pregnancies. *American Journal of Obstetrics and Gynecology*, 114, 34–8.

Quetel, T. A., Mejides, A. A., Salman, F. A. & Torres-Rodriguez, M. M. (1992). Amnioinfusion: an aid in the ultrasonographic evaluation of severe oligohydramnios in pregnancy. *American Journal of Obstetrics and Gynecology*, 167, 333–6.

Rabinowitz, R., Peters, M. T., Vyas, S., Campbell, S. & Nicholaides, K. H. (1989). Measurement of fetal urine production in normal pregnancy by real-time ultrasonography. *American Journal of Obstetrics and Gynecology*, 161, 1264–6.

Respondek, M., Weil, S. R. & Huhta, J. C. (1995). Fetal echocardiography during indomethacin treatment. *Ultrasound in Obstetrics and Gynecology*, 5, 86–9.

Reuss, A., Wladimiroff, J. W., Stewart, P. A. & Scholtmeijer, R. J. (1988). Non-invasive management of fetal obstructive uropathy. *Lancet*, ii, 949–51.

Reuss, A., Wladimiroff, J. W., Wijngaard, J. A., Pijpers, L. & Stewart, P. A. (1987). Fetal renal anomalies, a diagnostic dilemma in the presence of intrauterine growth retardation and oligohydramnios. *Ultrasound in Medicine and Biology*, 10, 619–24.

Rivett, L. C. (1933). Hydramnios. *Journal of Obstetrics and Gynaecolology of the British Empire*, 40, 522–5.

Roberts, A. B. & Mitchell, J. M. (1990). Direct ultrasonographic measurment of fetal lung length in normal pregnancies and pregnancies complicated by prolonged rupture of membranes. *American Journal of Obstetrics and Gynecology*, 163, 1560–6.

Robillard, J. E., Weitzam, R. E., Burmeister, L. & Smith, F. G. (1981). Development aspects of the renal response to hypoxemia in the fetal lamb *in utero*. *Circulation Research*, 48, 128–38.

Robson, S. C., Crawford, R. A. & Spencer, J. A. D. (1994). Intrapartum amniotic fluid index and its relationship to fetal distress. *American Journal of Obstetrics and Gynecology* , 166, 78–82.

Romero, R., Cullen, M., Grannum, P., Jeanty, P., Reece, E. A., Venus, I. & Hobbins, J. C. (1985). Antenatal diagnosis of renal anomalies with ultrasound, III. Bilateral renal agenesis. *American Journal of Obstetrics and Gynecology*, 151, 38–43.

Ross, M. G., Ervin, M. G., Leake, R. D., Oakes, G., Hobel, C. & Fisher, D. A. (1983). Bulk flow of amniotic fluid water in response to maternal osmotic challenge. *American Journal of Obstetrics and Gynecology*, 147, 697–701.

Ross, M. G., Sherman, D. J., Ervin, M. G., Day, L. & Humme, J. (1989). Stimuli for fetal swallowing: systemic factors. *American Journal of Obstetrics and Gynecology*, 161, 1559–65.

Rotschild, A., Ling, E. W., Puterman, M. L. & Farquharson, D. (1990). Neonatal outcome after prolonged preterm rupture of the membranes. *American Journal of Obstetrics and Gynecology*, 162, 46–52.

Sadovsky, Y., Amon, E., Bade, M. E. & Petrie, R. H. (1989). Prophylactic amnioinfusion during labor complicated by meconium: a preliminary report. *American Journal of Obstetrics and Gynecology*, 161, 613–17.

Schroder, H., Gilbert, R. D. & Power, G. G. (1984). Urinary and hemodynamic responses to blood volume changes in fetal sheep. *Journal of Development Physiology*, 6, 131–41.

Sepulveda, W., Stagiannis, K. D., Flack, N. J. & Fisk, N. M. (1995). Prenatal diagnosis of renal agenesis using color flow imaging in severe second-trimester oligohydramnios. *American Journal of Obstetrics and Gynecology*, 173, 1788–92.

Seyberth, H., Rascher, W., Hackenthal, R. & Wille, L. (1983). Effect of prolonged indomethacin therapy on renal function and selected vasoactive hormones in very low birth weight infants with symptomatic patent ductus arteriosus. *Journal of Pediatrics*, 103, 979–84.

Shalev, E., Battino, S., Romano, S., Blondhaim, O. & Ben-Ami, M. (1994). Intra-amniotic infection with *Candida albicans* succcessfully treated with trans-cervical amnioinfusion of amphotericin. *American Journal of Obstetrics and Gynecology*, 170, 1271–2.

Shields, L. E. & Brace, R. A. (1993). Fetal electrolyte and acid base responses to amnioinfusion: lactated Ringer's versus normal saline. *American Journal of Obstetrics and Gynecology*, 168, 300.

Sherer, D. M., Cullen, J. B. H., Thompsom, H. O. & Woods, J. R. (1990). Transient oligohydramnios in a severely hypovolemic gravid woman at 35 weeks'

gestation, with fluid reaccumulating immediately after intravenous hydration. *American Journal of Obstetrics and Gynecology*, 162, 770–1.

Slater, D. M., Berger, L. C., Newton, R., Moore, G. E. & Bennett, P.R. (1995). Expression of cyclo-oxygensase types 1 and 2 in human fetal membranes at term. *American Journal of Obstetrics and Gynecology*, 172, 77–82.

Stevens, A. D. & Lumbers, E. R. (1985). The effect of maternal fluid intake on the volume and com-position of fetal urine. *Journal of Developmental Physiology*, 7, 161–6.

Stevenson, K. M. & Lumbers, E. R. (1992). Effects of indomethacin on fetal renal function, renal and umbilicoplacental blood flow and lung liquid production. *Journal of Developmental Physiology*, 17, 257–64.

Strong, T. H. (1993). Reversal of olighydramnios with subtotal immersion: a report of five cases. *American Journal of Obstetrics and Gynecology*, 169, 1595–7.

Tabor, B. L. & Maier, J. A. (1987). Polyhydramnios and elevated intrauterine pressure during amnioinfusion. *American Journal of Obstetrics and Gynecology*, 156, 130–1.

Urig, M. A., Clewell, W. H. & Elliott, J. P. (1990). Twin–twin transfusion syndrome. *American Journal of Obstetrics and Gynecology*, 163, 1522–6.

van der Heijden, B. J., Carlus, C., Narcy, F., Bavoux, F., Deezoide, A. K & Gubler, M. C. (1994). Persistent anuria, neonatal death, and renal microcystic lesions after prenatal exposure to indomethacin. *American Journal of Obstetrics and Gynecology*, 171, 617–23.

van Eyck, J., van der Mooren, K. & Wladimiroff, J. W. (1990). Ductus arteriosus flow velocity modulation by fetal breathing movements as a measure of fetal lung development. *American Journal of Obstetrics and Gynecology*, 163, 558–66.

van Otterlo, L. C., Wladimiroff, J. W. & Wallenburg, H. C. S. (1977). Relationship between fetal urine production and amniotic fluid volume in normal pregnancy and pregnancy complicated by diabetes. *British Journal of Obstetrics and Gynaecology*, 84, 205–9.

Vergani, P., Ghidini, A., Locatelli, A., Cavallone, M., Ciarla, I., Cappellini, A. & Lapinski, R. H. (1994). Risk factors for PH in second-trimester premature rupture of membranes. *American Journal of Obstetrics and Gynecology*, 170, 1359–64.

Vintzileos, A. M., Campbell, W. A., Nochimson, D. J. & Weinbaum, P. J. (1985a). Degree of oligohydramnios and pregnancy outcome in patients with premature rupture of the membranes. *Obstetrics and Gynecology*, 66, 162–7.

Vintzileos, A. M., Campbell, W. A., Rodis, J. F., Nochimson, D. J., Pinette, M. G. & Petrikovsky, B. M. (1989). Comparison of six different ultra-sonographic methods for predicting lethal fetal PH. *American Journal of Obstetrics and Gynecology*, 161, 606–12.

Vintzileos, A. M., Turner, G. W., Campbell, W. A., Weinbaum, P. J., Ward, S. M. & Nochimson, D. J. (1985b). Polyhydramnios and obstructive renal failure. *American Journal of Obstetrics and Gynecology*, 152, 883–5.

Walker, M. P., Moore, T. R. & Brace, R. A. (1994). Indomethacin and arginine vasopressin interaction in the fetal kidney: a mechanism of oliguria. *American Journal of Obstetrics and Gynecology*, 171, 1234–41.

Wenstrom, K. D. & Parson, M. T. (1989). The prevention of meconium aspiration in labor using amnioinfusion. *Obstetrics and Gynecology*, 73, 647–651.

Wigglesworth, J. S. & Desai, R. (1982). Is fetal respiratory function a major determinant of perinatal survival? *Lancet*, i, 264–7.

Wladimiroff, J. W. (1975). Effect of furosemide on fetal urine production. British Journal of *Obstetrics and Gynaecology*, 82, 221–4.

14 Feto-fetal transfusion

GEORGE R. SAADE, ABRAHAM LUDOMIRSKY AND NICHOLAS M. FISK

Introduction

The finding of markedly increased amniotic fluid in one twin and the virtual absence of fluid in the co-twin is a devastating complication of monochorionic, diamniotic twin pregnancy. Because of the belief that this derangement is caused by placental vascular communications, the condition has been referred to as twin–twin transfusion syndrome. Since this condition also occurs in high-order multiple monochorionic pregnancies, feto-fetal transfusion syndrome (FFTS) has been suggested as a more appropriate term than twin–twin transfusion syndrome. The actual shunting of blood between fetuses, however, cannot be documented in every case which fulfils the ultrasonographic criteria (Tanaka *et al.*, 1992; Bruner & Rosemond, 1993; Wiener & Ludomirsky, 1994). Conversely, not all cases complicated by feto–fetal blood transfusion have the associated findings classically regarded as a hallmark of the twin–twin transfusion syndrome (King *et al.*, 1995). Indeed, the majority of monochorionic (MC) twins have placental vascular anastomoses, but do not develop FFTS. For this reason, some investigators prefer descriptive terms such as *stuck twin syndrome* or *oligohydramnios–polyhydramnios sequence* to those of twin–twin transfusion syndrome or FFTS.

Monozygous twinning occurs in approximately 4 in 1000 births (Little & Thompson, 1988). This incidence is relatively constant throughout the world irrespective of age, parity, ethnicity or the use of advanced reproductive technologies, although emerging epidemiological data suggest that it may be increased by *in vitro* fertilization. Because of a lack of agreement regarding the diagnostic criteria, the estimated incidence of FFTS varies greatly from 4 to 35% of diamniotic, MC twin pregnancies (Robertson & Neer, 1983; Patten *et al.*, 1989; Radestad & Thomassen, 1990; Urig, Clewell & Elliot, 1990; Weiner & Ludomirski, 1994). Since two-thirds of monozygotic twins are MC, FFTS would be expected to occur in 0.1 to 0.9 per 1000 births. Despite this low incidence in the general obstetrical population, FFTS is responsible for 15 to 17% of perinatal deaths in twins (Weir, Raten & Beisher, 1979; Steinberg *et al.*, 1990) and continues to occupy more time, on a per patient basis, than any other fetal disease state. Lack of understanding of its underlying pathophysiology and the resultant absence of uniform criteria for diagnosis have hampered development of more rational therapies.

Pathophysiology

An understanding of the pathophysiology of FFTS is prerequisite to the development of a therapeutic approach. Much of the available literature can be criticized for being based on inappropriate inclusion criteria such as neonatal weight and haemoglobin parameters, as discussed on p. 230. Even in carefully selected cases, research in FFTS is hampered by the relative inaccessibility of the human fetus to both invasive monitoring and radiological investigation. Animal studies have contributed little, largely because of the lack of a suitable model.

Classic hypothesis

The classic hypothesis of the pathogenesis of FFTS revolves around placental vascular communications, with shunting of blood volume from the donor fetus to the recipient. The donor ultimately becomes anaemic and develops growth restriction, oliguria, and oligohydramnios while the recipient develops polycythaemia, increased intravascular volume, polyuria and polyhydramnios. In severe cases, the recipient fetus undergoes cardiovascular decompensation and develops hydrops. The literature abounds with reports to support this hypothesis. Except for a few published cases that may have resulted from discordant growth retardation, the syndrome does not occur in the absence of placental vascular communications (Reisner et al., 1993).

Fluid imbalance

Abnormal urine production has been reported in donor and recipient fetuses (Rosen et al., 1990). Differences in atrial natriuretic peptide (ANP), anti-diuretic hormone (ADH), and renin between the fetuses reflect their discordance in intravascular volume. ANP has been found to be higher in the recipient while ADH and renin are higher in the donor (Nageotte et al., 1989; Wieacker et al., 1992). The concentration of these hormones was found to be concordant in the few control MC pregnancies studied. An increase in ANP would produce polyuria and polyhydramnios, while an increase in ADH and renin produces oliguria and oligohydramnios. The extent to which the increase in ANP is secondary to an elevated right atrial pressure or is secondary to hypoxia is unknown (Moya et al., 1990). ANP has been shown to rise with the increased volume of intravascular transfusion in some but not all fetuses (Panos et al., 1989; Fisk et al., 1990b), while in sheep, acute hypoxia appears to be the more potent stimulus for its release (Cheung & Brace, 1988).

Cardiac dysfunction

Ultrasonographic and fetal echocardiographic examinations suggest that myocardial dysfunction occurs in the recipient fetus. Doppler studies in severe cases show venous waveform patterns consistent with raised central venous pressure (Rizzo, Arduini & Romanini, 1994; Hecher, Ville & Nicolaides, 1995). Zosmer and co-workers (1994) noted tricuspid regurgitation in five recipient twins studied echocardiographically, reflecting

a high right ventricular pressure secondary to increased right ventricular afterload. Four of these five recipient fetuses with FFTS diagnosed in the mid-trimester who proceeded beyond 30 weeks' gestation developed pathological right ventricular outflow obstruction (Zosmer et al., 1995). This study supports a previous report of right ventricular outflow tract pathology showing pulmonary valve calcification both radiographically and at autopsy examination in neonates with FFTS (Popek et al., 1993). Finally, umbilical venous pressure has been shown to be elevated in some but not all recipient twins with hydrops, implicating heart failure as the cause of hydrops in the recipient twin (Weiner & Ludomirski, 1994). Right ventricular outflow obstruction may be secondary to increased preload and/or afterload. Plasma levels of endothelin-1, a potent vasoconstrictor, are two- to three-fold higher in recipient fetuses compared with donor or control fetuses (Bajoria, Sullivan & Fisk, 1996). This suggests increased afterload and is consistent with observations of relative hypertension in recipient twins in the neonatal period (Tolosa et al., 1993).

Placental vascular anatomy

Placental vascular communications are not the only requirement for the development of FFTS. Pooled results from six studies indicated that anastomoses were present in 83% of 296 MC placentas. This figure appears to be an underestimate, as the search for deep anastomoses was incomplete in over half the cases (Schatz, 1900; Bleisch, 1965; Strong & Corney, 1966; Benirschke & Driscoll, 1967; Cameron, 1968; Robertson & Neer, 1983). Placental vascular communications occur in almost all MC placentas and yet only a small minority develop FFTS (Robertson & Neer, 1983; Patten et al., 1989). In contrast, FFTS has not been reported in monoamniotic gestations (Carr, Aronson & Coustan, 1990; Tessen & Zlatnik, 1991; Moise, 1993; Belfort et al., 1993). It seems likely that the intertwin transfer of blood through vascular communications is a normal event in MC multiple pregnancies.

Pathological findings that have been recently reported may explain why some MC pregnancies develop FFTS while others do not. Bajoria, Wigglesworth & Fisk (1995) found that in the majority of patients with FFTS only one placental vascular anastomosis could be demonstrated. In the vast majority of cases this was arteriovenous in nature, located deep within the placenta and exhibited flow from the donor to the recipient. In contrast, MC placentas from normal pregnancies had significantly more than one vascular anastomosis per placenta. These were more likely to be superficial, located along the chorionic plate and were venovenous and/or arterioarterial in nature. In addition, arteriovenous anastomoses in the control group of twins were multiple and bi-directional, such that the number of anastomoses in the direction of one twin was always within one of the number running in the opposite direction. Superficial anastomoses, arterioarterial or venovenal, have previously been suggested to allow flow in either direction to compensate for haemodynamic imbalance caused by deeper arteriovenous anastomoses. It, therefore, appears that an additional placental vascular abnormality is required which, independently or in conjunction with the usual placental vascular anastomoses seen in all MC placentas, leads to more blood flowing from donor to recipient than blood returning in the opposite direction. The resultant net imbalance in the intravascular volumes between the twins leads to the clinical findings of FFTS.

Lack of flow along superficial anastomoses (i.e. artery to artery or vein to vein) implies completely balanced pressures between the communicating vessels, which for an arterioarterial anastomosis would require the unlikely combination of equal systolic and diastolic blood pressures in addition to identical fetal heart rates. Superficial arterioarterial anastomoses can be visualized by colour Doppler ultrasound (Hecher *et al.*, 1994). Bizarre bi-directional flow velocity waveforms in the watershed area have been recently shown by computer analysis to reflect the summation of arterial waveforms of different heart rates from opposing directions in two uncomplicated MC twin gestations.

Hydro-osmotic gradients

Because of the lack of an animal model, Talbert *et al.* (1996) have developed a computerized model of dynamic fetal and placental physiological variables to determine if the clinical features of FFTS can be explained by intertwin transfusion along placental vascular anastomoses. Two identical copies of a singleton program

were run simultaneously linked only by common amniotic pressure in addition to maternal blood hydrodynamic and osmotic pressures. Various experimental combinations of interplacental arteriovenous connections were then introduced.

With unidirectional anastomoses, disease severity, characterized by disparity in blood volumes, depended on the donor arterial pressure but not the number of anastomoses. Unidirectional flow along the arteriovenous anastomoses continued until the resultant fall in arterial pressure in the donor, together with the resultant rise in venous pressure in the recipient, negated the anastomotic pressure gradient. Flow stopped until the resultant hydrostatic water shifts into the donor and out of the recipient partially restored the anastomotic pressure gradient, at which point flow returns and the cycle continues. In the chronic state, such water movement was balanced by elevated osmotic pressure in the recipient and reduced osmotic pressure in the donor, producing a hydro-osmotic pressure equilibrium regulating anastomotic flow.

With bi-directional anastomoses, recirculation between the twins reduced discordance in colloids and haematocrit, and the clinical picture was determined by the degree of asymmetry in the number of connections. There were no clinical manifestations when the number of anastomoses in one direction matched that in the other direction.

In summary, modelling of the resultant interrelated haemodynamic filtration and metabolic variables in the MC twins reproduced the clinical manifestations of FFTS. The direction and symmetry of arteriovenous anastomoses in the model determined the net hydrostatic and osmotic gradients and the severity of the FFTS, a finding in keeping with the reported angioarchitectural associations of FFTS (Bajoria *et al.*, 1995).

Diagnostic criteria

The diagnostic criteria for FFTS remain controversial but have evolved considerably with better understanding of the disease.

Discordant weight and haemoglobin

Initially, when access to the fetuses *in utero* was limited, diagnosis relied on neonatal criteria. These included discordance in cord blood haemoglobins and birthweights with the presumed donor having a lower haemoglobin and birthweight compared with the presumed recipient. The most widely accepted thresholds were >5 g/dl difference in haemoglobin and ≥20% difference in birthweight (Rausen, Seki & Strauss, 1965; Abraham, 1967; Tan *et al.*, 1979). Although widely adopted in the 1970s and 1980s, these diagnostic criteria are now considered invalid for three reasons. First, the initial data on which the criteria were based were far from robust. Rausen *et al.* (1965) found that 19 of 130 MC twins had a cord blood haemoglobin difference >5 g/dl, in contrast to a difference <3.3 g/dl in all 46 dichorionic twin pairs. Eight of the twins in the series, however, were not discordant for weight. Tan *et al.* (1979) found that 9 of 35 twin sets with the required haemoglobin difference had a birthweight difference of >20%, but they did not report placentation. The second reason for no longer accepting discordance in haematocrit or birthweight as diagnostic of FFTS is that these parameters can be present with discordant fetal growth restriction without any evidence of feto–fetal blood transfusion. Impaired fetal growth is associated with polycythaemia. Fetal acidosis is a known cause of erythroblastosis, and increased erythropoietin concentrations in growth-retarded fetuses have been correlated with the degree of umbilical venous hypoxaemia and acidaemia (Snijders *et al.*, 1993). Thus, discordance in acid–base status between the fetuses may well explain the discordance in cord blood haemoglobins. Indeed, polycythaemia was found in the smaller twin in one third of the cases reported by Tan and co-workers (1979). Even in cases with known MC placentas and discordance for both haemoglobin and birthweight, one third of the smaller twins in another series had the higher cord blood haemoglobin (Wenstrom *et al.*, 1992). Danskin and Neilson (1989) found that 7 of 13 cases with a cord haemoglobin discordance >5 g/dl and 14 of 26 cases with birthweight discordance >20% had dichorionic placentation. Of the four pregnancies exhibiting both a haemoglobin difference of >5 g/dl and a birthweight difference of >20%, only one had a MC placenta.

Finally, fetal blood sampling studies have shown that the previously accepted requisite haemoglobin difference is rarely present *in utero* in cases of FFTS (Fisk *et al.*, 1990a; Saunders, Snijders & Nicolaides, 1991). While umbilical cord and neonatal blood haemoglobin concentration may be influenced by labour and cord clamping methods, results obtained *in utero* more accurately reflect the fetal haematological status. Figure 14.1 describes data on the haemoglobin difference obtained by fetal blood sampling at the Centre for Fetal Care at Queen Charlotte's Hospital in London (Fisk, 1995). A haemoglobin difference of >5 g/dl was present in approximately 20% of cases of FFTS. The situation also appears relatively dynamic as we have anecdotally observed changes in haemoglobin within periods as short as 1 to 14 days.

Another problem with the prenatal diagnosis of FFTS relates to the use of ultrasound for the prenatal detection of size discordance. Percentage difference in estimated fetal weight (100 × [weight of larger twin − weight of smaller twin]/weight of larger twin) and absolute difference in abdominal circumference have both been used (Blickstein, 1990). Most cases of FFTS do exhibit fetal weight discordance *in utero* (Fisk *et al.*, 1990a; Bajoria *et al.*, 1995). Classically, the postnatal criterion of more than a 20% difference in fetal weight has been applied to the prenatal diagnosis of FFTS (Patten *et al.*, 1989). In a study of 43 consecutive twins who had biometry measured within two weeks of delivery, a difference in abdominal circumference of ≤20 mm was found to have the same sensitivity, 80%, but a lower specificity, 85% vs 93% when compared with the estimated fetal weight for the prediction of birthweight discordance of ≥20% (Storlazzi *et al.*, 1987). Ultrasonographic estimates of fetal size are, however, subject to a 10 to 15% error and accordingly are difficult to use diagnostically. In addition, there is no consensus as to which threshold value should be used for the prenatal diagnosis of weight discordance. In a study not restricted to patients with FFTS, Cheung, Bocking and Dasilva (1995) found that 28 out of 122 sets of twins delivered between 25 and 34 weeks' gestation had a birthweight discordance of ≥20%. Only those with a discordance >30% were at increased risk for adverse perinatal outcome. While weight discordance may be common in fetuses without FFTS, pregnancies with this syndrome

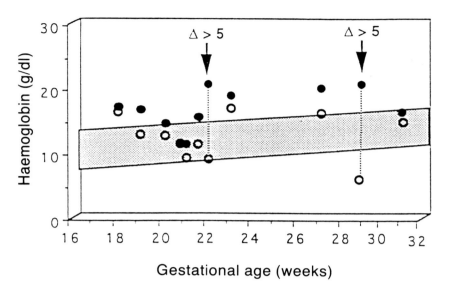

Fig. 14.1 In utero umbilical venous blood haemoglobin concentration in nine sets of twins and one set of triplets with FFTS. (After Fisk, 1995, with permission of the author.)

have been documented with birthweight discordance of much less than 20% (Bajoria *et al.*, 1995).

Placental anastomoses

Another criterion for FFTS has been the demonstration of placental vascular communications between the fetuses. Reliance on postnatal documentation of anastomoses to confirm or exclude the diagnosis may not be simple. Vascular anastomoses have been demonstrated in virtually all MC placentas, the majority of which were not associated with FFTS (Robertson & Neer, 1983). However, failure to document vascular anastomoses by casual macroscopic inspection of the placenta is insufficient. Unless proper perfusion and preparation of the placenta immediately after birth with a search for both deep and superficial anastomoses is undertaken, vascular communications may be missed (Bajoria *et al.*, 1995).

Intertwin transfusion

Because of the limitations outlined above, direct evidence of feto–fetal transfusion has been proposed by some to confirm the diagnosis of FFTS. This can be achieved by the intravascular injection of either a neuromuscular-blocking agent or red cells containing adult haemoglobin into the presumed donor and noting paralysis or the presence of haemoglobin A in the presumed recipient. The use of pancuronium bromide has been reported in two sets of twins with suspected FFTS (Tanaka *et al.*, 1992). In addition to fetal paralysis of both fetuses, changes in the heart rate of the recipient twin consisting of baseline tachycardia and a reduction in variability and reactivity were observed in one set but not the other. Others have used the Kleihauer–Betke stain to detect red cells containing adult haemoglobin in a blood sample obtained by fetal blood sampling from the presumed recipient twin following the intravascular injection of 20 to 30 ml of 70% haematocrit type O-negative adult blood into the presumed donor (Fisk *et al.*, 1990b; Bruner & Rosemond, 1993; Weiner & Ludomirski, 1994). The transfer of adult red blood cells was documented in some but not all sets of twins studied. These diagnostic tests as well as others that rely on the transfer of blood from one twin to the other may be misleading. The transfer of blood between the fetuses may be bi-directional or intermittent. Infusion and sampling at one period in time may not reflect the dynamic process of this condition. Furthermore, experience with this diagnostic technique is based on small numbers of predominantly monochorionic pregnancies with FFTS. The frequency of intertwin transfusion in MC pregnancies uncomplicated by FFTS remains unknown. Therefore, the sensitivity and specificity of these tests is uncertain.

Recommended diagnostic evaluation

Faced with the above difficulties and limitations, we have modelled our diagnostic evaluation to reflect therapeutic options. The diagnosis of FFTS is initially suspected based on the ultrasonographic finding in the mid-trimester of the polyhydramnios–oligohydramnios sequence, regardless of the presence or degree of fetal weight discordance. The next step is to exclude other aetiologies for the discordance in amniotic fluid volume.

A targeted ultrasound is performed to exclude fetal anomalies and dichorionic placentation. Unlike-sex fetuses, separate placentas and a thick interfetal membrane are indicative of dichorionic twinning (see Chapter 6). In 33 consecutive pregnancies with the polyhydramnios/oligohydramnios sequence, Reisner *et al.* (1993) reported that six had a dichorionic placenta on pathologic examination. Using the discordant amniotic fluid volume criteria alone would, therefore, lead to a false positive diagnosis in 20% of cases.

The role of invasive testing remains controversial. This is partly because causes other than FFTS for the oligohydramnios/polyhydramnios sequence seem rare. If invasive testing is undertaken, chromosomal and infectious aetiologies should be excluded in fetal samples. The tests performed on the fetus will depend on the extent of oligohydramnios. Whenever accessible, amniotic fluid is obtained from both sacs and sent for karyotype. Amniotic fluid is preferred over fetal blood since the latter can be chimaeric in the case of cytogenetic discordance and admixture of blood secondary to shunting through vascular anastomoses. At Baylor College of Medicine in Houston we also test for the presence of various viral nucleic acids (enterovirus, adenovirus, cytomegalovirus, herpes simplex virus, parvovirus, Epstein–Barr virus, and respiratory syncytial virus) using the polymerase chain reaction, based on our recent finding of positive viral DNA in 40% of 25 cases (I. B. Van den Veyver, personal communication). In the majority of cases, the stuck fetus has no accessible amniotic fluid and fetal blood sampling is used instead.

Treatment

Outcome data on perinatal mortality are also affected by lack of consistency in diagnosis. The prognosis is poor in cases diagnosed in the second trimester and untreated, perinatal mortality approaching 100% (Weir *et al.*, 1979; Chescheir & Seeds, 1987; Saunders, Snijders & Nicolaides, 1992). For this reason, several aggressive, even desperate treatment modalities have been attempted, including selective fetocide (Wittman *et al.*, 1986; Weiner, 1987; Chescheir & Seeds, 1987), hysterotomy for umbilical cord ligation or extirpation of one twin (Benirschke & Kim, 1973; Urig *et al.*, 1988), blood letting from a placental vessel (Vetter & Schneider, 1988) and maternal digoxin therapy (De Lia *et al.*, 1985a; Roman & Hare, 1995). None have gained wide acceptance.

Indomethacin has been successfully used in the treatment of polyhydramnios in singleton and twin pregnancies (Lange *et al.*, 1989; Kirshon, Mari & Moise, 1990). However, it is relatively contraindicated in FFTS because of its harmful effects on renal function in the already oliguric donor fetus. More recently, laser ablation under fetoscopic guidance of placental vessels has been reported in an attempt to improve survival (De Lia, Cruikshank & Keye, 1990; 995; Ville *et al.*, 1995). Serial drainage amniocenteses or amnioreduction, however, remains the most widely used therapy.

Amnioreduction

The technical aspects of this procedure are discussed in detail in Chapter 13. In a review of the available literature comprising 252 fetuses from 26 reports, Moise (1993) concluded an overall perinatal survival rate after serial amnioreduction in FFTS of 49%. However, many of these cases were reported in the 1930s and 1940s when amniocenteses were performed without ultrasound assistance with drainage of only small volumes of amniotic fluid. Uncontrolled series employing modern aggressive amnioreduction in which amniotic fluid volume is reduced to normal have been associated with perinatal survival rates from 37 to 83% (Mahoney *et al.*, 1990; Urig *et al.*, 1990; Elliot, Urig & Clewell, 1991; Radestad & Thomassen, 1990; Saunders *et al.*, 1992; Pinette *et al.*, 1993; Reisner *et al.*, 1993); in all but two of these series, the perinatal survival exceeding 60%, as illustrated in Table 14.1.

Amnioreduction aims primarily to control polyhydramnios to allow prolongation of gestation, although

Table 14.1 *Series of feto–fetal transfusion symdromes treated with aggressive amnioreduction*

Author	No. of patients	Gestation at diagnosis (weeks)	No. of procedures (mean)	Amniotic volume removed at each amnio reduction (ml)	Gestation at delivery (mean; weeks)	Survival (% of fetuses)
Urig *et al.*, 1990	5	21–25	1–7 (4)	1000–5000	27.3	60
Mahoney *et al.*, 1990	8	16–28	2–6 (3.5)	300–5500	31.4	69
Radestad & Thomassen, 1990	18	21–32	1–4 (2)	125–5000	30.1	53
Elliot *et al.*, 1991	17	16–28	1–10 (4)	225–5000	33.2	79
Saunders *et al.*, 1992	19	17–25	1–6 (3)	500–6700	28.3	37
Pinette *et al.*, 1993	9	20–26	1–9 (3.5)	300–8500	32.6	83
Reisner *et al.*, 1993	27	16–30	1–6 (3.5)	250–5500	31.5	74

there is some evidence that it may ameliorate the fetal condition. Amniotic fluid pressure is raised in severe polyhydramnios and is restored to normal by amnioreduction (Fisk *et al.*, 1990c; Weiner & Ludomirsky, 1994). Several authors have suggested that raised amniotic pressure may impair uteroplacental perfusion (Tabor & Maier, 1987; Elliot *et al.*, 1991) and that normalization of amniotic pressure may alter the haemodynamics of FFTS and improve fetal condition. Using Doppler ultrasound, Mari, Wasserstrum & Kirshon (1992) found that the pulsatility index of the middle cerebral artery decreased in both twins following decompression amniocentesis. This finding is consistent with a fetal cerebral vasodilatory response. Polyhydramnios is associated with impaired fetal acid–base status in both singleton and twin pregnancies; fetal hypoxaemia and acidaemia correlate linearly with the degree of elevation in amniotic pressure (Fisk, Vaughan & Talbert, 1994). Anecdotal observation of one case showed a dramatic improvement in fetal pO_2 and pH following amnioreduction (Fisk *et al.*, 1994). It is likely that such effects on the fetoplacental circulation are mediated through uteroplacental perfusion, as raised amniotic pressure in labour transiently impairs uteroplacental but not fetoplacental blood flow with contractions. Decompression amniocentesis has been shown to improve uterine artery blood flow significantly, as shown in Fig. 14.2 (Bower *et al.*, 1995).

In patients treated with amnioreduction, repeated decompressions are usually required. Occasionally,

however, resolution of FFTS can occur following a single amnioreduction. Prolonged equalization and restoration of normal amniotic fluid volumes following a single amnioreduction was first reported by Wax *et al.* (1991) in a patient with a stuck twin syndrome diagnosed at 27 weeks' gestation. Amniotic fluid volumes in both sacs remained normal following a single large volume amnioreduction until delivery at 35 weeks. On careful review of published series, it is not uncommon to find patients in whom the classical features of FFTS resolve after a single amniocentesis or after the last of a series of amniocenteses, with no subsequent need for therapy (Radestad & Thomassen, 1990; Elliot *et al.*, 1991; Saunders *et al.*, 1992; Pinette *et al.*, 1993). The latter, however, may be an effect of gestational age, as severe polyhydramnios caused by FFTS is unusual in the third trimester. Several authors have observed rapid reaccumulation of amniotic fluid volume in the donor twin's sac soon after amnioreduction. However, in the few studies where fetal urinary output was measured, urine production in the stuck twin did not increase in all cases after amnioreduction (Rosen *et al.*, 1990; Weiner & Ludomirski, 1994).

Fetoscopic laser ablation

Interruption of the vascular anastomoses between the fetuses seems a logical therapy for FFTS. Fetoscopic laser ablation of placental vessels was first attempted in animals (De Lia, Rogers & Dixon, 1985b; De Lia *et al.*,

Fig. 14.2 *The change in mean velocity of uterine blood flow after amnioreduction in eight patients with severe polyhydramnios. (Adpaped from Bower et al., 1995.)*

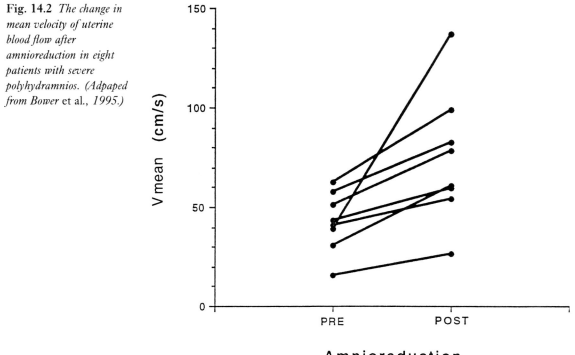

Amnioreduction

1989) and then used in human pregnancies with FFTS (De Lia *et al.*, 1990). Since this first report, a total of 71 patients have been described by two groups of investigators (Ville *et al.*, 1995; De Lia *et al.*, 1995). In each series, 53% of the fetuses survived to delivery. In general, both fetuses survived in one third of cases, one fetus survived in another third and both fetuses died in the remaining third. These results do not compare favourably with amnioreduction, a less invasive and more readily available therapy.

Without contrast studies, it is only the superficial and not the deep anastomoses that could be visualized fetoscopically. Both groups advocating laser therapy describe identifying and ablating multiple communicating vessels. However, the recent demonstration that FFTS placentas lack superficial anastomoses (Bajoria *et al.*, 1995) suggests that those workers are instead largely ablating normal chorionic plate vessels, which would explain the full thickness placental necrosis that has been described after this therapy (De Lia *et al.*,

1990). This would also explain why 50% of procedures are complicated by intrauterine death within 24 hours of the procedure (Ville *et al.*, 1995).

Notwithstanding the poor initial results with laser therapy, isolation of the two circulations would seem a logical aim of FFTS therapy. However, further application of ablative therapies will require better methods of identifying the responsible deep arteriovenous anastomosis(es).

Future developments

Despite the improved perinatal survival with modern aggressive serial amnioreduction, cardiac, neurological and renal sequelae remain common in survivors. There remains a clear need for a more effective treatment.

It seems unlikely that drug therapy will play a major role in the treatment of FFTS, as the desirable effect of a drug in one twin may have deleterious effects in the other. Even if selective delivery systems to an individual fetus could be developed, the sharing of their circulation would render the confinement of the drug effect to one twin problematic.

Better diagnostic techniques, such as contrast angiography or magnetic resonance imaging, for the identification of the responsible deep arteriovenous anastomoses warrant further investigation. If successful, these would allow targeted ablation, ideally by needling techniques obviating the need for fetoscopy. In the meantime, interest focuses on palliative techniques. One such approach, amniotic septostomy (Saade *et al.*, 1995) may be useful in the long-term control of amniotic fluid volume.

Amniotic septostomy

The sudden resolution of the FFTS after one or more amnioreductions and the lack of increased urine production in the stuck twin are not consistent with the explanation that the increase in the amniotic fluid around the stuck twin following the procedure is the direct result of improved fetal renal perfusion. We have hypothesized that, in such cases, the amnion separating the twins is inadvertently punctured at the time of amniocentesis (Saade *et al.*, 1995). Amniotic pressure is raised in the recipient's sac and is likely to be reduced in the donor's sac, based both on experience with aberrant amniotic volumes in singleton gestations (Fisk *et al.*, 1990c) and physiological principles related to diminished volume within a semi-distensible membrane. Disruption of the dividing membrane would, therefore, cause fluid to move along a hydrostatic pressure gradient from the sac with polyhydramnios into the sac with oligohydramnios. The following cases are described briefly to illustrate this point.

We intentionally punctured the amniotic septum at the time of amnioreduction for FFTS (Saade *et al.*, 1995). In two cases, this represented the first procedure at 25 and 32 weeks, respectively, while the third underwent septal perforation at the fifth amnioreduction at 24 weeks. In each case, amniotic fluid volume equilibrated within 30 minutes of the procedure, and the septum returned entirely to the midline by the following day (Fig.14.3). Normal and equal amniotic fluid volumes were monitored thereafter for 2 to 12 weeks until delivery.

Similar findings have been reported by another group (Hubinont *et al.*, 1996), although one of their two cases resulted in an intrauterine death. The latter was not obviously related to cord entanglement, although this remains a risk following the creation of functionally monoamniotic twins. Cord entanglement has been reported to occur in up to 70% of spontaneous mono amniotic twins, contributing to perinatal mortality rates of 28–47% (Salerno, 1959; Lumme & Saarikoski, 1986; Baldwin, 1994). Notwithstanding this, spontaneous rupture of the intervening twin membrane has been reported, as has unintentional rupture at the time of diagnostic amniocentesis utilizing a single needle insertion technique in twins (Jeanty, Shah & Roussis, 1990; Gilbert *et al.*, 1991). A recent series of 27 cases of diagnostic amniocenteses with septal puncture reported no case of cord entanglement (van Vugt, Nieuwint & van Geijn, 1995). We suggest that these complications occur less frequently after deliberate puncture with a small gauge needle and only minor disruption to the intervening membrane.

In these five cases, the intervening membrane was deliberately punctured. An explanation for the normalization of amniotic fluid volumes in amnioreduction cases where the dividing membrane was not intentionally punctured is more problematic. As shown by the needle position 1 in Fig.14.4, we speculate that in such cases the operator may be unaware that the intervening membrane is being traversed by the needle, as it is flattened against the uterine wall. This configuration would not be obvious ultrasonographically but has been observed during endoscopic laser treatment for FFTS (De Lia *et al.*, 1990). Under this hypothesis, normalization of volume in the donor sac would not occur after procedures in which the needle is introduced away from the septum, shown as needle position 2 in Fig.14.4.

The mechanism for the observed prolonged normalization of amniotic fluid volume in the recipient after septostomy remains unclear. It may reflect restitution of swallowing and/or intramembranous amniotic fluid absorption into the donor. It might also affect fetoplacental haemodynamics, either directly or secondary to improved fluid resorption and, thus, intravascular volume in the donor. In this light, it is interesting to note that FFTS does not appear to occur in MC monoamniotic twin pregnancies despite the presence of vascular

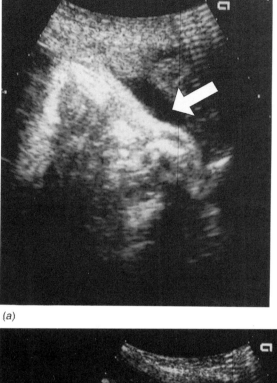

(a)

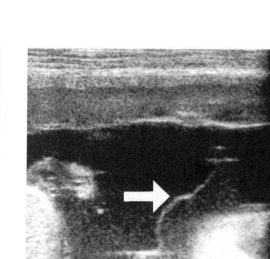

(c)

(b)

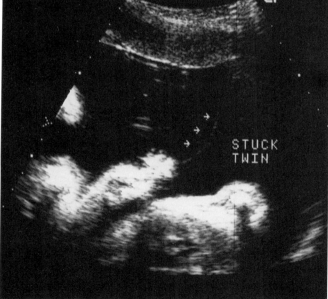

Fig. 14.3 *Changing amniotic fluid volume distribution after amnioreduction.* (a) *Amniotic fluid (arrow) beginning to re-accumulate around the stuck twin shortly after removal of the needle.* (b) *A significant volume of amniotic fluid is now noted on the stuck twin's side 30 minutes after the procedure. Note that the intervening membrane (arrows) is still bulging toward the twin with oligohydramnios.* (c) *By the next day the intervening membrane (arrow) appears to be floating freely between the two sacs indicating equal pressure on either side.*

anastomoses (Carr *et al.*, 1990; Tessen & Zlatnik, 1991; Moise, 1993; Belfort *et al.*, 1993).

Amniotic septostomy warrants formal evaluation in the treatment of FFTS. Any randomized trial against amnioreduction would need to take into account the possibility of unintentional septostomy during amnioreduction.

Twin reversed arterial perfusion sequence

Incidence

Twin reversed arterial perfusion sequence (TRAP), also referred to as acardiac twinning or chorioangiopagus parasiticus, is the most extreme manifestation of the

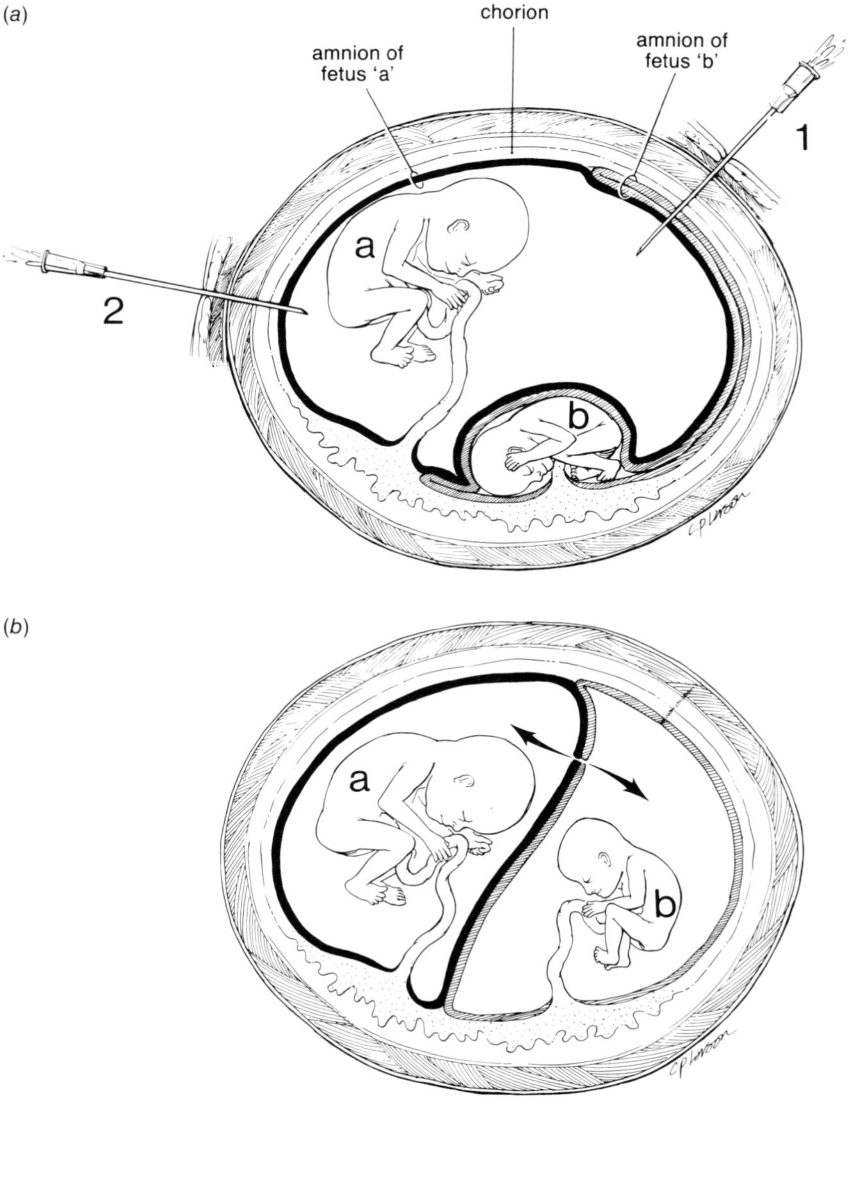

Fig. 14.4 *Needle location during amnioreduction.* (a) *The position of the dividing membrane in a pregnancy complicated by FFTS. Despite the fact that on ultrasound, the tip appears to be away from the membrane overlying the stuck twin, a needle inserted at site 1 results in puncture of the dividing membrane. A needle inserted at site 2, however, will only puncture the amniotic sac of twin 'a'.* (b) *Resolution of the stuck twin syndrome and the resulting defect (arrows) in the intervening membrane following amniocentesis performed at site 1.*

feto–fetal transfusion syndrome. It occurs in about 1% of MC gestations or 0.3 cases per 10 000 births (Gillim & Hendricks, 1953; Napolitani & Schreiber, 1960; Benirschke & des Roches Harper, 1977; James, 1977; Kaplan & Benirschke, 1979). Most cases with the TRAP sequence have been reported in MC pregnancies, but some have been reported in dichorionic and dizygotic pregnancies with fused placentas (Schinzel, Smith & Miller, 1979; Van Allen, Smith & Shepard, 1983). In a recent literature review, Healey (1994) found that 92% of 184 reported cases occurred in twins and 8% in triplets. Twenty-four per cent were monoamniotic, monochorionic; 74% were diamniotic, monochorionic; and 2% were diamniotic, dichorionic.

Pathophysiology

The term TRAP is preferred to describe this condition as it reflects the pathophysiology more accurately. The affected or *perfused* fetus has no direct vascular connection to the placenta, but rather obtains all of its blood supply through an arterioarterial communication from the unaffected or *pump* fetus. Blood enters the perfused fetus through its umbilical artery or arteries and exits through its umbilical vein, hence the term *reversed arterial perfusion*. In the review by Healey (1994), 66% of affected fetuses had one artery and one vein and 26% had two arteries and one vein. Reversed arterial perfusion can be documented by Doppler ultrasound (Pretorius, *et al.*, 1988; Benson *et al.*, 1989).

Associated anomalies

Uniformly, the perfused fetus has major structural anomalies that are incompatible with neonatal survival. The classification of Das (1902) is still used to describe these anomalies, although they are of little practical significance. Of the cases reviewed by Healey (1994), karyotype results were available in both fetuses in 22 cases, only in the pump fetus in 12 cases, and only in the perfused fetus in 11 cases. Thirty-three per cent of perfused fetuses had an abnormal karyotype, including monosomy, trisomy, deletions, mosaics and polyploidy. Trisomy was found in 9% of pump fetuses. No specific inheritance pattern or familial recurrence has been identified (Van Allen *et al.*, 1983; Deacon *et al.*, 1980).

Furthermore, the reported abnormalities do not correspond to any phenotypic expression of the associated genetic anomalies. TRAP twin pairs have been shown to be monozygous, even in the presence of discordant aneuploidy (Fisk *et al.*, 1996).

Since the blood to the perfused fetus enters through the hypogastric arteries, the organs of the lower trunk are more likely to be developed while those of the upper trunk are more likely to be absent or rudimentary. Those body parts that are present are usually abnormal secondary to perfusion with deoxygenated blood. The embryogenesis of TRAP remains controversial. One view is that the abnormalities are secondary to poor tissue oxygenation resulting from the anomalous circulation, suggesting a disruption type of anomaly. Alternatively, genetic and/or anatomical defects arising in early embryogenesis might result in circulatory reversal, or rather only survive in the presence of circulatory reversal. Except for a few case reports, the pump fetus is usually genetically and structurally normal and does not seem to be at any higher risk for congenital anomalies than that reported in monozygotic twinning.

As with the donor fetus in classic FFTS, the pump fetus may be predisposed to structural cardiac defects that are secondary to intrauterine congestive heart failure. Calcification of the pulmonary valve has been noted in one fetus (Popek *et al.*, 1993) and a heart murmur with right ventricular hypertrophy noted in five survivors of the TRAP sequence (Van Allen *et al.*, 1983), which points to a cardiomyopathy and right ventricular outflow tract obstruction similar to that seen in FFTS.

Perinatal morbidity and mortality

Fifty-one per cent of TRAP sequences are complicated by polyhydramnios and 75% by preterm labour (Healey, 1994). Perinatal mortality in the pump fetus is increased, mostly secondary to intrauterine heart failure, hydrops fetalis and preterm delivery. Early delivery may be indicated because of intrauterine decompensation or result from spontaneous preterm labour secondary to polyhydramnios and/or intrauterine crowding. In the review by Healey (1994), congestive cardiac failure in the pump fetus occurred in 28% of cases and intrauterine demise in 25%. The perinatal mortality of 29% inversely correlated with gestational age at delivery. The larger the size

Table 14.2 *Predictive value of twin weight ratio >50%*

	Hydramnios	Preterm delivery	Pump-twin death
Sensitivity (%)	83	86	64
Specificity (%)	56	67	42
Positive predictive value (%)	56	71	45
Negative predictive value (%)	83	83	62

of the perfused relative to the size of the pump fetus, the higher the risk of congestive heart failure, hydramnios and preterm delivery (Healey, 1994). Seventy per cent of cases reviewed by Moore, Gale & Benirschke (1990) had a ratio of perfused to pump fetal weight of >50%. The frequency of hydramnios, congestive heart failure, and prematurity in these cases was 44%, 25% and 94%, respectively, compared with 18%, 0% and 35%, respectively, in those cases with a ratio of ≤50%. The sensitivity, specificity and predictive values of a fetal weight ratio >50% for polyhydramnios, preterm delivery and death of the pump fetus are delineated in Table 14.2. Of interest is that all 13 pregnancies with a ratio ≥80% developed congestive heart failure in the pump fetus. In addition, the gestational age at delivery was negatively correlated with the fetal weight ratio. It is clear from the reviews of Healey (1994) and Moore *et al.* (1990) that perinatal morbidity and mortality correlate with the size of the perfused fetus in relation to the size of the pump fetus. It is important to note that these recommendations regarding risks to the pump fetus were based on neonatal weights. Prenatal estimates of these weights would, therefore, be helpful in determining prognosis and the need for intervention. The weight of the pump fetus can be estimated using standard fetal biometry with ultrasound. For the perfused fetus, the weight can be estimated prenatally using the following second-order regression equation derived by Moore *et al.* (1990): Weight (g) $= 1.21L^2 - 1.7L$, where L is the length of the perfused fetus in centimetres. The validity of these tenets utilizing fetal weights determined by ultrasound requires further verification. This is espe-

cially true in the rare case where the perfused twin has some autonomous partial circulation such as a rudimentary heart (Fouron *et al.*, 1994).

Treatment

Digoxin

Digoxin crosses the placenta readily in the absence of hydrops and therapeutic levels have been achieved in the fetus following maternal administration (Chapter 12). In pregnancies complicated by the TRAP sequence, transplacental therapy with digoxin has been used prophylactically in two cases and in a third case resulted in resolution of subcutaneous oedema in the pump fetus (Simpson *et al.*, 1983; Donnenfeld *et al.*, 1991). All three pump fetuses survived, albeit one with neurological sequelae. The dose of digoxin given to the mother was 0.25 mg twice daily for three days followed by a daily maintenance dose of 0.25 mg. Digoxin levels in the pump fetus were lower than maternal levels. As with fetal tachyarrhythmias, high maternal concentrations of digoxin may be required to achieve therapeutic fetal levels (see Chapter 12).

Prostaglandin synthetase inhibitors

Indomethacin has been used as a tocolytic agent in cases complicated by the TRAP sequence. Another desired effect includes decreased fetal urine production. Unlike the case of classic FFTS where concern exists for the deleterious effects of prostaglandin synthetase inhibitors on urine production in the stuck twin, the TRAP sequence represents a situation where only one twin is viable. In cases of polyhydramnios in association with the pump twin, indomethacin may have a therapeutic effect on urine production. Indomethacin, 50 mg orally four times a day, has been used in one case to treat symptomatic polyhydramnios without preterm contractions (Ash, Harman & Gritter, 1990). Despite discontinuation of the medication at 30 weeks, the amniotic fluid volume continued to decrease and the pregnancy was delivered at 34 weeks because of oligohydramnios. Whether indomethacin contributed to a successful outcome in this pregnancy may be debatable as the pump fetus had no evidence of cardiac failure and the ratio of perfused to pump fetal weight at birth was only 42%. The effect of indomethacin on the ductus arteriosus, however, may be detrimental to an already compromised cardiovascular system, especially in the neonatal period. Sulindac, as discussed in Chapter 13, may, therefore, be preferable to control polyhydramnios, although there is as yet no experience with its use in TRAP.

Sectio parva

Hysterotomy with selective delivery of the perfused fetus has been reported in seven pregnancies, with fetal death from placental abruption in one case and neonatal survival in six (Robie, Payne & Morgan 1989; Fries, Goldberg & Golbus, 1992; Ginsberg *et al.*, 1992). These cases were complicated by preterm labour and aggressive tocolysis was required, including the use of indomethacin. All patients except one delivered preterm at 20 to 35 weeks' gestation. In the only patient to deliver at term (Ginsberg *et al.*, 1992), the indication for the procedure was questionable as blood flow to the perfused fetus had spontaneously ceased before the hysterotomy. Other complications included placental abruption, maternal pulmonary oedema, haemorrhage and need for blood transfusion. The fetoscopic or ultrasound-guided alternatives which follow appear far safer and, therefore, preferable.

Cord occlusion

It would seem logical that occlusion of the umbilical vessels leading to the perfused fetus would prevent or reverse congestive heart failure in the pump fetus and thereby decrease perinatal mortality and morbidity. All techniques described in the literature are invasive in nature and by themselves carry some risk, such as preterm labour and prelabour rupture of the membranes. Whatever method is used, it is essential that all vascular communications between the pump and perfused fetuses be occluded simultaneously and completely to prevent a significant portion of the pump fetus's blood volume from becoming trapped in the perfused fetus. Faced with these potential complications, the treating physician has to decide whether the benefits of an invasive procedure outweigh the risks of non-intervention or preterm delivery. In addition, the timing of the procedure may have a significant effect on outcome. Waiting until the pump fetus decompensates before occluding the umbilical vessels may not be desirable. Conversely, prophylactic cord occlusion before the

development of congestive heart failure, polyhydramnios and/or preterm labour may subject a pregnancy otherwise destined for a good outcome to the unnecessary morbidity of an invasive procedure. The size of the perfused fetus relative to the pump fetus may facilitate decision making but, as mentioned earlier, the validity of the size algorithms has not been tested prenatally. Better understanding of the echocardiographic findings preceding fetal cardiac failure, such as tricuspid regurgitation and vena caval pulsations, may improve our ability to predict which pump fetus is at risk of complications and, therefore, in need of treatment.

Ligation of the perfused fetus's umbilical cord has been reported in three cases with present or impending cardiac failure in the pump fetus (McCurdy, Childers & Seeds, 1993; Quintero *et al.*, 1994; Foley *et al.*, 1995). In one case (McCurdy *et al.*, 1993), intrauterine visualization at 18 weeks' gestation was achieved with an endoscope introduced through a 5 mm port under general anaesthesia. A separate 3 mm port was used to insert grasping forceps to pull the cord through the loop of a prefabricated knot introduced through a third 3 mm port. The ligation was successful but the pump fetus died within 24 hours. Quintero *et al.* (1994) used a 1.9 mm endoscope and a suture introduced through a second 12-gauge trocar sleeve to ligate the umbilical cord at 19 weeks' gestation. In this case, the knot was tied extracorporeally. Despite some amniotic fluid leakage at 22 weeks, she delivered a healthy infant at 36 weeks. Foley *et al.* (1995) performed a laparotomy under epidural anaesthesia and inserted a manually controlled spring-wired device designed for manipulating the umbilical cord during difficult fetal blood sampling procedures. The cord of the perfused fetus was grasped with the instrument, pulled to the anterior uterine wall, and exteriorized through a 2.5 cm incision. The cord was then ligated, replaced into the uterine cavity, and the incision closed. The patient was delivered by caesarean section at 35 weeks because of suboptimal fetal heart rate tracing; the neonate was alive and well at three months of age.

An ultrasound-guided approach would have the advantage of avoiding the risks of endoscopy. In this regard, Lemery *et al.* (1994) have described a single puncture ultrasound-guided approach to cord ligation in TTTS, using biopsy forceps to encircle the cord and then tighten the extracorporeally tied knot. This has not to our knowledge yet been tried in TRAP.

The use of neodymium:yttrium-aluminum-garnet laser light via fetoscopy to occlude the umbilical vessels of the perfused fetus is an attractive therapeutic option. Ville *et al.* (1994) attempted this in four TRAP perfused twins. Laser successfully occluded blood flow in two fetuses at 17 and 20 weeks but failed in two others at 26 and 28 weeks. This is not surprising as, in the sheep model, vessels larger than 1 cm in diameter could not be completely occluded even at high energy levels (De Lia *et al.*, 1985b). In humans, the umbilical vessels reach a diameter of 1 cm at approximately 23 weeks of gestation. It appears as if the cord is too large to be occluded by laser in the presence of hydrops or after the mid-trimester. This suggests that laser tratment would need to be done in the mid-trimester before the development of hydrops. Prophylactic usage, however, would expose all TRAP pregnancies to the risks of the procedure, not just those at risk of complications.

Percutaneous intravascular injection of a thrombogenic material under ultrasound guidance has been used to occlude blood flow to the perfused fetus. The materials are those used by interventional radiologists and include helical metal coils, pieces of surgical suture soaked in alcohol, and absolute alcohol (Porreco, Barton & Haverkamp, 1991; Holzgreve *et al.*, 1994; Sepulveda *et al.*, 1995). Porecco *et al.* (1991) reported the percutaneous insertion of a thrombogenic coil into the umbilical artery of an acardiac fetus at 24 weeks' gestation. The polyhydramnios slowly resolved and the pump fetus was delivered by elective caesarean section at 39 weeks with an uneventful neonatal course. However, in two further cases, the pump twin also died (Roberts *et al.*, 1991; Grab *et al.*, 1992). Using a similar approach, Holzgreve *et al.* (1994) injected 10 mm lengths of standard surgical suture material soaked in 96% ethanol into the umbilical cord. Again, the polyhydramnios resolved and a healthy infant was delivered at term. Sepulveda *et al.* (1995) injected absolute alcohol into an acardiac fetus's single umbilical artery at 23 weeks' gestation. Polyhydramnios and cardiac insufficiency resolved. However, the patient developed chorioamnionitis and delivered 11 days after the procedure. On pathologic examination, the artery supplying the acardiac fetus was thrombosed but the vein was patent. The pump fetus

was discharged home after several months with no evidence of embolic phenomena.

These therapeutic modalities raise a few concerns. Occlusion of the vein before or without occlusion of the artery must be prevented otherwise the pump fetus may exsanguinate into the circulation of the acardiac fetus. This can be accomplished by occluding the easily identified intra-abdominal portion of the umbilical artery, as reported by Sepulveda *et al.* (1995). Another concern is vessel re-canalization. In one case managed with thrombogenic coils by one of us, pulsatile flow ceased after injection of the coil into the umbilical artery only to return within minutes.

The optimal occlusive treatment for TRAP is not yet clear. Fetoscopic cord ligation appears the most effective of the minimally invasive techniques at present. In the long term, however, ultrasound-guided approaches, provided they can be as effective, may prove both preferable and more readily available.

Single intrauterine death in MC pregnancy

Background

The antenatal death of one fetus in a multiple pregnancy is one of the most difficult situations to confront the obstetrician. Accurate estimates of its incidence are not available, most reports comprising single cases or case series from referral centres where selection bias may occur. One twin dies in the first trimester in 21% of twin pregnancies with documented double cardiac activity on ultrasound (Landy *et al.*, 1986). Experience in high-order multiple gestations after spontaneous loss or fetal reduction indicates that the loss of one fetus early in gestation is not associated with increased maternal or fetal morbidity (Prompeler *et al.*, 1994). For this reason, further discussion will concentrate on single fetal demise in multiple gestations after 20 weeks' gestation. The incidence of fetal demise in all multiple gestations after 20 weeks is 2 to 6% (Carlson & Towers, 1989; Prompeler *et al.*, 1994; Kilby, Govind & O'Brien, 1994; Santema, Swaak & Wallenburg, 1995) and monochorial placentation is found in 35 to 70%. Structural abnormalities occur in approximately 25% of cases of fetal demise, a significantly higher incidence than in multiple gestations without fetal demise (Rydhstrom, 1994; Kilby et al., 1994; Santema et al., 1995).

The major concerns with the death of one fetus in a multiple gestation are the effect on the remaining fetus(es), the management of the pregnancy and the psychological impact on the mother. Until recently, most published data on this subject have consisted of case reports, in many of which the timing of death or chorionicity were not known. Most publications included both dichorionic and monochorionic pregnancies, further confusing outcome data. Even reports with more than a few cases lack comparison to an appropriate control group (Carlson & Towers, 1989; Cattanach et al., 1990; Fusi & Gordon, 1990; Goldberg et al., 1991; Prompeler et al., 1994; Gaucherand, Rudigoz & Piacenza, 1994). Publication bias may, therefore, have resulted in the risk of fetal morbidity after single intrauterine death being overestimated in the literature. In this light, more favourable outcomes have been reported in more recent relatively large case-controlled studies (Santema et al., 1995; Kilby et al., 1994).

Maternal coagulation

The main maternal complication feared in association with prolonged retention of a dead fetus is disseminated intravascular coagulopathy (DIC), coagulopathy developing in 25% of pregnant patients with a singleton dead fetus retained for ≥4 weeks (Pritchard, 1959; Pritchard & Ratnoff, 1955). This does not, however, appear to be a problem in multiple gestations complicated by single intrauterine death. No evidence of maternal coagulopathy was noted in a total of 117 pregnancies reported in eight recent series (Carlson & Towers 1989; Cattanach et al., 1990; Fusi & Gordon 1990; Van den Veyver et al., 1990; Goldberg et al., 1991; Kilby et al., 1994; Gaucherand et al., 1994; Santema et al., 1995). Further reassurance was provided by Evans et al. (1994) who reviewed the experience with second-trimester selective termination for fetal abnormalities from nine centres in four countries to report no case of maternal coagulopathy in 183 cases, including 64 patients >20 weeks' at the time of the procedure. Finally, the coagulopathy that was reported in two cases (Romero et al., 1984; Skelly et al., 1982) was limited to depressed plasma fibrinogen levels without clinical manifestation.

Fetal morbidity

With the exception of prematurity, many of the complications observed in surviving fetuses occur almost exclusively in MC pregnancies. The most commonly reported sequelae include cerebral necrotic lesions such as multicystic encephalomalacia, renal cortical necrosis and occasionally other end-organ effects such as aplasia cutis and gangrene of the distal limbs (Moore, McAdams & Sutherland, 1969; Dimmick, Hardwick & Ho-Yuen, 1971; Mannino, Jones & Benirschke, 1977; Melnick, 1977; Yoshioka et al., 1979; Hughes & Miskin, 1986; Fusi & Gordon, 1990; Dawkins, Marshall & Rogers, 1995). In reviewing the available literature, Fusi and Gordon (1990) found a 26% incidence of neurological morbidity in the surviving twin of MC pregnancies complicated by a single fetal demise. However, a recent series of 29 single survivors after intrauterine death of their co-twins, 13 of which were MC, noted no sequelae (Santema et al., 1995).

These lesions are considered to have a vascular basis. Historically they were attributed to DIC, largely in the same way that the mothers were similarly presumed to be at risk of DIC, or to thrombo-embolic events. These abnormalities are now thought to result from the acute haemodynamic imbalance that occurs at the time of intrauterine death of one of the twins (Fusi et al., 1991; Okamura et al., 1994) for several reasons. First, DIC has not been reported in a surviving twin, either at fetal blood sampling or cord blood studies at birth. Second, the complications appear not to be delayed but to occur at around the time of the intrauterine death (Fusi et al., 1991). Third, anaemia has been demonstrated in the surviving twin at fetal blood sampling (Okamura et al., 1994). This suggests that the surviving twin is at risk for hypotensive damage as it haemorrhages into the dying twin's circulation, presumably by way of superficial vascular anastomoses. Superficial anastomoses are present in almost all MC twins, which explains why all are at risk of this complication, not just those with FFTS.

Similar abnormalities have been reported in MC pregnancies in the absence of fetal death (Mahoney et al., 1990; Bejar et al., 1990; Bromley et al., 1992; Reisner et al., 1993; Grafe, 1993; Hecher et al., 1994a; Dawkins et al., 1995). Haemodynamic imbalance resulting from anastomotic flow is presumably also the mechanism. Indeed, Bejar *et al.* (1990) found evidence of antenatally acquired cerebral white matter lesions in 25% of MC twins delivered preterm, in the absence of single IUD or FFTS. Haemodynamic imbalance is likely also to be the mechanism for one MC twin dying shortly after its co-twin, estimated to occur in 22% of MC pregnancies complicated by intrauterine death (L. Fusi, personal communication).

In addition to abnormalities of haemodynamic imbalance, these fetuses are at risk for preterm delivery, admission to special care units, intrauterine growth abnormalities and perinatal mortality (Kilby *et al.*, 1994; Santema *et al.*, 1995; Prompeler *et al.*, 1994). Whether these complications are higher than those in MC pregnancies without demise of one fetus has not been determined. In the series by Santema *et al.* (1995), neonatal mortality was twice that of the control group (18.5% vs 9.5%), but the difference did not reach statistical significance. Prematurity appears to be the main determinant of adverse perinatal outcome in such series. The adverse results of an older series (D'Alton, Newton & Cetrulo, 1984) using a protocol of immediate delivery, appear to support the more recent trend towards expectant management.

Suggested management

Maternal and fetal morbidity do not appear increased if the demise occurs at ≤20 weeks and the patient can be managed routinely. The management of a MC multiple pregnancy complicated by single intrauterine death after 20 weeks is based on the recognition that (i) maternal DIC is not a concern; (ii) any insult to the surviving fetus occurs at the time of the intrauterine death; and (iii) prematurity is the main determinant of outcome. In giving the following management principles, we acknowledge that the gestational age thresholds or antepartum fetal surveillance techniques will differ in various centres, depending on neonatal intensive care facilities, practice patterns and available resources.

Knowledge of chorionicity is important to the management of any multiple pregnancy with fetal compromise, as the prevention of the haemodynamic complications of MC single intrauterine death necessarily involves delivery of both twins before the intrauterine death. This is different from the situation in dichorionic twins, whereby non-intervention may be a more acceptable option at early gestational ages or very low fetal weights to avoid the complications of prematurity in the healthy survivor. In general we advise delivery in the presence of fetal compromise two to four weeks earlier in MC than in dichorionic twin pregnancies. However, even this is not appropriate at gestational ages ≤26–27 weeks, and it needs to be borne in mind that the 26% incidence of neurological sequelae reported by Fusi & Gordon (1990) may well be an overestimate, with prematurity instead being the greater risk. The practice at these gestational ages at Queen Charlotte's and Chelsea Hospital in London is not to intervene in the presence of fetal compromise in one MC twin but to admit the patient to hospital for continuous monitoring around the time of impending intrauterine death, to allow the option of delivery of the other twin if it manifests fetal distress. The theory is that this prevents exposing the healthy twin to the risks of prematurity unless needed to prevent its death or neurological damage.

If single intrauterine death has already occurred, there is no justification for routine delivery of the remaining twin providing that fetal and maternal condition remain adequate. Any resultant neurological damage has already occurred and should not be compounded by risks of iatrogenic prematurity. It seems logical that gross cerebral cavitatory lesions may become manifest on ultrasound over the ensuing weeks, assisting with prognostication and raising the possibility of late therapeutic termination of pregnancy in those countries such as the UK or France where such practice is legal. Otherwise management follows standard obstetric principles of monitoring fetal condition, suppressing premature uterine activity and promoting fetal lung maturity as appropriate, with the pregnancy continuing to 37 weeks or the attainment of fetal lung maturity.

Conclusions

Feto–fetal transfusion syndrome presenting in the midtrimester is associated with an extremely high perinatal morbidity and mortality. Serial aggressive amnioreduction has substantially improved perinatal survival rates to ≥60% in most series. This empirically compares with a

53% survival rate reported in both series of fetoscopic laser ablation of placental vessels plus amnioreduction. The validity of laser treatment has recently been questioned by the demonstration that FFTS placenta are associated with a paucity of superficial anastomoses, which might explain its high procedure-related fetal death rate. Neurological, renal and cardiac sequelae of FFTS remain high, such that there is need for evaluation of novel therapies, including targeted ablation and amniotic septostomy.

TRAP sequence is associated with high prenatal mortality and morbidity in the pump twin, in proportion to the size of the perfused twin. Limited case reports describe success in some but not all attempts at cord occlusion, using either fetoscopic or ultrasound-guided approaches.

Single intrauterine death of one MC twin carries a risk of neurological damage and/or death to the co-twin. The mechanism is acute haemodynamic imbalance at the time of intrauterine death as the healthy twin transfuses blood into the dying twin. Accordingly, routine delivery is not recommended after the death has occurred, and prematurity is the main determinant of perinatal outcome.

FFTS, TRAP sequence and death of a fetus in a MC gestation are rare complications of multiple gestation, but they continue to generate considerable debate. The lack of large prospective studies has significantly contributed to the confusion. Until such studies are available, therapy must be individualized according to the wishes of the informed patient and the available resources at each centre.

References

Abraham, J. M. (1967). Intrauterine feto–fetal transfusion syndrome. *Clinical Pediatrics* 6, 405–10.

Ash, K., Harman, C. R. & Gritter, H. (1990). TRAP sequence – successful outcome with indomethacin treatment. *Obstetrics and Gynecology*, 76, 960–2.

Bajoria, R., Sullivan, M. & Fisk, N. (1996). Raised endothelin levels in association with cardiac dysfunction in the recipient fetus of twin–twin transfusion syndrome. *American Journal of Obstetrics and Gynecology*, submitted.

Bajoria, R., Wigglesworth, J. & Fisk, N. (1995). Angioarchitecture of monochorionic placentas in relation to the twin–twin transfusion syndrome. *American Journal of Obstetrics and Gynecology*, 172, 856–63.

Baldwin, V. J. (1994). *Pathology of Multiple Pregnancy*, pp. 207–9. New York: Springer-Verlag.

Bejar, R., Vigliocco, G., Gramajo, H. & Solana (1990). Antenatal origin of neurologic damage in newborn infants. II. Multiple gestations. *American Journal of Obstetrics and Gynecology*, 162, 1230–6.

Belfort, M. A., Moise, K. J., Saade, G. R. & Kirshon, B. (1993). The use of color flow Doppler to diagnose umbilical cord entanglement in mono-amniotic twin gestation. *American Journal of Obstetrics and Gynecology*, 168, 601–4.

Benirschke, K. & des Roches Harper, V. (1977). The acardiac anomaly. *Teratology*, 15, 311–16.

Benirschke, K. & Driscoll, S. G. (1967). *Pathology of the Human Placenta*. New York: Springer-Verlag.

Benirschke, K. & Kim, C. K. (1973). Multiple pregnancy. *New England Journal of Medicine*, 288, 1276–84.

Benson, C. B., Bieber, F. R, Genest, D. R. & Doubilet, P. M. (1989). Doppler demonstration of reversed umbilical blood flow in an acardiac twin. *Journal of Clinical Ultrasound*, 17, 291–5.

Bleisch, V. (1965). Placental circulation of human twins. *American Journal of Obstetrics and Gynecology*, 91, 862–70.

Blickstein, I. (1990). The twin–twin transfusion syndrome. *Obstetrics and Gynecology*, 76, 714–22.

Bower, S. J., Flack, N. J., Sepulveda, W., Talbert, D. & Fisk, N. M. (1995). Uterine artery blood flow response to correction of amniotic fluid volume. *American Journal of Obstetrics and Gynecology*, 173, 502–7.

Bromley, B., Frigoletto, F. D., Estroff, J. A. & Benacerraf, B. R. (1992). The natural history of oligohydramnios/polyhydramnios sequence in monochorionic diamniotic twins. *Ultrasound Obstetrics and Gynecology*, 2, 317–20.

Bruner, J. P. & Rosemond, R. L. (1993). Twin-to-twin transfusion syndrome: a subset of the twin oligohydramios–polyhydramnios sequence. *American Journal of Obstetrics and Gynecology*, 169, 925–30.

Cameron, A. H. (1968). The Birmingham twin survey. *Proceedings of the Royal Society of Medicine*, 61, 229–34.

Carlson, N. J. & Towers, C. V. (1989). Multiple gestation complicated by the death of one fetus. *Obstetrics and Gynecology* 73, 685.

Carr, S. R., Aronson, M. P. & Coustan, D. R. (1990). Survival rates of monoamniotic twins do not decrease after 30 weeks' gestation. *American Journal of Obstetrics and Gynecology*, 163, 719–22.

Cattanach, S. A., Wedel, M., White, S. & Young, M. (1990). Single intrauterine fetal death in a suspected monozygotic twin pregnancy. *Australian and New Zealand Journal of Obstetrics and Gynaecology*, 30, 137–40.

Chescheir, N. C. & Seeds, J. W. (1988). Polyhydramnios and oligohydramnios in twin gestations. *Obstetrics and Gynecology*, 71, 882–4.

Cheung, C. Y. & Brace, R. A. (1988). Fetal hypoxia elevates plasma atrial natriuretic factor concentration. *American Journal of Obstetrics and Gynecology*, 159, 1263–8.

Cheung, V. Y., Bocking, A. D. & Dasilva, O. P. (1995). Preterm discordant twins: what birth weight difference is significant? *American Journal of Obstetrics and Gynecology*, 172, 955–9.

D'Alton, M. E., Newton, E. R. & Cetrulo, C. L. (1984). Intrauterine fetal demise in multiple gestation. *Acta Geneticae Medicae et Gemellologiae*, 33, 43–9.

Danskin, F. H. & Neilson, J. P. (1989). Twin-to-twin transfusion syndrome: what are appropriate diagnostic criteria? *American Journal of Obstetrics and Gynecology*, 161, 365–9.

Das, K. (1902). Acardiacus anceps. *Journal of Obstetrics and Gynaecology of the British Empire*, 2, 341–55.

Dawkins, R. R., Marshall, T. L. & Rogers, M. S. (1995). Prenatal gangrene in association with twin–twin transfusion syndrome. *American Journal of Obstetrics and Gynecology*, 172, 1055–7.

Deacon, J. S., Machin, G. A., Martin, J. M., Nicholson, S., Nwankwo, D. C. & Wintemute, R. (1980). Investigation of acephalus. *American Journal of Medical Genetics*, 5, 85–99.

De Lia, J. E., Cruikshank, D. P. & Keye, W. R. (1990). Fetoscopic neodymium: YAG laser occlusion of placental vessels in severe twin–twin transfusion syndrome. *Obstetrics and Gynecology*, 75, 1046–53.

De Lia, J. E., Cukierski, M. A., Lundergan, D. K. & Kochenour, N. K. (1989). Neodymium–yttrium–aluminum–garnet laser occlusion of rhesus placental vasculature via fetoscopy. *American Journal of Obstetrics and Gynecology* 160, 485–9.

De Lia, J. E., Emery, M. G., Sheafor, S. A. & Jennison, T. A. (1985a). Twin transfusion syndrome: Successful *in utero* treatment with digoxin. *International Journal of Gynaecology and Obstetrics*, 23, 197–201.

De Lia, J. E., Kuhlmann, R. S., Harstad, T. W. & Cruikshank, D. P. (1995). Fetoscopic laser ablation of placental vessels in severe previable twin–twin transfusion syndrome. *American Journal of Obstetrics and Gynecology*, 172, 1202–11.

De Lia, J. E., Rogers, J. G. & Dixon, J. A. (1985b). Treatment of placental vasculature with a neodymium–yttrium–aluminum–garnet laser via fetoscopy. *American Journal of Obstetrics and Gynecology*, 151, 1126–7.

Dimmick, J. E., Hardwick, D. F. & Ho-Yuen, B. (1971). A case of renal necrosis and fibrosis in the immediate newborn period. *American Journal of Diseases of Children* 122, 345–7.

Donnenfeld, A. E., van de Woestijne, J., Craparo, F., Smith, C. S, Ludomirsky, A. & Weiner, S. (1991). The normal fetus of an acardiac twin pregnancy: perinatal management based on echocardiographic and sonographic evaluation. *Prenatal Diagnosis*, 11, 235–44.

Elliot, J. P., Urig, M. A. & Clewell, W. H. (1991). Aggressive therapeutic amniocentesis for treatment of twin–twin transfusion syndrome. *Obstetrics and Gynecology*, 77, 537–40.

Evans, M. I., Goldberg, J. D., Dommergues, M., Wapner, R. J., Lynch, L., Dock, B. S., Horenstein, J., Golbus, M. S., Rodeck, C. H., Dumez, Y., Holzgreve, W., Timor-Tritsch, I., Johnson, M. P., Isada, N. B., Monteagudo, A. & Berkowitz, R. L. (1994). Efficacy of second-trimester selective termination for fetal abnormalities: international collaborative experience among the world's largest centers. *American Journal of Obstetrics and Gynecology*, 171, 90–4.

Fisk, N. M. (1995). The scientific basis of feto–fetal transfusion syndrome. In *Multiple Pregnancy*, ed. R. H. Ward & M. Whittle, pp. 235–50. London: RCOG Press.

Fisk, N. M., Borrell, A., Hubinont, C., Tannirandorn, Y., Nicolini, U. & Rodeck, C. H. (1990a). Fetofetal transfusion syndrome: do the neonatal criteria apply in utero? *Archives of Disease in Childhood*, 65, 657–61.

Fisk, N. M., Tannirandorn, Y., Nicolini, U., Hubinont, C., Rodeck, C. H. & Meliagros, L. (1990b). Atrial natriuretic peptide in fetal disease. *British Journal of Obstetrics and Gynaecology*, 97, 545–6.

Fisk, N. M., Tannirandorn, Y., Nicolini, U., Talbert, D. G. & Rodeck, C. H. (1990c). Amniotic pressure in disorders of amniotic fluid volume. *Obstetrics and Gynecology*, 76, 210–14.

Fisk, N. M., Vaughan, J. & Talbert, D. (1994). Impaired fetal blood gas status in polyhydramnios and its relation to raised amniotic pressure. *Fetal Diagnosis and Therapy*, 9, 7–13.

Fisk, N. M., Ware, M., Stanier, P., Moore, G. E. & Fisk N. M. (1996). Molecular genetic etiology of twin reversed arterial perfusion sequence. *American Journal of Obstetrics and Gynecology*, in press.

Foley, M. R., Clewell, W. H., Finberg, H. J. & Mills, M. D. (1995). Use of the Foley Cordostat grasping device for selective ligation of the umbilical cord of an acardiac twin: a case report. *American Journal of Obstetrics and Gynecology*, 17, 212–14.

Fouron, J. C., Leduc, I., Grigon, A., Maragnes, P., Lessard, M., & Drblik, S. P. (1994). Importance of meticulous ultrasonographic investigation of the acardiac twin. *Journal of Ultrasound in Medicine*, 13, 1001–4.

Fries, M. H., Goldberg, J. D., & Golbus, M. S. (1992). Treatment of acardiac-acephalus twin gestation by hysterotomy and selective delivery. *Obstetrics and Gynecology*, 79, 601–4.

Fusi, L. & Gordon, H. (1990). Twin pregnancy complicated by single intrauterine death. Problems and outcome with conservative mangement. *British Journal of Obstetrics and Gynaecology*, 97, 511–16.

Fusi, L., McParland, P., Fisk, N. M., Nicolini, U. & Wigglesworth, J. (1991). Acute twin–twin transfusion: a possible mechanism for brain-damaged survivors after intrauterine death of a monochorionic twin. *Obstetrics and Gynecology*, 78, 517–20.

Gaucherand, P., Rudigoz, R. C. & Piacenza, J. M. (1994). Monofetal death in multiple pregnancies: risks for the co-twin, risk factors and obstetrical management. *European Journal of Obstetrics and Gynecology and Reproductive Biology*, 55, 111–15.

Gilbert, W. M., Davis, S. E., Kaplan, C. Pretorius, D., Merrit, T. A. & Bernirschke, K. (1991). Morbidity associated with prenatal disruption of the dividing membrane in twin gestations. *Obstetrics and Gynecology*, 78, 623–30.

Gillim, D. L. & Hendricks, C. H. (1953). Holoacardius: review of the literature and a case report. *Obstetrics and Gynecology*, 12, 647–50.

Ginsberg, N. A., Applebaum, M., Rabin, S. A., Caffarelli, M. A., Kuuspalu, M., Daskal, J. L., Verlinsky, Y., Strom, C. M. & Barton, J. J. (1992). Term birth after midtrimester hysterotomy and selective delivery of an acardiac twin. *American Journal of Obstetrics and Gynecology*, 167, 33–7.

Goldberger, S. B., Rosen, D. J., Shulman, A., Bahary, C. & Fejgin, M. D. (1991). Conservative approach to multiple pregnancy with intrauterine fetal death of one or more fetuses. *American Journal of Obstetrics and Gynecology*, 34, 367–72.

Grab, D., Schneider, V., Keckstein, J., & Terinde, R. (1992). Twin, acardiac, outcome. *Fetus*, 2, 11–13.

Grafe, M. R. (1993). Antenatal cerebral necrosis in monochorionic twins. *Pediatric Pathology*, 13, 15–19.

Hecher, K., Jauniaux, E., Campbell, S., Deane, C. & Nicolaides, K. H. (1994). Artery-to-artery anastomosis in monochorionic twins. *American Journal of Obstetrics and Gynecology*, 171, 570–2.

Healey, M. G. (1994). Acardia: predictive risk factors for the co-twin's survival. *Teratology*, 50, 205–13.

Holzgreve, W., Tercanli, S., Krings, W. & Schuierer, G. A. (1994). A simpler technique for umbilical-cord blockade of an acardiac twin. *New England Journal of Medicine*, 331, 56–7.

Hubinont, C., Bernard, P., Magritte, J. P. & Donnez, J. (1996). YAG laser disruption of the interfetal septum: a possible therapy in severe twin–twin transfusion syndrome. *Journal of Gynecologic Surgery*, in press.

Hughes, H. E. & Miskin, M. (1986). Congenital microcephaly due to vascular disruption: *in utero* documentation. *Pediatrics*, 78, 85–7.

James, W. H. (1977). A note on the epidemiology of acardiac monsters. *Teratology*, 16, 211–16.

Jeanty, P., Shah, D. & Roussis, P. (1990). Single-needle insertion in twin amniocentesis. *Journal of Ultrasound in Medicine*, 9, 511–17.

Kaplan, C. & Benirschke, K. (1979). The acardiac anomaly, new case reports and current status. *Acta Geneticae Medicae et Gemellologiae*, 28, 51–9.

Kilby, M. D., Govind, A. & O'Brien, P. M. (1994). Outcome of twin pregnancies complicated by a single intrauterine death: a comparison with viable twin pregnancies. *Obstetrics and Gynecology*, 84, 107–9.

King, A. D., Soothill, P. W., Montemagno, R., Young, M. P., Sams, V. & Rodeck, C. H. (1995). Twin-to-twin blood transfusion in a dichorionic pregnancy without the oligohydramnios–polyhydramnios sequence. *British Journal of Obstetrics and Gynaecology*, 102, 334–5.

Kirshon, B., Mari, G. & Moise, K., (1990). Indomethacin therapy in the treatment of symptomatic polyhydramnios. *Obstetrics and Gynecology*, 75, 202–5.

Landy, H. L., Weiner, S., Corson, S. L., Batzer, F. R. & Bolognese, R. J. (1986). The vanishing twin; ultrasonographic assessment of fetal disappearance in the first trimester. *American Journal of Obstetrics and Gynecology*, 155, 14–19.

Lange, I. R., Harman, C. R., Ash, K. M., Manning, F. A. & Menticoglou, S. (1989). Twin with hydramnios: treating premature labor at source. *American Journal of Obstetrics and Gynecology*, 160, 552–7.

Lemery, D. J., Vanlieferinghen, P., Gasq, M., Finkeltin, F., Beaufrere, A. M. & Beytout, M. (1994). Fetal umbilical cord ligation under ultrasound guidance. *Ultrasound in Obstetrics and Gynecology*, 4, 399–401.

Little, J. & Thompson, B. (1988). Descriptive epidemiology. In *Twinning and Twins*, ed. I. MacGillvray, D. M. Campbell & B. Thomson, pp. 37–66. Chichester: John Wiley.

Lumme, R. H. & Saarikoski, S. V. (1986). Monoamniotic twin pregnancy. *Acta Geneticae Medicae et Gemellologiae*, 35, 99–105.

McCurdy, C. M., Childers, J. M. & Seeds, J. W. (1993). Ligation of the umbilical cord of an acardiac-acephalus twin with an endoscopic intrauterine technique. *Obstetrics and Gynecology*, 82, 708–11.

Mahoney, B. S., Petty, C. N., Nyberg, D. A., Luthy, D. A., Hickok, D. E. & Hirsch, J. H. (1990). The 'stuck twin' phenomenon: ultrasonographic findings, pregnancy outcome, and management with serial amniocentesis. *American Journal of Obstetrics and Gynecology*, 163, 1513–22.

Mannino, F. L., Jones, K .L. & Benirschke. K. (1977). Congenital skin defects and fetus papyraceus. *Journal of Pediatrics*, 91, 559–64.

Mari, G., Wasserstrum, N. & Kirshon, B. (1992). Reduction in the middle cerebral artery pulsatility index after decompression of polyhydramnios in twin gestation. *American Journal of Perinatology*, 9, 381–4.

Melnick, M. (1977). Brain damage in survivor after *in utero* death of monozygous co-twin. *Lancet*, ii, 1287.

Moise, K. J. (1993). Polyhydramnios: problems and treatment. *Seminars in Perinatology*, 17, 197–209.

Moore, C. M., McAdams, J. A. & Sutherland, J. (1969). Intrauterine disseminated intravascular coagulation: a syndrome of multiple pregnancy with a dead twin fetus. *Journal of Pediatrics*, 74, 523–8.

Moore, T. R., Gale, S. & Benirschke, K. (1990). Perinatal outcome of forty-nine pregnancies complicated by acardiac twinning. *American Journal of Obstetrics and Gynecology*, 163, 907–12.

Moya, F. R., Grannum, P. A., Riddick, L., Robert, J. A. & Pinheiro, J. (1990). Atrial natriuritic factor in hydrops fetalis caused by Rh isoimmunization. *Archives of Disease in Childhood*, 65, 683–6.

Nageotte, M. P., Hurwitz, S. R, Kaupke, C. J., Vaziri, N. D. & Pandian, M. R. (1989). Atriopeptin in the twin transfusion syndrome. *Obstetrics and Gynecology*, 73, 867–70.

Napolitani, F. & Schreiber, I. (1960). The acardiac monster. *American Journal of Obstetrics and Gynecology*, 8, 582–9.

Okamura, K., Murotsuki, J., Tanigawara, S., Uehara, S. & Yajima, A. (1994). Funipuncture for evaluation of hematologic and coagulation indices in the surviving twin following co-twin's death. *Obstetrics and Gynecology*, 83, 975–8.

Panos, M. Z., Nicolaides, K. H., Anderson, J. V., Economides, D. L., Rees, L. & Williams, R. (1989).

Plasma atrial natriuretic peptide in human fetus: response to intravascular blood transfusion. *American Journal of Obstetrics and Gynecology*, 161, 357–61.

Patten, R. M., Mack, L. A., Harvey, D., Cyr, D. R. & Pretorius, D. H. (1989). Disparity of amniotic fluid volume and fetal size: problem of the stuck twin – US Studies. *Radiology*, 172, 153–7.

Pinette, M. G., Pan, Y., Pinette, S. G. & Stubblefield, P. G. (1993). Treatment of twin–twin transfusion syndrome. *Obstetrics and Gynecology*, 82, 841–6.

Popek, E. J., Strain, J. D., Neumann, A. & Wilson, H. (1993). In utero development of pulmonary artery calcification in monochorionic twins: a report of three cases and discussion of the possible etiology. *Pediatric Pathology*, 57, 597–611.

Porreco, R. P., Barton, S. M. & Haverkamp, A. D. (1991). Occlusion of umbilical artery in acardiac, acephalic twin. *Lancet*, 337, 326–27.

Pretorius, D. H., Leopold, G. R., Moore, T. R., Benirschke, K. & Sivo, J. J. (1988). Acardiac twin report of Doppler sonography. *Journal of Ultrasound in Medicine* 7, 413–16.

Pritchard, J. A. (1959). Fetal death in utero. *Obstetrics and Gynecology*, 14, 573–80.

Pritchard, J. A. & Ratnoff, O. D. (1955). Studies of fibrinogen and other hemostatic factors in women with intrauterine death and delayed delivery. *Surgery, Gynecology and Obstetrics*, 101, 467–77.

Prompeler, H. J., Madja, R. H., Klosa, W., du Bois, A., Zahradnik, H. P., Schillinger, H. & Breckwoldt, M. (1994). Twin pregnancies with single fetal death. *Acta Obstetricia et Gynecologica Scandinavica*, 73, 205–8.

Quintero, R. A., Reich, H., Puder, K. S., Bardicef, M., Evans, M. I., Cotton, D. B. & Romero, R. (1994). Brief report: umbilical-cord ligation of an acardiac twin by fetoscopy at 19 weeks of gestation. *New England Journal of Medicine*, 330, 469–71.

Radestad, A. & Thomassen, P. A. (1990). Acute polyhydramnios in twin pregnancy. A retrospective study with special reference to therapeutic amniocentesis. *Acta Obstetricia et Gynecologcica Scandinavic,* 69, 297–300.

Rausen, A. R., Seki, M. & Strauss, L (1965). Twin transfusion syndrome. *Journal of Pediatrics,* 66, 613–27.

Reisner, D. P., Mahoney, B. S., Petty, C. N., Nyberg, D. A., Porter, T. F., Zingheim, R. W., Williams, M. A. & Luthy, D. A. (1993). Stuck twin syndrome: outcome in 37 consecutive cases. *American Journal of Obstetrics and Gynecology,* 169, 991–5.

Rizzo, G., Arduini, D. & Romanini, C. (1994). Cardiac and extracardiac flows in discordant twins. *American Journal of Obstetrics and Gynecology,* 170, 1321–7.

Roberts, R. M., Shah, D. M., Jeanty, P. & Beattle, J. F. (1991). Twin, acardiac, ultrasound guided embolization. *Fetus,* 1, 5–10.

Robertson, E. G. & Neer, K. J. (1983). Placental injection studies in twin gestation. *American Journal of Obstetrics and Gynecology,* 147, 170–4.

Robie, G. F., Payne, G. G. & Morgan, M. A. (1989). Selective delivery of an acardiac acephalic twin. *New England Journal of Medicine,* 320, 512–13.

Roman, J. D. & Hare, A. A. (1995). Digoxin and decompression amniocentesis for treatment of feto–fetal transfusion. *British Journal of Obstetrics and Gynaecology,* 102, 421–3.

Romero, R., Duffy, T. P., Berkowitz, R. L., Chang, E. & Hobbins, J. C. (1984). Prolongation of a preterm pregnancy complicated by death of a single twin *in utero* and disseminated intravascular coagulation: effects of treatment with heparin. *New England Journal of Medicine,* 10, 772–4.

Rosen, D. J. D., Rabinowitz, R., Beyth, Y., Fejgin, M. D. & Nicolaides, K. H. (1990). Fetal urine production in normal twins and in twins with acute polyhydramnios. *Fetal Diagnosis and Therapy,* 5, 57–60.

Rydhstrom, H. (1994). Discordant birthweight and late fetal death in like-sexed and unlike-sexed twin pairs: a population-based study. *British Journal of Obstetrics and Gynaecology,* 101, 765–9.

Saade, G. R., Olson, G., Belfort, M. A. & Moise, K. J. (1995). Amniotomy: a new approach to the 'stuck twin' syndrome. *American Journal of Obstetrics and Gynecology,* 172, 429.

Salerno, L. J. (1959). Monoamniotic twinning. A survey of the American literature since 1935 with a report of four new cases. *Obstetrics and Gynecology,* 14, 205–13.

Santema, J. G., Swaak, A. M. & Wallenburg, H. C. S. (1995). Expectant management of twin pregnancy with single fetal death. *British Journal of Obstetrics and Gynaecology,* 102, 26–30.

Saunders, N. J., Snijders, R. J. & Nicolaides, K. H. (1991). Twin–twin transfusion syndrome during the 2nd trimester is associated with small intertwin haemoglobin differences. *Fetal Diagnosis and Therapy,* 6, 34–6.

Saunders, N. J., Snijders, R. J. & Nicolaides, K. H. (1992). Therapeutic amniocentesis in twin–twin transfusion syndrome appearing in the second trimester of pregnancy. *American Journal of Obstetrics and Gynecology* 166, 820–4.

Schatz, F. (1900). *Klinische Beitruge zur Physiologie des Fetus.* Berlin: Hirschwald.

Schinzel, A. A, Smith, D. W. & Miller, J. R. (1979). Monozygotic twinning and structural defects. *Journal of Pediatrics,* 95, 921–30.

Sepulveda, W., Bower, S., Hassan, J. & Fisk, N. M. (1995). Ablation of acardiac twin by alcohol injection into the intra-abdominal umbilical artery. *Obstetrics and Gynecology,* 86, 680–1.

Simpson, P. C., Trudinger, B. J., Walker, A. & Baird, P. J. (1983). The intrauterine treatment of fetal cardiac failure in a twin pregnancy with an acardiac, acephalic monster. *American Journal of Obstetrics and Gynecology,* 147, 842–5.

Skelly, H., Marivate, M., Norman, R., Kenoyer, G. & Martin, R. (1982). Consumptive coagulopathy following fetal death in a triplet pregnancy. *American Journal of Obstetrics and Gynecology,* 142, 595–6.

Snijders, R. J., Abbas, A., Melby, O., Ireland, R. M. & Nicolaides, K. H. (1993). Fetal plasma erythropoietin concentration in severe growth retardation. *American Journal of Obstetrics and Gynecology*, 168, 615–19.

Steinberg, L. H., Hurley, V. A., Desmedt, E. & Beischer, N. A. (1990). Acute polyhydramnios in twin pregnancies. *Australian and New Zealand Journal of Obstetrics and Gynaecology*, 30, 196–200.

Storlazzi, E., Vintzileos, A. M., Campbell, W., Nochimson, D. J. & Weinbaum, P. J. (1987). Ultrasonic diagnosis of discordant fetal growth in twin gestations. *Obstetrics and Gynecology*, 69, 363–7.

Strong, S. J. & Corney, G. (1966). *The Placenta in Twin Pregnancy*. Oxford: Pergamon Press.

Tabor, B. L. & Maier, J. A. (1987). Polyhydramnios and elevated intrauterine pressure during amnioinfusion. *American Journal of Obstetrics and Gynecology*, 156, 130–1.

Talbert, D., Bajoria, R., Sepulveda, W., Bower, S. & Fisk, N. (1996). Hydrostatic and osmotic pressure gradients produce manifestations of feto-fetal transfusion syndrome in a computerized model of monochorial twin pregnancy. *American Journal of Obstetrics and Gynecology*, in press.

Tan, K. L., Tan, R., Tan, S. H. & Tan, A. M. (1979). The twin transfusion syndrome. Clinical observations on 35 affected pairs. *Clinical Pediatrics*, 18, 111–14.

Tanaka, M., Natori, M., Ishimoto, H., Kohno, H., Kobayashi, T. & Nozawa, S. (1992). Intravascular pancuronium bromide infusion for prenatal diagnosis of twin–twin transfusion syndrome. *Fetal Diagnosis and Therapy*, 7, 36–40.

Tessen, J. A. & Zlatnik, F. J. (1991). Monoamniotic twins: a retrospective controlled study. *Obstetrics and Gynecology*, 77, 832–4.

Tolosa, J., Zoppini, C., Ludomirsky, A., Bhutani, V., Weil, S. & Huhta, J. A. (1993). Fetal hypertension and cardiac hypertrophy in the discordant twin syndrome. *American Journal of Obstetrics and Gynecology*, 168, 292.

Urig, M. A., Clewell, W. H. & Elliot, J. P. (1990). Twin–twin transfusion syndrome. *American Journal of Obstetrics and Gynecology*, 163, 1522–6.

Urig, M. A., Simpson, G. F., Elliot, J. P. & Clewell, W. H. (1988). Twin-twin transfusion syndrome: the surgical removal of one twin as a treatment option. *Fetal Therapy*, 3, 185–8.

Van Allen, M. T., Smith, D. W. & Shepard, T. H. (1983). Twin reversed arterial perfusion (TRAP) sequence: a study of 14 twin pregnancies with acardius. *Seminars in Perinatology*, 7, 285–93.

Van den Veyver, I. B., Schatteman, E., Vanderheyden, J. S., Van Wiemeersch, J. V. & Meulyzer, P. (1990). Antenatal fetal death in twin pregnancies; a dangerous condition mainly for the surviving co-twin; a report of four cases. *European Journal of Obstetrics and Gynecology and Reproductive Biology*, 1, 69–73.

van Vugt, J. M., Nieuwint, A. & van Geijn, H. P. (1995). Single-needle insertion: an alternative technique for early second-trimester genetic twin amniocentesis. *Fetal Diagnosis and Therapy*, 10, 178–81.

Vetter, K. & Schneider, K. T. (1988). Iatrogenic remission of twin transfusion syndrome. *American Journal of Obstetrics and Gynecology*, 158, 221.

Ville, Y., Hyett, J., Hecher, K. & Nicolaides, K. H. (1995). Preliminary experience with endoscopic laser surgery for severe twin-twin transfusion syndrome. *New England Journal of Medicine*, 332, 224–7.

Ville, Y., Hyett, J. A., Vandenbussche, F. P. H. A. & Nicolaides, K. H. (1994). Endoscopic laser coagulation of umbilical cord vessels in twin reversed arterial perfusion sequence. *Ultrasound in Obstetrics and Gynecology*, 4, 396–8.

Wax, J. R., Blakemore, K. J., Blohm, P. & Callan, N. A. (1991). Stuck twin with co-twin nonimmune hydrops: successful treatment by amniocentesis. *Fetal Diagnosis and Therapy*, 6, 126–31.

Weiner, C. P. (1987). Diagnosis and treatment of twin to twin transfusion in the mid-second trimester of pregnancy. *Fetal Therapy*, 2, 71–4.

Weiner, C. P. & Ludomirski, A. (1994). Diagnosis, pathophysiology, and treatment of chronic twin-to-twin transfusion syndrome. *Fetal Diagnosis and Therapy*, 9, 283–90.

Weir, P. E., Raten, G. J. & Beisher, N. A. (1979). Acute polyhydraminos – a complication of monozygous twin pregnancy. *British Journal of Obstetrics and Gynaecology*, 86, 849–53.

Wenstrom, K. D., Tessen, J. A., Zlatnik, F. J. & Sipes, S. L. (1992). Frequency, distribution, and theoretical mechanisms of hematologic and weight discordance in monochorionic twins. *Obstetrics and Gynecology*, 80, 257–61.

Wieacker, P., Wilhelm, C., Prömpeler, H., Petersen, K. G., Schillinger, H. & Breckwoldt, M. (1992). Pathophysiology of polyhydramnios in twin transfusion syndrome. *Fetal Diagnosis and Therapy*, 7, 87–92.

Wittmann, B. K., Farquharson, D. F., Thomas, W. D., Baldwin, V. J. & Wadsworth, L. D. (1986). The role of feticide in the management of severe twin transfusion syndrome. *American Journal of Obstetrics and Gynecology*, 155, 1023–6.

Yoshioka, H., Kadamato, Y., Mino, M., Morikawa, Y., Kasubuchi, Y. & Kusunoki, T. (1979). Multicystic encephalomalacia in liveborn twin with a stillborn macerated co-twin. *Journal of Pediatrics*, 95, 798–800.

Zosmer, N., Bajoria, R., Weiner, E., Rigby, M., Vaughan, J. & Fisk, N. M. (1994). Clinical and echographic features of *in utero* cardiac dysfunction in the recipient twin in twin–twin transfusion syndrome. *British Heart Journal*, 72, 74–9.

15 Goitre

J. GUY THORPE-BEESTON

Introduction

Thyroid hormones play a vital role in fetal growth, neural development and maturation. A fetal goitre may occur as a consequence of either hypo- or hyperthyroidism, both of which may be associated with persistent neurological and developmental abnormalities. Until recently, direct *in utero* assessment of fetal thyroid function has not been possible. The advent of high-resolution ultrasonography has allowed the prenatal diagnosis of goitre, and fetal blood sampling now facilitates direct evaluation of fetal thyroid hormone status. Knowledge of the cause and severity of abnormal fetal thyroid function permits rational treatment. Evidence of thyroid dysfunction in the presence of fetal goitre should be aggressively managed, either by treatment of the maternal condition or direct fetal therapy.

Thyroid function in normal fetuses

In the human, failure of the orderly maturation of the hypothalamic–pituitary–thyroid axis results in well recognised clinical sequelae, manifest at their extreme by cretinism. Until recently our knowledge of pituitary and thyroid development in human fetuses was largely based in early pregnancy on histological studies of abortuses or blood samples obtained at hysterotomy, and in later pregnancy on blood samples obtained at delivery (Greenberg *et al.*, 1970, Fisher *et al.*, 1970, Fisher & Klein, 1981). However, results from samples obtained at hysterotomy or caesarean section may be influenced by maternal fasting or hypotension, which might alter placental perfusion and, therefore, the supply of oxygen

and nutrients to the fetus (Morriss *et al.*, 1975). Furthermore, samples obtained after preterm delivery may not represent normal prelabour values, as the condition causing preterm delivery itself might influence fetal thyroid stimulating hormone (TSH) and thyroid hormone levels; in addition fetuses delivered before 37 weeks' gestation cannot truly be described as normal. Despite their limitations, such studies indicated that the thyroid gland begins to produce thyroxine (T_4) at 10 to 12 weeks' gestation (Shepard, 1967; Rosen & Ezrin, 1966). The gestation at which the fetal pituitary–thyroid axis becomes functionally mature is controversial. Some authors suggest that TSH secretion is responsive to changes in serum free T_4 concentration as early as 11 weeks (Greenberg *et al.*, 1970); others that such maturation occurs largely during the last half of pregnancy (Fisher *et al.*, 1977).

Ultrasound-guided fetal blood sampling, has permitted investigation of relatively undisturbed physiology in normal fetuses. Such studies have shown that serum TSH, thyroxine-binding globulin (TBG) and both free and total thyroxine and triiodothyronine (T_3) concentrations rise with gestation (Ballabio *et al.*, 1989, Thorpe-Beeston *et al.*, 1991a) (Figs. 15.1 and 15.2). Fetal and maternal serum concentrations of thyroid hormones and TSH were not related, suggesting that the human fetal pituitary–thyroid axis develops independently from that of the mother.

Total and free T_4 serum concentrations in the fetus reach adult levels by 36 weeks' gestation, whereas total and free T_3 concentrations are always less than the respective mean adult concentrations, suggesting that in intrauterine life the mechanisms necessary for peripheral conversion of T_4 to T_3 are either immature or lack the necessary stimulus for their activation (Thorpe-Beeston et al., 1991a). Animal studies provide support for this hypothesis, showing that the conversion rate of T_4 to T_3 and reverse T_3 (rT_3) in liver and kidney increases with advancing gestation (Brezezomska-Slebodzinska & Krysin, 1990). The increase in the fetal serum thyroid hormone and TBG concentrations with gestation reflect increasing maturation of the fetal thyroid gland and liver. The lack of correlation between TSH and thyroid hormones suggests that the thyroid gland matures independently of the influence of TSH. Although a study of infants with severe congenital hypothyroidism suggested that T_4 is transferred from mother to fetus (Vulsma et al., 1989), the cord blood levels of T_4 at term were only a quarter to half of normal values. Therefore, it is likely that the bulk of fetal T_4 is derived from fetal thyroid secretion and not from improved placental transfer. As fetal serum TSH increases significantly with gestation, the fetal pituitary appears either relatively insensitive to negative feedback from thyroid hormones or increasingly sensitive to stimulation by thyrotrophin releasing hormone (Thorpe-Beeston et al., 1991a,b).

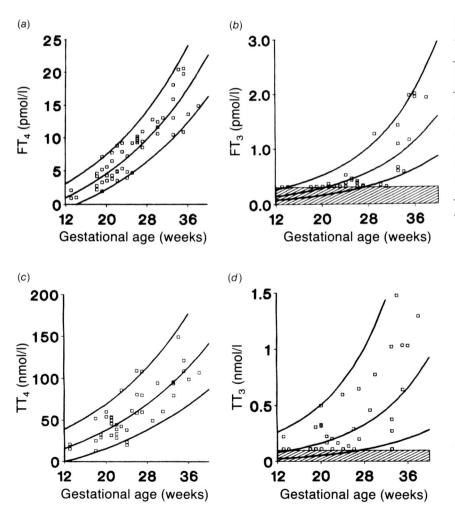

Fig. 15.1 *Individual fetal values of serum free T_4 (a), free T_3 (b), total T_4 (c) and total T_3 (d) in normal fetuses plotted on the fetal reference ranges (mean, 5th and 95th centiles). Hatched areas represent the lower limits of sensitivity for the assays; GA, gestational age. (Reprinted, with permission from the* New England Journal of Medicine.)

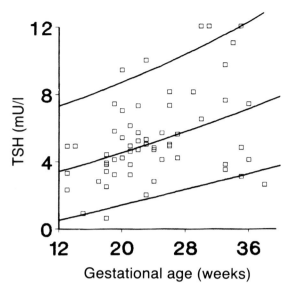

Fig. 15.2 *Individual fetal values of serum TSH concentration in normal fetuses plotted on the fetal reference ranges (mean, 5th and 95th centiles). (Reprinted with permission from the* New England Journal of Medicine.)

Aetiology

Severe abnormalities in fetal thyroid function may result in the development of goitre.

Hypothyroidism

Congenital hypothyroidism occurs in 1 in 4000–5000 births (Trainer & Howard, 1983) and is classified as either permanent or transient. Thyroid dysgenesis is the most common form of permanent hypothyroidism, accounting for 80 to 90% of cases of fetal goitre, and may be sub-classified by the presence or absence of functioning thyroid tissue at normal or ectopic sites. Athyreosis is the absence of thyroid tissue, typically associated with an absence of detectable thyroglobulin in serum, whereas the presence of small amounts of appropriately sited tissue is termed hypoplastic dysgenesis. Ectopic thyroid refers to thyroid tissue sited within the region from the foramen caecum, the site of origin of the thyroglossal

duct on the tongue, to the anterior mediastinum. Goitre may also rarely be associated with biochemical defects in one or other of the steps involved in thyroid hormone synthesis, or with TSH resistance, congenital absence of the pituitary gland or the inadvertent use of ^{131}I, which is contraindicated in pregnant women.

Fetal goitre caused by transient hypothyroidism is most frequently associated with maternal antithyroid drug ingestion, commonly propythiouracil or carbimazole in pregnant women with Graves' disease, although occasionally it is caused by amiodarone or lithium (Matsumura *et al.*, 1992). The thionamides propythiouracil and carbimazole inhibit thyroid synthesis by blocking iodination of the tyrosine molecule. In women with Graves' disease on antithyroid drugs, maternal T_4 should be kept in the upper normal range to minimize the chance of fetal hypothyroidism. Excessive maternal iodine intake has also been associated with the development of fetal goitre. Idiopathic transient hypothyroidism is defined as abnormal thyroid function in a newborn which spontaneously recovers within a few weeks (Delange *et al.*, 1978). This syndrome is more common in acutely ill preterm infants, and similar abnormalities in thyroid function tests, such as low T_4 and elevated TSH, have been described in growth-retarded fetuses (Thorpe-Beeston *et al.*, 1991c).

Postnatally, universal screening identifies most neonates at risk of hypothyroidism and treatment is usually effective in preventing long-term consequences such as mental retardation (New England Congenital Hypothyroid Collaborative, 1990). However, despite early postnatal therapy, some infants still exhibit impaired language, perceptual motor and visual spatial development (Rovet *et al.*, 1987). In this light, uncorrected antenatal deficiency of thyroid hormone is known to impair maturation of the fetal central nervous system (Glorieux *et al.*, 1985).

Hyperthyroidism

A thyrotoxic goitre in the fetus or newborn is almost invariably secondary to maternal autoimmune disorders, principally Graves' disease. Because only 1.5 to 12% of infants from mothers with Graves' disease suffer from neonatal thyrotoxicosis (Bruinse *et al.*, 1988), the incidence of neonatal hyperthyroidism has been variously estimated to be 1 in 4000 to 40 000 (Ramsey, 1991; Fort *et al.*, 1988; Fisher, 1986). The condition is characterized by the presence of several thyroid-stimulating immunoglobulins, including those directed against TSH receptors in the thyroid gland. The fetal thyroid reacts to these antibodies, which are of the IgG subclass and, therefore, cross the placenta. It is noteworthy that transplacental transfer of these antibodies may occur in euthyroid mothers who have undergone partial thyroidectomy for Graves' disease. In such cases, the prematurity rate may be as high as 90% and the perinatal death rate 50% (Bruinse *et al.*, 1988).

Fetal effects

In addition to the endocrine abnormalities, a fetal goitre may cause significant mechanical problems, including hyperextension of the fetal neck and dystocia. Polyhydramnios may develop secondary to oesophageal compression and is associated with malpresentation and preterm delivery. After delivery, there can be respiratory embarrassment and feeding difficulties.

Fetal hypothyroidism, in addition to producing a goitre, is associated with intrauterine growth retardation, congenital heart block, delayed skeletal maturation and cardiomegaly (Utiger, 1991; Belfar *et al.*, 1991). Neonatal clinical manifestations include mental and growth retardation, feeding problems, constipation, inactivity, hypotonia, umbilical hernia, enlarged tongue, skin mottling, open posterior fontanelle and typical facies (Letarte *et al.*, 1981).

Fetal hyperthyroidism, however, may cause tachycardia, hydrops secondary to cardiac failure, hyperactivity, growth retardation and craniosynostosis (Fisher, 1986). Visceromegaly, pulmonary hypertension, generalized adenopathy and a reduction in subcutaneous fat have also been described at autopsy (Page *et al.*, 1988). Typical neonatal features include exophthalmos, feeding intolerance, frontal bossing, high output cardiac failure, jaundice and liver dysfunction (Skelton & Gans, 1955; Riggs *et al.*, 1972). Subsequent development may be impaired by perceptual motor difficulties (Daneman & Howard, 1980). Overall, neonatal hyperthyroidism has a 12 to 26% mortality rate, most

deaths being secondary to cardiac failure (Hollingsworth & Mabry, 1976).

Investigation

Timely recognition and treatment of congenital hypo- and hyperthyroidism is essential if affected children are to achieve optimal growth and intellectual development. A fetus should be considered at risk of thyroid disease if the mother has a history of Graves' disease or autoimmune thyroiditis, is using antithyroid medication or, less commonly, if there is a known genetic predisposition. The maternal thyroid hormone and thyroid-stimulating antibody status of such women should be investigated. Maternal hyperthyroidism may also occur for the first time during pregnancy but may be missed because its symptoms of emotional lability, heat intolerance, nervousness, irritability, increased perspiration and appetite are common to many normal pregnancies. The presence of maternal TSH receptor antibodies is associated with neonatal thyroid dysfunction (Southgate *et al.*, 1984; Mitsuda *et al.*, 1993), but their measurement does not directly assess fetal thyroid function. Thyroid-stimulating immunoglobulins are capable of inducing fetal thyrotoxicosis only after 22 weeks' gestation (Dove & Johnston, 1985).

The various manifestations of fetal thyroid disease, including goitre, have increasingly been detected by ultrasound. Although the normal sonographic appearance of the fetal thyroid gland has been described (Bromley *et al.*, 1992), few goitres are diagnosed by 'routine' scanning. Only a quarter of antenatally diagnosed goitres are detected in women without a history of thyroid disease, in which case polyhydramnios was the usual indication for detailed ultrasonography. Three-quarters of fetal goitres are detected in women with a past history of thyroid disease, in whom monthly fetal ultrasound assessment is recommended to look for the development of goitre, polyhydramnios or fetal tachycardia. Although the diagnosis of fetal goitre by ultrasound is usually straightforward (Fig. 15.3) there is an extensive differential diagnosis, including hygroma, teratoma and haemangioma (Rempen & Feige, 1985). Diagnosis of a fetal goitre warrants a thorough search for other manifestations of fetal thyroid dysfunction, such as tachycardia or growth retardation.

Physical examination and laboratory investigation of the mother are unreliable in assessing fetal well-being. Although there may be ultrasound evidence of fetal compromise, the picture may be confused, for example appropriately grown fetuses may be thyrotoxic (Page *et al.*, 1988; Lamberg *et al.*, 1981); similarly, a fetal goitre in a woman with Graves' disease may be caused either by hyperthyroidism or by hypothyroidism secondary to excessive antithyroid medication (Davidson *et al.*, 1991). Monitoring the fetal heart rate is an insensitive means of assessing fetal thyroid function, not only because of wide variation in the normal rate but also because of the influence of factors other than thyroid hormone concentrations. Abnormalities of fetal thyroid function may arise independently of maternal thyroid status (Hollingsworth, 1983). Ultrasonography and the investigation of maternal thyroid status remain, therefore, indirect methods of assessing fetal thyroid function.

Direct assessment of fetal thyroid function has been attempted by amniocentesis. Amniotic fluid thyroid hormone levels, however, do not reliably predict fetal thyroid status (Hollingsworth & Alexander, 1983; Sack *et al.*, 1975). Fetal blood sampling is the only direct method of accurately assessing fetal thyroid function.

Normal ranges for fetal thyroid function have been established (Thorpe-Beeston *et al.*, 1991a) and several reports attest to the value of fetal blood sampling in fetuses with thyroid dysfunction (Avni *et al.*, 1992; Davidson *et al.*, 1991; Johnson *et al.*, 1989; Porreco & Bloch, 1990; Wenstrom *et al.*, 1990; Sagot *et al.*, 1991; Noia *et al.*, 1992; Hatjis, 1993). Fetal serum may be assayed for thyroid hormones and TSH concentrations and the results of assays interpreted against established reference ranges (Figs. 15.1 and 15.2). If the volume of serum is limited, measurement of T_4 and TSH concentrations are sufficient for diagnosis, as T_3 and free thyroid hormones may only be present in very low concentrations. TSH is markedly elevated or reduced in cases of hypothyroid or hyperthyroid goitre, respectively (Noia *et al.*, 1992; Hatjis, 1993). In experienced hands, the small risks of fetal blood sampling (Chapter 2) seem acceptable given the importance of correct diagnosis of thyroid status to successful treatment. It is unlikely that trials of sufficient power will be undertaken to determine the precise value of blood sampling in fetal goitre. Nonetheless, this investigation should be considered in cases of suspected fetal thyroid disease; first, because ultrasonic assessment of fetal thyroid size is not diagnostic and, second, because neonatal diagnosis based on

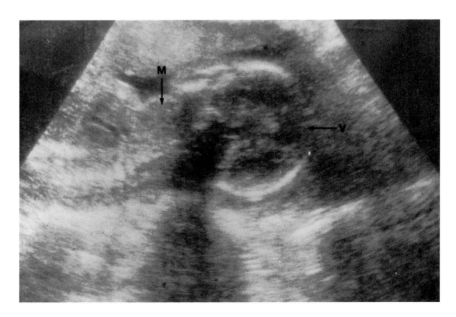

Fig. 15.3 *Saggital ultrasound scan of fetal head and upper thorax showing an anterior neck mass, which was subsequently shown to be a goitre. M, neck mass; v, skull vertex. (Reprinted with permission from* Ultrasound in Obstetrics and Gynecology.*)*

cord blood at delivery may occur too late to prevent intellectual impairment. Fetal blood sampling to assess fetal thyroid function in the absence of goitre has not been reported but may be of value in the investigation of fetuses with growth retardation or fetal heart rate abnormalities in women with a past history of thyroid disease.

Therapy

Transplacental treatment

Prior to the advent of fetal blood sampling, maternal therapy had to be instituted on the presumption that the fetus was suffering from either hyper- or hypothyroidism (Ramsay 1976; Weiner et al., 1980). Determination of exact fetal thyroid status is now considered an essential prerequisite to treatment in two situations. The first is when fetal goitre is detected in a euthyroid mother. If the fetus is found to be thyrotoxic, this will usually respond to maternal administration of antithyroid drugs (Hollingsworth, 1988). Porreco et al. (1990) reported a case of fetal thyrotoxicosis resulting from maternal Graves' disease previously treated by radioactive iodine. Fetal blood sampling confirmed elevated T_4, and maternal treatment with antithyroid medication led to a good outcome. In this situation, the mother may require T_4 if not already on supplementation. The second is when fetal goitre is detected in a mother with Grave's disease who is already on antithyroid drugs. Fetal blood sampling here is crucial to determine whether the goitre is the result of transplacental passage of the antithyroid drugs or transplacental passage of thyroid-stimulating antibodies. If the former, the dose of maternal PTU should be reduced, although repeat fetal blood sampling may be necessary to monitor therapy if the goitre does not resolve (Davidson et al., 1990). If, however, the fetus is found to be hyperthyroid, an increase in maternal antithyroid drug dose is indicated. Again, the mother may require additional T_4 supplementation. A sustained fetal heart rate 160 beats/minute is indicative of hyperthyroidism and can be used to monitor therapy (Bruinse et al., 1988).

Direct fetal treatment

The placenta essentially does not permit maternal to fetal T_4 transport (Roti et al., 1983; Vulsma et al., 1989), and, therefore, must be bypassed. Direct administration of thyroid hormones to the fetus by intra-amniotic, intravascular and intramuscular routes are all theoretically possible. Intramuscular injections of T_4 were first reported in 1975 (Van Herle et al., 1975) in a fetus at risk of hypothyroidism, following maternal thyroid radioablation at 13 weeks' gestation. After direct fortnightly injections from 32 weeks' gestation, the cord blood TSH at birth was nevertheless elevated and the T_4 concentration undetectable, suggesting inadequate thyroid replacement. It was suggested that the dose of T_4 required for adequate replacement would be too great for intramuscular injection. Direct intravascular injection would have similar disadvantages in being technically difficult, requiring frequent dosing and posing a significant cumulative risk to the fetus.

The intra-amniotic route is, therefore, generally preferred because of the relative ease of the technique and the longer intervals between administration. The daily requirement of a hypothyroid fetus has been estimated at 50 μg/day (Van Herle et al., 1975) although there is little information available on the pharmacokinetics of fetal absorption of T_4 from amniotic fluid. Johnson et al. (1989) successfully treated a fetus with acute polyhydramnios and goitrous hypothyroidism with serial 500 mg doses of intra-amniotic thyroxine at 10 to 14 day intervals. Other reports testify to the success of a lower weekly dose of 250 mg (Noia et al., 1992; Davidson et al., 1991). An overdose at these dosages has yet to be described and, therefore, 250 to 500 mg at 7–10 day intervals seems a reasonable regimen based on the limited information available.

The benefits of treatment may be assessed by observing a diminution in the size of the goitre and a return of the fetal heart rate to normal. If there is any doubt regarding its efficacy, such as with a worsening of the fetal condition, failure of the goitre to resolve or the development of polyhydramnios, serial fetal blood sampling may be required, permitting the fetus the comparable assessment to that performed in the infant after birth and allowing effective monitoring of treatment (Porreco & Bloch, 1990; Hatjis, 1993). The rationale for such an aggressive approach is that effective prenatal treatment may offset the risk of subsequent neurological impairment. It is important to institute therapy as soon as a definitive diagnosis is made because, although a lack of thyroid hormones only seems detrimental to fetal nervous system maturation after 32 weeks (Glorieux *et al.*, 1985), fetal goitre is still associated with polyhydramnios and preterm labour, the risks of which should be reduced by early institution of therapy.

Conclusion

Fetal goitres are either hypo- or hyperthroid in aetiology and most are diagnosed in women with a history of thyroid disease. Fetal blood sampling is often necessary to determine fetal thyroid status, and in particular in women with Grave's disease, to find out whether goitre is secondary to transplacental passage of antithyroid drugs or of thyroid-stimulating antibodies. Treatment to render the fetus euthyroid is indicated to prevent complications of the goitre itself, such as polyhydramnios and dystocia, and to ensure normal neurological development. The fetus may be treated by optimizing maternal thyroid status, by transplacental antithyroid drugs, or by direct administration of thyroid hormones to the fetus.

Maternal therapy usually corrects fetal hyperthyroidism and direct fetal therapy cases of hypothyroid goitre. Based on limited case reports, adequate fetal thyroid replacement therapy can be achieved by intra-amniotic administration of 250 to 500 mg at 7 to 10 day intervals. Treatment efficacy is assessed by non-invasive techniques, although serial fetal blood sampling may be indicated if these show no improvement.

References

Avni, E. D., Rodesch, F., Vandermerckt, C. & Vermeylen, D. (1992). Detection and evaluation of fetal goitre by ultrasound. *British Journal of Radiology*, 65, 302–5.

Ballabio, M., Nicolini, U., Jowett, T., Ruiz de Elvira, M. C., Ekins, R. P. & Rodeck, C. H. (1989). Maturation of thyroid function in normal human foetuses. *Clinical Endocrinology*, 31, 565–71.

Belfar, H. L., Foley, T. P., Hill, L. M. & Kislak, S. (1991). Sonographic findings in maternal hyperthyroidism. *Journal of Ultrasound in Medicine*, 10, 281–4.

Bromley, B., Frigoletto, F. D., Cramer, D., Osathanondh, R. & Benacerraf, B. R. (1992). The fetal thyroid: normal and abnormal sonographic measurements. *Journal of Ultrasound in Medicine*, 11, 25–8.

Bruinse, H. W., Vermeulen-Meiners, C. & Wit, J. M. (1988). Fetal treatment for thyrotoxicosis in non-thyrotoxic pregnant women. *Fetal Therapy*, 3, 152–7.

Brzezinska-Slebodzinska, E. & Krysin, E. (1990). Investigation of thyroxine monodeiodinase activity in the liver, kidney and brown adipose tissue of foetal and neonatal rabbit. *Journal of Developmental Physiology*, 13, 309–14.

Daneman, D. & Howard, N. J. (1980). Neonatal thyrotoxicosis: intellectual impairment and craniostenosis in later years. *Journal of Pediatrics*, 97, 257–62.

Davidson, K. M., Richards, D. S., Schatz, D. A. & Fisher, D. A. (1991). Successful *in utero* treatment of fetal goitre and hypothyroidism. *New England Journal of Medicine*, 324, 543–6.

Delange, F., Dodion, J., Wolter, R., Bourdoux, P., Dalkem, A., Glinoer, D. & Ermanans, A. M. (1978). Transient hypothyroidism in the newborn infant. *Journal of Pediatrics*, 92, 974.

Dove, D. H. & Johnston, P. (1985). Fetal hyperthyroidism: experience of treatment of four siblings. *Lancet*, i, 430–2.

Fisher, D. A. (1986). Neonatal thyroid disease in offspring of women with autoimmune thyroid disease. *Thyroid Today*, 9, 1–7.

Fisher, D. A., Dussault, J. H., Sack, J. & Chopra, I. J. (1977). Ontogenesis of hypothalamic–pituitary–thyroid function and metabolism in man, sheep and rat. *Recent Progress in Hormone Research*, 33, 59–116.

Fisher, D. A., Hobel, C. J., Garzra, R. & Pierce, C. A. (1970). Thyroid function in the preterm fetus. *Pediatrics*, 46, 208–16.

Fisher, D. A. & Klein, A. H. (1981). Thyroid development and disorders of thyroid function in the newborn. *New England Journal of Medicine*, 304, 702–12.

Fort, P., Lifshitz, F., Pugliese, M. & Klein, I. (1988). Neonatal thyroid disease: differential expression in three successive offspring. *Journal of Clinical Endocrinology and Metabolism*, 66, 645–7.

Glorieux, J., Dussault, J. H., Marissette, J., Desjardins, M., Letarte, J. & Guyda, H. (1985). Follow-up of ages 5 and 7 years on mental development in children with hypothyroidism detected by Quebec screening program. *Journal of Pediatrics*, 107, 913–15.

Greenberg, A. H., Czernichow, P., Reba, R. C., Tyson, J. & Blizzard, R. M. (1970). Observations on the maturation of thyroid function in early fetal life. *Journal of Clinical Investigation*, 49, 1790–3.

Hatjis, C. G. (1993). Diagnosis and successful treatment of fetal goitrous hyperthyroidism caused by maternal Graves' disease. *Obstetrics and Gynecology*, 81, 837–90.

Hollingsworth, D. R. (1983). Grave's disease. In *Clinical Obstetrics and Gynecology*, ed. R. M. Pitkin. pp. 615–34, Philadelphia: W. B. Saunders.

Hollingsworth, D. R. (1988). Hyperthyroidism in pregnancy. In *The Thyroid*, ed. S. H. Ingebar, pp. 1049–51. Philadelphia: W. B. Saunders.

Hollingsworth, D. R. & Alexander, N. M. (1983). Amniotic fluid concentrations of iodothyronines and thyrotropin do not reliably predict fetal thyroid status in pregnancies complicated by maternal thyroid disorders or anencephaly. *Journal of Clinical Endocrinology and Metabolism*, 57, 349–55.

Hollingsworth, D. R. & Mabry, C. C. (1976). Congenital Graves' disease. Four familial cases with long-term follow-up and perspective. *American Journal of Diseases of Children*, 130, 148–156.

Johnson, R. L., Finberg, H. J., Perelman, A. H. & Clewell, W. H. (1989). Fetal goitrous hypothyroidism. *Fetal Therapy*, 4, 141–5.

Lamberg, B. A., Ikonen, E., Teramo, K., Wager. G., Osterlund, K., Makinen, T. & Perkonen, F. (1981). Treatment of maternal hypothyroidism with anti-thyroid agents and changes in thyrotropin and thyroxine in the newborn. *Acta Endocrinologica*, 97, 186–95.

Letarte, J., Dussault, J. H. & Guyda, H. (1981). Clinical and laboratory investigation of early detected hypothyroid infant. In *Pediatric Endocrinology*, ed. J. H. Dussault & P. Walker, p. 433. New York: Raven Press.

Matsumura, L. K., Born, D., Kunii, I. S., Franco, D. B. & Maciel, R. M. (1992). Outcome of thyroid function in newborns from mothers treated with amiodarone. *Thyroid*, 2, 279–81.

Mitsuda, N., Tamaki, H., Amino, N, Hosono, T., Miyai, K. & Tanizana, O. (1993). Risk factors for developmental disorders in infants born to women with Graves' disease. *Obstetrics and Gynecology*, 80, 359–64.

Morriss, F. H., Makowski, E. L., Meschia, G., Battaglia, F. C. (1975). The glucose/oxygen quotient of the term human fetus. *Biology of the Neonate*, 25, 44–52.

New England Congenital Hypothyroidism Collaborative (1990). Elementary school performance of children with congenital hypothyroidism. *Journal of Pediatrics*, 116, 27–32.

Noia, G., De Santis, M., Tocci, A., Maussier, M. L., D'Errico, G., Bianchi, A., Romagnoli, C., Masini, L., Caruso, A. & Mancuso, S. (1992). Early prenatal diagnosis and therapy of fetal hypothyroid goitre. *Fetal Diagnosis and Therapy*, 7, 138–43.

Page, D. V., Brady, K., Mitchell, J., Pehrson, J. & Wade, G. (1988). The pathology of intrauterine thyrotoxicosis. *Obstetrics and Gynecology*, 72, 479–81.

Porreco, R. P. & Bloch, C. A. (1990). Fetal blood sampling in the management of intrauterine thyrotoxicosis. *Obstetrics and Gynecology*, 76, 509–12.

Ramsey, I. (1976). Attempted prevention of neonatal thyrotoxicosis. *British Medical Journal*, ii, 1110.

Ramsey, I. (1991). Fetal and neonatal hyper-thyroidism. *Contemporary Reviews in Obstetrics and Gynaecology*, 3, 74–8.

Rempen, A. & Feige, A. (1985). Differential diagnosis of sonographically detected tumours in the cervical region. *European Journal of Obstetrics, Gynecology and Reproductive Biology*, 20, 89–105.

Riggs, W., Wilroy, S. & Etteldorf, J. N. (1972). Neonatal hyperthyroidism with accelerated skeletal maturation, craniosynostosis, and brachydactyly. *Radiology*, 105, 621.

Rosen, F. & Ezrin, C. (1966). Embryology of the thyrotroph. *Journal of Clinical Endocrinology and Metabolism*, 26, 1343–5.

Roti, E., Gnudi, A. & Braverman, L.E. (1983). The placental transport, synthesis and metabolism of hormones and drugs which affect thyroid function. *Endocrinology Reviews*, 4, 131–49.

Rovet, J., Ehrlich, R. & Sorbara, D. (1987). Intellectual outcome in children with fetal hypo-thyroidism. *Journal of Pediatrics*, 110, 700–4.

Sack, J., Fisher, D. A., Hobel, C. J. & Lam, R. (1975). Thyroxine in human amniotic fluid. *Journal of Pediatrics*, 87, 364–8.

Sagot, P., David, A., Yvinec, M., Pousset, P., Papon, V., Mouzard, A. & Boog, G. (1991). Intrauterine treatment of thyroid goiters. *Fetal Therapy*, 6, 28–33.

Shepard, T. H. (1967). Onset of function in the human fetal thyroid: biochemical and radioautographic studies from organ culture. *Journal of Clinical Endocrinology and Metabolism*, 27, 945–58.

Skelton, M. O. & Gans, B. (1955). Congenital thyrotoxicosis, hepatosplenomegaly, and jaundice in two infants of exophthalmic mothers. *Archives of Disease in Childhood*, 30, 460.

Southgate, K., Creagh, F., Teece, M., Kinswood, C. & Rees Smith, B. (1984). A receptor assay for the measurement of TSH receptor antibodies in un-extracted serum. *Clinical Endocrinology*, 20, 539–43.

Thorpe-Beeston, J. G., Nicolaides, K. H., Felton, C. V., Butler, J. & McGregor, A. M. (1991a). Maturation of the secretion of thyroid hormone and thyroid stimulating hormone in the fetus. *New England Journal of Medicine*, 324, 532–6.

Thorpe-Beeston, J. G., Nicolaides, K. H., Snijders, R. J. M., Butler, J. & McGregor, A. M. (1991b). Fetal response to the maternal administration of TRH. *American Journal of Obstetrics and Gynecology*, 164, 1244–5.

Thorpe-Beeston, J. G., Nicolaides, K. H., Snijders, R. J. M., Felton, C. V. & McGregor, A. M. (1991c). Thyroid function in small for gestational age fetuses. *Obstetrics and Gynecology*, 77, 701–6.

Trainer, T. D. & Howard, P. L. (1983). Thyroid function tests in thyroid and non-thyroid disease. *CRC Critical Reviews Clinical Laboratory Science*, 19, 135–71.

Utiger, R. D. (1991). Recognition of thyroid disease in the fetus. *New England Journal of Medicine*, 324, 559–61.

Van Herle, A. J., Young, R. T., Fisher, D. A., Uller, R. P. & Brinkman, C. R. (1975). Intrauterine treatment of a hypothyroid fetus. *Journal of Clinical Endocrinology and Metabolism*, 40, 474–7.

Vulsma, T., Gons, M. H. & de Vijlder, J. J. M. (1989). Maternal–fetal transfer of thyroxine in congenital hypothyroidism due to a total organification defect or thyroid agenesis. *New England Journal of Medicine*, 321, 13–16.

Weiner, S., Scarf, J. I., Bolognese, R. J. (1980). Antenatal diagnosis and treatment of a fetal goiter. *Journal of Reproductive Medicine*, 24, 39–42.

Wenstrom, K. D., Weiner, C. P., Williamson, R. A. & Grant, S. S. (1990). Prenatal diagnosis of hyper-thyroidism using funipuncture. *Obstetrics and Gynecology*, 76, 513–17.

16 Pleural effusions

HEVERTON N. PETTERSEN AND KYPROS H. NICOLAIDES

Introduction

Pleural effusions, found in approximately 1 per 10 000 deliveries, may be an isolated finding or may occur in association with hydrops fetalis where in addition to the effusions there is generalized skin oedema and ascites.

Isolated pleural effusions may occur primarily when they are often attributed postnatally to clylothorax. Chylothorax, the commonest cause in neonates, is diagnosed after alimentation by demonstrating chylomicrons in pleural fluid (Chernick & Reed, 1970). Primary fetal pleural effusions, however, often resolve after birth before this diagnosis can be confirmed. Some groups have made the implausible claim that this diagnosis can be made *in utero* by showing high mononuclear cell counts in aspirated pleural fluid (Elser *et al.*, 1983; Benacerraf, Frigoletto & Wilson, 1986), although lymphocyte counts and lipoprotein electrophoresis in aspirated pleural fluid is similar in fetuses confirmed postnatally to have chylothoraces and those with hydrothoraces from other causes (Fisk & Rodeck, 1990). Isolated pleural effusions may also be caused by congenital pulmonary lymphangiectasia, which is generally fatal in the neonatal period and may have a familial occurrence (Scott-Emuakpor *et al.*, 1981). Isolated fetal pleural effusions may also occur secondary to structural abnormalities. Congenital diaphragmatic hernia may present ultrasonically as a fetal hydrothorax when the hernial sac, which only occurs in about 20% of all diaphragmatic hernias, fills with fluid and envelops the lung. Pleural effusions may also be secondary to local lung or mediastinal tumours such as extralobar sequestration, thyroid teratoma and congenital goitre.

Hydrops is a non-specific finding in a wide variety of fetal and maternal disorders, including haematological, chromosomal, cardiovascular, pulmonary, gastrointestinal, hepatic and metabolic abnormalities, congenital infection, neoplasms and malformations of the placenta or umbilical cord (Machin, 1989). Cardiac and anaemic causes for non-immune hydrops are less likely in the presence of fetal pleural effusions than in their absence (Salztman *et al.*, 1989; Skoll, Sharland & Allan, 1991). While in many instances the underlying cause may be determined by detailed ultrasound scanning and investigations of maternal and fetal blood, frequently the abnormality remains unexplained even after expert postmortem examination. It has, therefore, been suggested that pleural effusions in cases of unexplained non-immune hydrops should be assumed *in utero* to be primary, with hydrops the consequence of raised intrathoracic pressure.

Pleural effusions are well recognised associations of Down syndrome (Foote & Vickers, 1986) and Turner syndrome (Chernick & Reed, 1970) in neonates. Although numbers are small, prenatal series report aneuploidy in approximately 10% of fetuses with isolated pleural effusions (Rodeck *et al.*, 1988; Nicolaides & Azar, 1990). This can also occur in association with hydrops.

Irrespective of the underlying cause, infants affected by pleural effusions usually present in the neonatal period with severe, and often fatal, respiratory insufficiency. This is either a direct result of pulmonary compression caused by the effusions, or the result of pulmonary hypoplasia secondary to chronic intrathoracic compression.

Table 16.1 *Reports on antenatally diagnosed pleural effusions managed conservatively in which the babies died*

Author	No. of babies	Site[a]	Hydrops	Age at diagnosis[b] (weeks)	Age at delivery[b] (weeks)	Outcome[c]
Carrol, 1977	1	R+L	Yes	36	36	IUD
Thomas & Anderson, 1979	1	R+L	No	32	35	NND
Bovicelli et al., 1981	1	R+L	No	35	38	NND
Jouppila et al., 1983	2	R+L	No	33	40	NND
		R	Yes	26	28	IUD
Peleg et al., 1985	3	R+L	Yes	34	35	NND
		R+L	Yes	33	33	NND
		R+L	No	34	34	NND
Castillo et al., 1987	6	R+L	Yes	26	32	NND
			Yes	26	40	NND
			No	30	38	NND
			Yes	26	27	NND
			Yes	25	28	IUD
			Yes	18	19	NND
Adams et al., 1988	1	L	No	25	39	NND
Longaker et al., 1989	10	R+L	Not stated	29 (18–35)	32 (22–37)	NND
Saltzman et al., 1989	9	R+L	Yes	28	Not stated	NND
		R+L	Yes	24	Not stated	IUD
		R+L	Yes	24	Not stated	IUD
		R+L	Yes	31	Not stated	NND
		R+L	Yes	34	Not stated	NND
		R+L	Yes	30	Not stated	NND
		R+L	Yes	26	Not stated	NND
		R+L	Yes	25	Not stated	IUD
		R+L	Yes	27	Not stated	NND
Moerman et al., 1993	5	R+L	Yes	29	29	NND
		R+L	Yes	40	40	IUD
		R+L	Yes	35	35	NND
		R+L	Yes	32	32	IUD
		R+L	Yes	30	30	NND

[a] Site of the effusion: R, right; L, left.

[b] Gestational age.

[c] IUD, babies died *in utero*; NND, babies died in the neonatal period.

Assessment

Fetal pleural effusions are non-specific entities. Detailed invesigation is essential to establish the primary aetiology, as this affects the clinical course and prognosis. Primary fetal hydrothorax is ultimately a diagnosis of exclusion.

Detailed ultrasonography is performed to exclude structural abnormalities associated with fetal pleural effusions and hydrops (Machin, 1989). More subtle abnormalities detected include fixed limb deformities, placental chorioangiomas and markers suggesting genetic syndromes. Next, fetal echocardiography is undertaken to exclude both structural abnormalities and arrhythmias, as these can account for up to 53% of non-immune hydrops (Skoll et al., 1991).

When a cause for the fetal pleural effusions cannot be determined on ultrasound, maternal and invasive fetal investigations are indicated.

Maternal serology is performed to exclude congenital infections (syphilis, toxoplasmosis, rubella, cytomegalovirus, herpes simplex and parvovirus B19). Maternal investigations are also done to exclude the possibility of anaemia in the fetus (Kleihauer–Betke test, group and antibody status, and haemoglobin electrophoresis).

The fetal karyotype and infection status are then determined. Although possible through amniocentesis, fetal blood sampling ensures more rapid results and has the advantage that the fetal haemoglobin and blood film may be assessed.

Conservative management

Isolated pleural effusions in the fetus may either resolve spontaneously or can be treated effectively after birth. Nevertheless, in some cases severe and chronic compression of the fetal lungs can result in pulmonary hypoplasia and neonatal death. In others, mediastinal compression leads to the development of hydrops and polyhydramnios, which are associated with a high risk of premature delivery and perinatal death.

There are at least four case reports of fetuses with isolated pleural effusions diagnosed at 16 to 32 weeks' gestation, where spontaneous resolution was documented within 2 to 12 weeks of diagnosis (Lien et al., 1990; Adams, Jones & Hayward, 1988; Sherer et al., 1992; Jaffe et al., 1986). In addition, spontaneous antenatal resolution occurred in a total of 5 (15%) of 33 fetuses (Longaker et al., 1989; Pijpers et al., 1989) in two series examining the natural history of antenatally diagnosed pleural effusions. All these babies survived.

There are also 24 published cases of pleural effusions, only four of which were untreated, that were managed conservatively and although the effusions did not resolve

the babies survived after appropriate postnatal treatment (Lange & Manning, 1981; Meizner, Carmi & Bar-Siv, 1986; Booth et al., 1987; Bruno et al., 1988; Adams et al., 1988; Longaker et al, 1989; Carmant & Guennec, 1989; Pijpers et al., 1989; Petrikovsky et al., 1991). In contrast, there are at least 39 reported cases of fetal pleural effusions that were managed conservatively and the outcome was either intrauterine or early neonatal death primarily as a result of pulmonary hypoplasia (Table 16.1). Therefore, overall perinatal survival was 46% in published reports of fetuses with hydrothoraces managed conservatively. Hydrops was present in 61% of fetuses that eventually died, compared with 33% of those that survived, suggesting that hydrops is a poor prognostic indicator.

Antenatal thoracocentesis

There are 17 reported cases of pleural effusions treated by antenatal thoracocentesis. In seven, the babies survived; this included all three in which there was spontaneous antenatal resolution of the pleural effusions after one to five thoracocenteses. Ten babies died either in utero or soon after birth as a result of pulmonary insufficiency. This survival rate is comparable to that of fetuses managed conservatively, although clearly selection criteria may have differed.

The data from fetuses with isolated pleural effusions suggest that certainly in some fetuses short-term decompression by thoracocentesis or temporary drainage may disrupt the underlying pathology. However, in the majority of cases the fluid reaccumulates within 24 hours, requiring repeated procedures which are likely to be more traumatic than pleuro-amniotic shunting.

Chronic antenatal drainage

Rationale

Studies in fetal lambs have demonstrated that progressive inflation of an intrathoracic balloon from day 100 of development resulted in respiratory insufficiency at birth, which was not improved by postnatal decompression. In contrast, prenatal decompression on day 120

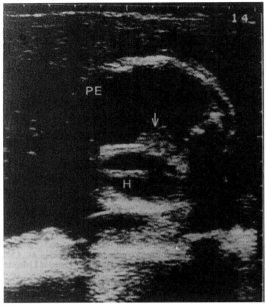

(a)

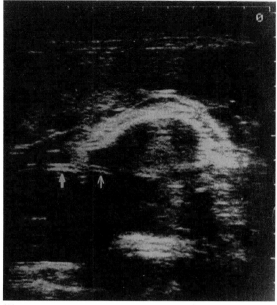

(b)

Fig. 16.1 *Ultrasound cross-sectional views of the fetal chest. (a) A large, right-sided pleural effusion (PE) with mediastinal shift, displacement of the heart (H) and a markedly compressed right lung (arrow). (b) At 24 hours after shunt insertion, the effusion has drained and the lung has re-expanded. Note the intrapleural (thin arrow) and extrapleural (thick arrow) portions of the catheter in situ. (From Rodeck et al., 1988, reproduced with permission of the authors.)*

was associated with normal respiratory function at birth because it prevented the development of pulmonary hypoplasia (Harrison *et al.*, 1980).

In addition to possible prevention of pulmonary hypoplasia, pleuro-amniotic shunting would facilitate neonatal resuscitation and could also potentially reverse hydrops and polyhydramnios.

Pleuro-amniotic shunt insertion

Shunting is usually performed as an out-patient procedure (Nicolaides & Azar, 1990), as described in Chapter 2. Under ultrasound guidance, the trochar and cannula is inserted through the fetal chest wall, in the

mid-thoracic region, into the effusion. After removing the trochar, a double pigtail catheter is positioned such that half of the catheter lies in the effusion and the other half of the catheter lies in the amniotic cavity (Fig. 16.1). If drainage of the contralateral lung is also needed, the appropriate fetal position is achieved by rotation of the fetal body using the tip of the cannula.

After shunting, serial scans are carried out at weekly intervals to determine if the effusions reaccumulate, in which case another shunt is inserted.

Results

Data are available from 16 published cases from other centres, as well as from our own extensive experience of 74 cases.

Other centres

Details of published cases are shown in Table 16.2. Roberts *et al.* (1986) inserted one end of an epidural catheter into the unilateral pleural effusion of a fetus at 25 weeks' gestation; the other end of the catheter was placed in a bag on the mother's abdomen. During the first 24 hours, 70 ml of bright yellow fluid was drained,

Table 16.2 *Reported cased of pleuro-amniotic shunting in centres other than the Harris Birthright Research Centre*

Author	No. of fetuses	Site[a]	Hydrops	Age at shunting[b] (weeks)	Age at delivery[b] (weeks)	Outcome[c]	Comments
Seeds & Bowes, 1986	1	R+L	Yes	30	31	Alive	
Weiner *et al.*, 1986	1	L	Yes	25+27+27	29	NND	Extralobar sequestration
Rodeck *et al.*, 1988	8	L	No	27	39	Alive	
		R+L	Yes	28	32	Alive	
		R	No	32	34	Alive	Trisomy 21
		R	No	25	39	Alive	
		R+L	Yes	35+36	39	Alive	
		R+L	Yes	31+32	34	Alive	
		R+L	Yes	31	32	NND	
		R+L	Yes	29	32	NND	
Longaker *et al.*, 1989	1	R+L	Yes	30+31	32	Alive	
King *et al.*, 1991	1	R+L	Yes	34	38	IUD	
Mandelbrot *et al.*, 1992	2	R+L	Yes	31	32	NND	Opitz
		R+L	Yes	31	34	Alive	Trigonocephaly
Ronderos-Dumit *et al.*, 1993	1	R+L	Yes	33	37	Alive	
Becker *et al.*, 1993	1	L	Yes	23+27	36	Alive	

[a] Site of the effusion: R, right; L, left.

[b] Gestational age.

[c] NND, babies died in the neonatal period; IUD, babies died *in utero*.

but only 30 ml drained over the next five days and subsequently the catheter was removed. The effusion did not reaccumulate and a healthy infant was delivered at term. Seeds & Bowes (1986) inserted pleuro-amniotic catheters in a fetus with large pleural effusions at 30 weeks' gestation. Postoperatively, fetal activity increased, polyhydramnios decreased and there was cessation of the uterine contractions that were present before shunting. However, after three days the effusions reaccumulated because one of the catheters had come out of the fetal chest, and the other catheter had been drawn under the fetal skin surface. Polyhydramnios increased and the infant, delivered 48 hours later, made a good recovery after drainage and ventilatory support. Weiner *et al.* (1986) performed pleuro-amniotic shunting at 25 weeks in a hydropic fetus with extralobar sequestration. Although there was resolution of the oedema and ascites, the infant born at 29 weeks died in the neonatal period.

Rodeck *et al.* (1988) reported eight cases with pleural effusions, including five with hydrops, that were shunted at 25 to 35 weeks' gestation. The infants were delivered at 32 to 39 weeks' gestation; six infants survived with good respiratory function and two died in the neonatal period as as result of pulmonary hypoplasia. In the latter two cases, the lungs did not expand after pleuro-amniotic shunting.

Harris Birthright Centre

During a 10 year period (1985–94), pleuro-amniotic shunting was performed in 74 singleton pregnancies. The data of the first 47 cases were reported previously (Blott, Nicolaides & Greenough, 1988; Nicolaides & Azar, 1990). Pleuro-amniotic shunting was considered if there was associated hydrops, polyhydramnios or major, progressive pulmonary compression and/or mediastinal shift. Fetal karyotyping was performed at the time of shunting and if abnormal, or if hydrops worsened, the option of termination was discussed with the parents. If intrathoracic fluid reaccumulated, further shunting was considered.

In five cases, the pregnancies were terminated at the request of the parents because the fetuses were found to have Down syndrome ($n = 3$), Turner syndrome ($n = 1$), or progressive hydrops despite successful drainage of the effusions ($n = 1$).

In the 69 cases where the pregnancies continued, the effusions were bilateral in 55% and unilateral with associated mediastinal shift in 45%. Fetal ascites and/or generalized skin oedema was present in 23% of the 31 with unilateral effusions and in 89% of the 38 with bilateral effusions. All had normal karyotypes, except for one fetus with trisomy 21.

Insertion of pleuro-amniotic shunts resulted in rapid expansion of the lungs in all but one fetus, which was subsequently found to have arthrogryposis. In cases with unilateral effusions, there was a simultaneous shift of the heart to its normal position within the thorax. In eight cases (12%), the effusions reaccumulated one to three weeks after shunting, presumably because the shunts blocked or the fetus pulled out the shunt; in these cases further shunts were inserted.

Polyhydramnios was present in 62% of the 69 cases and this resolved within one to three weeks after shunting in 65%. Similarly, hydrops resolved in 46% of the 41 affected pregnancies.

All 28 non-hydropic fetuses survived (Table 16.3), but in the hydropic group 19 (46%) of the 41 babies survived and 22 (54%) died *in utero* or in the neonatal period (Table 16.4). The six intrauterine deaths occurred one to eight weeks after shunting, which was effective in draining the pleural effusions but did not prevent progressive increase in skin oedema. In the group of neonatal deaths, there were two cases of diaphragmatic hernia and one case each of major cardiac defect, arthrogryposis, pseudomonas septicaemia and disseminated intravascular coagulation; in 10 cases death was caused by a combination of respiratory, cardiovascular and renal failure.

In the 47 surviving infants, seven (15%) required surgery for atrioventricular septal defect, coarctation of the aorta, thyroid teratoma, congenital porto-caval shunt, congenital diaphragmatic hernia, pulmonary extralobar sequestration or cystic hygroma.

Booth *et al.* (1987) examined the neonatal course of two babies from our centre with hydrops fetalis associated with pleural effusions. One baby that was treated by pleuro-amniotic shunting had no effusion at birth and required less resuscitation than the baby with no antenatal intervention. Thompson, Greenough & Nicolaides (1993) examined the respiratory status at 3 to 60 months of age in 17 of these infants who had undergone pleuro-amniotic shunting. Although six (35%) suffered from recurrent respiratory symptoms, this incidence is similar to that found in healthy infants born at term (Greenough, Maconochie & Yuksel, 1990). The mean functional residual capacity of these 17 infants was normal, suggesting that pleuro-amniotic shunting may have permitted normal lung growth (Thompson *et al.*, 1993); infants with impaired lung growth have small volume lungs (Helms, 1982).

Overall results

Table 16.5 summarizes perinatal survival results after conservative management, antenatal thoracocentesis or pleuro-amniotic shunting in fetuses with pleural effusions. Although these data are uncontrolled, shunting was associated with higher survival rates than thoracocentesis and conservative management in both hydropic and non-hydropic fetuses. Nevertheless, shunting was associated with perinatal survival in only 50% of hydropic fetuses, confirming that hydrops is a major adverse prognostic variable. Polyhydramnios independent of the presence or absence of hydrops does not appear to influence the chance of survival.

The data on pleuro-amniotic shunting also demonstrate the value of this technique in diagnosis and assessment. First, the diagnosis of an underlying cardiac abnormality or other intrathoracic lesion may become apparent only after effective decompression and return of the mediastinum to its normal position. Second, it may be useful in the prenatal diagnosis of pulmonary hypoplasia because in such cases the lungs often fail to expand after shunting. Third, it may help distinguish between hydrops caused by primary accumulation of pleural effusions, in which case the ascites and skin oedema may resolve after shunting, and other causes of hydrops such as infection, in which drainage of the effusions does not prevent worsening of the hydrops.

Table 16.3 *Results of pluero-amniotic shunting at the Harris Birthright Research Centre in fetuses with pleural effusions in the absence of hydrops*

Case	Site[a]	AFV[b]	Age at shunt[c] (weeks)	Age at delivery[c] (weeks)	Outcome	Comments
1	L	N	20	32	Alive	
2	L	N	20	36	Alive	
3	L	N	20	39	Alive	
4	L	N	20	41	Alive	
5	R+L	N	21	37	Alive	
6	L	N	21	41	Alive	
7	R	N	22	38	Alive	Diaphragmatic hernia
8	L	N	22	39	Alive	
9	R	P[d]	24	39	Alive	
10	L	P[d]	24+26	39	Alive	
11	L	P	27	32	Alive	
12	R+L	N	27	37	Alive	
13	L	N	27	39	Alive	
14	L	N	28	39	Alive	
15	R	N	29	31	Alive	
16	R	N	29	41	Alive	
17[e]	L	P	30	30	Alive	
18	L	P[d]	30	34	Alive	
19	R	P[d]	30	34	Alive	
20	L	N	31	36	Alive	Extralobar sequestration
21	R	N	31	38	Alive	
22	R	P[d]	31	38	Alive	
23	R	P[d]	32	35	Alive	Atrioventricular septal defect, trisomy 21
24	R	P	32+34	35	Alive	
25	R	P	33	35	Alive	Cystic hygroma
26	L	P[d]	33	39	Alive	
27	R+L	P[d]	34	37	Alive	
28	R+L	P[d]	35	39	Alive	

[a] Site of effusion: R, right; L, left.
[b] AFV, amniotic fluid volume is either normal (N) or polyhydramnios (P).
[c] Gestational age.
[d] Resolution of polyhydramnics after shunting.
[e] Presented in labour.

Table 16.4 *Pleuro-amniotic shunting at the Harris Birthright Research Centre in hydropic fetuses with pleural effusions*

Case	Site[a]	Ascites[b]	Oedema[b]	AFV[c]	Age at shunt[d] (weeks)	Age of delivery[d] (weeks)	Outcome[e]	Comments
1	R+L	++	++	N	20	33	Alive	Congenital porto-caval shunt
2	R+L	++	+	N	21	37	Alive, R	
3	R+L	+	+	P[f]	22	38	Alive, R	
4	R+L	+	+	N	24+26+29	39	Alive, R	
5	R+L	++	−	N	25	38	Alive, R	
6	R	+	+	P[f]	26	37	Alive, R	
7	R+L	+	++	P[f]	30	36	Alive, R	
8	R+L	+	+	P[f]	30+32	38	Alive, R	
9	R+L	++	+	P[f]	31	37	Alive, R	
10	R+L	+	+	N	32	33	Alive, R	
11	R+L	+	+	P	32	33	Alive	
12	R+L	++	+	P[f]	32	35	Alive, R	
13	L+R	++	−	P[f]	32	39	Alive, R	
14	L	+	++	P[f]	32	40	Alive, R	
15	R	−	++	P	33	34	Alive	Thyroid teratoma
16	R+L	++	++	P[f]	33	37	Alive, R	
17	R	++	++	P[f]	33	38	Alive, R	Supraventricular tachycardia
18	R	+	++	P[f]	33	38	Alive, R	Coarctation of the aorta
19	L	++	+	P	34	36	Alive	
20	R+L	++	+	N	22	23	IUD	Mucopolysacharoidosis VII
21	R+L	++	++	N	22	30	IUD	
22	R+L	+	++	N	23	25	IUD	Recurrent unexplained hydrops
23	R+L	++	++	P[f]	24	26	IUD	
24	R+L	+	++	P[f]	26	27	IUD	
25	R+L	+	++	P[f]	35	36	IUD	
26	R+L	++	++	N	20	29	NND	
27	R+L	+	++	P	25	32	NND, R	Recurrent unexplained hydrops
28	R+L	++	++	O	26	35	NND	
29	R+L	−	++	P	28	32	NND	
30	R+L	+	++	Pf	2?–32	33	NND, R	
31	R+L	++	+	P[f]	29–30	31	NND	
32	R+L	++	++	P[f]	29	32	NND	Disseminated intravascular coagulation
33	R+L	++	++	P[f]	29–32	35	NND	Pseudomonas septicaemia
34	R+L	+	++	Pf	30	31	NND	
35	R+L	++	++	P	30	31	NND, R	
36	R+L	++	+	N	30	35	NND, R	Diaphragmatic hernia
37	R+L	+	+	P	31	32	NND	
38	R+L	+	++	P	31–32	35	NND	Arthrogryposis
39	R+L	−	++	P	33	34	NND	Univentricular heart
40	R+L	+	++	P	35	36	NND	
41	R	+	++	P	35	37	NND	Diaphragmatic hernia

[a] Site of effusion: R, right; L, left.
[b] Associated ascites and oedema classified as mild/moderate (+) or severe (++).
[c] AFV, amniotic fluid volume: N, normal; P, polyhydramnios, O, oligohydramnios.
[d] Gestational age.
[e] Outcome: IUD, intrauterine death; NND, neonatal death; R, resolution of hydrops after shunting.
[f] Resolution of polyhydramnics after shunting.

Table 16.5 *Perinatal survival in non-hydropic and hydropic fetuses with pleural effusions, by mode of treatment* [a]

Management	Non-hydrops		Hydrops	
	Total	Alive	Total	Alive
Conservative	35	29 (83%)	26	3 (12%)
Thoracocentesis	8	4 (50%)	9	3 (33%)
Pleuro-amniotic shunting	31	31 (100%)	54	27 (50%)

[a] Includes published reports and data from the Harris Birthright Centre.

Delivery

In fetuses that have not been shunted intrapartum, thoracocentesis can be performed to facilitate neonatal resuscitation. This is of particular importance for those units without constant availability of highly trained neonatal staff and the appropriate equipment to perform drainage within seconds of delivery. Petres, Redwine & Cruikshank (1982), drained the right pleural effusion of a fetus at 36 weeks' gestation, but this reaccumulated within 24 hours. At 37 weeks, when the mother was in labour, the effusion was again drained and the infant was born in good condition. Similarly, Schmidt, Harms & Wolf (1985) reported the successful intrapartum thoracocentesis and paracentesis in a hydropic fetus at 35 weeks' gestation; the infant required assisted ventilation until the 20th day after birth and survived. One problem with this approach is reaccumulation before delivery, and chronic pleuro-amniotic shunting can be used to ensure that the lung remains expanded until labour ensures. After delivery, the chest drains are immediately clamped and removed to avoid the development of pneumothorax.

Maternal morbidity

Ronderos-Dumit *et al.* (1993) described a case of bilateral pleural effusions, hydrops and polyhydramnios in which pleuro-amniotic shunting was complicated by the development of massive maternal ascites and oligohydramnios. This was presumably the result of amniotic fluid leakage through the uterine wall. After 24 hours, there was resolution of maternal ascites and reaccumulation of amniotic fluid. Subsequently, the pregnancy progressed uneventfully and a healthy infant was delivered at 37 weeks' gestation, four weeks after shunting.

Becker *et al.* (1993) performed pleuro-amniotic shunting in a hydropic fetus at 23 weeks' gestation. However, the shunt got stuck in the uterine wall. A further shunt was introduced a few day later. Serial scans demonstrated effective drainage of the effusions and resolution of the hydrops. However, ultrasound examination at 36 weeks, after spontaneous onset of labour, failed to demonstrate any of the shunts. Abdominal X-ray was performed which identified one of the catheters in the uterine wall and the other in the upper maternal abdomen. After delivery, one of the catheters was found in the amniotic membranes and the second was removed by laparoscopy. The infant was well.

Conclusions

Pleuro-amniotic shunting is an effective and apparently safe method of chronic drainage of fetal pleural effusions. It can reverse fetal hydrops, resolve polyhydramnios and thereby reduce the risk of preterm delivery, and may prevent pulmonary hypoplasia. The alternative management of pleural effusions by thoracocentesis, immediately before or after delivery, could prevent respiratory distress in the neonate if this is the result of simple mechanical compression of the otherwise normally developed lung. However, such treatment would not prevent pulmonary hypoplasia, caused by prolonged intrathoracic compression, or indeed progressive disease from pleural effusions to hydrops fetalis and intrauterine death. Nevertheless, in approximately half of the hydropic fetuses pleuro-amniotic shunting does not prevent their ultimate death, which is presumably the consequence of the underlying disease causing the hydrops.

References

Adams, H., Jones, A. & Hayward, C. (1988). The sonographic features and implications of fetal pleural effusions. *Clinical Radiology*, 39, 398–401.

Becker, R., Arabin B., Novak A., Entezami, M. & Weitzel, H. K. (1993). Successful treatment of primary fetal hydrothorax by long-time drainage from week 23. *Fetal Diagnosis and Therapy*, 8, 331–7.

Benacerraf, B. R., Frigoletto, F. D. Jr & Wilson, M. (1986). Successful midtrimester thoracentesis with analysis of the lymphocyte population in the pleural effusion. *American Journal of Obstetrics and Gynecology*, 155, 398–9.

Blott, M., Nicolaides, K. H. & Greenough, A. (1988). Pleuroamniotic shunting for decompression of fetal pleural effusions. *Obstetrics and Gynecology*, 71, 798–800.

Booth, P., Nicolaides, K. H., Greenough, A. & Gamsu, H. R. (1987). Pleuro-amniotic shunting for fetal chylothorax. *Early Human Development*, 15, 365–7.

Bovicelli, L., Rizzo, N., Orsini, L. F. & Calderoni, P. (1981). Ultrasonic real-time diagnosis of fetal hydrothorax and lung hypoplasia. *Journal of Clinical Ultrasound*, 9, 253–4.

Bruno M., Iskra L., Dolfin, G. & Farina, D. (1988). Congenital pleural effusion: prenatal ultrasonic diagnosis and therapeutic management. *Prenatal Diagnosis*, 8, 157–9.

Carmant, L. & Guennec, J. C. (1989). Congenital chylothorax and persistent pulmonary hypertension of the neonate. *Acta Paediatrica Scandinavica*, 78, 789–92.

Carrol, B. (1977). Pulmonary hypoplasia and pleural effusions associated with fetal death in utero: ultrasonic findings. *American Journal of Roentgenology*, 129, 749–50.

Castillo, R. A., Devoe, L. D., Falls, G., Holzman, G. B., Hadi, H. A. & Fadel, H. E. (1987). Pleural effusion and pulmonary hypoplasia. *American Journal of Obstetrics and Gynecology*, 157, 1252–5.

Chernick, V. & Reed, M. H. (1970). Pneumothorax and chylothorax in the neonatal period. *Journal of Pediatrics*, 76, 624–32.

Elser, H., Borutto, F., Schneider, A. & Schneider, K. (1983) Chylothorax in a twin pregnancy of 34 weeks – sonographically diagnosed. *European Journal of Obstetrics, Gynaecology and Rerproductive Biology*, 16, 205–11.

Fisk, N. M. & Rodeck, C. H. (1991). Antenatal diagnosis and fetal medicine. In *Textbook of Neonatology*, 2nd edn, ed. N. C. Roberton, pp. 121–50. Edinburgh: Churchill Livingstone.

Foote, K. D. & Vickers, D. W. (1986). Congenital pleural effusion in Down's syndrome. *British Journal of Radiology*, 59, 609–10.

Greenough, A., Maconochie, I. & Yuksel, B. (1990). Recurrent respiratory symptoms in the first year of life following preterm delivery. *Journal of Perinatal Medicine*, 8, 489–94.

Harrison, M. R., Bressack, M. A., Churg, A. M. & Lorimier, A. A. (1980). Correction of congenital diaphragmatic hernia in utero. II Simulated correction permits fetal lung growth with survival at birth. *Surgery*, 88, 260–8.

Helms, P. (1982). Lung function in infants with congenital pulmonary hypoplasia. *Journal of Paediatrics*, 101, 918–22.

Jaffe, R., Segni, E. D., Altaras, M., Loebel, R. & Aderet, N. B. (1986). Ultrasonic real-time diagnosis of transitory fetal pleural and pericardial effusion. *Diagnostic Imaging in Clinical Medicine*, 55, 373–5.

Jouppila, P., Kirkinen, P., Herva, R. & Koivisto, M. (1983). Prenatal diagnosis of pleural effusions by ultrasound. *Journal of Clinical Ultrasound*, 11, 516–19.

King, P. A., Ghosh, A., Tang, M. H. Y. & Lam, S. K. (1991). Recurrent congenital chylothorax. *Prenatal Diagnosis*, 11, 809–11.

Lange, I. R. & Manning, F. A. (1981). Antenatal diagnosis of congenital pleural effusions. *American Journal of Obstetrics and Gynecology*, 140, 839–40.

Lien, J. M., Colmorgen, G. H. C., Gehret, J. F. & Evantash, A. B. (1990). Spontaneous resolution of fetal pleural effusion diagnosed during the second trimester. *Journal of Clinical Ultrasound*, 18, 54–6.

Longaker, M. T., Laberge, J. M., Dansereau, J., Langer, J. C., Crombleholme, T. M., Callen, P. W., Golbus, M. S. & Harrison, M. R. (1989). Primary fetal hydrothorax: natural history and management. *Journal of Pediatric Surgery*, 24, 573–6.

Machin, G. A. (1989). Hydrops revisited: literature review of 1414 cases published in the 1980s. *American Journal of Medical Genetics*, 34, 366–90.

Mandelbrot, L., Dommergues, M., Aubry, M. C., Mussat, P. & Dumez, Y. (1992). Reversal of fetal distress by emergency in utero decompression of hydrothorax. *American Journal of Obstetrics and Gynecology*, 167, 1278–83.

Meizner, I., Carmi, R. & Bar-Siv, J. (1986). Congenital chylothorax – prenatal ultrasonic diagnosis and successful post partum management. *Prenatal Diagnosis*, 6, 217–21.

Moerman, P., Vandenberghe, K., Devlieger, H., Hole, C. V., Fryns, J. P. & Lauweryns, J. M. (1993). Congenital pulmonary lymphangiectasis with chylothorax: a heterogeneous lymphatic vessel abnormality. *American Journal of Medical Genetics*, 47, 54–8.

Nicolaides, K. H. & Azar, G. B. (1990). Thoraco-amniotic shunting. *Fetal Diagnosis and Therapy*, 5, 153–64.

Peleg, D., Golichowski, A. M. & Ragan, W. D. (1985). Fetal hydrothorax and bilateral pulmonary hypoplasia. *Acta Obstetricia et Gynecologica Scandinavica*, 64, 451–3.

Petres, R. E., Redwine, F. O. & Cruikshank, D. P. (1982). Congenital bilateral chylothorax. Antepartum diagnosis and successful intrauterine surgical management. *Journal of the American Medical Association*, 248, 1360–1.

Petrikovsky, B. M., Shmoys, S. M., Baker, D. A. & Monheit, A. G. (1991). Pleural effusion in aneuploidy. *American Journal of Perinatology*, 91, 214–16.

Pijpers, L., Reuss, A., Stewart, P. A. & Wladimiroff, J. W. (1989). Noninvasive management of isolated bilateral fetal hydrothorax. *American Journal of Obstetrics and Gynecology*, 161, 330–2.

Roberts, A. B., Clarkson, P. M., Pattison, N. S., Jamieson, M. G. & Mok, P. M. (1986). Fetal hydrothorax in the second trimester of pregnancy: successful intra-uterine treatment at 24 weeks' gestation. *Fetal Therapy*, 1, 203–9.

Rodeck, C. H., Fisk, N. M., Fraser, D. I. & Nicolini U. (1988). Long-term in utero drainage of fetal hydrothorax. *New England Journal of Medicine*, 319, 1135–8.

Ronderos-Dumit, D., Nicolini, U., Vaughan, J., Fisk, N. M., Chamberlain, P. F. & Rodeck, C. H. (1991). Uterine-peritoneal amniotic fluid leakage: an unusual complication of intrauterine shunting. *Obstetrics and Gynecology*, 78, 913–15.

Saltzman, D. H., Frigoletto, F. D., Harlow, B. L., Barss, V. A. & Benacerraf, B. R. (1989). Sonographic evaluation of hydrops fetalis. *Obstetrics and Gynecology*, 74, 106–11.

Seeds, J. W & Bowes, W. A., Jr (1986). Results of treatment severe feral hydrothorax with bilateral pleuroamniotic catheters. *Obstetrics and Gynecology*, 68, 577–9.

Schmidt, W., Harms, E. & Wolf, D. (1985). Successful prenatal treatment of non-immune hydrops fetalis due to congenital chylothorax. Case report. *British Journal of Obstetrics and Gynaecology*, 92, 685–7.

Scott-Emuakpor, A. B., Warren, S. T., Kapur, S., Quiachon, E. B. & Higgins, J. V. (1981). Familiar occurrence of congenital pulmonary lymphan-giectasis. Genetic implications. *American Journal of Diseases in Children*, 135, 532–4.

Sherer, D. M., Abramowicz, J. S., Eggers, P. C. & Woods, J. R., Jr (1992). Transient severe unilateral and subsequent bilateral primary fetal hydrothorax with spontaneous resolution at 34 weeks' gestational associated with normal neonatal outcome. *American Journal of Obstetrics and Gynecology*, 166, 169–70.

Skoll, M. A., Sharland, G. K. & Allan, L. D. (1991). Is the ultrasound definition of fluid collections in non immune hydrops fetalis helpful in defining the underlying cause or predicting outcome? *Ultrasound in Obstetrics and Gynecology*, 1, 309–12.

Thomas, D. B. & Anderson, J. C. (1979). Antenatal detection of fetal pleural effusion and neonatal management. *Medical Journal of Australia*, 2, 435–6.

Thompson, P. J., Greenough, A. & Nicolaides, K. H. (1993). Respiratory function in infancy following pleuro-amniotic shunting. *Fetal Diagnosis and Therapy*, 8, 79–83.

Weiner, C. P., Varner, M., Pringle, K., Hein, H., Williamson, R. & Smith W. L. (1986). Antenatal diagnosis and palliative treatment of nonimmune hydrops fetalis secondary to pulmonary extralobar sequestration. *Obstetrics and Gynecology*, 68, 275–80.

17   Urinary tract obstruction

DAVID C. MERRILL AND CARL P. WEINER

Introduction

Developmental abnormalities of the genitourinary tract are among the most common sonographically identified anomalies, with an incidence of 1 in 250 to 1 in 1000 pregnancies. Obstructive uropathies account for the majority of cases. The obstruction may be at the level of the ureteropelvic junction (UPJ), the ureterovesical junction (UVJ) or the urethra. An obstruction can be either unilateral or bilateral. UPJ and UVJ obstructions are typically unilateral, whereas those at the level of the urethra are by definition bilateral. The prognosis for the fetus with urinary obstruction at the level of either the UPJ or UVJ is generally quite good unless other anomalies are present. There is rarely a need for early obstetrical intervention with unilateral obstruction. In cases of bilateral severe obstruction, preterm delivery with postnatal relief of the obstruction may on occasion be indicated. However, in the majority of cases, routine obstetrical care is not altered.

It is in the fetus with a urethral obstruction that antenatal intervention may be an acceptable option since perinatal mortality can be high. Considerable investigation has been undertaken both to help elucidate the pathophysiology of severe urethral obstruction utilizing animal models and to identify fetuses who may be candidates for antenatal therapy. In this chapter, we will focus on urethral level obstruction, reviewing the current understanding of the pathophysiology and natural history of this condition, the antenatal diagnosis and suggested workup of such cases, the types of antenatal intervention which have been attempted, the short-term and long-term outcomes utilizing such interventions, and a proposed management scheme.

Natural history

Knowledge of the natural history of any clinical condition is essential not only for accurate counselling of patients but also to assess the efficacy of intervention. The natural history of bladder outlet obstruction proved difficult if not impossible to elucidate prior to the advent of routine antenatal sonography.

The most common aetiology of bladder outlet obstruction is posterior urethral valves in males followed by urethral atresia (Steinhardt et al., 1990) and prune belly syndrome (Cullen et al., 1989). A review of the paediatric urology literature (Churchill et al., 1990; Williams, 1977) suggests that the prognosis for infants with posterior urethral valves has improved dramatically, declining from 25% in the 1960s to 3% in the 1970s, to nearly 0% in the 1980s. However, it is estimated that 25 to 30% of children who survive the neonatal period subsequently develop end-stage renal disease necessitating dialysis, transplantation, or both. (Parkhouse et al., 1988; Warshaw, Edelbrook & Ettinger, 1982). Therefore, any assessment of the efficacy of antenatal therapy requires long-term follow-up. The mortality associated with bladder outlet obstruction is probably much higher than that reported in the paediatric literature because of early neonatal and fetal deaths which are never seen by the paediatric urologist.

Long-term urethral obstruction is associated with cystic renal dysplasia, decreased renal function, oligohydramnios, pulmonary hypoplasia, Potters facies, and limb abnormalities secondary to extrinsic compression. Although most series are small, a clearer picture of the natural history of urethral obstruction (Barss, Benacerraf & Frigoletto, 1984; Bastide et al., 1986) is forming with the emergence of routine sonography. Thomas *et al.* (1985) reported 18 infants with bilateral obstruction detected antenatally. The mortality rate was 33%, and 56% had coexistent abnormalities. Despite prompt postnatal treatment, only 22% of the infants were felt to have a good prognosis for renal function. Mahoney *et al.* (1985) reviewed 40 fetuses with antenatally diagnosed urethral obstruction. Overall mortality in this series was 63%; if the pregnancy had been associated with oligohydramnios, the mortality was 80%. Although normal to increased amounts of amniotic fluid did not guarantee survival, the associated mortality was much lower at 25%. Nakayama *et al.* (1986) reported 11 fetuses with posterior urethral valves diagnosed shortly after birth. Mortality was 45%. Three infants died of pulmonary hypoplasia and two died of rapidly progressive renal disease. Of the six survivors, three ultimately developed renal failure. Hayden *et al.* (1988) reviewed 11 cases of fetal urethral obstruction managed expectantly. Only 9% of the infants survived beyond five weeks. Reuss *et al.* (1988) reported 43 cases of fetal obstructive uropathy also managed expectantly; survival was 28%. Consistent with prior observations (Hellstrom, Kogan & Jeffrey, 1984), only 1 of the 12 survivors was noted to have reduced amniotic fluid. From these retrospective, descriptive studies, the clinical consequences of significant urethral obstruction are obvious.

Pathophysiology in animal models

Several animal models in various species, including the lamb, rabbit, chick and opossum, have been developed in an attempt to elucidate the pathophysiological mechanisms associated with congenital obstructive uropathy (Adzick *et al.*, 1985b; Beck, 1971; Bermann & Maizels, 1982; Bussieres *et al.*, 1993; Glick *et al.*, 1983; 1984; Harrison *et al.*, 1982b; 1983; Maizels & Simpson, 1983; Peters *et al.*, 1991a,b; 1992). Their relevance to spontaneous disease remains controversial. Beck (1971) first demonstrated in fetal sheep that the consequences of ureteral ligation are dependent on the gestational age when the obstruction occurs. Simple hydronephrosis always results when ureteral ligation is performed in the last half of gestation. However, ureteral obstruction,

either unilateral or bilateral, performed during the first half of gestation results in small, hydronephrotic kidneys with histological features similar to human dysplasia. Histological changes noted include primitive ductules, undifferentiated mesenchymal stroma, and ducts lined with cuboidal to columnar epithelium and surrounded by mesenchymal collars. This work was confirmed by Glick and Harrison (1983) who created their obstructions in fetal sheep at 55–65 days' gestation (term is 145 days).

In other studies, Glick *et al.* (1984) addressed the question of whether antenatal decompression of the urinary obstruction could prevent or reverse renal damage. In these studies, fetal sheep underwent decompression of the unilateral obstruction 20, 40 or 60 days after the initial procedure. They reported that the recovery of renal function is directly proportional to the duration of *in utero* decompression and is inversely proportional to the duration of obstruction. In addition, *in utero* decompression reduced the severity of the renal histological changes.

Despite these studies, the applicability of animal models to the human fetus remains controversial, since it is unclear whether or not the renal dysplasia seen in the human fetus in cases of severe bladder outlet obstruction is caused solely by the mechanical obstruction (Bernstein, 1971). Though some continue to believe that dysplasia is caused by increased pressure secondary to the mechanical obstruction, other evidence indicates that it may be caused by an abnormal interaction between the ureteral bud and its metanephrogenic mesenchyme. The work of Berman and Maizels (1982) is often quoted as evidence against mechanical obstruction being the primary mechanism for the renal damage. To study very early ureteral obstruction, these investigators developed an *in vitro* model using early chick embryonic metanephric rudiments and ureters. The ureter and blastema were transplanted onto chick chorioallantoic membranes, and the ureter ligated. Hydronephrosis was the only pathological result associated with early ligation. However, when the model was modified by stripping away some of the mesenchyme of the metanephric rudiments, dysplastic changes were observed. These results suggest that mechanical obstruction is not the sole explanation for the renal dysplasia noted in cases of obstructive uropathy. In addition, the model created by

Harrison *et al.* (1983) of bladder outlet obstruction in the fetal lamb did not produce the histological changes of renal dysplasia commonly observed with severe urethral obstruction in the human fetus. This stands in contrast to their result with ureteral ligation, where the fetus does develop pulmonary hypoplasia and renal lesions that are partially corrected by *in utero* decompression. Another issue is the point in gestation when the obstruction occurs. Even if obstruction is the sole cause of renal damage in the human fetus, it is possible that any harm may not be reversible when discovered several months later.

Despite this controversy and the potential lack of applicability to the human condition, these animal studies provide the basis for clinical trials to evaluate the potential for *in utero* therapy in the human fetus. However, it is important to consider the results of these animal studies when attempting to understand or explain the success or failure of attempts of *in utero* urinary diversion procedures in the human fetus.

Sonographic diagnosis

Sonography is relatively sensitive in the detection of fetal urinary tract obstruction (Arger *et al.*, 1985; Chinn & Filly, 1982; Glazer, Filly & Callen, 1982; Gruenewald *et al.*, 1984; Helin & Persson, 1986; Hobbins *et al.*, 1984; Reuss *et al.*, 1987; Seeds, Mittelstaedt & Mandell, 1986; Stiller, 1989). Portions of the fetal urinary system can be seen as early as 12 weeks of gestation. The sonographic criteria for the diagnosis of hydronephrosis is less clear in the fetus than the child since many fetuses normally have a small amount of pyelectasis. Arger *et al.* (1985) suggested that hydronephrosis should not be diagnosed unless either the renal pelvic diameter is >10 mm in the anterior posterior dimension or the pelvic to kidney ratio is >O.5. The latter criterium is not widely accepted. If hydronephrosis is detected, a complete evaluation of the fetal urinary tract usually permits localization of the level of urinary tract obstruction. A complete anomaly scan should be performed since urinary malformations are often associated with abnormalities of other organ systems and karyotype abnormalities (Brumfield *et al.*, 1991; Hirata, Medearis & Platt, 1990).

Hydronephrosis can result from obstruction at the level of the UPJ, UVJ or the urethra. Obstruction at the level of the UVJ is the rarest of the three. It is commonly associated with ureteral duplication and an ectopic ureterocoele. Sonographically, it appears as a dilated upper pole with a normal appearing lower pole, and/or a dilated ureter with an ectopic ureterocoele protruding into the lumen of the fetal bladder (see Fig. 17.1). UPJ obstruction, the most common of the three, is usually a diagnosis of exclusion. The diagnosis is made sonographically when there is evidence of fetal hydronephrosis and no evidence of either ureterectasis, vesicomegaly, ectopic ureterocoele, or posterior urethral dilatation (see Fig. 17.2). The diagnosis of bladder outlet or urethral obstruction is easily made with ultrasound. The main sonographic findings associated with urethral obstruction include dilatation of the fetal urinary bladder, proximal urethral dilatation, and thickening of the urinary bladder wall. Caliectasis and ureterectasis, however, are inconsistent findings in cases of urethral obstruction (see Fig. 17.3).

It is important to differentiate true urethral obstruction from megacystis microcolon intestinal hypoperistalsis syndrome (MMIHS). MMIHS is a rare disorder characterized by functional intestinal obstruction and an enlarged nonobstructed bladder. This condition is generally associated with a poor prognosis for long-term survival; the aetiology is unknown. The sonographic differentiation of true obstruction from MMIHS can at times be difficult. The presence of a fetus, especially a female, with evidence of urinary obstruction and increased amniotic fluid volume suggests MMIHS as opposed to true urethral obstruction.

Antenatal assessment

In any fetus with bladder outlet obstruction in whom *in utero* therapy is contemplated, a detailed anomaly scan and determination of the fetal karyotype are obligatory. Overall, karyotypic abnormalities and congenital malformations of other organ systems are observed in 15 to 40% of cases of fetal obstructive uropathy (Holzgreve & Evans, 1993). A sample for the fetal karyotype can be obtained by means of amniocentesis, chorionic villus

Fig. 17.1 *Sonogram of fetus with ureterovesical junction obstruction secondary to ureterocoele. The short arrow points to the ureterocoele within the bladder. The long arrow points to the dilated ureter.*

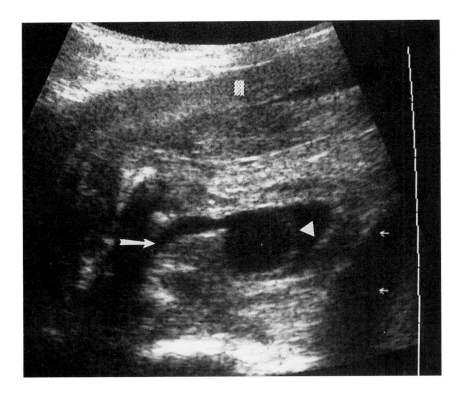

Fig. 17.2 *Sonogram of fetus with bilateral hydronephrosis secondary to mid-ureteral obstruction. The triangle (left panel) is in the dilated pelvis of the left kidney. The long arrow (right panel) demonstrates the dilated loops of the ureter proximal to the obstruction.*

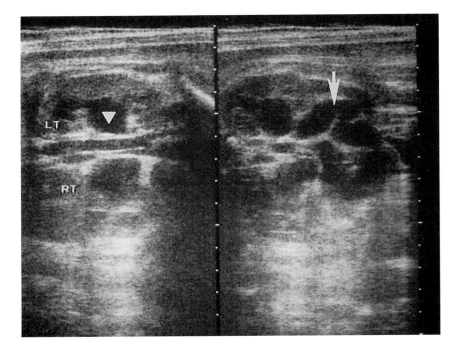

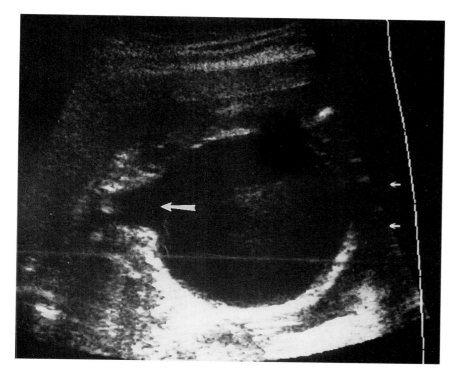

Fig. 17.3 *Sonogram of fetus at 22 weeks' gestation with bladder outlet obstruction secondary to posterior urethral valves. The arrow within the bladder points to the dilated posterior urethra.*

sampling or fetal blood sampling. Even the uroepithelium can be cultured for a karyotype if the urine is drained.

Assuming a normal karyotype and the availability of effective therapy, the perfect candidate for antenatal intervention would be the fetus whose obstruction is severe enough to compromise pulmonary and renal development but not so severe that the damage is irreversible after antenatal relief of the obstruction.

There is general agreement there is no highly sensitive technique to assess the risk of development of pulmonary hypoplasia. Three modalities have been utilized in the assessment of fetal and subsequent long-term neonatal renal function. Urine in the fetal bladder can be drained under sonographic guidance and analyzed for various electrolytes and microproteins. Fetal kidneys are carefully examined sonographically for any evidence of renal dysplasia which would signify that long-term, irreversible damage has already occurred. Finally, the volume of amniotic fluid is assessed.

Fetal urine

Numerous investigations have evaluated various urinary parameters in an effort to predict the potential for long-term normal renal function (Adzick *et al.*, 1985a; Burghard *et al.*, 1987; Elder *et al.*, 1990; Glick *et al.*, 1985; Grannum *et al.*, 1989; Holzgreve *et al.*, 1989; 1991; Jonasson, Ervin & Wibell, 1974; Lenz *et al.*, 1985; Lipitz *et al.*, 1993; Mandelbrot *et al.*, 1991; Muller *et al.*, 1993; Nicolaides *et al.*, 1992; Nicolini *et al.*, 1991; Nicolini, Fisk & Rodeck, 1992; Nolte, Mueller & Pringsheim, 1991; Reuss *et al.*, 1987; Quintero *et al.*, 1995; Wilkins *et al.*, 1986). Glick *et al.* (1985) presented retrospective experience measuring electrolytes in fetuses with bilateral congenital hydronephrosis. They observed that fetuses with hypotonic urine were later noted to have good renal function after birth; those with isotonic urine tended to have poor renal function. They proposed that a urinary sodium above 100 mmol/l, chloride level above 90 mmol/l and osmolarity above 210 mOsm were associated with insufficient tubular reabsorption capacity and irreversible renal damage after birth. Based on this experience, they suggested that only those fetuses with values consistent with good renal function be considered candidates for antenatal intervention. Similar findings were reported by Grannum *et al.* (1989). Unfortunately, these initial studies failed to consider the normal ontogeny of renal tubular function.

Other investigators have subsequently challenged the value of urinary electrolytes in forecasting long-term renal function (Berkowitz *et al.*, 1982; Elder *et al.*, 1990; McFadyen, Wigglesworth & Dillon, 1983; Weiner *et al.*, 1986; Wilkins *et al.*, 1987). Wilkins *et al.* (1987) sampled nine fetuses with obstructive uropathy. Five fetuses were predicted to have good renal function using the above criteria, three developed renal failure after birth and one had renal dysplasia discovered at autopsy after elective termination. Only one child was alive and well at the time of the report. Nicolini *et al.* (1987) reported a fetus in which sampling from the bladder suggested poor function. However, separate sampling of urine from both kidneys suggested good function in the left kidney and poor function in the right kidney. A vesicoamniotic shunt was placed and the newborn had good function of the left kidney and renal dysplasia in the right kidney. Based on their case, these authors suggested sampling from both kidneys may provide more accurate information regarding long-term prognosis. Others (Evans *et al.*, 1991; Nicolini *et al.*, 1991) have suggested that repeat sampling of the fetal urine may provide more reliable information, although this approach has not been systematically investigated.

Because of the above discrepancies, others have suggested using urinary microproteins as indicators of renal damage (Burghard *et al.*, 1987; Holzgreve *et al.*, 1989, 1991; Jonasson *et al.*, 1974; Lenz *et al.*, 1985; Nolte *et al.*, 1991). In postnatal studies, an increase in urinary proteins with a molecular weight of 000 indicates impairment in tubular reabsorption (Pesce, Boreisha & Pollak, 1972). Holzgreve *et al.* (1989; 1991) used a similar approach antenatally using a SDS polyacrylamide gel electrophoresis. In 21 fetuses, they observed that the electrolyte and osmolarity evaluations incorrectly predicted renal function in four instances whereas the protein levels were accurate in all cases. Others (Jonasson *et al.*, 1974; Nolte *et al.*, 1991) have suggested

that urinary β_2-microglobulin may be useful for evaluating renal function *in utero*.

Recently, several larger series have been published evaluating a variety of urinary parameters in cases of obstructive uropathy (Lipitz *et al.*, 1993; Mandelbrot *et al.*, 1991; Muller *et al.*, 1993; Nicolaides *et al.*, 1992; Nicolini *et al.*, 1992). Nicolini *et al.* (1992) reported normal values for urinary sodium and chloride in 26 control fetuses from 16 to 33 weeks' gestation. Sodium concentration decreased with advancing gestation. Serial urine samples from fetuses with obstruction demonstrated a more pronounced deviation from normal with increasing gestation when renal dysplasia was present. Utilizing gestational age-appropriate norms, they observed that the test with the highest sensitivity for the detection of renal dysplasia was urinary calcium, with a sensitivity of 100%. Unfortunately, its specificity was only 60%. Urinary sodium had the highest specificity at 80%, with a reasonable sensitivity of 87%. Nicolaides *et al.* (1992) reported that, based on 60 untreated fetuses, the best predictor of ultimate renal failure was the presence of either a high urinary calcium or a high urinary sodium content. This was found to have a positive predictive value of 91% and negative predictive value of 78% when corrected for gestational age. Similar results were reported by Lipitz *et al.* (1993), who also noted that a urinary β_2-microglobulin 13 mg/l was almost invariably associated with a fatal outcome.

Dumez's group (Mandelbrot *et al.*, 1991; Muller *et al.*, 1993) have presented two important cohort studies of fetuses with antenatally diagnosed but untreated urinary obstruction. The first report included 100 consecutive patients. Antenatal findings were matched to renal function of survivors at one to two years of life. Renal insufficiency was diagnosed if the serum creatinine exceeded 50 mol/l by the second year of life. Fetal urinary concentrations of sodium, chloride, calcium, phosphorus, ammonium, urea, creatinine, glucose, proteins and β_2-microglobulin were measured. A β_2-microglobulin >2 mg/l yielded a sensitivity of 80% and specificity of 83% for the prediction of renal insufficiency. The urinary sodium concentration of fetuses with normal renal function at two years of life was much lower than the cut off originally proposed by Glick *et al.* (1985). In their most recent investigation, they measured amino acids using proton nuclear magnetic resonance spectroscopy (Eugène *et al.*, 1994). A two-dimensional representation of alanine/valine and valine/threonine concentration provided a clear separation of fetuses into normal function compromised function, and renal failure. In this series, amino acid measurement was superior to any of the other electrolytes or β_2-microglobulin.

Renal appearance

Mahoney *et al.* (1984) sought sonographic features which might be predictive of renal dysplasia in fetuses with obstructive uropathy. Renal cysts invariably signified the presence of dysplasia, with a predictive value of 100%. Renal cysts were only seen in dysplastic kidneys. Unfortunately, renal cysts were seen in only 44% of dysplastic fetal kidneys and only 44% of kidneys without cysts were free of dysplastic changes. The other sonographic feature predictive of renal dysplasia was echogenicity. Increased echogenicity is thought to be caused by fibrosis. In the Mahoney series, assessment of renal echogenicity was a less reliable predictor than renal cysts.

Amniotic fluid volume

Ultrasonographic assessment of amniotic fluid volume has also been utilized as a crude index of fetal renal function. In many series of fetuses with obstructive uropathy, amniotic fluid volume has been described as 'normal,' 'decreased' or 'absent' with no real quantification. Oligohydramnios in association with obstructive uropathy is thought to signify a high-grade obstruction to urinary flow whereas normal or only slightly decreased amniotic fluid volume is thought to represent minimal or incomplete obstruction.

Treatment modalities

Vesicoamniotic shunts

The most commonly used method to relieve urinary obstruction *in utero* is the placement of a double pigtailed vesicoamniotic catheter, as described in detail in Chapter 2. Preliminary amnioinfusion is often necessary to correct oligohydramnios to allow placement of the intra-amniotic portion of the shunt.

Complications do occur. A 4.8% procedure-related fetal mortality was reported in the International Fetal Surgery Registry (Manning *et al.*, 1986). Elder *et al.* (1987) reviewed 57 vesicoamniotic shunts and found that some complication occurred in 25 (44%). The most common problem was unsatisfactory drainage by the shunt after it became occluded or migrated. In seven patients, preterm labour occurred within 48 hours of the procedure. Occlusion is no longer common with the current shunt design. Robichaux *et al.* (1991) reported two fetuses with traumatic abdominal wall defects secondary to vesicoamniotic shunt placement. The authors suggest two potential mechanisms for abdominal wall defects induced by shunt placement. In cases where the fetus inadvertently removed the shunt, fetal intestines and mesentery may become entangled in the shunt and be pulled through the abdominal wall. Another proposed explanation was that increased fetal intra-abdominal pressure caused by persistent hydronephrosis may cause the bowel to eviscerate alongside the shunt at the point of entry through the abdominal wall. These authors recommend that placement of the shunt be limited to the fetal midline in the suprapubic region.

Harrison *et al.* (1991) question whether long-term drainage can be reliably achieved with vesicoamniotic shunts. It has been our experience (Weiner *et al.*, 1986) and the experience of others (Evans *et al.*, 1992; Holzgreve & Evans, 1993) that prolonged decompression is possible and can be reliably accomplished, as judged by normalization of amniotic fluid volume.

Open fetal surgery

Harrison and coworkers (1982a) have applied open fetal surgery techniques to cases of congenital hydronephrosis. The first surgery was performed in 1981; since then, a total of eight fetuses have undergone correction of their urinary obstruction (Crombleholme *et al.*, 1988; Harrison *et al.*, 1982a). The overall survival has been 38%. One of the three survivors ultimately required a renal transplant. The potential risk to the mother from open fetal surgery cannot be disputed. At least two separate laparotomies during the index pregnancy will be required, one for fetal surgery and the second for delivery. In addition, these women must be delivered by caesarean section in future pregnancies. Finally, the immediate postoperative course after fetal surgery is almost uniformly complicated by preterm labour necessitating extensive tocolytic use.

Fetoscopic surgery

The inherent risk and limited success of open fetal surgery coupled with the potential problems of catheter migration and inadequate drainage have stimulated interest in the development of fetoscopic techniques to treat congenital anomalies. Estes *et al.* (1992) have successfully corrected bladder obstruction in fetal sheep by endoscopically placing a wire mesh shunt. Quintero *et al.* (1995a) fulgurated a human fetus with posterior ureteral valves utilizing an endoscopic approach. More recently, the same group positioned one of two vesicoamniotic shunts at fetal cystoscopy (Quintero *et al.*, 1995b). This early experience suggests that such approaches to therapy may be technically feasible.

Outcome

The efficacy of antenatal intervention for obstructive uropathy is difficult to assess for several reasons. First, the multiple case reports or small series reported use different criteria for fetal selection and different surgical techniques. Second, there is often a lack of documentation of amniotic fluid volume both before and after intervention. This information is important in order to determine the extent of obstruction prior to intervention and the adequacy of the relief of the obstruction after intervention. Third, there are multiple aetiologies of obstructive uropathy, including posterior urethral valves, urethral atresia (Steinhardt *et al.*, 1990), prune belly syndrome (Cullen *et al.*, 1989) and MMIHS (Vintzileos *et al.*, 1986). The natural history of fetal urinary obstruction is likely to be influenced by the aetiology of the obstruction. Fourth, the duration of the obstruction and the magnitude of the back pressure on the renal parenchyma are impossible to determine yet are likely to be critical. And fifth, many untreated fetuses are aborted, biasing reports of perinatal outcome.

The results of the International Fetal Surgery Registry were published in 1986 as an early attempt to consolidate outcome data (Manning *et al.*, 1986). Seventy-three fetuses with a treated obstructive uropathy were included, with an overall survival of 45%. However, 11 of the 73 pregnancies were terminated after placement of the catheter; therefore, the survival rate of ongoing pregnancies was 48%. Long-term follow-up was inadequate, with only limited observation of the 30 survivors. Two had chronic illnesses, one with chronic renal failure and one with persistent cloacal syndrome requiring surgery. Harrison's group (Crombleholme *et al.*, 1990) summarized 40 fetuses with fetal obstructive uropathy who underwent diagnostic evaluation and selective treatment. They retrospectively assigned the fetuses to either a good or poor prognosis group based on urinary parameters and ultrasonographic evidence of dysplasia. Survival was higher in the good-prognosis group than in the poor-prognosis group, 87% vs 30%. In the group of fetuses not undergoing intervention, 70% of the good-prognosis group survived compared with no survivors in the poor-prognosis group. In fetuses undergoing intervention, 89% of the good-prognosis group survived compared with a 30% rate of survival in the poor-prognosis group. This would seem to suggest that treatment has its greatest effect when the prognosis is poor. However, these statistics may be somewhat misleading since 11 of the 14 fetuses in the poor-prognosis group without intervention died as a result of elective termination. Fetal intervention successful restored amniotic fluid volume in 9 of 17 cases complicated by oligohydramnios; 89% of these fetuses survived. Failure of the amniotic fluid volume to return to normal in the remaining eight pregnancies was associated with a very poor outcome, with death secondary to pulmonary hypoplasia in the five fetuses delivered at term. The long-term success of therapy, judged by renal function in these same patients (Fries *et al.*, 1992) is even less optimistic. Of the 10 fetuses that survived, seven were treated with vesicoamniotic shunt replacement and three with open fetal surgery. Renal transplantation has been performed or is planned in four of these. Therefore, out of the original group of 29 pregnancies allowed to continue, only six have renal function consistent with survival. We too have observed similar findings in our treated fetuses with long-term follow-up. Of the five fetuses considered to have a good prognosis who under-

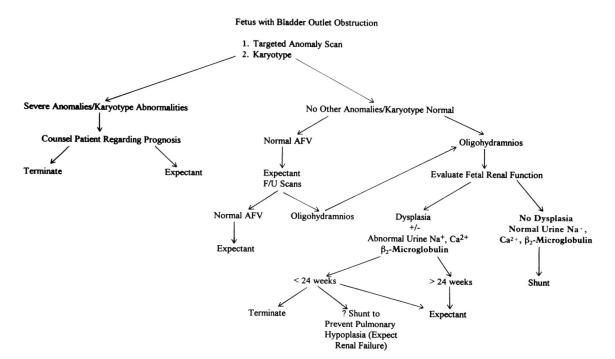

Fig. 17.4 *Proposed management scheme for the fetus presenting with bladder outlet obstruction.*

went a vesicoamniotic shunt with correction of amniotic fluid volume, four survived. One newborn died secondary to pulmonary hypoplasia. The four survivors all have findings of severe renal dysfunction and will probably require renal transplantation in the future.

Management

A proposed management scheme is outlined in Fig. 17.4 for fetuses with obstructive uropathy. Available information supports a consideration for intervention only when the obstruction is associated with oligohydramnios and the parents understand the current state of knowledge regarding long-term prognosis. A comprehensive ultrasound for associated anomalies should be performed. The fetal kidneys should be carefully evaluated for echogenicity or renal cysts that would indicate renal dysplasia. Karyotype evaluation should be performed by amniocentesis or aspiration of fetal urine. It is important

to sample the fetal urine to assess renal function. If studies reveal normal fetal anatomy, normal karyotype, no evidence of renal dysplasia, and urine studies consistent with good prognosis, vesicoamniotic shunting should be undertaken at less than 32 weeks' gestation. Placement of a shunt in fetuses prior to 24 weeks' gestation with sonographic or urinary evidence of renal dysfunction is certainly controversial. However, death from pulmonary hypoplasia may be prevented if the volume is restored. Based on published series, the performance of urinary diversion in a fetus with obstructive uropathy and oligohydramnios is associated with the development of renal failure in surviving neonates and the requirement for transplantation.

Conclusion

In cases of lower obstructive uropathy, urinary diversion has been attempted *in utero* to restore amniotic fluid volume, allow normal lung development and prevent renal damage. Despite a sound experimental basis from animal studies, clinical results have proved disappointing. Although there are technical difficulties with both the open and closed approaches to intervention, the major difficulty has been that of case selection. At present, vesicoamniotic shunting is restricted to otherwise normal fetuses with normal renal function and oligohydramnios prior to 24 weeks' gestation. Whatever technical advances occur, real progress can only come with better methods of predicting long-term renal function and selecting fetuses that might benefit from intrauterine therapy.

References

Adzick, N. S., Harrison, M. R., Flake, A. W. & Laberge, J. M. (1985a). Development of fetal renal function test using endogenous creatinine clearance. *Journal of Pediatric Surgery*, 20, 602–7.

Adzick, N. S., Harrison, M. R., Glick, P. L. & Flake, A. W. (1985b). Fetal urinary tract obstruction: experimental pathophysiology. *Seminars in Perinatology*, 9, 79–90.

Arger, P. H., Coleman, B. G., Mintz, M. C., Snyder, H. P., Camardese, T., Arenson, R. L., Gabbe, S. G. & Aquino, L. (1985). Routine fetal genitourinary tract screening. *Radiology*, 156, 485–9.

Barss, V. A., Benacerraf, B. R. & Frigoletto, F. D., Jr (1984). Second trimester oligohydramnios, a predictor of poor fetal outcome. *Obstetrics and Gynecology*, 64, 608–10.

Bastide, A., Manning, F., Harman, C., Lang, I. & Morrison, I. (1986). Ultrasound evaluation of amniotic fluid: outcome of pregnancies with severe oligohydramnios. *American Journal of Obstetrics and Gynecology*, 154, 895–900.

Beck, A. D. (1971). The effect of intra-uterine urinary obstruction upon the development of the fetal kidney. *Journal of Urology*, 105, 784–9.

Berkowitz, R. L., Glickman, M. G., Smith, G. J. W., Siegal, N. J., Weiss, R. M., Mahoney, M. J. & Hobbins, J. C. (1982). Fetal urinary tract obstruction: what is the role of surgical intervention in-

utero? *American Journal of Obstetrics and Gynecology*, 144, 367–75.

Berman, D. J. & Maizels, M. (1982). The role of urinary obstruction in the genesis of renal dysplasia. A model in the chick embryo. *Journal of Urology*, 128, 1091–6.

Bernstein, J. (1971). The morphogenesis of renal parenchymal maldevelopment (renal dysplasia). *Pediatric Clinics of North America*, 18, 395–407.

Brumfield, C. G., Davis, R. O., Joseph, D. B. & Cosper, P. (1991). Fetal obstructive uropathies. Importance of chromosomal abnormalities and associated anomalies to perinatal outcome. *Journal of Reproductive Medicine*, 36, 662–6.

Burghard, R., Pallacks, R., Gordjani, N., Leititis, J. U., Hackeloer B. J. & Brandis, M. (1987). Microproteins in amniotic fluid as an index of changes in fetal renal function during development. *Pediatric Nephrology*, 1, 574–80.

Bussières, L., Wieckowski, J., Revillon, Y., Chourrout, Y., Sachs, C. & Laborde, K. (1993). Creation of experimental urethral obstruction *in utero*: evaluation of fetal renal function. *European Journal of Pediatric Surgery*, 3, 161–5.

Chinn, D. H. & Filly, R. A. (1982). Ultrasound diagnosis of fetal genitourinary tract anomalies. *Urologic Radiology*, 4, 115–23.

Churchill, B. M., McLorie, G. A., Khoury, A. E., Merguerian, P. A. & Houle, A. M. (1990).

Emergency treatment and long-term follow-up of posterior urethral valves. *Urologic Clinics of North America*, 17, 343–60.

Crombleholme, T. M., Harrison, M. R., Golbus, M. S., Longaker, M. T., Langer, J. C., Callen, P. W., Anderson, R. L., Goldstein, R. B. & Filly, R. A. (1990). Fetal intervention in obstructive uropathy: prognostic indicators and efficacy of intervention. *American Journal of Obstetrics and Gynecology*, 162, 1239–44.

Crombleholme, T. M., Harrison, M. R., Langer, J. C., Longaker, M. T., Anderson, R. L., Slotnick, N. S., Filly, R. A., Callen, P. W., Goldstein, R. B. & Golbus, M. S. (1988). Early experience with open fetal surgery for congenital hydronephrosis. *Journal of Pediatric Surgery*, 23, 1114–21.

Cullen, M. T., Athanassiadis, A. A., Grannum, P., Green, J. J. & Hobbins, J. C. (1989). In utero intravesicular pressure and the prune belly syndrome. *Fetal Therapy*, 4, 73–7.

Elder, J. C., Duckett, J. W., Jr & Snyder, H. M. (1987). Intervention for fetal obstructive uropathy: Has it been effective? *Lancet*, ii, 1007–10.

Elder, J. S., O'Grady, J. P., Ashmead, G., Duckett, J. W. & Philipson, E. (1990). Evaluation of fetal renal function: unreliability of fetal urinary electrolytes. *Journal of Urology*, 44, 574–8.

Estes, J. M., MacGillivray, T. E., Hedrick, M. H., Adzick, N. S. & Harrison, M. R. (1992). Fetoscopic surgery for the treatment of congenital anomalies. *Journal of Pediatric Surgery*, 27, 950–4.

Eugène, M., Muller, F., Dommergues, M., Le Moyec, L. & Dumez, Y. (1994). Evaluation of postnatal renal function in fetuses with bilateral obstructive uropathies by proton nuclear magnetic resonance spectroscopy. *American Journal of Obstetrics and Gynecology*, 170, 595–602.

Evans, M. I., Harrison, M. R., Nicolaides, K. H., Johnson, M. P. & Holzgreve, W. (1992). Fetal therapy. In *Genetic Disorders and the Fetus: Diagnosis, Prevention, and Treatment*, ed. A. Milunsky, pp. 771–97. Baltimore, MD: Johns Hopkins University Press.

Evans, M. I., Sacks, A. J., Johnson, M. P., Robichaux, A. G., May, M. & Moghissi, K. S. (1991). Sequential invasive assessment of fetal renal function and the intrauterine treatment of fetal obstructive uropathies. *Obstetrics and Gynecology*, 77, 545–50.

Fries, M. H., Norton, M., Goldberg, J., Harrison, M., Filly, R., Callen, P. & Goldstein, R. & Golbus, M. (1992). Renal function after in-utero intervention for fetal obstructive uropathy. *American Journal of Obstetrics and Gynecology*, 166, 357.

Glazer, G. M., Filly, R. A. & Callen, P. W. (1982). The varied sonographic appearance of the urinary tract in the fetus and newborn with urethral obstruction. *Radiology*, 144, 563–8.

Glick, P. L., Harrison, M. R., Adzick, N. S., Noall, R. A. & Villa, R. L. (1984). Correction of congenital hydronephrosis in utero. IV: In utero decompression prevents renal dysplasia. *Journal of Pediatric Surgery*, 19, 649–57.

Glick, P. L., Harrison, M. R., Golbus, M. S., Adzick, N. S., Filly, R. A., Callen, P. W., Mahoney, B. S., Anderson, R. L. & de Lorimier, R. A. (1985). Management of the fetus with congenital hydronephrosis. II: prognostic criteria and selection for treatment. *Journal of Pediatric Surgery*, 20, 376–87.

Glick, P. L., Harrison, M. R., Noall, R. A. & Villa, R. L. (1983). Correction of congenital hydronephrosis in utero. III. Early mid-trimester ureteral obstruction produces renal dysplasia. *Journal of Pediatric Surgery*, 18, 681–7.

Grannum, P. A., Ghidini, A., Scioscia, A., Copel, J. A., Romero, R. & Hobbins, J. C. (1989). Assessment of fetal renal reserve in low level obstructive uropathy. *Lancet*, i, 281–2.

Gruenewald, S. M., Crocker, E. F., Walker, A. G. & Trudinger, B. J. (1984). Antenatal diagnosis of urinary tract abnormalities: correlation of ultrasound appearance with postnatal diagnosis. *American Journal of Obstetrics and Gynecology*, 148, 278–83.

Harrison, M. R. & Filly, R. A. (1990). The fetus with obstructive uropathy: Pathophysiology, natural history, selection, and treatment. In *The Unborn*

Patient: Prenatal Diagnosis and Treatment, 2nd edn, ed. M. R. Harrison, M. S. Golbus & R. A. Filly, pp. 328–93. Philadelphia, PA: W. B. Saunders.

Harrison, M. R., Golbus, M. S., Filly, R. A., Callen, P. W., Katz, M., de Lorimar, A. A., Rosen, M. & Jonsen, A. R. (1982a). Fetal surgery for congenital hydronephrosis. *New England Journal of Medicine*, 306, 591–3.

Harrison, M. R., Nakayama, D. K., Noall, R. & de Lorimier, A. A. (1982b). Correction of congenital hydronephrosis *in utero*. II. Decompression reverses the effects of obstruction on the fetal lung and urinary tract. *Journal of Pediatric Surgery*, 17, 965–74.

Harrison, M. R., Ross, N., Noall, R. & de Lorimier, A. A. (1983). Correction of congenital hydro-nephrosis in-utero. I. The model: fetal urethral obstruction produces hydronephrosis and pulmonary hypoplasia in fetal lambs. *Journal of Pediatric Surgery*, 18, 247–56.

Hayden, S. A., Russ, P. D., Pretorius, D. H., Manco-Johnson, M. L. & Clewell, W. H. (1988). Posterior urethral obstruction: prenatal sonographic findings and clinical outcome in 14 cases. *Journal of Ultrasound in Medicine*, 7, 371.

Helin, I. & Persson, P. H. (1986). Prenatal diagnosis of urinary tract abnormalities by ultrasound. *Pediatrics*, 78, 879–83.

Hellstrom, W. J., Kogan, B. A., Jeffrey, R. B., Jr & McAninch, A. L. (1984). The natural history of prenatal hydronephrosis with normal amounts of amniotic fluid. *Journal of Urology*, 132, 947–50.

Hirata, G. I., Medearis, A. L. & Platt, L. D. (1990). Fetal abdominal abnormalities associated with genetic syndromes. *Clinical Perinatology*, 17, 675–702.

Hobbins, J. C., Romero, R., Grannum, P., Berkowitz, R. L., Cullen, M. & Mahoney, M. (1984). Antenatal diagnosis of renal anomalies with ultrasound. I. Obstructive uropathy. *American Journal of Obstetrics and Gynecology*, 148, 868–77.

Holzgreve, W. & Evans, M. (1993). Nonvascular needle and shunt placements for fetal therapy. *Western Journal of Medicine*, 159, 333–40.

Holzgreve, W., Lison, A. & Bulla, M. (1989). SDS–PAGE as an additional test to determine fetal kidney function prior to intrauterine diversion of urinary tract obstruction. *Fetal Therapy*, 4, 93–6.

Holzgreve, W., Lison, A., Bulla, M. & Evans, M. (1991). Protein analysis to determine fetal kidney function. *American Journal of Obstetrics and Gynecology*, 164, 336.

Jonasson, L. E., Evrin, P. E. & Wibell, L. (1974). Content of β_2-microglobulin and albumin in human amniotic fluid. A study of normal pregnancies complicated by haemolytic disease. *Acta Obstetricia et Gynecologica Scandinavica*, 53, 49–58.

Lenz, S., Lund-Hansen, T., Bang, J. & Christensen, E. (1985). A possible antenatal evaluation of renalfunction by amnio acid analysis on fetal urine. *Prenatal Diagnosis*, 5, 259–67.

Lipitz, S., Ryan, G., Samuell, C., Haeusler, M. C., Robson, S. C., Dhillon, H. K., Nicolini, U. & Rodeck, C. H. (1993). Fetal urine analysis for the assessment of renal function in obstructive uropathy. *American Journal of Obstetrics and Gynecology*, 168, 174–9.

Mahoney, B. S., Callen, P. W. & Filly, R. A. (1985). Fetal urethral obstruction: US evaluation. *Radiology*, 157, 221–4.

Mahoney, B. S., Filly, R. A., Callen, P. W., Hricak, H., Golbus, M. S. & Harrison, M. R. (1984). Fetal renal dysplasia: sonographic evaluation. *Radiology*, 152, 143–6.

Maizels, M. & Simpson, S. B., Jr (1983). Primitive ducts of renal dysplasia induced by culturing of ureteral buds denuded of condensed renal mesenchyme. *Science*, 219, 509.

Mandelbrot, L., Dumez, Y., Muller, F. & Dommergues, M. (1991). Prenatal prediction of renal function in fetal obstructive uropathies. *Journal of Perinatal Medicine*, 19, 283–97.

Manning, F. A., Harrison, M. R. & Rodeck, C. (1986). Catheter shunts for fetal hydronephrosis and hydrocephalus. Report of the International

Fetal Surgery Registry. *New England Journal of Medicine*, 315, 336–40.

McFadyen, I. R., Wigglesworth, J. S. & Dillon, M. J. (1983). Fetal urinary tract obstruction: is active intervention before delivery indicated? *British Journal of Obstetrics and Gynaecology*, 90, 342–9.

Muller, F., Dommergues, M., Mandelbrot, L., Aubry, M. C., Fekete, C. & Dumez, Y. (1993). Fetal urinary biochemistry predicts postnatal renal function in children with bilateral obstructive uropathies. *Obstetrics and Gynecology*, 82, 813–20.

Nakayama, D. K., Harrison, M. R. & de Lomimier, A. A. (1986). Prognosis of posterior urethral valves presenting at birth. *Journal of Pediatric Surgery*, 21, 43–5.

Nicolaides, K. H., Cheng, H. H., Snijders, R. J. & Moniz, C. F. (1992). Fetal urine biochemistry in the assessment of obstructive uropathy. *American Journal of Obstetrics and Gynecology*, 166, 932–7.

Nicolini, U., Fisk, N. M. & Rodeck, C. (1992). Fetal urine biochemistry: an index of renal maturation and dysfunction. *British Journal of Obstetrics and Gynaecology*, 99, 46–50.

Nicolini, U., Rodeck, C. H. & Fisk, N. M. (1987). Shunt treatment for fetal obstructive uropathy (Letter). *Lancet*, ii, 1338–9.

Nicolini, U., Tannirandorn, Y., Vaughan, J., Fisk, N. M., Nicolaidis, P. & Rodeck, C. H. (1991). Further predictors of renal dysplasia in fetal obstructive uropathy: bladder pressure and biochemistry of 'fresh' urine. *Prenatal Diagnosis*, 11, 159–66.

Nolte, S., Mueller, B. & Pringsheim, W. (1991). Serum alpha 1-microglobulin and beta 2-microglobulin for the estimation of fetal glomerular renal function. *Pediatric Nephrology*, 5, 573–7.

Parkhouse, H. F., Barratt, T. M., Dillon, M. J., Duffy, P. G., Fay, J., Ransley, P. G., Woodhouse, C. R. & Williams, D. I. (1988). Long term outcome of boys with posterior urethral valves. *British Journal of Urology*, 62, 59–62.

Pesce, A. J., Boreisha, I. & Pollak, V. E. (1972). Rapid differentiation of glomerular and tubular proteinuria by sodium dodecyl sulfate polyacryclamide gel electrophoresis. *Clinica Chimica Acta*, 40, 27–34.

Peters, C. A., Carr, M. C., Lais, A., Retik, A. B. & Mandell, J. (1992). The response of the fetal kidney to obstruction. *Journal of Urology*, 148, 503–9.

Peters, C. A., Docimo, S. G., Luetic, T., Reid, L. M., Retik, A. B. & Mandell, J. (1991a). Effect of *in utero* vesicostomy on pulmonary hypoplasia in the fetal lamb with bladder outlet obstruction and oligohydramnios: a morphometric analysis. *Journal of Urology*, 146, 1178–83.

Peters, C. A., Reid, L. M., Docimo, S., Luetic, T., Carr, M., Retik, A. B. & Mandell, J. (1991b). The role of the kidney in lung growth and maturation in the setting of obstructive uropathy and oligo-hydramnios. *Journal of Urology*, 146, 597–600.

Quintero, R. A., Hume, R., Smith, C., Johnson, M. P., Cotton, D. B., Romero, R. & Evans, M. I. (1995a). Percutaneous fetal cystoscopy and endoscopic fulguration of posterior urethral valves. *American Journal of Obstetrics and Gynecology* 172, 206–9.

Quintero, R. A., Johnson, M. P., Romero, R., Smith, C., Arias, F., Guevara-Zuloaga F., Cotton, D. B. & Evans, M. I. (1995b). *In utero* percutaneous cystoscopy in the management of fetal lower obstructive uropathy. *Lancet*, 346, 537–40.

Reuss, A., Wladimiroff, J. W. & Niermeijer, M. F. (1987a). Antenatal diagnosis of renal tract anomalies by ultrasound. *Pediatric Nephrology*, 1, 546–52.

Reuss, A., Wladimiroff, J. W., Pijpers, L. & Provoost, A. P. (1987b). Fetal urinary electrolytes in bladder outlet obstruction. *Fetal Therapy*, 2, 148–53.

Reuss, A., Wladimiroff, J. W., Stewart, P. A. & Scholtmeijer, R. J. (1988). Non-invasive management of fetal obstructive uropathy. *Lancet*, ii, 949–51.

Robichaux, A. G., III, Mandell, J., Greene, M. F., Benacerraf, B. R. & Evans, M. T. (1991). Fetal abdominal wall defect: a new complication of vesicoamniotic shunting. *Fetal Diagnosis and Therapy*, 6, 11–13.

Seeds, J. W., Mittelstaedt, C. A. & Mandell, J. (1986). Pre- and postnatal ultrasonographic diagnosis of congenital obstructive uropathies. *Urologic Clinics of North America*, 13, 131–54.

Steinhardt, G., Hogan, W., Wood, E., Weber, T. & Lynch, R. (1990). Long-term survival in an infant with urethral atresia. *Journal of Urology*, 143, 336–7.

Stiller, R. J. (1989). Early ultrasonic appearance of fetal bladder outlet obstruction. *American Journal of Obstetrics and Gynecology*, 160, 584–5.

Thomas, D. F., Irving, H. C. & Arthur, R. J. (1985). Pre-natal diagnosis: how useful is it? *British Journal of Urology*, 57, 784–7.

Vintzileos, A. M., Eisenfeld, L. I., Herson, V. C., Ingardia, C. J., Feinstein, S. J. & Lodeiro, J. G. (1986). Megacystis-microcolon-intestinal hypo-peristalsis syndrome. Prenatal sonographic findings and review of the literature. *American Journal of Perinatology*, 3, 297.

Warshaw, B. L., Edelbrock, H. H. & Ettenger, R. B. (1982). Progression to end-stage renal disease in children with obstructive uropathy. *Journal of Pediatrics*, 100, 183–7.

Weiner, C., Williamson, R., Bonsib, S. M., Erenberg, A., Pringle, K., Smith, W. & Abu-Yousef, M. (1986). In utero bladder diversion – problems with patient selection. *Fetal Therapy*, 1, 196–202.

Wilkins, I. A., Chitkara, U., Lynch, L., Goldberg, J. D., Mehalek, K. E. & Berkowitz, R. L. (1987). The nonpredictive value of fetal urinary electrolytes: preliminary report of outcomes and correlations with pathologic diagnosis. *American Journal of Obstetrics and Gynecology*, 157, 694–8.

Williams, D. I. (1977). Urethral valves: a hundred cases with hydronephrosis. *Birth Defects, Original Article Series*, 13, 55–62.

18 Diaphragmatic hernia

W. D. ANDREW FORD

Introduction

Background

Congenital diaphragmatic hernia (CDH) is a common lethal anomaly. It occurs in approximately 1 in 2000 pregnancies, but only in 1 in 5000 live births (de Lorimier, Tierney & Parker, 1967; Pringle, 1991), demonstrating that the majority of fetuses with CDH die before they get to a neonatal surgical or intensive care unit. Therefore, more than 80% of fetuses found to have CDH on antenatal ultrasound will die, during pregnancy, at birth or soon after (Harrison et al., 1978; Adzick et al., 1985a; Harrison, 1990; Pringle, 1991). While approximately 35% of these have other major anomalies that could preclude survival (Harrison, 1990), 60–70% of those with only a hernia still die (Nakayama et al., 1985; Pringle, 1991; Sharland et al., 1992; Harrison et al., 1993b).

This low fetal/neonatal survival has not improved in parallel with improvements in survival both for other major anatomical defects and for other respiratory problems in the newborn. Overall results have possibly even deteriorated, as more severely affected neonates now survive transport into surgical centres (Harrison, 1990). Even prolonged heart–lung by-pass using extracorporeal membrane oxygenation (ECMO) for up to two weeks after birth improves results only marginally for those that get to an ECMO centre alive (Langham et al., 1987; Vacanti et al., 1988; Harrison, 1990; Breaux et al., 1991, Wilson et al., 1992; Harrison et al., 1993b).

Rationale for fetal surgery

Apart from those fetuses with additional lethal anomalies, the major causes of death in babies born alive with a CDH are: (i) pulmonary hypoplasia (PH) (Pringle, 1989; Harrison, 1990), (ii) delayed lung maturation (Pringle, 1989), and (iii) pulmonary vasculature changes leading to pulmonary hypertension (Shochat, 1987). These have all been assumed to be the result of viscera herniated through a defect in the diaphragm and pressing on the lungs from early gestation (Harrison, 1990). This pressure has then been assumed to prevent further development of the lungs (Kent et al., 1972).

Therefore, intrauterine correction of diaphragmatic defects by open fetal surgery has evolved on the assumption that removing viscera from the chest early in gestation would improve survival rates after birth. Such a procedure would relieve pressure on the lungs and allow the lungs to grow and mature to a point where they could support the neonate at birth (Kent et al., 1972; Harrison, 1990; Harrison et al., 1993b).

Animal studies

To test the hypothesis that removing viscera from the chest improves fetal survival in human fetuses with CDH, an animal model that closely mimics the changes seen in human CDH has been developed and refined over a period of years in fetal sheep (de Lorimier et al., 1967; Pringle, 1984; Harrison et al., 1980a; Harrison,

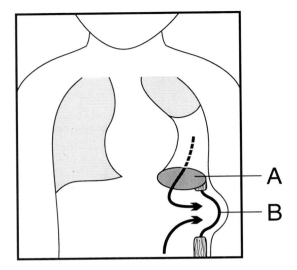
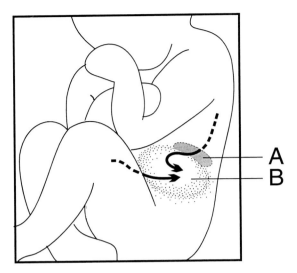

Fig. 18.1 *The abdominoplasty. AP and lateral views of the fetus. Viscera are withdrawn from the chest and the defect closed with a patch (A). Abdominal contents are allowed to herniate partially into an incisional hernia that contains another domed patch in its deep layer (B). Note the lateral approach as the fetal thigh prevents access to the left upper quadrant.*

Jester & Ross, 1980b; Adzick *et al.*, 1985b). This model has been used extensively to devise methods of repair applicable to the human fetus.

Initial animal studies demonstrated that there were marked reductions in lung volume and lung compliance in fetal sheep subjected to the creation of a hernia by incising the diaphragm. In addition, the lungs were immature, and both these changes were more marked the earlier the defect was created (de Lorimier *et al.*, 1967; Kent *et al.*, 1972). Severe pulmonary hypertension was also produced when the lesions were created early in gestation (Kent *et al.*, 1972; Adzick *et al.*, 1985b). A comparison was made with the human fetus, where the lungs are assumed to be completely differentiated to the point in time that the hernia appears, but pressure then slows lung growth and arrests maturation, giving credence to the possibility of *in utero* repair of a human hernia (Kent *et al.*, 1972).

Correction of CDH in the animal model, and subsequently in the human fetus, has evolved from the obser-

vation that introducing a balloon into one hemithorax of a fetal sheep at 100 days' gestation produced lethal PH at birth. If that balloon was deflated at 120 days' gestation, the newborn lamb survived (Harrison *et al.*, 1980a,b).

In fetal sheep, diaphragmatic herniae were then induced by the surgical creation of a defect in the diaphragm ((Harrison *et al.*, 1980b), and these were corrected *in utero*, in a similar manner to the surgical corrections used in the human neonate. This did not succeed, as the reduction of viscera from the chest into the abdomen created such an increase in intra-abdominal pressure that blood flow from the placenta was obstructed at the level of the umbilical vein (Harrison, Ross & de Lorimier, 1981).

The next step in the development of fetal surgery for CDH in the animal model was the deliberate production of a ventral hernia in the abdominal incision to create more space for the returning intestine and less pressure within the abdomen at the end of the procedure. The lamb fetuses survived (Harrison *et al.*, 1981). Similar procedures were then attempted in human fetuses with CDH (Fig. 18.1), with limited success (Harrison *et al.*, 1990b,c; 1993a). Often the cause of the failure in the human fetus was that a large volume of liver was found in the chest, and reduction of this liver into the abdomen compressed and angulated the ductus venosus as it coursed through the liver, resulting in intra-operative fetal death (Harrison *et al.*, 1990c). Nevertheless, this form of surgery has been the mainstay of open fetal surgery for CDH in humans to date, with modifications involving a two-step approach (Harrison *et al.*, 1990c; 1993a) and, where possible, partial amputation of the liver (Harrison, 1993b).

In an attempt to deal with fetuses with a large volume of liver in the chest, an alternative procedure has been developed in the fetal sheep to reduce intestine, and potentially liver, slowly back into the abdomen (Ford, Cool & Derham, 1992; Ford *et al.*, 1993) (Fig. 18.2). In this procedure, a silastic chimney is placed around the viscera in the chest with no attempt made to reduce them. As the fetus grows the silastic chimney does not increase in internal volume so that there is a gradual reduction in the relative size of the hernia, allowing the lungs to grow. The approach is through the lateral chest wall and the exposure of the viscera in the chest is better than through the abdomen (Ford *et al.*, 1992; Harrison *et al.*, 1993b). The incision in the uterus is smaller and the operative time potentially less. The procedure should, therefore, be less stressful to the fetus and might reduce present loss rates (Ford *et al.*, 1993). Furthermore, when fetal lambs were deliberately delivered prematurely after this procedure, lung compliance had increased whereas those undergoing primary repair with abdominoplasty had no improvement in comparison with uncorrected fetuses. As many of the human fetuses undergoing CDH surgery have delivered prematurely,

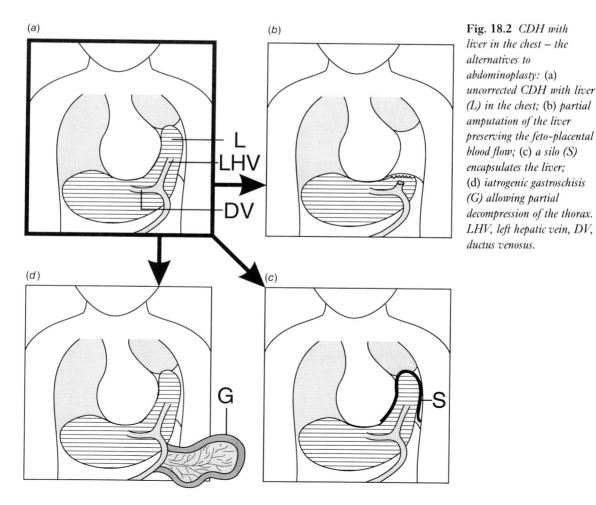

Fig. 18.2 *CDH with liver in the chest – the alternatives to abdominoplasty:* (a) *uncorrected CDH with liver (L) in the chest;* (b) *partial amputation of the liver preserving the feto-placental blood flow;* (c) *a silo (S) encapsulates the liver;* (d) *iatrogenic gastroschisis (G) allowing partial decompression of the thorax. LHV, left hepatic vein, DV, ductus venosus.*

this early improvement in compliance could be an additional advantage for the silo procedure (Parsons *et al.*, 1994). Nevertheless, with the surgically created fetal lamb model at 75 days' gestation, the liver does not migrate into the chest to any significant degree, so whether or not the silo procedure will actually reduce the liver slowly, without obstructing feto–placental blood flow, has not been thoroughly tested, even in the sheep (Ford *et al.*, 1992; 1993), and has yet to be attempted in the human fetus.

The fetal sheep model has also been used to investigate tocolytic drugs, fetal stress, methods of fetal monitoring (Fenton *et al.*, 1992; Harrison *et al.*, 1993b; Levin, Mills & Weinberg, 1979; Sabik, Assad & Hanley, 1993; Jennings *et al.*, 1993a) and the development of less invasive endoscopic methods of fetal surgery (Estes, Szabo & Harrison, 1992; Copeland *et al.*, 1993; Deprest *et al.*, 1994), as discussed in Chapter 3.

Human experience

Results of fetal surgery

The experience with antenatal correction of CDH in humans has been disappointing. The results from San Francisco have shown that for the three years 1991–93, 4 of 14 fetuses survived, two further fetuses surviving only for short periods after preterm delivery, one for seven weeks, and one for five weeks after correction *in utero* (Harrison *et al.*, 1990c; 1993b). Thereafter, the perinatal survival is still approximately only 30%.

There have been many technical difficulties encountered during the development of fetal surgery in the human. The most significant is the immediate death of the fetus when a large volume of herniated liver is reduced from the chest into the fetal abdomen. This liver contains the ductus venosus, which kinks during reduction with disastrous results (Harrison *et al.*, 1990c; Ford *et al.*, 1992). Other technical difficulties include: (i) blood loss from the uterine wall, (ii) loss of amniotic fluid, and (iii) monitoring the fetus both during and after the procedure (Chapter 3). Despite the initial difficulties, the last problems have been effectively overcome to the point that the surgery itself can be carried out with a reasonable chance of success (Harrison *et al.*, 1993b).

To improve methods of dealing with the liver, the viscera in the chest are now first approached through the lateral chest wall rather than the abdomen (Harrison *et al.*, 1993b). This improves exposure (Ford *et al.*, 1992) and allows for either partial amputation of the liver (Harrison *et al.*, 1993b) or a two-step procedure to facilitate reduction of the viscera using a further incision in the abdomen (Harrison *et al.*, 1993a), or even a combination of the two. Partial amputation of the liver (Fig. 18.2) introduces a theoretical risk of obstructing the ductus venosus at a point close to the amputation, although this has not happened in practice (Jennings *et al.*, 1992).

Less invasive approaches have also been used. One has been the aspiration of pleural effusions often associated with CDH and other space-occupying lesions in the thorax (Chapter 16). One of three fetuses with a CDH and pleural effusion survived at birth (Nicolaides & Azar, 1990). Pleural effusions are not, however, a common feature in early gestation and do not reflect the usual circumstances where there is a hernia alone. They are in fact a feature of a fetus with severe cardiovascular compromise facing imminent demise (Nicolaides & Azar, 1990).

Another approach has been to create a fetal gastroschisis in the human with a CDH (Fig. 18.2) so that the intestine could herniate out through the abdominal wall defect and relieve the pressure on the lungs. Two fetuses have undergone this procedure before birth (Porreco *et al.*, 1994). One survived, but with major intestinal problems at birth, and is now nine months old and off all therapy. The other fetus with a large volume of liver in the chest died four days after birth (J. H. T. Chang, personal communication).

Despite the technical progress made in open fetal surgery (Fig. 18.3), fetal mortality rates remain unacceptably high. Therefore, there is little chance that these procedures will gain widespread acceptance as a solution for all antenatally detected CDH. As the natural survival for a fetus with a CDH and no other detectable abnormality is approximately 40% (Harrison *et al.*, 1994), fetal surgery will require further development until it offers at least a 70–80% chance of survival at birth, if that is achievable. In the meantime, to justify further procedures on the human fetus, attempts have been made to identify subgroups with a mortality greater than the

60–70% seen in those with a hernia alone (Pringle, 1991). Ideally this group should have an *a priori* mortality approaching 100%.

Patient selection

The following groups of fetuses appear to have mortality rates 60 to 70%: (i) those detected before 25 weeks (Adzick *et al.*, 1989; Harrison *et al.*, 1990c); (ii) those with a large distended stomach in the chest (Goodfellow *et al.*, 1987; Adzick *et al.*, 1989; Burge, Atwell & Freeman, 1989; Harrison *et al.*, 1990c); (iii) those with cardiac ventricular disproportion (Crawford *et al.*, 1986; 1989; Sharland *et al.*, 1992); (iv) those with a small lung to thoracic area ratio (Kamata *et al.*, 1992); (v) those with a large volume of liver in the chest (Adzick *et al.*, 1989; Pringle, 1991; Harrison *et al.*, 1993a); and (v) those with polyhydramnios (Harrison *et al.*, 1993b). Unfortunately, none of these attempts at prediction have been entirely successful. Detection of a CDH before 25 weeks' gestation is not a reliable predictor of mortality. A high mortality rate in one report was not borne out by others (Adzick *et al.*, 1989; Pringle, 1991; Sharland *et al.*, 1992).

Initially, cardiac ventricular disproportion seen before 24 weeks' gestation appeared to indicate a mortality rate of 100% (Crawford *et al.*, 1986; 1989). With further experience, however, two cases diagnosed before 24 weeks with cardiac ventricular disproportion suggesting a poor outcome survived (Sharland *et al.*, 1992). This left an 84% mortality for fetuses with CDH and an abnormally low left:right ventricular ratio. Gestational age at diagnosis made little difference in this series, although progressive deterioration of the left ventricular development was predictive of poor outcome. The cause of poor left heart development is uncertain (Siebert, Haas & Beckwith, 1984), but the presence of right-sided underdevelopment in a right-sided hernia suggests that it is pressure related (Sharland *et al.*, 1992), although neither of these observations rule out a field defect (Iritani, 1984; Kluth, Petersen & Zimmerman, 1982; Kluth *et al.*, 1990; 1993), as discussed later.

Estimation of the fetal lung area:thoracic area ratio in the four chamber view (Kamata *et al.*, 1992) initially suggested that a ratio >0.18 predicted 100% survival. A ratio <0.18 did not, however, predict who would die, as two of six with this small lung area survived. Therefore, the ratio is no better a predictor of mortality than simple antenatal detection of CDH. Furthermore, the two

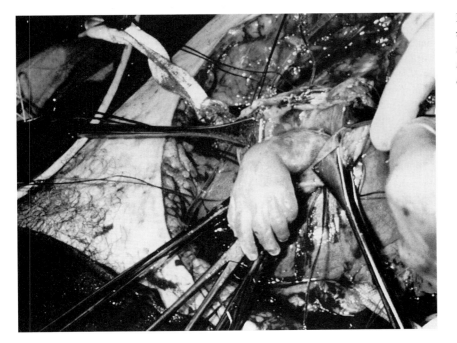

Fig. 18.3 *The fetal hand visible through a small uterine incision prior to correction of the diaphragmatic defect.*

fetuses with the smallest lungs measured in this manner actually survived. This ratio appears more useful in predicting neonatal survival than in identifying those suitable for fetal surgery.

Polyhydramnios is a good indicator of poor prognosis but is of little practical value as it occurs too late in gestation to allow for intervention before 25 to 27 weeks' gestation (Adzick *et al.*, 1989; Harrison *et al.*, 1993b). After 25 to 27 weeks, the uterus becomes more irritable and the time for lung growth and maturation becomes shorter. Therefore, intervention after this stage in gestation is unlikely to be of benefit (Harrison *et al.*, 1990c).

A review of published mortality rates in these subgroups is difficult to interpret as the reports are from different units, the postnatal treatments are different, and the numbers in each group are small (Pringle, 1991). The subgroup with the highest mortality, however, appears to be that group with a large volume of liver in the chest, especially where the ductus venosus is above the diaphragm, and gestational age is <25 weeks. Here, expected mortality exceeds 90% (Pringle, 1991). Remembering that fetal surgery after 25 weeks is more likely to induce preterm labour (Harrison *et al.*, 1993b), this combination is, therefore, the one with the greatest justification for fetal surgery, at a time when fetal surgery is still possible.

The major drawback for intervention in fetuses with liver in the chest is that this is also the most technically difficult group to correct antenatally. Because the ductus venosus is pulled above the remnants of the diaphragm with the liver, reducing the liver back into the abdomen kinks the ductus venosus and the fetus dies (Harrison *et al.*, 1990c; 1993a,b). Despite these technical difficulties, the candidate for further development of clinical trials for fetal correction of CDH appears to be the fetus with a large volume of liver in the chest detected before 25 weeks' gestation. Those picked up early in gestation without liver in the chest may also become future candidates for fetal surgery, if postoperative management can be improved and surgical techniques made successful to the point that 70–80% of these fetuses survive after fetal surgery.

Present limitations

At present, two major hurdles face fetal surgery for CDH. One is the inability to control uterine contractions and the other is the shut down in fetoplacental blood flow during and after surgery (Harrison *et al.*, 1981; 1982; 1990b,c; 1993a,b; Adzick *et al.*, 1986; Nakayama *et al.*, 1984; Ford *et al.*, 1992; 1993). Another major theoretical barrier is whether or not surgical techniques allow the lungs to grow sufficiently to function at birth. So far no animal study of surgical correction *in utero* has mimicked the early onset of severe CDH, especially as the underlying cause may be a defective lung rather than a simple hole in the diaphragm (see below).

Maternal risks

The fetus is not the only consideration. High-risk surgery cannot be justified solely on the basis that the fetus would die without intervention, especially if the potential improvement in survival, seen only in selected groups, is little better than the natural history. The risks to the mother are not inconsiderable in both current and future pregnancies (Longaker, Golbus & Filly, 1991). In Adelaide we have found that mothers who consider fetal surgery are older and subfertile, whereas those who terminate are often younger and have had no difficulties with conception. The older mothers are more likely to have other medical problems which contribute to infertility, to the risks of surgery and, for example in the case of diabetes, to the risk of the abnormality in the first place. Indeed, diabetes itself has been cited as a contraindication to fetal surgery for CDH (F. Bargy, personal communication). Obviously, where the results of fetal surgery are poor, the balance of risk is often against an intervention. So far, however, there have been no reported fatalities and little morbidity (Harrison *et al.*, 1993b).

Associated anomalies

Before embarking on intervention, the fetus has to be assessed. Obviously, other major lesions that are lethal preclude intervention. The more common include trisomies 18 and 13, neural tube and cardiac defects (Puri, 1989; Thorpe-Beeston, Gosden & Nicolaides, 1989; Sharland *et al.*, 1992). Those stillborn have a high frequency of chromosomal defects, whereas those who are born alive but die before transfer to a neonatal surgical unit have a high frequency of major cardiac defects (Sweet & Puri, 1993). Nevertheless, virtually all of these can be ruled out by present antenatal diagnostic methods (Harrison, 1990). Therefore, the workup should include detailed ultrasound, karyotyping and fetal echocardiography. Furthermore, for fetuses with liver in the chest, colour Doppler helps determine the position of the ductus venosus to warn of the potentially fatal difficulties with liver reduction.

Fetal risks

The fetus itself is also at increased risk in circumstances where the mother's health is less than ideal, so that the results of fetal surgery to date may well have been unfavourably biased by the type of patient involved. For example, in one case of fetal intervention for CDH attempted in Adelaide, the patient was diabetic, obese, infertile and towards the end of her reproductive years. The surgery on the fetus was uneventful (Fig. 18.3), but the fetus died *in utero* two days later. Abnormal variations in blood sugar levels may have contributed to this, as surgery, diabetes and b-mimetics all increase blood sugar levels (Keirse, Grant & King, 1989) and jeopard-ize diabetic control, which in turn may have produced fetal acidaemia (Lawrence, Brown & Parsons, 1982). In addition, postmortem changes in this fetus were similar to those seen in fetal lambs in right heart failure after indomethacin administration (Levin *et al.*, 1979), again implying that there had been disruption of fetoplacental blood flow. Myocardial depression associated with the use of halothane possibly also contributed to the demise (Sabik *et al.*, 1993).

Even if the fetus survives the immediate risks of open surgery, the major problem after fetal intervention for CDH remains the inability to maintain uterine quies-cence, and fetoplacental blood flow (Harrison *et al.*, 1993b). This in turn appears to have a large contribution from fetal stress, which can also produce circulatory shutdown, fetal demise and preterm labour (Fenton *et al.*, 1992). Present methods have been unsuccessful in preventing this chain of events (Harrison *et al.*, 1993b) and, unless they can be prevented, the development of fetal surgery will be limited.

Is the lesion correctable?

To date, the assumption has been that the primary defect is one in the diaphragm, and the resultant PH, pulmo-nary immaturity and vascular changes are all the direct result of pressure, preventing the lung on the affected side from growing, pushing the mediastinum across and preventing the lung on the opposite side from growing (Harrison, 1980a,b; Anderson, 1986; Pringle, 1984; 1989). This may not be the case. The lungs may not have grown because they are part of a field defect. Viscera entering the chest would then be a passive event (Kimbrough *et al.*, 1974; Costlow & Manson, 1981; Iritani, 1984; Kluth *et al.*, 1982; 1990; 1993) and any antenatal correction of the defect in the diaphragm would be unlikely to induce growth and maturation in the defective lungs, and any postnatal salvage procedure such as ECMO would similarly be unlikely to work (Langham *et al.*, 1987; O'Rourke, Lillehei & Crone, 1991; Wilson *et al.*, 1991; 1992).

Therefore, the possibility of a field defect becomes central to whether or not fetal correction of CDH will work. There are observations for and against the concept of a field defect being the cause of severe forms of CDH. The evidence for a field defect occurring at the stage of lung budding, at least in those with liver in the chest, is as follows. First, the similarity to the field defects produced by teratogens given to the embryo at the time of lung budding and early formation of the septum transversum, but not at the time of closure of the pleuro-peritoneal canals (Iritani, 1984; Kluth *et al.*, 1990), implies that development of the lung and septum transversum is impaired, not the closure of the diaphragm. Therefore, when nitrofen or bisdiamine (Momma *et al.*, 1992) is administered to fetal rats, they develop CDH similar to those seen in human neonates with liver in the chest. These induced lesions are equivalent to the most severe form of human CDH (Kluth *et al.*, 1993). In this animal model, there is a field defect affecting the lung bud, medial portion of the diaphragm, liver and, possibly, the heart itself (Kluth *et al.*, 1990; Momma *et al.*, 1992). Surprisingly, however, despite the expectation that the lung will be abnormal from the earliest stages, the lung appears normal until such time as the liver moves up into the chest (Kluth *et al.*, 1993), suggesting that fetal surgery may still have the potential to correct PH in this situation.

Whether a teratogen is involved in the human embryo that develops CDH is unknown and, therefore, chemically induced CDH cannot be considered entirely analogous to the human situation. Nevertheless, if CDH in animals secondary to chemically induced field defects can be ameliorated by fetal surgery with subsequent neonatal survival, it would imply that the most affected lungs could also recover in the human.

Another observation that supports the concept of the lungs being the major defect is that other malformations of disordered lung budding are also associated with CDH (Savic et al., 1979; Jaubert & Daniel, 1991; Chavrier, 1991). For example, in a review of 56 extra-lobar sequestrations there was a 30% incidence of CDH, and in 400 intralobar sequestrations, there was a 3% incidence (Savic et al., 1979).

Evidence against a field defect, and in favour of simple pressure on the lungs, is that other mass lesions in the chest also interfere with lung growth and development. In the fetus, large cystic adenomatoid malformations (CAM) of the lung can increase in size to produce mediastinal shift, polyhydramnios, marked pulmonary hypoplasia in the remaining lung and fetal hydrops (Dumez et al., 1993), similar to the effects of CDH. If the CAM is removed antenatally, or after birth, the residual lung will recover (Chapter 19) (Harrison, 1990; Kuller et al., 1992). If there is fetal cardiomegaly, then there is also PH (Kleinman & Copel, 1992; Chaoui et al., 1994). Furthermore, the presence of viscera in a left CDH can also produce reversible hypoplasia of the left side of the heart (Crawford et al., 1986), implying that this part of the complex, at least, is the result of direct pressure and is not a field defect (Siebert et al., 1984; Kluth et al., 1993).

Children who survived the postnatal correction of CDH 10 to 20 years ago have been shown to have almost normal lungs by adolescence (Simson & Eckstein, 1985; Falconer et al., 1990), demonstrating the capacity to recover from pressure effects similar to those seen in the first animal model of a balloon occupying one hemithorax (Harrison et al., 1980a). In more recent studies, more severely affected survivors have shown far less capacity for lung growth and recovery. Where ECMO has been used, respiratory cripples are being seen (Langham et al., 1987; O'Rourke et al., 1991; Wilson et al., 1991; 1992), suggesting that the more severely affected neonates may be suffering from a different disease, such

as a field defect, to those who survived with normal lung function in the past, i.e. a failure of closure of the pleuro-peritoneal canal at a later stage of development. Therefore, there remains some doubt that CDH is a simple easily correctable mechanical defect that merely prevents development of the lungs by pressure alone.

So far human experience with fetal surgery for CDH has failed to clarify the issue. After surgery, most fetuses have not died of unremitting PH after many weeks in utero (which would have allowed the lungs to grow). Rather they have died immediately or within days of the surgery because of failure to achieve uterine quiescence, or they have died because of interference with fetoplacental blood flow, as a result of either compression of the ductus venosus (Harrison et al., 1993b; Ford et al., 1993), or right heart failure, as seen in lamb fetuses after indomethacin and halothane (Levin et al., 1979; Kleinman & Copel, 1992; Sabik et al., 1993). Until such time as the fetus with the liver and ductus venosus in the chest can be operated on with relative impunity, leaving the fetus in utero for several weeks to recover, the advisability of correcting those with a potential field defect remains uncertain.

Future developments

Reducing fetal stress

Because of the disappointing results achieved to date with fetal surgery, other less invasive methods of in utero correction are being developed in the laboratory animal. The observation that high spinal anaesthesia during heart–lung bypass in fetal sheep prevents placental shutdown (Fenton et al., 1992) implies that if fetal pain or physiological stress can be avoided then there might be more chance of the fetus remaining in utero after surgery. This has led to the concept of a 'fetal intensive care unit' where the fetus is intensively monitored and analgesia provided as needed (Harrison et al., 1993b; Jennings et al., 1993a). If this includes more invasive techniques that involve direct access to the fetus, and more prolonged fetal stress, however, then those techniques might themselves initiate labour.

Nevertheless, procedures with less stress apparently induce less preterm labour. When urinary catheters are placed in the fetus, the procedure-related mortality rate is 6% (Manning, Harrison & Rodeck, 1986), whereas open fetal surgery for CDH has a rate of 70% (Harrison et al., 1993b).

Minimally invasive fetal surgery

This has led to the concept of attempting 'laparoscopic' or minimally invasive procedures on the fetus (Estes et al., 1992; Copeland et al., 1993; Deprest et al., 1994), as discussed in Chapter 3. If the mortality for CDH could be reduced even to 20–30% employing minimally invasive surgery, then there would be greater acceptance of antenatal intervention for this condition. Nevertheless, the creation of a laparoscopic 'window' within the fetus will be a limiting factor, or even an impossible barrier, as the pressure created could obstruct the umbilical vein. Therefore, techniques may be limited to those that can be employed by operating on the outer surface of the fetus or on its superficial tissues using the uterus and amniotic fluid as the 'window' (McMahon et al., 1992; Deprest et al., 1994; Montgomery et al., 1995).

There are two potential techniques for the correction of CDH that lend themselves to operating from outside the fetus: the PLUG ('plug the lung until it grows'), and the creation of a fetal gastroschisis.

The PLUG technique

A procedure being developed in fetal sheep, at the University of California at San Francisco and in Boston (Harrison et al., 1993a; Wilson et al., 1993; M. H. Hedrick, personal communication), may succeed in reducing fetal stress, but it might also cause further damage to the lung. Although the procedure obstructs the trachea of fetuses with CDH, it would only necessitate operating on the superficial tissues of the fetus and could also deal with the problem of liver in the chest.

The lungs of fetuses with CDH are both small and immature (Pringle, 1989), but if the trachea is ligated and obstructed there is the possibility that both volume and maturation could be improved (Wilson et al., 1993). The procedure relies on the observation that the fetus forms lung fluid throughout most of pregnancy (Kitterman et al., 1979), and this lung fluid flows out of the lungs at a low but positive pressure (Nicolini et al., 1989;

Wilson et al., 1993). Any obstruction to the outflow of this fluid would increase the pressure within the lungs, which would in turn increase the volume of the lungs themselves, pushing the viscera back out of the chest (Wilson et al., 1993). One such study in sheep established a CDH at 90 days' gestation and ligated the trachea at the same time: the lung expanded to the point that it entered the abdomen (Wilson et al., 1993). Ligating the trachea may produce a big lung that is ineffective and, even where the lung is normal at the time of ligation in the fetal lamb, the end result is a larger alveolus, with reduced type II cells and reduced lamellar bodies (Alcorn et al., 1977).

In the human fetus with CDH, the lungs may be affected from so early in gestation that they are incapable of secreting sufficient fluid to 'inflate' the lung to a more normal size and accelerate maturation. In the human neonate with Fraser syndrome, for example, a completely blocked airway produces potentially ineffective lungs with delayed alveolization (Labbe et al., 1992) and maturation, despite animal experiments suggesting accelerated maturation (Wilson et al., 1993). Where there is complete laryngeal atresia in this syndrome, the lungs are large despite the absence of functioning kidneys. Where there is stenosis, the associated absence of kidneys and amniotic fluid produced lungs that were hypoplastic (Boyd, Keeling & Lindenbaum, 1988; Gattuso, Patton & Barraitser, 1987), suggesting that complete obstruction would have to be maintained if the lungs were to become larger and more mature in CDH. Similar changes have been noted in non-syndromal atresias (Wigglesworth, Desai & Hislop, 1987; Furness, Donnelly & Lipsett, 1991; Choong et al., 1992).

Nevertheless, tracheal ligation with a CDH in the fetal sheep appears to produce an acceleration of maturation as well as lung growth, so hopefully a procedure that blocks off the trachea from early in gestation could improve both the PH and the immaturity seen in human fetuses with a CDH (Wilson et al., 1993). So, despite possible drawbacks, the PLUG is potentially the best method for further development of fetal surgery for CDH. Technical problems which need to be addressed include atraumatic blockage of the trachea without ligation, maintenance of the blockage with tracheal growth, and rapid relief of the blockage at birth.

Iatrogenic gastroschisis

If the maldevelopment of the lungs is entirely the result of pressure of herniated viscera, relieving the pressure generated by those viscera could improve lung function at birth. Allowing the intestine to herniate out of the abdominal cavity could relieve that pressure. While creating an artificial gastroschisis works effectively in surgically created CDH in fetal sheep (Montgomery *et al.*, 1995), the potential gastrointestinal complications of that gastroschisis remain. In addition, it has the same potential drawbacks as all other methods of correction if the lung is primarily at fault. Nevertheless, this procedure has been carried out in two human fetuses with mixed results (Porecco *et al.*, 1994).

Neonatal lung transplantation

If a reliable technique for intervention is developed and fetuses subsequently remain *in utero* for several weeks, failure of the lung to recover would imply that there is an underlying lung defect that is uncorrectable. Either a field defect or the marked delay in maturation and growth precludes short-term recovery. Then, part lung transplantation at birth may be the most logical method of salvaging these fetuses. The lung that is directly compressed by the CDH could be removed and part of an adult lung might be transplanted into the newborn (Adzick *et al.*, 1992). Obviously that raises its own ethical, technical and financial questions, which will have to be addressed.

Single segments of adult lungs have been transplanted into neonatal animals. They exchange gas effectively and are more compliant than the whole neonatal lung (Crombleholme *et al.*, 1990; Adzick, 1992). The most suitable segment for transplantation has been determined for the human (Jennings *et al.*, 1993b), and one neonatal transplant has been performed at Stanford University using the left upper lobe and lingula of a cadaveric donor (Adzick, 1992). That transplant failed at eight months because of massive rejection.

Can the adult segment grow and can rejection be controlled? Transplantation of segments of adult beagle lungs from living related donors to puppies showed that there was still acute and chronic rejection despite immunosuppression. In addition, there was stenosis of the pulmonary artery, pulmonary vein and bronchus in these animals. But, in the 10% that survived long term, lung function of the transplanted segment alone was adequate to support the animal for up to 330 days after transplant when they are almost fully grown (Backer *et al.*, 1991). In the clinical setting, one 12-year-old girl has received a segment of her mother's lung and was doing well one year later (Adzick, 1992).

The possibility of inducing tolerance to engraftment in the fetal recipient has been studied in the neonatal swine, the dog and the mouse to improve the prospects of transplantation without rejection of the graft (Adzick, 1992; West, Morris & Wood, 1994). In one study, fetal liver haematopoietic cells were used to induce tolerance to subsequent cardiac allografts in neonatal mice (immunologically immature at birth) without evidence of graft-versus-host disease (GVHD), and without the need for immunosuppression (West *et al.*, 1994). Furthermore, the 'unresponsiveness was found not to be donor-specific with prolongation of third-party allografts as well as donor-type grafts'. To date, the donor had to be semi-allogeneic to the recipient to avoid GVHD and had to share major and minor histocompatibility antigens to establish this type of tolerance, but when the donor and the recipient are both immunologically immature, then fully allogeneic donors may be used (West *et al.*, 1994). Therefore, tolerance to lung grafts might be induced *in utero* by using fetal stem cells from a donor, with transplantation from that living donor after birth. The use of anencephalics is, however, controversial, but the possibility exists that grafting from other species may be feasible.

Furthermore, an allogeneic segment of transplanted lung may not have to be a permanent fixture, as the contralateral lung may still have the potential to grow and mature, assuming that it is not involved in a field defect that would prevent such growth. Therefore, the transplanted lung segment may be no more than a temporary assist device while that occurs (Adzick, 1992).

Parental choice

Finally, the wishes of the parents have to be paramount for any fetus detected with a major defect when termination of pregnancy can still be offered. In many cases, the parents will wish to terminate rather than embark on the highly stressful pathway of fetal intervention, no matter what its form. In addition, cost will become a factor, as expensive technology for an abnormality that occurs in 1:2000 fetuses will be impractical for all. Nevertheless, if the results improve to the point that fetal surgery is simple and applicable in many centres, then costs would be contained and might be far less than the alternatives of ECMO and other expensive treatment options after birth.

Perinatal management of uncorrected CDH

If the fetus with a CDH does not undergo intervention, then the place and timing of delivery needs careful consideration. Should the neonate undergo emergency surgery, or should surgery be delayed to allow lung function to improve? Emergency surgery may well decrease chest wall compliance and gas exchange (Sakai et al., 1987). So far, there is no definite answer, but delayed surgery with aggressive decompression of the GI tract (to prevent the pressure of gas in the herniated intestine from producing further pulmonary compromise) is at least as effective as emergency surgery. Prolonged delay, even to the point of letting the neonate die without surgery gives at least as good an overall survival rate as emergency surgery (Cartlidge, Mann & Kapila, 1986; Sakai et al., 1987; Langer et al., 1988; Charlton, Bruce & Davenport, 1991; Goh et al., 1992). Therefore, those faced with an unexpected CDH in the delivery room can initiate treatment as effective, or possibly more effective than emergency surgery.

Should the mother be given steroids and thyroid-releasing hormone in an attempt to improve surfactant production? Should the fetus be given a course of prophylactic surfactant as soon as it is born on the basis that the lungs are immature? In the animal model, the lungs are surfactant deficient (Glick et al., 1992). The answer is unclear from the anecdotal reports and limited experience.

Whether or not the mother is transferred to a unit that has ECMO capability will depend on availability, but the impact of these units on the outcome for CDH has not been as great as in other neonatal respiratory diseases (Wilson et al., 1992). Early delivery for immediate extra-uterine repair does not improve survival and should not be attempted (Harrison, 1990).

Conclusion

Isolated congenital diaphragmatic hernia is associated with a high perinatal mortality rate of 60 to 70% if untreated, largely owing to pulmonary hypoplasia. Despite a sound basis for correction validated in animal experiments, human experience with open fetal surgery has been disappointing. In addition to technical difficulties, the major limiting factor remains iatrogenic preterm labour. Minimally invasive techniques are being developed which may be adapted to the in utero amelioration of diaphragmatic hernia.

References

Adzick, N. S. (1992). On the horizon: neonatal lung transplantation. *Archives of Disease in Childhood*, 67, 455–7.

Adzick, N. S., Harrison, M. R., Glick, P. L., Anderson, J., Villa, R. L., Flake, A. W. & Laberg, J.-M. (1986). Fetal surgery in the primate. III. Maternal outcome after fetal surgery. *Journal of Pediatric Surgery*, 21, 477–80.

Adzick, N. S., Harrison, M. R., Glick, P. L., Nakayama, D. K., Manning, F. A. & de Lorimier, A. A. (1985a). Diaphragmatic hernia in the fetus: prenatal diagnosis and outcome in 94 cases. *Journal of Pediatric Surgery*, 20, 357–61.

Adzick, N. S., Outwater, K. M., Harrison, M. R., Davies, P., Glick, P. L., de Lorimier, A. A. & Reid, L. (1985b). Correction of congenital diaphragmatic hernia in utero. IV. An early gestation fetal lamb model for pulmonary vascular morphometric analysis. *Journal of Pediatric Surgery*, 20, 673–80.

Adzick, N. S., Vacanti, J. P., Lillehei, C. W., O'Rourke, P. P., Crone, R. K. & Wilson, J. M. (1989). Fetal diaphragmatic hernia: ultrasound diagnosis and clinical outcome in 38 cases. *Journal of Pediatric Surgery*, 24, 654–8.

Alcorn, D., Adamson, T. M., Lambert, T. F., Maloney, J. E., Ritchie, B. C. & Robinson, P. M. (1977). Morphological effects of chronic tracheal ligation and drainage in the fetal lamb lung. *Journal of Anatomy*, 123, 649–60.

Anderson, K. D. (1986). Congenital diaphragmatic hernia. In *Pediatric Surgery*, 4th edn, ed. K. J. Welch, J. G. Rudolph, M. M. Ravitch, J. A. O'Neill & M. I. Rowe, pp. 589–601. Chicago: Year Book Medical Publications.

Backer, C. L., Ohtake, S., Zales, V. R., LoCicero, J., Michaelis, L. L. & Idriss, F. S. (1991). Living-related lobar lung transplantation in beagle puppies. *Journal of Pediatric Surgery*, 26, 429–33.

Boyd, P. A., Keeling, J. W. & Lindenbaum, R. H. (1988). Fraser syndrome (cryptophthalmos-syndactyly syndrome): a review of 11 cases with post-mortem findings. *Journal of Anatomy*, 31, 159–68.

Breaux, C. W., Rouse, T. M., Cain, W. S. & Georgeson, K. E. (1991). Improvement in survival of patients with congenital diaphragmatic hernia utilizing a strategy of delayed repair after medical and/or extracorporeal membrane oxygenation stabilization. *Journal of Pediatric Surgery*, 26, 333–8.

Burge, D. M., Atwell, J. D. & Freeman, N. V. (1989). Could the stomach site help predict outcome in babies with left-sided congenital diaphragmatic hernia diagnosed antenatally? *Journal of Pediatric Surgery*, 24, 567–9.

Cartlidge, P. H. T., Mann, N. P. & Kapila, L. (1986). Preoperative stabilization in congenital diaphragmatic hernias. *Archives of Disease in Childhood*, 61, 1226–8.

Chaoui, R., Bollmann, R., Goldner, B., Heling, K. S. & Tennstedt, C. (1994). Fetal cardiomegaly: echocardiographic findings and outcome in 19 cases. *Fetal Diagnosis and Therapy*, 9, 92–104.

Charlton, A. J., Bruce, J. & Davenport, M. (1991). Timing of surgery in congenital diaphragmatic hernia. Low mortality after pre-operative stabilisation. *Anaesthesia*, 46, 820–3.

Chavrier, P. M. (1991). Intrapulmonary lesions. In *Pediatric Thoracic Surgery*, ed. J. C. Fallis, R. M. Filler & G. Lemoine, pp. 75–83. New York: Elsevier.

Choong, K. K. L., Trudinger, B., Chow, C. & Osborn, R. A. (1992). Fetal laryngeal obstruction: sonographic detection. *Ultrasound in Obstetrics and Gynecology*, 2, 357–9.

Copeland, M. L., Bruner, J. P., Richards, W. O., Sundell, H. W. & Tulipan, N. B. (1993). A model of *in utero* endoscopic treatment of myelomeningocele. *Neurosurgery*, 33, 542–5.

Costlow, R. D. & Manson, J. M. (1981). The heart and diaphragm: target organs in the neonatal death induced by bitroren (2,4-dichlorophenyl-*p*-nitrophenyl ether). *Toxicology*, 20, 209–27.

Crawford, D. C., Drake, D. P., Kwaitkowski, D. K., Chapman, M. G. & Allan, L. D. (1986). Prenatal diagnosis of reversible cardiac hypoplasia associated with congenital diaphragmatic hernia: implications for post-natal management. *Journal of Clinical Ultrasound*, 14, 718–21.

Crawford, D. C., Wright, V. M., Drake, D. P. & Allan, L. D. (1989). Fetal diaphragmatic hernia: the value of fetal echocardiography in the prediction of postnatal outcome. *British Journal of Obstetrics and Gynaecology*, 96, 705–10.

Crombleholme, T. M., Adzick, N. S., Hardy, K., Longaker, M. T., Bradley, S. M., Duncan, B. W., Verrier, E. D. & Harrison, M. R. (1990). Pulmonary lobar transplantation in neonatal swine: a model for treatment of congenital diaphragmatic hernia. *Journal of Pediatric Surgery*, 25, 11–18.

de Lorimier, A. A., Tierney, D. F. & Parker, H. R. (1967). Hypoplastic lungs in fetal lambs with surgically created congenital diaphragmatic hernia. *Surgery*, 62, 12–17.

Deprest, J. A., Luks, F. I., Vandenberghe, K., Lerut, T., Brosens, I. A., Van Asche, F. A. (1994). Intra-uterine video-endoscopic creation of lower urinary tract obstruction in the fetal lamb. *American Journal of Obstetrics and Gynecology*, 170, 274.

Dumez, Y., Mandelbrot, L., Radunovic, N., Revillon, Y., Dommergues, M., Aubry, M. C., Narcy, F. & Sonigo, P. (1993). Prenatal management of congenital cystic adenomatoid malformation of the lung. *Journal of Pediatric Surgery*, 28, 36–41.

Estes, J. M., Szabo, Z. & Harrison, M. R. (1992). Techniques for *in utero* endoscopic surgery. A new approach for fetal intervention. *Surgical Endoscopy*, 6, 215–18.

Falconer, A. R., Brown, R. A., Helms, P., Gordon, I. & Baron, J. A. (1990). Pulmonary sequelae in survivors of congenital diaphragmatic hernia. *Thorax*, 45, 126–9.

Fenton, K. N., Heinemann, M. K., Hickey, P. R. & Hanley, F. L. (1992). The stress of fetal surgery is blocked by total spinal anaesthesia. *Surgical Forum*, 43, 631–2.

Ford, W. D. A., Cool, J. & Derham, R. (1992). Intrathoracic silo for the potential antenatal repair of diaphragmatic herniae with liver in the chest. *Fetal Diagnosis and Therapy*, 7, 75–81.

Ford, W. D. A., Martin, A. J., Cool, J. C., Parsons, D. W. & Kennedy, J. D. (1993). Intrathoracic silo for fetal diaphragmatic hernia: lung growth and slow reduction of abdominal viscera. *Journal of Pediatric Surgery*, 28, 1006–8.

Furness, M. E., Donnelly, B. W. & Lipsett, J. (1991). Larynx, atresia. *Fetus*, 1, 74–83.

Gattuso, J., Patton, M. A. & Baraitser, M. (1987). The clinical spectrum of the Fraser syndrome: report of three cases, and a review. *Journal of Medical Genetics*, 24, 549–55.

Glick, P. L., Stannard, V. A., Leach, C. L., Rossman, J., Hosada, Y., Morin, F. C., Cooney, D. R., Allen, J. E. & Holm, B. (1992) Pathophysiology of congenital diaphragmatic hernia. II. The fetal lamb CDH model is surfactant deficient. *Journal of Pediatric Surgery*, 27, 382–8.

Goh, D. W., Drake, D. P., Brereton, R. J., Kiely, E. M. & Spitz, L. (1992). Delayed surgery for congenital diaphragmatic hernia. *British Journal of Surgery*, 79, 644–6.

Goodfellow, T., Hyde, I., Burge, D. M. & Freeman, N. V. (1987). Congenital diaphragmatic hernia: the prognostic significance of the site of the stomach. *British Journal of Radiology*, 60, 993–5.

Harrison, M. R. (1990). The fetus with a diaphragmatic hernia: pathophysiology, natural history, and surgical management. In *The Unborn Patient*, 2nd edn, ed. M. R. Harrison, M. S. Golbus & R. A. Filly, pp. 295–313. Philadelphia: W. B. Saunders.

Harrison, M. R., Adzick, N. S., Estes, J. M. & Howell, L. J. (1994). A prospective study of the outcome for fetuses with diaphragmatic hernia. *Journal of the American Medical Association*, 271, 382–4.

Harrison, M. R., Adzick, N. S., Flake, A. W. & Jennings, R. W. (1993a). The CDH two-step, a dance of necessity. *Journal of Pediatric Surgery*, 28, 813–16.

Harrison, M. R., Adzick, N. S., Flake, A. W., Jennings, R. W., Estes, J. M., MacGillivray, T. E., Chueh, J. T., Goldberg, J. D., Filly, R. A., Goldstein, R. B., Rosen, M. A., Cauldwell, C., Levine, A. H. & Howell, L. J. (1993b). Correction of congenital diaphragmatic hernia *in utero*. VI. Hard-earned lessons. *Journal of Pediatric Surgery*, 28, 1411–18.

Harrison, M. R., Adzick, N. S., Jennings, R. W., Duncan, B. W., Rosen, M. A., Filly, R. A., Goldberg, R. A., de Lorimier, A. A. & Golbus, M. S. (1990a). Antenatal intervention for congenital cystic adenomatoid malformation. *Lancet*, 336, 965–7.

Harrison, M. R., Adzick, N. S., Longaker, M. T., Goldberg, J. D., Rosen, M. A., Filly, R. A., Evans, M. I. & Golbus, M. S. (1990b). Successful repair *in utero* of a fetal diaphragmatic hernia after removal of herniated viscera from the left thorax. *New England Journal of Medicine*, 332, 1582–4.

Harrison, M. R., Anderson, J., Rosen, M. A., Ross, N. A. & Henricks, A. G. (1982). Fetal surgery in the primate. I. Anesthetic, surgical, and tocolytic management to maximize fetal-neonatal survival. *Journal of Pediatric Surgery*, 17, 115–22.

Harrison, M. R., Bjordal, R. I., Langmark, R. I. & Knutrud, O. (1978). Congenital diaphragmatic hernia: the hidden mortality. *Journal of Pediatric Surgery*, 13, 227–30.

Harrison, M. R., Bressack, M. A., Churg, A. M. & de Lorimier, A. A. (1980a). Correction of congenital diaphragmatic hernia *in utero*. II. Simulated correction permits fetal lung growth with survival at birth. *Surgery*, 88, 260–8.

Harrison, M. R., Jester, J. A. & Ross, N. A. (1980b). Correction of congenital diaphragmatic hernia *in utero*. I. The model: intrathoracic balloon produces fatal pulmonary hypoplasia. *Surgery*, 88, 174–82.

Harrison, M. R., Langer, J. C., Adzick, N. S., Golbus, M. S., Filly, R. A., Anderson, R. L., Rosen, M. A., Callen, P. W., Goldstein, R. B. & de Lorimier, A. A. (1990c). Correction of congenital diaphragmatic hernia *in utero*. V. Initial clinical experience. *Journal of Pediatric Surgery*, 25, 47–57.

Harrison, M. R., Ross, N. A. & de Lorimier, A. A. (1981). Correction of congenital diaphragmatic hernia *in utero*. III. Development of a successful surgical technique using abdominoplasty to avoid compromise of umbilical blood flow. *Journal of Pediatric Surgery*, 16, 934–42.

Iritani, I. (1984). Experimental study on embryo-genesis of congenital diaphragmatic hernia. *Anatomy and Embryology*, 169, 133–9.

Jaubert, F. & Danel, C. (1991). Intrathoracic malformations of the foregut derivatives. In *Pediatric Thoracic Surgery*, ed. J. C. Fallis, R. M. Filler & G. Lemoine, pp.72–74. New York: Elsevier.

Jennings, R. W., Adzick, N. S., Longaker, M. T., Lorenz, H. P., Estes, J. M. & Harrison, M. R. (1993a). New techniques in fetal surgery. *Journal of Pediatric Surgery*, 27, 1329–33.

Jennings, R. W., Lorenz, H. P., Duncan, B. W., Bradley, S. M., Harrison, M. R. & Adzick, N. S. (1993b). Adult-to-neonate lung transplantation: anatomical considerations. *Journal of Pediatric Surgery*, 27, 1285–90.

Jennings, R. W. MacGillivray, T. E., Rudolph, A. M., Ring, E. J., Adzick, N. S. & Harrison, M. R. (1992). Vascular changes in correction of congenital diaphragmatic hernia. *Surgical Forum*, 43, 629–31.

Kamata, S., Hasegawa, T., Ishikawa, S., Usui, N., Okuyama, H., Kawahara, H., Fukuzawa, M., Imura,

K. & Okada, A. (1992). Prenatal diagnosis of congenital diaphragmatic hernia and perinatal care: assessment of lung hypoplasia. *Early Human Development*, 29, 375–79.

Kent, G. M., Olley, P. M., Creighton, R. E., Dobbinson, T., Bryan, M. H., Symchych, M. H., Zingg, W. & Cummings, J. N. (1972). Hemodynamic and pulmonary changes following surgical creation of a diaphragmatic hernia in fetal lambs. *Surgery*, 72, 427–33.

Keirse, M. J. N. C., Grant, A. & King, J. F. (1989). Preterm labour. In *Effective Care in Pregnancy and Childbirth*. vol. I: *Pregnancy*, ed. I. Chalmers, M. Erkin & J. N. C. Keirse, pp. 694–745. Oxford: Oxford University Press.

Kimbrough, R. D., Gaines, T. B., Linder, R. E. & Ga, C. (1974). 2,4-Dichlorophenyl-*p*-nitrophenyl ether (TOK). Effects on the lung maturation of the rat fetus. *Archives of Environmental Health*, 28, 316–20.

Kitterman, J. A., Ballard, P. L., Clements, J. A., Meschner, J. E. & Tooley, W. H. (1979). Tracheal fluid in fetal lambs: spontaneous decrease prior to birth. *Journal of Applied Physiology*, 47, 985–9.

Kleinman, C. S. & Copel, J. A. (1992). Fetal cardiovascular physiology and therapy. *Fetal Diagnosis and Therapy*, 7, 147–57.

Kluth, D., Kangah, R., Reich, P., Tenbrick, R., Tibboel, D. & Lambrecht, W. (1990). Nitrofen-induced diaphragmatic hernia in rats: an animal model. *Journal of Pediatric Surgery*, 25, 850–4.

Kluth, D., Petersen, C. & Zimmermann, H. J. (1982). The developmental anatomy of congenital diaphragmatic hernia. *Paediatric Surgery International*, 2, 322–6.

Kluth, D., Tenbrick, R., von Ekesparre M., Kangah, R., Reich, P., Brandsma, A., Tibboel, D. & Lambrecht, W. (1993). The natural history of congenital diaphragmatic hernia and pulmonary hypoplasia in the embryo. *Journal of Pediatric Surgery*, 28, 456–63.

Kuller, J. A., Yankowitz, J., Goldberg, J. D., Harrison, M. R., Adzick, N. S., Filly, R. A., Callen, P. W. & Golbus, M. S. (1992). Outcome of antenatally diagnosed cystic adenomatoid malformations. *American Journal of Obstetrics and Gynecology*, 167, 1038–41.

Labbe, A., Dechelotte, P., Lemery, D. & Malpuech, G. (1992). Pulmonary hyperplasia in Fraser syndrome. *Pediatric Pulmonology*, 14, 131–4.

Langer, J. C., Filler, R. M., Bohn, D. J., Shandling, B., Ein, S., Wesson, D. E. & Superina, R. A. (1988). Timing of surgery for congenital diaphragmatic hernia: is emergency operation necessary? *Journal of Pediatric Surgery*, 23, 731–4.

Langham, M. R., Krummel, T. M., Bartlett, R. H., Drucker, D. E. M., Tracey, T. F., Toomasian, J. M., Greenfield, L. J. & Salzberg, A. M. (1987). Mortality with extracorporeal membrane oxygenation following repair of congenital diaphragmatic hernia in 93 infants. *Journal of Pediatric Surgery*, 22, 1150–4.

Lawrence, G. F., Brown, V. A. & Parsons, R. J. (1982). Feto–maternal consequences of high dose glucose infusion during labour. *British Journal of Obstetrics and Gynaecology*, 89, 27–32.

Levin, D. L., Mills, L, J, & Weinberg, A. G. (1979). Hemodynamic, pulmonary vascular, and myocardial abnormalities secondary to pharmacologic constriction of the fetal ductus arteriosus: a possible mechanism for persistent pulmonary hypertension in transient tricuspid insufficiency in the newborn infant. *Circulation*, 60, 360–6.

Longaker, M. Y., Golbus, M. S. & Filly, R. A. (1991). Maternal outcome after open fetal surgery: a review of the first 17 cases. *Journal of the American Medical Association*, 265, 737–41.

MacMahon, R. A., Renou, P. M., Shekelton, P. A. & Paterson, P. J. (1992). In utero cystostomy. *Lancet*, 340, 1234.

Manning, F. R., Harrison, M. R. & Rodeck, C. (1986). Catheter shunts for fetal hydronephrosis and hydrocephalus. Report of the International Fetal Surgery Registry. *New England Journal of Medicine*, 315, 336–40.

Momma, K., Ando, M., Mori, Y. & Ito, T. (1992). Hypoplasia of the lung and heart in fetal rats with diaphragmatic hernia. *Fetal Diagnosis and Therapy*, 7, 46–52.

Montgomery, L. D., Belfort, M. A., Saade, G. R., Baker, B. W., Pokorny, W., Minifee, P., Langston, C., Jevon, G., Van den Veyver, I., Robie, D., Longmire, S., Palacios, Q. & Moise, K. J. Jr (1995). Iatrogenic gastoschisis decreases pulmonary hypoplasia in an ovine congenital diaphragmatic hernia model. *Fetal Diagnosis and Therapy*, 10, 119–26.

Nakayama, D. K., Harrison, M. R., Chinn, D. H., Callen, P. W., Filly, R. A., Golbus, M. S. & de Lorimier, A. A. (1985). Prenatal diagnosis and natural history of the fetus with a congenital diaphragmatic hernia: initial clinical experience. *Journal of Pediatric Surgery*, 29, 118–24.

Nakayama, D. K., Harrison, M. R., Serron-Ferre, M. & Villa, R. L. (1984). Fetal surgery in the primate. II. Uterine electromyographic response to operative procedure and pharmacologic agents. *Journal of Pediatric Surgery*, 19, 333–9.

Nicolaides, K. H. & Azar, G. B. (1990). Thoraco-amniotic shunting. *Fetal Diagnosis and Therapy*, 5, 153–64.

Nicolini, U., Fisk, N. M., Rodeck, C. H., Talbert, D. G. & Wigglesworth, J. S. (1989). Low amniotic pressure in oligohydramnios – is this the cause of pulmonary hypoplasia? *American Journal of Obstetrics and Gynecology*, 161, 1098–1101.

O'Rourke, P. P., Lillehei, C. W. & Crone, R. K. (1991). The effect of extracorporeal membrane oxygenation (ECMO) on the survival of neonates with high risk congenital diaphragmatic hernia: 45 cases from a single institution. *Journal of Pediatric Surgery*, 26, 147–52.

Parsons, D. W., Ford, W. D. A., Cool, J. C., Martin, A. J., Staugas, R. E. M. & Kennedy, J. D. (1994). Fetal lung compliance in premature and term lambs after two methods of *in utero* repair of diaphragmatic hernia. *Thorax*, 49, 1015–19.

Porreco, R. P., Chang, J. H. T., Quissell, B. J. & Morgan, M. A. (1994). Palliative fetal surgery for diaphragmatic hernia. *American Journal of Obstetrics and Gynecology*, 170, 833–4.

Pringle, K. C. (1984). Fetal lamb and fetal lamb lung growth following creation and repair of a diaphragmatic hernia. In *Animal Models in Fetal Medicine*, ed. P. W. Nathanielz, pp. 109–48. New York: Perinatology Press.

Pringle, K. C. (1989). Lung development in congenital diaphragmatic hernia. In *Modern Problems in Paediatrics*, vol. 24, *Congenital Diaphragmatic Hernia*, ed. P. Puri, pp. 28–53. Basel: Karger.

Pringle, K. C. (1991). Fetal surgery: practical considerations and current status: where do we go from here with Bochdalek diaphragmatic hernia? In *Pediatric Thoracic Surgery*, ed. J. C. Fallis, R. M. Filler & G. Lemoine, pp. 333–43. New York: Elsevier.

Puri, P. (1989). Epidemiology of congenital diaphragmatic hernia. In *Modern Problems in Paediatrics*, vol. 24, *Congenital Diaphragmatic Hernia*, ed. P. Puri, pp. 22–7. Basel: Karger.

Sabik, J. F., Assad, R. S. & Hanley, F. L. (1993). Halothane as an anesthetic for fetal surgery. *Journal of Pediatric Surgery*, 28, 542–7.

Sakai, H., Tamura, M., Hosakawa, Y., Bryan, A. C., Barker, G. A. & Bohn, D. J. (1987). Effect of surgical repair on respiratory mechanics in congenital diaphragmatic hernia. *Journal of Pediatrics*, 111, 432–8.

Savic, B., Birtel, F. J., Tholen, W., Funke, H. D. & Knoche, R. (1979). Lung sequestration: report of seven cases and review of 540 published cases. *Thorax*, 34, 96–101.

Sharland, K. G., Lockhart, S. M., Heward, A. J. & Allan, L. D. (1992). Prognosis in fetal diaphragmatic hernia. *American Journal of Obstetrics and Gynecology*, 166, 9–13.

Shochat, S. J. (1987). Pulmonary vascular pathology in congenital diaphragmatic hernias. *Pediatric Surgery International*, 2, 331–5.

Siebert, J. R., Haas, J. E. & Beckwith, J. B. (1984). Left ventricular hypoplasia in congenital diaphragmatic hernia. *Journal of Pediatric Surgery*, 19, 567–71.

Simson, J. N. L. & Eckstein, H. B. (1985). Congenital diaphragmatic hernia: a 20 year experience. *British Journal of Surgery*, 72, 733–6.

Sweet, Y. & Puri, P. (1993). Congenital diaphragmatic hernia: influence of associated malformations on survival. *Archives of Disease in Childhood*, 69, 68–70.

Thorpe-Beeston, J. G., Gosden, C. M. & Nicolaides, K. H. (1989). Prenatal diagnosis of congenital diaphragmatic hernia: associated malformations and chromosomal defects. *Fetal Diagnosis and Therapy*, 4, 21–28.

Vacanti, J. P., O'Rourke, P. P., Lillehei, C. W. & Crone, R. K. (1988). The cardiopulmonary consequences of high-risk congenital diaphragmatic hernia. *Pediatric Surgery International*, 3, 1–5.

West, L. J., Morris, P. J. & Wood, K. J. (1994). Fetal liver haematopoietic cells and tolerance to organ allografts. *Lancet*, 343, 148–9.

Wigglesworth, J. S., Desai, R. & Hislop, A. A. (1987). Fetal lung growth in congenital laryngeal atresia. *Pediatric Pathology*, 7, 515–25.

Wilson, J. M., Di Fiore, J. W. & Peters, C. A. (1993). Experimental fetal tracheal ligation prevents the pulmonary hypoplasia associated with fetal nephrectomy: possible application for congenital diaphragmatic hernia. *Journal of Pediatric Surgery*, 28, 1433–40.

Wilson, J. M., Lund, D. P., Lillehei, C. W., O'Rourke, P. P. & Vacanti, J. P. (1992). Delayed repair and preoperative ECMO does not improve survival in high-risk congenital diaphragmatic hernia. *Journal of Pediatric Surgery*, 27, 368–75.

Wilson, J. M., Lund, D. P., Lillehei, C. W. & Vacanti, J. P. (1991). Congenital diaphragmatic hernia: predictors of severity in the ECMO era. *Journal of Pediatric Surgery*, 26, 1028–34.

19   Other surgical conditions

N. SCOTT ADZICK AND MARC H. HEDRICK

Introduction

After considerable initial investigation in animal models, we reported five cases of human fetal surgery by open hysterotomy in 1990 (Harrision et al., 1990). Although our early experience was limited to the treatment of congenital diaphragmatic hernia, it soon became apparent that the lessons learned in open hysterotomy and fetal surveillance could be applied to the correction of other major congenital defects. Surgery has been attempted in fetuses with cystic adenomatoid malformation, sacrococcygeal teratoma, stuck twin syndrome and congenital heart block in an effort to ameliorate these life-threatening lesions *in utero*. Correction of congenital hydrocephalus by transcutaneous shunt placement has also been undertaken in an effort to improve neonatal morbidity. Fetal surgery has proven beneficial for meningomyelocele in animal models but has yet to be undertaken in humans.

Congenital cystic adenomatoid malformation

Background

Prenatal diagnosis provides new insight into the natural history, pathophysiology, and management of fetuses with congenital cystic adenomatoid malformation (CCAM) of the lung (Adzick et al., 1985a; MacGillivray et al., 1993). The overall prognosis depends on the size of the lung mass and the secondary physiological derangement: a large mass causes mediastinal shift, hypoplasia of normal lung tissue, polyhydramnios and

cardiovascular compromise leading to fetal hydrops and death (Fig. 19.1). Hydrops is a harbinger of fetal or neonatal demise and manifests itself as fetal ascites, pleural and pericardial effusions, and skin and scalp oedema. The hydrops is secondary to obstruction of the fetal vena cava and direct cardiac compression from huge tumours that cause an extreme mediastinal shift. Smaller thoracic lesions can cause respiratory distress in the newborn period, and the smallest masses may be asymptomatic until later in childhood or adult life, when infection or malignant degeneration may occur (Halloran, Silverberg & Salzberg, 1972; Murphy et al., 1992).

Types of lesion

CCAM is almost always unilateral and is usually confined to one pulmonary lobe. Stocker et al. defined three types of CCAM based primarily on cyst size (Stocker, Manewell & Drake, 1977), whereas other authors have separated CCAM into two groups based on whether the predominant component of the lesion is cystic or solid (Oster & Fortune, 1979). We have classified CCAM lesions diagnosed in the fetus into two categories based on gross anatomy and ultrasound findings (Adzick et al., 1985c). Macrocystic lesions contain single or multiple cysts that are 5 mm in diameter, appear cystic on ultrasound, are not usually associated with hydrops and have a more favourable prognosis. Microcystic lesions are more solid, appear echogenic on ultrasound and are more commonly associated with pulmonary hypoplasia, fetal hydrops and death. Differences in perinatal survival in fetuses with CCAM have been previously ascribed to the histologic type of the lesion, but our experience and

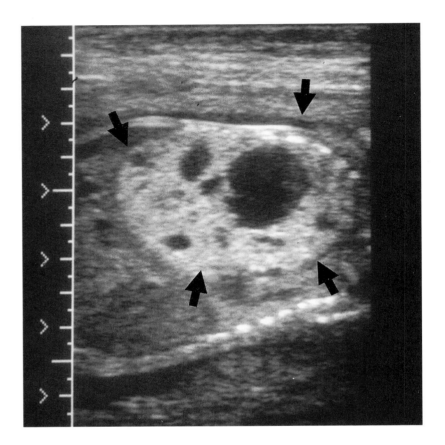

Fig. 19.1 *Sagittal sonogram of the fetal thorax and abdomen at 23 weeks' gestation demonstrates a large multicystic mass in the left hemithorax.*

that of others demonstrates that an unfavourable outcome is associated most closely with the size of the lesion and the presence of hydrops (Adzick *et al.*, 1985b; Harrison *et al.*, 1990a).

Differential diagnosis

Although a large pulmonary lesion diagnosed *in utero* might appear to be an ominous finding, the natural history of these lesions is variable. Some large fetal lung lesions can decrease in size and even 'disappear' before birth. We have followed 12 fetuses with large pulmonary lesions, four with CCAMs and eight with extralobar pulmonary sequestrations, associated with contralateral mediastinal shift that dramatically decreased in size over the course of the pregnancy (MacGillivray *et al.*, 1993). None of these fetuses had signs of hydrops. Other groups have also reported the partial involution of large

fetal pulmonary lesions, as determined by serial ultrasound examinations (Fine, Adzick & Doubilet, 1988; Saltzman, Adzick & Benacerraf, 1988; Kuller *et al.*, 1992). It would, therefore, appear that the natural history of fetal pulmonary lesions is dynamic and variable. Initial impressions concerning the prognosis of large pulmonary lesions should be tempered with the understanding that they can occasionally decrease in size.

Although sonographic prenatal diagnosis is becoming increasingly sophisticated, diagnostic errors are possible. Pulmonary sequestrations are masses of nonfunctioning lung tissue supplied by an anomalous systemic artery. The ultrasonographic appearance of pulmonary sequestration in the fetus is a well-defined, echodense, homogeneous mass in the lower chest or abdomen. Detection by colour flow Doppler of a systemic artery arising from the aorta and supplying the fetal lung lesion is a pathognomonic feature of pulmonary sequestration

(Hernanz-Schulman *et al.*, 1991), although pulmonary sequestrations that contain tissue with histologic changes of cystic adenomatoid malformation have been reported (Morin, Filiatrault & Russo, 1989). A diaphragmatic hernia can be distinguished either by careful sonographic assessment or by an amniography with or without CT scan. Other possibilities in the ultrasonographic differential diagnosis of fetal thoracic masses include bronchogenic and enteric cysts (Avni *et al.*, 1986), mediastinal cystic teratoma (Golladay & Mollitt, 1984), and bronchial atresia or stenosis.

Natural history

Large fetal lung tumours are frequently associated with polyhydramnios, which serves as a diagnostic marker. The increased amount of amniotic fluid makes the mother large for dates, which is a common obstetrical indication for ultrasonography. Polyhydramnios is likely to be caused by oesophageal compression by the thoracic mass with subsequent interference with fetal swallowing of amniotic fluid. Support for this concept comes from the absence of fluid in the fetal stomach in some of these cases, and the alleviation of polyhydramnios with the appearance of fluid in the fetal stomach after effective *in utero* treatment (Nicolaides & Azar, 1990). Although there is some association of both polyhydramnios and hydrops with fetal CCAM, our studies indicate that either can occur independently of one another.

Fifty-two fetal CCAM patients were referred to the University of California, San Francisco (UCSF) Fetal Treatment Center over an 11 year period from 1 January, 1983 to 1 January, 1994. All patients had evaluation of their sonographic findings at UCSF, and patient management was subsequently performed either in San Francisco or at the referring institution. In the absence of nonimmune hydrops, serial prenatal sonography was performed to monitor the size of the lesion and to look for the early presence of hydrops. In any fetus where prenatal intervention was considered, fetal echocardiography was used to rule out cardiac defects, and karyotyping was performed.

Forty-six women elected to continue their pregnancies after their fetus was diagnosed with a CCAM lesion. Six women underwent pregnancy termination: four fetuses had hydrops, one had multiple structural abnormalities and hydrops, and one had no other evidence of anomalies.

There were 26 fetuses with CCAM lesions that were not associated with hydrops. Three fetuses had *in utero* pleuroamniotic shunts placed; the remaining 23 fetuses were managed with maternal transport, planned delivery near or at term, and resection of the mass by lobectomy during the neonatal period. Several of these babies required substantial ventilatory support, with one requiring treatment with extracorporeal membrane oxygenation (ECMO). All of these neonates survived. In this group, four CCAM lesions appeared large at 20 to 26 weeks' gestation with an associated contralateral mediastinal shift, but they then decreased in size during the third trimester with return of the heart back toward the midline. Although two of these 'shrinking' lesions were initially associated with polyhydramnios and one case was associated with ascites, these phenomena resolved as the masses decreased in size.

Twenty cases were associated with hydrops. Only one had an associated anomaly, tetralogy of Fallot. Early in our experience, 11 hydropic fetuses were followed expectantly. All died after preterm labour and delivery at 28 to 36 weeks' gestation; five mothers had associated placentomegaly and preeclampsia.

Experimental studies: rationale for fetal surgery

Experimental studies have elucidated the pathophysiological consequences of fetal intrathoracic masses and have demonstrated that fetal pulmonary resection is straightforward. Simulation of the thoracic mass effect with an intrathoracic balloon in the third trimester fetal lamb resulted in pulmonary hypoplasia and death at term as a result of respiratory insufficiency (Harrison, Jester & Ross, 1980). In contrast, lambs that underwent simulated resection of the mass by balloon deflation in the middle of the third trimester had sufficient lung growth to permit survival at birth (Harrison *et al.*, 1980). In addition, intrauterine pneumonectomy in fetal lambs is technically feasible at early and midgestation and can induce compensatory growth of the remaining lung by term (Adzick *et al.*, 1985c).

In order to study the aetiology of hydrops associated with huge fetal lung masses, a fetal sheep model was

Table 19.1 *Pleuroamniotic shunts for CCAM*

Case	Fetal hydrops	Age at shunt placement (weeks)	Prenatal course	Age at delivery (weeks)	Outcome	Lesion location
1	Yes	22	Membranes ruptured 3 days after shunt; stillborn fetus	22	–	Entire right lung
2	No	30	Catheter migration at 32 weeks prompted delivery	32	High frequency ventilation for 2 weeks; surgery twice; alive and well at 3 years	Entire left lung
3	No	28	Catheter functioned for 10 weeks and polyhydramnios resolved	38	Resection at 1 h of age; postop. ECMO for 4 days; alive and well at 2 years	RUL RML
4	No	25	Catheter functioned for 11 weeks	36	Resected at 3 days; alive and well at 1 year	RLL

RML, right middle lobe; RUL, right upper lobe.

created in which a surgically implanted intrathoracic tissue expander was gradually inflated over several days. Fetal arterial, venous, intrathoracic and intraamniotic pressures and the sonographic appearance of hydrops were closely monitored (Rice *et al.*, 1994). Balloon inflation resulted in hydrops as a consequence of cardiac venous obstruction and increasing central venous pressure. Simulation of prenatal resection of the fetal thoracic mass by deflating the expander resulted in complete resolution of the hydrops and return of the venous pressure to normal. This model may be used to evaluate further the pathophysiological and sonographic features of large fetal chest masses.

Human fetal surgery experience

The knowledge that hydrops is a predictor of poor neonatal outcome led us to offer fetal surgical resection in cases of massive multicystic or predominantly solid CCAM lesions. Fetuses with life-threatening CCAM were selected for prenatal treatment according to predetermined guidelines, including the gestational age of the fetus, the size of the intrathoracic lesion, maternal health and the presence of fetal hydrops. The finding that fetuses with large tumours and hydrops are at high risk for fetal or neonatal demise led to several therapeutic manoeuvres in 12 fetuses. The first six fetal

surgery patients have been reviewed in detail (Adzick, Harrison & Flake, 1993). Fetal thoracentesis alone was ineffective because of rapid reaccumulation of cyst fluid. Pleuroamniotic shunts are difficult to place, may lead to membrane rupture and are prone to migration and occlusion. Successful shunt placement has been reported in two fetuses with unilocular CCAM lesions; resolution of hydrops after three weeks of catheter drainage has been documented in an additional case (Nicolaides, Blott & Greenough, 1987; Clark *et al.*, 1987). Multicystic or predominantly solid CCAM lesions do not lend themselves to catheter decompression and require resection.

At UCSF, four fetuses with large solitary cysts had placement of pleuroamniotic shunts percutaneously under ultrasound guidance (Table 19.1). Fetal thoracentesis alone was ineffective. One hydropic fetus died after prelabour premature rupture of membranes three days following shunt placement at 22 weeks' gestation. Three other nonhydropic fetuses with large cystic lesions and severe mediastinal shift had shunts placed at 25, 28, and 30 weeks' gestation that functioned for 11, 10, and 2 weeks, respectively. All three patients survived and underwent lobectomy immediately after birth although one required ECMO support for four days and another required high-frequency ventilation for two weeks.

Fetal surgical resection by lobectomy of the massively

Table 19.2 *CCAM resections*

Case	Fetal hydrops	Age at surgery (weeks)	Prenatal course	Age of delivery (weeks)	Outcome	Lesion location
1	Yes	27	Preterm labour and 'mirror' syndrome	28	Died from lung hypoplasia at 40 h	RML
2	Yes	23	Hydrops resolved 1 week after surgery	30	Ventilated for 2 days; left pneumothorax; alive and well at 4 years	LLL
3	Yes	26	Failed shunt at 25 weeks; hydrops resolved 2 weeks after surgery	34	Ventilated for 6 days; alive and well at 2½ years	LLL
4	Yes	26	Hydrops resolved 1 week after surgery	33	Ventilated for 2 days; alive and wlel at 2½ years	LLL
5	Yes	24	Postop. indomethacin-induced ductus arteriosus constriction; preterm labour/delivery 2 weeks postop.	26	Ventilated for 4 weeks; right pneumothorax; PDA ligation; alive and well at 2 years	RML
6	Yes	21	Fetal demise 8 h postop.; autopsy: no known cause of death	21	–	RML, RLL
7	Yes	25	Intra-op. fetal demise secondary to uterine contractions	–	–	RUL
8	Yes	24	Minimal uterine activity on nitroglycerin; hydrops resolved 1 week after surgery	30	Ventilated for 10 days; alive and well at 1 year	RML, RLL

RML, right middle lobe; LLL, left lower lobe; RUL, right upper lobe.

enlarged pulmonary lobe was performed at 21 to 27 weeks' gestation in eight patients with five survivors (Adzick *et al.*, 1993) (Table 19.2). In the first fetus, resection was too late, since preterm labour and maternal preeclampsia persisted postoperatively, leading to premature delivery of a nonviable infant. Therefore, the maternal hyperdynamic state referred to as the 'mirror syndrome' cannot be reversed solely by treatment of the underlying fetal condition. This preeclamptic state is also associated with molar pregnancies and fetal conditions that cause placentomegaly. It may be caused by a factor released by poorly perfused placental tissue that leads to endothelial cell injury (Roberts *et al.*, 1989; Goodlin, 1979; Langer *et al.*, 1989). Until the pathophysiology of the maternal 'mirror syndrome' is understood, earlier intervention before the onset of placentomegaly and the related maternal preeclamptic

state may be the only approach to salvage these doomed fetuses.

In the five patients who survived, CCAM resection led to resolution of the hydrops, impressive *in utero* lung growth and normal postnatal development, with a follow-up period of 12 to 48 months (Fig. 19.2). After resection, fetal hydrops resolved over a period of one to two weeks, and the mediastinum returned to the midline within three weeks. Right middle and lower lobe resection in the sixth fetus at 21 weeks' gestation was successful, but a subsequent unexplained fetal demise highlights the need for improved postoperative fetal monitoring and treatment. The seventh case was unsuccessful because of uncontrolled intraoperative uterine contractions leading to fetal death. The clinical focus must now shift from the technical details of the fetal surgical procedure to the crucial need for better

Fig. 19.2 *Fetal anatomy preoperatively at 24 weeks' gestation and 6 weeks postoperatively after fetal left lower lobectomy (case 2 in Table 19.2). Postoperatively, the fetal ascites resolved, the mediastinum returned to the midline, and the remaining left upper lobe and right lung showed remarkable growth. (Reprinted with permission; Harrison et al., 1990.)*

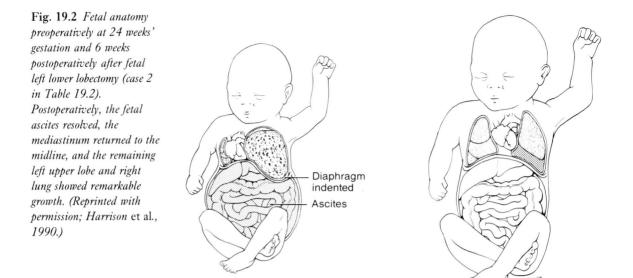

Pre-op   6 weeks post-op

postoperative maternal and fetal monitoring (Jennings *et al.*, 1992), reliable long-term fetal intravascular access for fetal blood sampling and infusions, noninvasive maternal and fetal haemodynamic assessment (Kleinman *et al.*, 1982) and effective detection and treatment of preterm labour (Jennings, MacGillivray & Harrison, 1993). As a result of ongoing work in fetal animal models, the concept of a fetal intensive care unit with a specially trained cadre of physicians and nurses is becoming a clinical reality.

Management protocol

An algorithm for management of the fetus with a CCAM is presented in Fig. 19.3. Initial evaluation begins with an ultrasound to confirm the diagnosis, amniocentesis or fetal blood sampling to exclude chromosomal anomalies, and a fetal echocardiogram to detect congenital heart disease. The natural history of prenatally diagnosed lung masses is variable, and associated anomalies are rare. If an associated life-threatening anomaly is present or if the mother is sick with the 'mirror syndrome,' then the family may choose to terminate the pregnancy. For isolated fetal thoracic masses, the fetus undergoes a prognostic evaluation since there is a wide spectrum of

severity. If the fetus is not hydropic, then the mother is followed with serial ultrasounds. Fetuses with CCAM who do not have hydrops have a good chance for survival in the setting of maternal transport, planned delivery and immediate resuscitation and surgery at a tertiary centre with ECMO capability. Occasionally some of these lesions will decrease in size. At birth, babies that are asymptomatic and had an antenatal 'shrinking' CCAM lesion should still be considered for surgical resection because of the long-term risks of infection and malignant degeneration (Halloran *et al.*, 1972; Murphy *et al.*, 1992; Benjamin & Cahill, 1991).

If the fetus is hydropic at presentation or if hydrops develops during serial follow-up, then management depends upon the gestational age. For those fetuses 32 weeks' gestation, early delivery should be considered so that the lesion can be resected after birth. For those fetuses <32 weeks' gestation, there is now a new therapeutic option, treatment of the lesion before birth.

Other conditions treated with open fetal surgery

The majority of cases of open fetal surgery at UCSF Fetal Treatment Center have been undertaken for

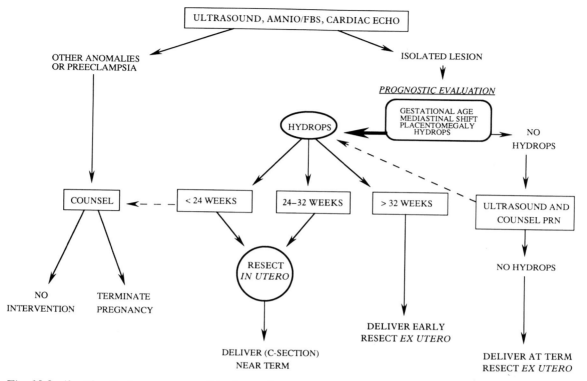

Fig. 19.3 *Algorithm for the management of the fetus with a CCAM. FBS, fetal blood sampling. (Reprinted with permission; Adzick et al., 1993).*

diaphragmatic hernia or CCAM. However, such fetal conditions as sacrococcygeal teratoma, congenital heart block and twin–twin transfusion syndrome have also been treated with this technique.

Sacrococcygeal teratoma

Sacrococcygeal teratoma (SCT) is the most common tumour of newborns. The majority of these tumours have a good prognosis, as they are commonly diagnosed in newborns when the malignant potential is low. More recently, sonography has helped to define the natural history of fetal SCT and to identify fetuses with tumours in whom hydrops from high output heart failure develops as a result of shunting through the tumour. Similar to CCAM, the development of nonimmune hydrops in fetuses with SCT appears to be a marker of

impending fetal demise and may be an indication for open fetal surgery. Fetal SCT with associated hydrops fetalis and placentomegaly has also been associated with the development of maternal 'mirror syndrome,' a potentially devastating illness in which the mother's condition begins to reflect that of the sick fetus.

We have operated on three fetuses with large SCTs associated with nonimmune hydrops by debulking the tumour mass and ligating the blood vessels that supplied the tumour. In the first case, the maternal hyperdynamic state prevented the use of tocolytic therapy and the fetus delivered prematurely and died in the early postoperative period. The second attempt was also complicated by preterm labour with delivery one week postoperatively. The neonate did well with minimal pulmonary support. Concerns regarding the potential malignant nature of the residual tumour in this baby prompted reexploration at two weeks of life. The infant suffered a fatal intraoperative cardiac arrest from a presumed air embolus. The third fetus died during fetal surgery as a result of cardiac dysfunction. Our experience indicates that fetal teratoma excision leads to resolution of hydrops, but resection must be undertaken before initiation of placentomegaly, end-stage cardiac failure and the associated maternal 'mirror syndrome'. Less-invasive intervention utilizing ultrasound guidance or videofetoscopy may soon be used to occlude selectively the vessels that supply the tumour, thereby interrupting the vascular shunt.

Fetal cardiac surgery

Fetuses with structurally normal hearts and complete heart block secondary to maternal collagen vascular disease may develop hydrops and die *in utero*. If the heart failure cannot be reversed by increasing the heart rate with the maternal administration of β-mimetics, placement of a pacemaker may be of benefit to the fetus. The transcutaneous placement of a pacemaker in a fetus with congenital heart block has been unsuccessfully attempted previously (Carpenter *et al.*, 1986), as discussed in Chapter 12. After establishing the efficacy of pacing for heart block in fetal lambs (Crombleholme, Harrison & Longaker, 1990), we successfully placed a pacemaker in a 22 week hydropic fetus with heart block. Unfortunately, the heart did not respond even to direct electrical pacing at the time of fetal thoracotomy. This indicated to us that the heart was already irreversibly damaged by more than six weeks of heart failure, and earlier intervention for this condition may be required. Recent advances in fetal cardiac bypass have led to the development in animals of additional procedures for correcting selected cardiac defects (Fenton, Heinemann & Hanley, 1993). Techniques for operating on the fetal heart may improve the management of such fetal cardiac diseases as pulmonary stenosis or critical aortic stenosis (Turley *et al.*, 1982).

Twin–twin transfusion syndrome

Open hysterotomy has been attempted as a treatment option for severe twin–twin transfusion in one case (Urig *et al.*, 1988). The smaller twin was removed at 21 weeks' gestation. Preterm prelabour rupture of the membranes occurred on the 21st postoperative day. Intractable preterm labour ensued at 28 weeks of gestation and the remaining twin was delivered by caesarean section. The infant died on the ninth day of life during surgery for congenital aortic stenosis.

Fetal hydrocephalus

Background
With the advent of widespread prenatal ultrasound, hydrocephalus is one of the more common fetal anomalies detected. In a recent Scandinavian study, 61 anomalies were detected during 16 763 second-trimester screening ultrasounds (Brocks & Bang, 1991). Twenty-seven (44%) of these anomalies involved the central nervous system; seven of these were hydrocephalus. Early shunting in the neonatal period has improved both the survival and long-term prognosis in these infants. This led to the hypothesis that *in utero* shunting could further improve the prognosis for this condition.

Animal models
Our group described the use of kaolin injection into the cisterna magna through the atlanto-occipital membrane to create an animal model for fetal hydrocephalus (Nakayama *et al.*, 1983). The technique proved successful in six lambs and two fetal rhesus monkeys. At birth, both the lateral and third ventricles were dilated secondary to obstruction of the outlet foramina of the fourth ventricle. Histopathology revealed that the grey matter of the animals was well preserved while white matter was noted to be attenuated, findings analogous to those seen in human neonates with congenital hydrocephalus. In a subsequent investigation, we attempted to reverse the effects of experimentally induced hydrocephalus by *in utero* shunting (Glick *et al.*, 1984). Twenty hydrocephalic lambs and eight fetal monkeys underwent placement of a variety of ventricular shunts. Shunted lambs exhibited a 70% rate of survival compared with a 14% survival in control animals with hydrocephalus that did not undergo shunting. Although a marked decompression of the lateral ventricles was noted in shunted lambs, the majority of animals demonstrated evidence of kaolin deposition in the lateral ventricles and subependymal zones. A severe inflammatory response to the kaolin was responsible for dense adhesions in the ventricular system as well as dense gliosis in white matter adjacent to these spaces. Similar findings were noted in shunted fetal monkeys but not in parallel controls. We concluded that the kaolin

demonstrated in the ventricular system above the aqueduct of Sylvius was probably the result of reflux at the time of *in utero* shunt placement. Therefore, the experimental induction of hydrocephalus by kaolin injection was not felt to represent a good animal model for the evaluation of *in utero* shunting of fetal hydrocephalus.

In a subsequent investigation, Michejda *et al.* (1986) successfully induced experimental hydrocephalus secondary to neural tube defects in 60 primate fetuses exposed to triamcinolone. CT scans of untreated fetuses revealed dilation of the lateral ventricles, porencephaly and loss of occipital parietal bone with encephalocele formation. At 115 to 125 days of gestation (term: 164 + 5 days), half of the fetuses underwent placement of an indwelling shunt that communicated between the posterior horn of the lateral ventricle and the amniotic cavity. Survival in the untreated group of fetuses was 77% compared with 93% in the treated group. Fetuses that underwent *in utero* shunting revealed normal gross anatomy with CT scanning; cytoarchitecture was also preserved in these fetuses.

Fetal registry

In 1982, an international group of authorities in fetal medicine met and adopted specific criteria for the *in utero* treatment of hydrocephalus (Harrison et al., 1982b). Initial evaluation was proposed to include a comprehensive ultrasound and amniocentesis for fetal karyotype, α-fetoprotein and viral studies. Appropriate criteria for possible *in utero* shunting were singleton gestation, ultrasonographic evidence of progressive ventriculomegaly in association with a decrease in the thickness of the cortical mantle, no ultrasonographic evidence of other CNS or extra CNS fetal anomalies, and a gestational age representing a fetus too immature for delivery with subsequent neonatal shunting. Centres engaged *in utero* shunting for fetal hydrocephalus were to have a high-risk obstetrical unit in conjunction with a tertiary neonatal intensive care unit. Access to bioethical and psychosocial consultation was recommended. A multidisciplinary team of specialists was to include an obstetrician experienced in intrauterine transfusion, an ultrasonographer experienced in the diagnosis of fetal anomalies, a pediatric surgeon and a neonatologist.

Between 1982 and 1989, a total of 45 cases of *in utero* shunting of fetal hydrocephalus had been reported to the International Fetal Surgery Registry (Evans *et al.*, 1989). The majority of cases involved aqueductal stenosis (32 of 44). However, five cases were associated with extra CNS anomalies, while one case each of holoprosencephaly, porencephaly, Dandy–Walker syndrome, and Arnold–Chiari malformation were reported. The procedure-related mortality was 9%. Overall survival for the series was 83% and was clearly related to diagnosis, with aqueductal stenosis achieving the highest rate of survival: 88%. Most distressing was the finding that only 12 of the 34 survivors were felt to be neurologically normal on follow-up; half of the survivors demonstrated severe neurological handicaps.

Several learning points became evident from this experience. First, the type of shunt, Denver variety, that was routinely used was problematic. Several cases of shunt failure related to occlusion or fetal removal were reported. Changes in shunt design such as the screw type device developed by Michejda *et al.* (1984) may have prevented these problems. Unfortunately, their device required open hysterotomy for placement. Second, patient selection was poor in many cases. Several centres had enrolled fetuses with karyotypic abnormalities and lethal CNS defects such as holoprosencephaly. The presence of extra CNS anomalies, a factor affecting long-term survival, was often missed by skilled ultrasonographers. Finally, even in the best of cases, fetal survival appeared improved but severe neurologic handicap was not averted.

Current status of in utero *shunting*

Based on these initial poor results, a *de facto* moratorium was called regarding the placement of further *in utero* ventricular shunts (Clewell *et al.*, 1986). In addition, the sole manufacturer of the one ventricular shunt available for clinical use has discontinued production of the device as a result of decreasing demand for its use.

Myelomeningocele

Myelomeningocele can be detected early in gestation by α-fetoprotein screening and sonography. There is some evidence that progressive neurologic impairment is caused by exposure of the spinal cord *in utero*. We have found that fetal sheep whose spinal cord is exposed to amniotic fluid early in gestation develop hemiplegia and a cystic spinal lesion remarkably similar to the human myelomeningocele. We have developed an *in utero* myocutaneous flap repair to determine whether prevention of long-term exposure of the fetal neural tissue will prevent or reverse the associated neurologic deficit. At birth, repaired animals had almost normal motor function of the hindlimbs in conjunction with a normally functioning bladder (Meuli*et al.*, 1995). Microscopic examination of the spinal cord revealed preservation of the cytoarchitecture. Copeland *et al.* (1993) have used a similar animal model for myelomeningocele and successfully corrected the defect utilizing endoscopic techniques. Split thickness skin grafts of fetal or maternal origin were held in place with fibrin glue as a temporary covering to prevent exposure of neural elements to amniotic fluid. The authors proposed that definitive therapy for the defect could then be undertaken after birth.

Conclusion

A variety of fetal anomalies have been successfully treated with surgery prior to birth. Whereas CCAM with hydrops has previously almost universally been associated with fetal death, current experience with open fetal surgery has resulted in survival in five of eight fetuses. The limited experience with *in utero* repair of SCT has yielded no long-term survivors. Experience with open fetal surgery for the removal of one twin in cases of stuck twin syndrome and placement of a pacemaker in cases of congenital heart block is limited to a single case each and cannot be recommended at this time. *In utero* shunt placement for severe fetal hydrocephalus has been associated with an increased survival of severely handicapped infants such that it is currently not recommended. Repair of meningomyeloceles, especially through the use of minimally invasive surgical techniques, holds promise in the future in decreasing the long-term morbidity associated with neural tube defects.

References

Adzick, N. S., Harrison, M. R. & Flake, A. W. (1993). Fetal surgery for cystic adenomatoid malformation of the lung. *Journal of Pediatric Surgery*, 28, 1–6.

Adzick, N. S., Harrison, M. R., Flake, A. W., Glick, P. L. & Bottles, K. (1985a). Automatic uterine stapling devices in fetal operation: Experience in a primate model. *Surgery Forum*, 36, 479–81.

Adzick, N. S., Harrison, M. R., Glick, P. L., Golbus, M. S., Anderson, R. L., Mahony, B. S., Callen, P. W., Hirsch, J. H., Luthy, D. A., Filly, R. A. & de Lorimier, A. A. (1985b). Fetal cystic adenomatoid malformation: prenatal diagnosis and natural history. *Journal of Pediatric Surgery*, 20, 483–8.

Adzick, N. S., Harrison, M. R., Hu, L. M., Davies, P., Flake, A. W. & Reid, L. M. (1985c). Compensatory growth after pneumonectomy in fetal lambs: a morphologic study. *Surgery Forum*, 37, 309–11.

Avni, E.F., Vanderolst, A., Van Gansbeke, D.V., Schils, J. & Rodesch, F. (1986). Antenatal diagnosis of pulmonary tumors: report of two cases. *Pediatric Radiology*, 16, 190–2.

Benjamin, D.R. & Cahill, J.L. (1991). Bronchioloalveolar carcinoma of the lung and congenital cystic adenomatoid malformation. *American Journal of Clinical Pathology*, 95, 889–92.

Brocks, V. & Bang, J. (1991). Routine examination by ultrasound for the detection of fetal malformations in a low risk population. *Fetal Diagnosis and Therapy*, 6, 37–45.

Carpenter, R. J., Strasburger, J. F., Garson, A., Smith, R. T., Deter, R. L., & Engelhardt, H. T. (1986). Fetal ventricular pacing for hydrops secondary to complete atrioventricular block. *Journal of the American College of Cardiology*, 8, 1434–6.

Clark, S. L., Vitale, D. J., Minton, S. D., Stoddard, R. A. & Sabey, P. L. (1987). Successful fetal therapy for cystic adenomatoid malformation associated with second trimester hydrops. *American Journal of Obstetrics and Gynecology*, 157, 294–7.

Clewell, W. H., Manco-Johnson, M. L. & Manchester, D. K. (1986). Diagnosis and management of fetal hydrocephalus. *Clinical Obstetrics and Gynecology*, 29, 514–22.

Copeland, M. L., Bruner, J. P., Richards, W. O., Sundell, H. W. & Tulipan, N. B. (1993). A model for *in utero* endoscopic treatment of myelomeningocele. *Neurosurgery*, 33, 542–5.

Crombleholme, T. M., Harrison, M. R., & Longaker, M. T. (1990). Complete heart block in fetal lambs I. Technique and acute physiologic response. *Journal of Pediatric Surgery*, 25, 587–93.

Evans, M. I., Drugan, A., Manning, F. A. & Harrison, M. R. (1989). Fetal surgery in the 1990s. *American Journal of the Diseases of Children*, 143, 1431–6.

Fenton, K. N., Heinemann, M. K., & Hanley, F. L. (1993). Exclusion of the placenta during fetal cardiac bypass augments a systemic flow and provides important information about the mechanism of placental injury. *Journal of Thoracic and Cardiovascular Surgery*, 105, 502–10.

Fine, C., Adzick, N. S. & Doubilet, P. M. (1988). Decreasing size of a congenital cystic adenomatoid malformation *in utero*: case report. *Journal of Ultrasound Medicine*, 7, 405–8.

Glick, P. L., Harrison, M. R., Halks-Miller, M., Adzick, N. S., Nakayama, D. K., Anderson, J. H., Nyland, T. G. & Edwards, M. S. (1984). Correction of congenital hydrocephalus *in utero* II. Efficacy of *in utero* shunting. *Journal of Pediatric Surgery*, 19, 870–81.

Golladay, E. S. & Mollitt, D. L. (1984). Surgically correctable hydrops. *Journal of Pediatric Surgery*, 19, 59–63.

Goodlin, R. C. (1979). Mirror syndromes. In *Care of the Fetus*, ed. R. C. Goodlin, pp. 48–50. New York: Masson.

Halloran, L. G., Silverberg, S. G. & Salzberg, A. M. (1972). Congenital cystic adenomatoid malformation of the lung. A surgical emergency. *Archives of Surgery*, 104, 715–9.

Harrison, M. R., Adzick, N. S., Jennings, R. W., Duncan, B. W., Rosen, M. A., Filly, R. A., Goldberg, J. D., de Lorimier, A. A. & Golbus, M. S. (1990a). Antenatal intervention for congenital cystic adenomatoid malformation. *Lancet*, 336, 965–7.

Harrison, M. R., Adzick, N. S., Longaker, M. T., Goldberg, J. D., Rosen, M. A., Filly, R. A., Evans, M. I. & Golbus, M. S. (1990b). Successful repair *in utero* of a fetal diaphragmatic hernia after removal of herniated viscera from the left thorax. *New England Journal of Medicine*, 322, 1582–4.

Harrison, M. R., Anderson, J., Rosen, M. A., Ross, N. A. & Hendrickx, A. G. (1982a). Fetal surgery in the primate I. Anesthetic, surgical, and tocolytic management to maximize fetal–neonatal survival. *Journal of Pediatric Surgery*, 17, 115–22.

Harrison, M. R., Filly, R. A., Globus, M. S., Berkowitz, R. L., Callen, P. W., Canty, T. G., Catz, C., Clewell, W. H., Depp, R., Edwards, M. S., Fletcher, J. C., Frigoletto, F. D., Garrett, W. J., Johnson, M. L., Jonsen, A., de Lorimier, A. A., Liley, W. A., Mahoney, M. J., Manning, F. D., Meier, P. R., Michejda, M., Nakayama, D. K., Nelson, L., Newkirk, J. B., Pringle, K., Rodeck, C., Rosen, M. A. & Schulman, J. D. (1982b). Fetal treatment 1982. *New England Journal of Medicine*, 307, 1651–2.

Harrison, M. R., Jester, J. A. & Ross, N. A. (1980). Correction of congenital diaphragmatic hernia *in utero* I. The model: intrathoracic balloon produces fatal pulmonary hypoplasia. *Surgery*, 88, 174–80.

Hernanz-Schulman, M., Stein, S. M., Neblett, W. W., Atkinson, J. B., Kirschner, S. G., Heller, R. M., Merrill, W. H. & Fleischer, A. C. (1991). Pulmonary sequestration: diagnosis with color flow sonography and a new theory of associated hydrothorax. *Radiology*, 180, 817–21.

Jennings, R. W., Adzick, N. S., Longaker, M. T., Lorenz, H. P., Estes, J. M. & Harrison, M. R. (1992). New techniques in fetal surgery. *Journal of Pediatric Surgery*, 27, 1329–33.

Jennings, R. W., MacGillivray, T. E. & Harrison, M. R. (1993). Nitric oxide inhibits preterm labor in the rhesus monkey. *Journal of Maternal Fetal Medicine*, 2, 170–5.

Kleinman, C. S., Donnerstein, R. L., DeVore, G. R., Jaffe, C. C., Lynch, D. C., Berkowitz, R. L., Talner, N. S. & Hobbins, J. C. (1982). Fetal echocardiography for evaluation of *in utero* congestive heart failure: a technique for study of nonimmune hydrops. *New England Journal of Medicine*, 306, 568–75.

Kuller, J. A., Laifer, S. A., Tagge, E. P., Nakayama, D. K. & Hill, L. M. (1992). Diminution in size of a fetal intrathoracic mass: caution against aggressive *in utero* management. *American Journal of Perinatology*, 9, 223–4.

Langer, J. C., Harrison, M. R., Schmidt, K. G., Silverman, N. H., Anderson, R. L., Goldberg, J. D., Filly, R. A., Crombleholme, T. M., Longaker, M. T. & Goldbus, M. S. (1989). Fetal hydrops and death from sacrococcygeal teratoma: rationale for fetal surgery. *American Journal of Obstetrics and Gynecology*, 160, 1145–50.

MacGillivray, T. E., Harrison, M. R., Goldstein, R. B. & Adzick, N. S. (1993). Disappearing fetal lung lesions. *Journal of Pediatric Surgery*, 28, 1321–5.

Meuli, M., Meuli-Simmen, C., Hutchins, G. M., Yingling, C. D., Hoffman, K. M., Harrison, M. R. & Adzick, N. S. (1995). In utero surgery rescues neurological function at birth in sheep with spina bifida. *Nature Medicine*, 1, 342–7.

Michejda, M., Patronas, N., Di Chiro, G. & Hodgen, G. D. (1984). Fetal hydrocephalus II. Amelioration of fetal porencephaly by *in utero* therapy in nonhuman primates. *Journal of the American Medical Association*, 251, 2548–52.

Michejda, M., Queenan, J. T. & McCullough, D. (1986). Present status of intrauterine treatment of hydrocephalus and its future. *American Journal of Obstetrics and Gynecology*, 155, 873–82.

Morin, C., Filiatrault, D. & Russo, P. (1989). Pulmonary sequestration with histologic changes of cystic adenomatoid malformation. *Pediatric Radiology*, 19, 130–2.

Murphy, J. J., Blair, G. K., Fraser, G. C., Ashmore, P. G., LeBlanc, J. G., Sett, S. S., Rogers, P., Magee, J. F., Taylor, G. P. & Dimmick, J. (1992). Rhabdomyosarcoma arising within congenital pulmonary cysts: report of three cases. *Journal of Pediatric Surgery*, 27, 1364–7.

Nakayama, D. K., Harrison, M. R., Berger, M. S., Chinn, D. H., Halks-Miller, M. & Edwards, M. S.

(1983). Correction of congenital hydrocephalus *in utero* I. The model: intracisternal kaolin produces hydrocephalus in fetal lambs and rhesus monkeys. *Journal of Pediatric Surgery*, 18, 331–8.

Nakayama, D. K., Harrison, M. R., Seron-Ferre, M. & Villa, R. L. (1984). Fetal surgery in the primate II. Uterine electromyographic response to operative procedure and pharmacologic agents. *Journal of Pediatric Surgery*, 19, 333–9.

Nicolaides, K. H. & Azar, G. B. (1990). Thoraco-amniotic shunting. *Fetal Diagnostic Therapy*, 5, 153–64.

Nicolaides, K. H., Blott, A. J. & Greenough, A. (1987). Chronic drainage of fetal pulmonary cyst. *Lancet*, i, 618.

Oster, A. G. & Fortune, D. W. (1979). Congenital cystic adenomatoid malformation of the lung. *American Journal of Clinical Pathology*, 70, 595–603.

Rice, H. E., Estes, J. M., Hedrick, M. H., Harrison, M. R. & Adzick, N. S. (1994). Congenital cystic adenomatoid malformation: a sheep model of fetal hydrops. *Journal of Pediatric Surgery*, 29, 692–6.

Roberts, J. M., Taylor, R. N., Musci, T. J., Rodgers, G. M., Hubel, C. A. & McLaughlin, M. K. (1989). Pre-eclampsia: an endothelial cell disorder. *American Journal of Obstetrics and Gynecology*, 161, 1200–4.

Saltzman, D. H., Adzick, N. S. & Benacerraf, B. R. (1988). Fetal cystic adenomatoid malformation of the lung: apparent improvement *in utero*. *Obstetrics and Gynecology*, 71, 1000–3.

Stocker, T. J., Manewell, J. E. & Drake, R. M. (1977). Congenital cystic adenomatoid malformation of the lung: classification and morphologic spectrum. *Human Pathology*, 8, 155–71.

Turley, K., Vlahakes, G. J., Harrison, M. R., Messina, L., Hanley, F., Uhlig, P. N. & Ebert, P. A. (1982). Intrauterine cardiothoracic surgery: the fetal lamb model. *Annals of Thoracic Surgery*, 34, 422–6.

Urig, M. A., Simpson, G. F., Elliot, J. P. & Clewell, W. H. (1988). Twin–twin transfusion syndrome: the surgical removal of one twin as a treatment option. *Fetal Therapy*, 3: 185–8.

Part four

Future developments

20 Stem cell transplantation

JEAN-LOUIS TOURAINE

Introduction

Many severe congenital disorders and a number of acquired haematological diseases can be successfully treated by bone marrow transplantation (Bortin & Rimm, 1977; De Koning et al., 1969; Gatti et al., 1968; Thomas et al., 1975; Touraine et al., 1987). However, a large proportion of patients have no perfectly matched HLA identical donor available and the incompatible transplant is responsible for severe graft-versus-host disease (GVHD). Since GVHD is induced by T lymphocytes which are present in the transplant and react with host tissues (Grebe & Streilen, 1976; Korngold & Sprent, 1982), transplants from a donor who is not genotypically HLA-identical frequently need to involve T cell depletion of the donor bone marrow. This manoeuvre reduces the incidence of GVHD but is associated with increased risks of graft failure as well as incomplete reconstitution, Epstein–Barr virus-induced lymphomas, or leukaemia relapse (Fischer et al., 1986; O'Reilly et al., 1983).

It is, therefore, of considerable interest that, because of the natural lack of T cells during the early phases of ontogeny, fetal liver stem cells can reconstitute the haemopoietic and lymphopoietic systems of experimental animals and humans without producing severe GVHD, even in cases of full donor–host incompatibility (Bortin & Salzstein, 1969; Champlin et al., 1987; Löwenberg, 1975; Prümmer et al., 1985; Touraine, 1983; Touraine et al., 1987). From the transplanted stem cells, the various cell lineages develop progressively and uneventfully.

Accordingly, fetal liver transplants in utero have been developed and demonstrated to be feasible and effective in the human fetus, when performed during the early stages of fetal development and immediately after prenatal diagnosis (Raudrant, Touraine & Rebaud, 1992; Touraine et al., 1989; 1992; Touraine, 1992). This chapter will concentrate both on the extensive experience in Lyon of postnatal transplantation with fetal stem cells and on intrauterine transplantation with fetal stem cells.

Rationale

The human fetal liver, between weeks 8 and 12 postfertilization, contains all haemopoietic stem cells and no T lymphocytes. These stem cells have earlier migrated from the yolk sac of the human embryo to the liver. After week 12, the fetal thymus produces thymocytes and T lymphocytes which migrate to the periphery. A few T cells are then present in the fetal liver and in the bone marrow. Later on, stem cells migrate from the fetal liver to the spleen and to the bone marrow, where T cells are always present. Fetal liver cells, obtained during the third month postfertilization, are therefore the only convenient source of a large number of haemopoietic stem cells naturally devoid of GVHD-inducing T lymphocytes.

Animal studies

Since the pioneering work of Uphoff (1958), much has been learned in the field of experimental and clinical fetal liver transplantation. Most of the studies have been carried out in mice (Boersma, 1983; Löwenberg, 1975). They have shown the effectiveness of fetal liver transplants in correcting the haematological and immunological consequences of lethal doses of irradiation (Aitouche & Touraine, 1993; Löwenberg, 1975; Uphoff, 1958). Such irradiation is the most frequent conditioning treatment given to mice in order to induce 'take' of allogeneic stem cells, stable chimaerism and, as a result, immunological tolerance to donor antigens (Aitouche & Touraine, 1993). Fetal liver transplantation can also cure the immunodeficiency of severe combined immunodeficiency (SCID) mice (Sanhadji, Négrier & Touraine, 1990), the leukaemia of AKR mice (Touraine, Royo & Gitton, 1990) and improve significantly the neurological manifestations and survival of mice which suffer with lysosomal storage disease (LSD), an inborn error of metabolism (Veyron & Touraine, 1990). Adding T cells from the same allogeneic donor can accelerate transplant 'take' and a similar effect, without the associated risk of GVHD, appears to be obtainable using factors released by T lymphocytes activated *in vitro* (Plotnicky & Touraine, 1993b). Fleischman and coworkers (Fleischman, Cluster & Mintz, 1982) and Mintz (1985) have shown that haemopoietic stem cells from the fetal liver can induce reconstitution of erythroid cells in genetically anaemic murine fetuses when injected via the placental circulation. By using computerized statistical models, the authors calculated that some animals must have been seeded by only a single donor stem cell, which has been sufficient for reconstitution. Fetal liver transplantation is also effective in reconstituting erythroid cells in rats (Crouch, 1959; Kelemen, Gulya & Szabo, 1980) as well as in larger and outbred animals: dogs (Prümmer *et al.*, 1985), horses (Perryman, 1980), sheep (Bunch, Wood & Kelly, 1985), mini-pigs (Andreani *et al.*, 1985), and monkey or sheep fetuses (Flake *et al.*, 1986; Harrison *et al.*, 1989).

Human studies

The unique and remarkable properties of fetal stem cells, including their considerable capacity for proliferation and differentiation, their ability to become tolerant to host antigens and to differentiate normally in a foreign host, have prompted the development of studies on human fetal liver transplantation. Good-quality reconstitution has been obtained in most patients treated, despite the lack of HLA matching between donor and recipient (Touraine, 1983; Touraine *et al.*, 1987). Infants with SCID have been successfully treated by transplants of fetal liver together with fetal thymus from the same allogeneic donor of less than 15 weeks' gestation (Touraine *et al.*, 1987; Touraine, 1989). Patients with severe forms of Di George syndrome have also benefited from fetal thymus transplants (J.-L. Touraine & M. G. Roncarolo, unpublished data). The condition of several patients with severe aplastic anaemia and other haematological diseases has shown improvement in some cases after fetal liver transplantation (Gale, 1987; Kochupillai *et al.*, 1987a,b). In patients with inborn errors of metabolism, a beneficial effect has been noted as a result of transplantation of both stem cells and prehepatocytes from the fetal liver (Touraine, 1991).

The main reasons for developing *in utero* fetal liver transplantation are summarized as follows:

1. increased probability of graft take and chimaerism, especially in diseases such as bare lymphocyte syndrome in which residual immunity can induce rejection, and even more so in diseases without immunodeficiency (provided that transplantation is performed very early in gestation)
2. improved isolation at the time of transplant, since the uterus is even better than a sterile bubble
3. better environment for fetal cell development compared with that in the infant.

Preparation of fetal cells for transplantation

Donor fetal cells can be prepared in a variety of ways. They can be used fresh or cryopreserved and then thawed before administration. The preparation described below is that employed in our institution from 1974.

Fetal organ procurement was organized in accordance with the recommendations of the French National Committee for Bioethics (Touraine, 1985). A few hours following fetal death, the liver and the thymus were removed aseptically. Only fresh tissues and cells were used for transplantation.

For transplants to immunodeficient patients and to fetal recipients, the ages of fetal donors ranged from 7 to 12.5 weeks postfertilization; for postnatal transplants to patients with inborn errors of metabolism, they ranged from 8 to 22 weeks. The fetal thymus and liver were gently disrupted using an homogenizer, and a single cell suspension was thus prepared in RPMI 1640 medium supplemented with gentamycin. The fetal liver was mainly a source of stem cells, the fetal thymus of epithelial cells.

The cells were counted and their viability checked using the Trypan blue exclusion method. Cell suspensions with insufficient viability, (i.e. less than 70% when fetuses were less than 12.5 weeks of age, and less than 40% above this age) were discarded. The total number of living nucleated cells that were transplanted from an individual fetal liver varied greatly with the age of the fetal donor (mean number: 8×10^8 cells). Thymuses which contained numerous thymocytes, i.e. 12.5-week-old thymuses, were irradiated with 40 Gy prior to transplantation into patients with SCID, when such thymuses were transplanted together with syngeneic, untreated fetal liver cells.

Maternal serum was tested for hepatitis B antigens and antibodies, and for antibodies against hepatitis C, cytomegalovirus (CMV), human immunodeficiency viruses (HIV1, HIV2) and human T lymphotropic viruses (HTLV 1, HTLV 2). Tissue was not used for transplantation when a risk of transmitting infectious disease, e.g. HIV infection, hepatitis B or C, septicaemia or other maternal infections, was identified. The tissues were also discarded in cases of certain tumours or in cases of known chromosomal abnormalities. Bacteriological tests were performed on the cell suspension, but the results were not available until after the transplant itself (in cases of bacterial contamination antibiotics could then be given to the transplant recipient). In recent years, a spleen cell suspension and a fibroblast cell line were routinely performed to determine the ABO blood group and the HLA phenotype by both serological and molecular methods. Before administration to the patient, the cell suspension was diluted in the appropriate volume of medium for intraperitoneal injection or intravenous infusion.

Postnatal transplantation of fetal stem cells

Immunodeficiency diseases

Transplantation of fetal liver cells, with syngeneic thymic cells, was used to treat every SCID child who had no available HLA identical donor for bone marrow transplantation. The first of these transplants was done using two fetal donors in 1976; in this male infant, immunological reconstitution has been very successful, the lethal disease completely cured and he is now a very healthy teenager, living a normal life, without sequelae or treatment. He is the oldest patient cured of SCID by fetal liver and thymus transplantation. Since then, 16 further children (ages 0 to 3 years) with SCID, including three with adenosine deaminase deficiency and two with bare lymphocyte syndrome (Touraine et al., 1978; Touraine, 1981), have also been treated by this method (Table 20.1).

In addition, six other children with severe forms of Di George syndrome and one with bare lymphocyte syndrome received fetal thymus transplants between 1974 and 1990. The first patient who had Di George syndrome and was treated with fetal thymus transplantation is now a perfectly healthy young man who has maintained normal immunity from the first few months following the transplant.

Altogether, 24 patients with severe immunodeficiency diseases have been treated by fetal cell transplantation, 12 of whom have been cured of their otherwise lethal disease (Fig. 20.1). Following reconstitution, the favourable clinical and immunological status of survivors remained stable after the first few years (Fig. 20.1). Despite complete HLA-mismatch between donor and recipient, normal cell-mediated and humoral immunities developed in most patients (Roncarolo, Touraine & Banchereau, 1986; Roncarolo et al., 1988; Touraine, 1983; Touraine et al., 1987), and immunological tolerance to alloantigens was total (Plotnicky & Touraine, 1993a).

The failures were mainly severe infections that were already apparent in the patients before transplantation: for example, meningitis with neurological consequences, resistant salmonella infection, bCG infection, and septicaemia associated with moderate and

Table 20.1 *Inherited immunodeficiencies and inborn errors of metabolism treated postnatally with fetal liver transplantation*

Diseases treated	No. of patients
Severe combined immunodeficiencies	
With adenosine deaminase deficiency	3
With bare lymphocyte syndrome	2
Others	12
Fabry	6
Gaucher	5
Familial amyloidosis	3
Fucosidosis	2
Niemann Pick A	1
Niemann Pick B	1
Niemann Pick C	2
Glycogenosis	2
Hurler	2
Metachromatic leukodystrophy	2
Adrenoleukodystrophy	1
Morquio B	1
San Filippo A	1
Hunter	1
Gangliosidosis (GM2)	1

delayed GVHD. In addition, one child had haemorrhages with renal failure and one infant who had Di George syndrome died of cardiomyopathy.

Inborn errors of metabolism

A variety of inborn errors of metabolism (IEM), without associated immunodeficiency, has been treated by fetal liver transplantation, in conjunction with prolonged immunosuppressive therapy at moderate doses comparable to those given in non-severe autoimmune diseases. No adverse effect of the treatment was observed. Thirty-one patients with IEM had transplants, as shown in Table 20.1.

Most patients are now in relatively good condition and display objective criteria of partial improvement (Touraine, 1991) (Fig. 20.1). By comparison with children with immunodeficiency diseases treated postnatally by fetal tissue transplantation, patients with inborn errors of metabolism were not completely cured by the fetal transplant, but their disease was stabilized for some time after each transplant. For example, stabilization for 5–10 years in three children with Gaucher disease enabled them to benefit later from glucocerebrosidase therapy. Patients with Fabry disease had diminished symptoms, with slower or halted disease progression. Fetal liver transplantation was repeated to maintain the clinical result, but some patients in an already advanced state of deterioration, especially of the central nervous system, eventually died. The serum levels of the defective enzymes were not increased dramatically, but the various substrates did decrease after fetal liver transplantation, and tissue deposits stabilized. Fetal donors for liver transplantation in IEM were relatively more advanced in gestation than those chosen for fetal liver and thymus transplantation in SCID. The respective part played by stem cells and prehepatocytes in the partial improvement seen after transplantation is under investigation. Coculture of fetal cells with normal enzyme activities together with defective cells from patients has shown how the latter benefit from the enzymes released by neighbouring normal cells. After transplantation, viability of the fetal liver cells in the host can be monitored by serial serum α-fetoprotein measurements; these levels rose sharply, then decreased progressively as the cells matured over 1–2 months.

Overall results

In both severe immunodeficiency diseases and IEM, fetal tissue transplantation into postnatal recipients has demonstrated beneficial effects. Two-thirds of children achieved cure or significant improvement as a result of treatment, and this effect seems long-lasting (Fig. 20.1). Without transplantation, the life expectancy of more than 80% of the patients was less than three years. Nevertheless, almost one-third of patients did not improve. In most cases, failure was the result of one of two

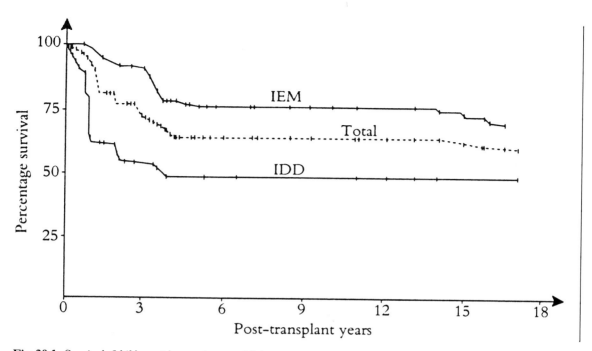

Fig. 20.1 *Survival of children with severe immunodeficiency diseases (IDD) or inborn errors of metabolism (IEM) treated by postnatal transplantation of fetal tissue. The global survival of all patients from these two groups is shown by the line 'total'. (Reproduced from Touraine, 1993.)*

factors: first, insufficient graft take in patients capable of rejection; second, late diagnosis of the initial disease with severe infection being present prior to transplantation. It is largely to overcome these difficulties, both in transplant take and in control of infection, that we have more recently developed *in utero* transplantation. Provided that the diagnosis can be performed at an early phase of pregnancy, such earlier transplants (before immune development and before exposure of the host to microorganisms) would lead to an increased probability of graft take and a lower risk of infection.

In utero transplantation of fetal stem cells

Immunodeficiencies

The first two patients treated by *in utero* fetal liver transplantation were fetuses with SCID diagnosed in mid-gestation. A third fetal patient with chronic granulomatous disease is also described.

The first fetal patient, designated A in Table 20.2, suffered from bare lymphocyte syndrome, a genetically transmitted form of combined immunodeficiency disease caused by lack of expression of HLA antigens (Touraine *et al.*, 1978; Touraine, 1981). Infections, especially with opportunistic microorganisms, lead to death in these infants unless they grow up isolated in a fully sterile atmosphere while being successfully reconstituted with stem cell transplants. When carried out postnatally, however, such stem cell transplants, in the form of either bone marrow or fetal liver transplant, are usually associated with graft failure as a result of allogeneic reactions in the host (persisting transplant immunity) and to high susceptibility to infections (defective immunity to infectious antigens). Prenatal diagnosis of bare lymphocyte syndrome can be performed by HLA analysis of lymphocytes in fetal blood (Durandy *et al.*, 1987).

The first child in this family had previously died of bare lymphocyte syndrome before the age of two, despite an attempted stem cell transplant which failed to result in stable graft take and immunological reconstitution. When the mother became pregnant again, she asked for

Table 20.2 *Conditions and results of* in utero *transplants in human fetuses*

Patient	Disease	Gestational age at transplant (weeks)	Gestational age of donor (weeks)	Route of cell infusion	Evidence for engraftment	Correction of initial disease	Clinical status
A	BLS[a]	30	9 and 9.5	Intravenous	HLA markers	Reconstitution of of T cells with normal function	Alive and well
B	SCID[b]	28	9.5	Intravenous	Y chromosome and HLA markers	Reconstitution of T cells with normal function	Alive and well
C	CGD[c]	19 23	15.5 16	Intravenous Intravenous	–	–	Bradycardia and fetal death
D	TM[d]	14	11.5	Intraperitoneal	Y chromosome	Presence of HbA coexisting with abnormal Hb	Alive and well
E	TM[d]	19	13.5	Intravenous	–	–	Bradycardia and fetal death

[a] Bare lymphocyte syndrome.
[b] Severe combined immunodeficiency disease.
[c] Chronic granulomatous disease.
[d] β^0 Thalassaemia major.

prenatal diagnosis, which demonstrated type III bare lymphocyte syndrome with virtually complete lack of expression of both class I and class II HLA antigens at the cell surface. Three choices were offered to this family: (i) therapeutic abortion; (ii) no treatment before birth and stem cell transplant after birth; (iii) *in utero* stem cell transplant followed by postnatal stem cell transplant. The parents were informed that the last option had not previously been attempted and that its efficacy was, therefore, uncertain. The mother and father opted for the earliest possible transplant. At 30 weeks' gestation, the transplant was carried out by infusing 7 ml culture medium containing a suspension of 16×10^6 fetal liver cells and fetal thymic epithelial cells into the umbilical vein (Berkowitz *et al.*, 1987; Raudrant *et al.*, 1992; Touraine *et al.*, 1989; 1992). The technique for intravenous infusion (Raudrant *et al.*, 1992; Touraine *et al.*, 1989) was comparable to that used for

intravascular intrauterine transfusion (Chapter 2). Liver and thymic cells were obtained from two dead fetuses of 9 to 10 weeks' gestation (Table 20.2). At birth, the diagnosis of bare lymphocyte syndrome was again confirmed, but some cells with class I HLA antigens became progressively detectable. As shown in Fig. 20.2, 10% of the lymphocytes had normal expression of class I HLA antigens at age one month (Touraine *et al.*, 1989), and these cells were of donor origin since their HLA specificities were of donor type and not inherited from the child's parents. In particular, these cells expressed the HLA-A9 specificity of donor origin, which made transplanted cells readily detectable in the initial test, at birth and in subsequent tests. These results demonstrated persisting engraftment of the fetal liver cells infused into the sick fetus. The expression of class II HLA antigens remained comparatively low at the surface of resting lymphocytes. This finding confirms that B cell differen-

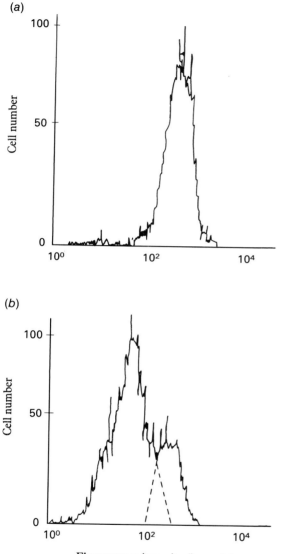

(a)

(b)

Fig. 20.2 *Cytofluorometric analysis of peripheral blood lymphocytes with W6/32 anti-HLA-ABC monoclonal antibody. (a) Normal HLA expression in cells from a normal patient. (b) Patient A one month after birth, i.e. three months after fetal liver transplantation and before additional cell infusion, shows two populations of cells, a larger one with HLA deficiency (patient's cells) and another, smaller, with normal HLA expression (donor-derived cells). (Reproduced from Touraine* et al., *1989.)*

tiation does not occur as rapidly as T cell differentiation from stem cell transplants in immunodeficient patients (Touraine *et al.*, 1987). As scheduled initially, the new-born was placed in a sterile bubble and, to accelerate reconstitution, received seven additional stem cell transplants from nine fetal donors. This complementary treatment was carried out after the tests demonstrating engraftment of *in utero* transfused stem cells.

No engraftment of the cells infused after birth could be demonstrated, confirming the 'resistance' to transplantation in these patients. However, the number of cells deriving from the *in utero* transplant increased and was found to be 26% among peripheral blood lymphocytes at one year. In parallel, T cell maturity and immunological reconstitution progressed significantly. Although this reconstitution cannot be considered absolutely complete, the proliferative responses to antigens (candida antigens, CMV antigens and tetanus toxoid) have occurred and progressed up to a normal degree. Immunoglobulin levels are still relatively low, a finding consistent with the previous observation of slow reconstitution of humoral immunity following fetal liver transplantation (Touraine *et al.*, 1987). Because of the T cell reconstitution from the cells transplanted *in utero*, and in view of good health, the child was allowed to leave the isolator at the age of 16 months. The child's present condition is excellent. He has not experienced any severe infection and lives a normal life at home. He continues to receive immunoglobulins every month until he produces sufficient amounts of IgM and IgG.

After the encouraging results of the first *in utero* fetal liver transplant, a second fetus, designated B, in which a complete form of SCID had been diagnosed prenatally was similarly treated (see Table 20.2). At birth, the female infant still had immunological manifestations of SCID. She was, therefore, maintained in sterile isolation and received additional infusions of fetal liver and thymus cells, with the aim of accelerating development of the *in utero* transplanted stem cells. Cell-mediated immunity progressed sufficiently to allow adequate immunity against microorganisms, so that the child was allowed to leave the isolator. She is now healthy, with satisfactory immunological reconstitution and lives normally at home, only receiving monthly immunoglobulin infusions.

By polymerase chain reaction (PCR) gene amplification techniques, Y chromosome-specific DNA sequences were demonstrated in DNA extracted from this girl's peripheral blood lymphocytes at 8 and 10 months. Engraftment has, therefore, been obtained and donor stem cells differentiated into T lymphocytes with adequate immune function. Recent analyses confirmed a progressively increasing number of peripheral blood T cells, derived from the cells transplanted *in utero*. Together with the development of a significant population of donor-derived T lymphocytes, satisfactory proliferative responses to various stimuli, including phytomitogens and specific antigens, appeared and grew up to virtually normal levels.

A further fetus (Table 20.2) received two fetal liver transplants to treat chronic granulomatous disease. An elder brother was known to have the disease and prenatal diagnosis in the current case was positive. The first transplant was carried out uneventfully by umbilical vein infusion at 19 weeks' gestation but the number of cells available for infusion was considered insufficient. A second transplant was, therefore, attempted at 23 weeks but unfortunately resulted in fetal bradycardia (possibly as a result of the relatively rapid infusion of a larger number of cells) and led to fetal death within one hour.

Beta-thalassaemia

The results obtained in the first two patients with severe immunodeficiency disease next prompted us to attempt *in utero* fetal liver transplantation in fetuses with severe non-immune haematological disorders. In such conditions, however, graft take may be more difficult in a fetal host with an intact immune system and we, therefore, assumed that grafting had to be carried out during the first trimester or the beginning of the second, at a time when normal fetuses have not yet developed cell-mediated immunity (Royo, Touraine & de Bouteiller, 1987).

In one case, designated D, the mother had a family history of thalassaemia and requested early prenatal diagnosis. The fetus was shown by molecular techniques to have β^0 thalassaemia major. The mother rejected the option of termination for religious reasons and instead requested *in utero* fetal liver transplantation. Fetal stem cell transplantation was carried out at 14 weeks' gestation by intraperitoneal injection of donor fetal liver cells (Table 20.2). Studies performed after birth confirmed

the presence of thalassaemia. However, there were a few cells of donor origin: PCR gene amplification techniques revealed Y chromosome-specific DNA fragments in peripheral blood lymphocytes of this girl. In addition, haemoglobin A was found to account for 0.9% of all haemoglobin at six months. No further transplant was needed in this infant who is presently in good general condition. At one year of age, during which she received only a single blood transfusion, her total haemoglobin level was slightly below normal and the haemoglobin A percentage, three months after blood transfusion, was 30% (Table 20.2). These data suggest that engraftment of a few donor cells has been followed by some cell proliferation, resulting in partial correction of this haematological disorder.

In a further fetal patient in whom a prenatal diagnosis of β^0 thalassaemia had also been made, stem cell transplantation with fetal liver was attempted by intravascular infusion at 19 weeks' gestation. A 4 ml sample of blood was drawn, and 10 ml medium containing fetal cells was infused. Unfortunately, fetal bradycardia resulted, possibly related to the relatively rapid infusion, leading to fetal death within one hour.

Overall results

The results of the above cases demonstrate the feasibility of fetal liver transplantation *in utero* (Touraine et al., 1991). They are in agreement with experimental data in animals (Harrison et al., 1989) and show that the procedure can be effective in humans with engraftment and correction of inherited immunodeficiencies. However, with regard to other IEM, such as thalassaemia, experience is too limited to determine whether transplantation leads to significant improvement. To improve further efficacy in non-immunodeficiency cases, it may be useful to increase the number of donor cells and to perform the transplantation earlier in gestation.

Recently, several groups have also attempted *in utero* stem cell transplantation, with a comparable method, to treat various congenital diseases. Although the results of these cases are not yet published, similar findings have been obtained. The beneficial effect of the earliest possible transplant has been confirmed, the superiority of fetal liver cells over bone marrow cells, at least in the present state of *in utero* transplantation, has been demonstrated, and in IEM the slow reconstitution and partial effect again observed.

The earlier the transplant is performed the greater the chance of full and rapid development of the transplanted cells. Whether the use of additional therapy in fetuses with normal immunity might be beneficial to increase the number of engrafted cells able to proliferate and to differentiate has not been investigated, although this would obviously have to be studied in animal models before use in humans.

Immune immaturity of the fetal donor prevents acute GVHD. Immune immaturity of the fetal recipient prevents rejection. Indeed, when stem cells are transplanted *in utero* before immune maturation in the recipient, rejection is prevented and tolerance readily obtained (Touraine *et al.*, 1994). Such results in humans confirm the early experimental data reported in the neonatal murine model by Billingham, Brent & Medawar (1953). However, because of the comparatively earlier immune development in the human fetus, the immunological tolerance that can be induced in the mouse newborn must be achieved by the end of the first trimester or the very beginning of the second trimester in humans to obtain the same result.

Until recently prenatal diagnosis of the severe genetic disorders most frequently resulted in a decision to terminate the pregnancy. This new option of *in utero* transplantation may represent a more satisfactory solution for the sick fetus. Stem cell transplantation *in utero* offers great promise and in future will share with somatic gene therapy the ability to cure many of these severe diseases.

Immunological studies in human chimaeras: tolerance to alloantigens and antigen recognition by T cells

Whether treated prenatally or postnatally, patients with engraftment of donor stem cells following fetal liver transplantation became human chimaeras with cells, especially T lymphocytes, of donor origin co-existing with the various host cells, despite major HLA mismatch.

Investigations have been carried out in our institution on peripheral blood lymphocytes from several of the above patients; most investigations have been carried out in postnatally treated patients, but comparable results have recently been obtained in patients treated *in utero*. In particular, the first patient with SCID cured by postnatal fetal liver and thymus transplants from two donors was studied repeatedly. T lymphocytes were shown to derive from the first (10–20%) as well as the second (80–90%) donor. In contrast, B lymphocytes, monocytes and natural killer cells were all shown to be of host type. There was a complete mismatch at the *A*, *B*, *C* and *DR* loci of the HLA regions between host, donor 1 and donor 2 (Roncarolo *et al.*, 1986; 1988). Other more recently treated patients have comparable results.

The results of these investigations may be summarized as follows. Progenitor T cells deriving from the transplant(s) mature in the host thymus homing into the recipient thymus at the same time as host prothymocytes. These influences of host and donor cells on the T lineage, during the differentiation of T cells from donor stem cells, result in mature T lymphocytes with exogenous and endogenous peptidic recognition restricted by recipient MHC and with immunological tolerance to antigens of the donor(s) and of recipient (Fig. 20.3).

Fetal livers of less than 14.5 weeks' gestation age contain only immature cells which do not induce GVHD when transplanted into allogeneic hosts. Despite HLA mismatch with the recipient, these cells can give rise to fully immunocompetent T lymphocytes with helper and cytotoxic functions. Host cells impose positive selection and donor cells impose negative selection during T cell maturation in these chimaeric patients.

Conclusion

Fetal liver is an efficient source of stem cells for transplantation in children with immunodeficiency diseases or inborn errors of metabolism. Despite HLA mismatch between donor and host, engraftment, chimaerism and tolerance are obtained, and immunological reconstitution occurs with long-term survival in excess of 60%. However, transplantation of stem cells *in utero* should be the optimal therapy for fetuses with a variety of immunological or haematological disorders diagnosed early in gestation. *In utero* fetal liver transplantation has several advantages over postnatal fetal liver transplantation:

Fig. 20.3 *Differentiation of T lymphocytes from stem cells of donors 1 and 2 within the host thymus, in contact with host and donor cells, resulting in cells with peptidic antigen recognition restricted by host MHC and with tolerance to host antigens and to both donors antigens. (Reproduced from Touraine et al., 1994.)*

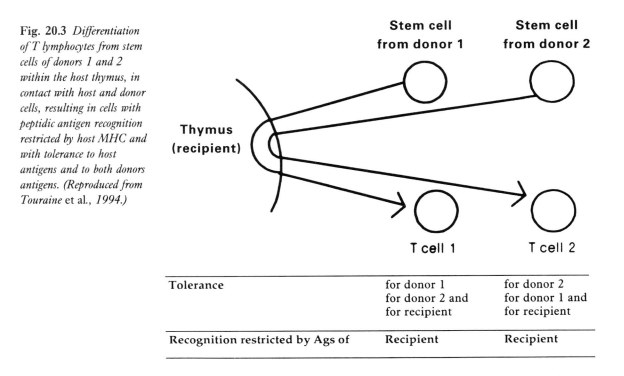

	T cell 1	T cell 2
Tolerance	for donor 1 for donor 2 and for recipient	for donor 2 for donor 1 and for recipient
Recognition restricted by Ags of	Recipient	Recipient

increased probability of graft take, ideal isolation of the patient in the uterus, and optimal environment for fetal cell development within the fetal host. Initial results are promising, and it can now be proposed as a real alternative to therapeutic abortion or to delayed, postnatal transplantation.

Acknowledgements

We are very grateful to R. Bacchetta, F. Barbier, H. Bétuel, D. Frappaz, F. Freycon, L. Gebuhrer, E. Goillot, S. Laplace, N. Philippe, H. Plotnicky, D. Raudrant, A. Rebaud, F. Rezzoug, M. G. Roncarolo, C. Royo, K. Sanhadji, G. Souillet, H. Spits, F. Touraine, J. E. de Vries, C. Vullo, H. Yssel and M. T. Zabot for their great contribution to patient care and to immunological studies.

References

Aitouche, A. & Touraine, J.-L. (1993). Accelerated rejection of H-2 incompatible skin allografts in the absence of specific antibodies. *Transplantation*, 56, 503–8.

Andreani, M., de Biagi, M., Centis, F., Manna, M., Agostinelli, F., Filipetti, A., Gaudenzi, G., Muretto, P., Grianti, C., Sotti, G., Rigon, A. & Lucarelli, G. (1985). Fetal liver transplantation in the mini-pig. In *Progress in Clinical and Biological Research: Fetal Liver Transplantation*, 193, ed. R. P. Gale, J.-L. Touraine & G. Lucarelli, pp. 205–17. New York: Alan R. Liss.

Berkowitz, R. L., Chitkara, U., Wilkins, I., Lynch, L. & Mehalek, K. E. (1987). Technical aspects of intravascular intrauterine transfusions: lessons learned from 33 procedures. *American Journal of Obstetrics and Gynecology*, 157, 4–9.

Billingham, R. E., Brent, L. & Medawar, P. B. (1953). Actively acquired tolerance of foreign cells. *Nature*, 172, 603–6.

Boersma, W. J. A. (1983). Prothymocytes in mouse fetal liver. *Thymus*, 5, 419–28.

Bortin, M. M. & Rimm, A. A. (1977). Severe combined immunodeficiency disease : characterization of the disease and results of transplantation. *Journal of the American Medical Association*, 238, 591–600.

Bortin, M. M. & Saltzstein, E. C. (1969). Graft-versus-host inhibition: fetal liver and thymus cells to minimise secondary disease. *Science*, 164, 316–18.

Bunch, C., Wood, W. G. & Kelly, S. J. (1985). Fetal haemopoietic cell transplantation in sheep: an approach to the cellular control of haemoglobin switching. In *Progress in Clinical and Biological Research: Fetal Liver Transplantation*, 193, ed. R. P. Gale, J.-L.Touraine & G. Lucarelli, pp. 219–33. NewYork : Alan R. Liss.

Champlin, R. E., Cain, G., Stitzel, K. & Gale, R. P. (1987). Sustained recovery of hematopoiesis and immunity following transplantation of fetal liver cells in dogs. *Thymus*, 10, 13–18.

Crouch, B. G. (1959). Transplantation of fetal haemopoietic tissues into irradiated mice and rats. In *Proceedings of the Seventh Congress of the European Society for Haematology*, p. 973.

De Koning, J., Van Bekkum, D. W., Dicke, A., Dooren, L. J., Van Rood, J. J. & Radl, J. (1969). Transplantation of bone marrow cells and fetal thymus in an infant with lymphopenic immunological deficiency. *Lancet*, i, 1223–7.

Durandy, A., Cerf-Bensussan, N., Dumez, Y. & Griscelli, C. (1987). Prenatal diagnosis of severe combined immunodeficiency with defective synthesis of HLA molecule. *Prenatal Diagnosis*, 7, 27–31.

Fischer, A., Griscelli, C., Friedrich, W., Kubaneck, B., Levinsky, R., Morgan, G., Vossen, J., Wagemaker, G. & Landais, P. (1986). Bone marrow transplantation for immunodeficiencies and osteopetrosis: European Survey, 1968–1985. *Lancet*, ii, 1080–3.

Flake, A. W., Harrison, M. R., Adzick, N. S. & Zanjani, E. D. (1986). Transplantation of fetal haemopoietic stem cells *in utero:* the creation of haemopoietic chimeras. *Science*, 233, 776–8.

Fleischman, R. A., Cluster, R. P. & Mintz, B. (1982). Totipotent hematopoietic stem cells: normal self-renewal and differentiation after transplantation between mouse fetuses. *Cell*, 30, 351–9.

Gale, R. P. (1987). Fetal liver transplantation in aplastic anemia and leukaemia. *Thymus*, 10, 89–94.

Gatti, R. A., Allen, H. D., Meuwissen, H. J., Hong, R. & Good, R. A. (1968). Immunological reconstitution in sex-linked lymphopenic immunological deficiency. *Lancet*, ii, 1366.

Grebe, S. C. & Streilen, J. (1976). Graft-versus-host reactions: a review. *Advances in Immunology*, 22, 119–22.

Harrison, M. R., Slotnick, R. N., Crombleholme, T. M., Globus, M. S., Tarantal, A. F. & Zanjani, E. D. (1989). *In utero* transplantation of fetal liver haemopoietic stem cells in monkeys. *Lancet*, ii, 1425–7.

Kelemen, E., Gulya, E. & Szabo, L. (1980). Xenogeneic transfer of fetal liver- and adult bone marrow-derived haemopoietic cells in rodents. In *Fetal Liver Transplantation. Current Concepts and Future Directions*, ed. G. Lucarelli, T. M. Fliedner & R. P. Gale, pp. 168–74. Amsterdam: Excerpta Medica.

Kochupillai, V., Sharma, S., Francis, S., Nanu, A., Mathew, S., Bhatia, P., Dua, H., Kumar, L., Aggarwal, S., Singh, S., Kumar, S., Karak, A. & Bhargava, M. (1987a). Fetal liver infusion in aplastic anemia. *Thymus*, 10, 95–102.

Kochupillai, V., Sharma, S., Francis, S., Nanu, A., Verma, I. C., Dua, H., Kumar, L., Aggarwal, S. & Singh, S. (1987b). Fetal liver infusion in acute myelogenous leukaemia. *Thymus*, 10, 117–24.

Korngold, R. & Sprent, J. (1982). Features of T-cells causing H-2 restricted lethal graft-versus-host disease across minor histocompatibility barrier. *Journal of Experimental Medicine*, 155, 182.

Löwenberg, B. (1975). Fetal liver cell transplantation. Thesis Erasmus University Rotterdam. (Rijswijk (ZH), The Netherlands Radiobiological Institute of the Organisation for Health Research TNO.

Mintz, B. (1985). Renewal and differentiation of totipotent hematopoietic stem cells of the mouse after transplantation into early fetuses. In *Progress in Clinical and Biological Research: Fetal Liver Transplantation*, 193, ed. R. P. Gale, J.-L.Touraine & G. Lucarelli, pp. 3–16. New York: Alan R. Liss.

O'Reilly, R. J., Kapoor, N., Kirkpatrick, D., Flomenberg, N., Pollack, M. S., Dupont, B., Good, R. A. & Reisner, Y. (1983). Transplantation of hematopoietic cells for lethal congenital immunodeficiencies. In *Primary Immunodeficiency Diseases. The March of Dimes Birth Defects Foundation*, ed. R. J. Wedgwood, F. S. Rosen & N. W. Paul, pp. 129–37. New York: Alan R. Liss.

Perryman, L. E. (1980). Use of fetal tissues for immunoreconstitution in horses with severe combined immunodeficiency. In *Fetal Liver Transplantation. Current Concepts and Future Directions*, ed. G. Lucarelli, T. M. Fliedner & R. P. Gale, pp. 183–97. Amsterdam: Excerpta Medica.

Plotnicky, H. & Touraine, J.-L. (1993a). Cytotoxic T cells from a human chimera induce regression of Epstein–Barr virus-infected allogeneic host cells. *International Immunology*, 5, 1413–20.

Plotnicky, H. & Touraine, J.-L. (1993b). Promotion of fetal liver cell engraftment in irradiated mice by activated T lymphocytes. *Bone Marrow Transplant*, 12, 307–14.

Prümmer, O., Raghavarvachar, A., Werner, C., Calvo, W., Carbonell, F., Steinbach, I. & Fliedner, T. M. (1985). Fetal liver transplantation in the dog. *Transplantation*, 39, 349–55.

Raudrant, D., Touraine, J-L. & Rebaud, A. (1992). *In utero* transplantation of stem cells in humans: technical aspects and clinical experience during pregnancy. *Bone Marrow Transplant.*, 9 (suppl. 1), 98–100

Roncarolo, M. G., Touraine, J.-L. & Banchereau, J. (1986). Co-operation between major histocompatibility complex mismatched mononuclear cells from a human chimera in the production of antigen-specific antibody. *Journal of Clinical Investigation*, 77, 673–80.

Roncarolo, M. G., Yssel, H., Touraine, J.-L., Bacchetta, R., Gebuhrer, L., de Vries, J.E. & Spits, H. (1988). Antigen recognition by MHC-incompatible cells of a human mismatched chimera. *Journal of Experimental Medicine*, 168, 2139–52.

Royo, C., Touraine, J.-L. & de Bouteiller, O. (1987). Ontogeny of T-lymphocyte differentiation in the human fetus: acquisition of phenotype and functions. *Thymus*, 10, 57–73.

Sanhadji, K., Négrier, M. S. & Touraine, J.-L. (1990). Fetal liver cell transplantation in SCID mice. *Thymus*, 15, 57–64.

Thomas, E. D., Stoeb, R., Clift, R. A., Fefer, A., Johnson, F. L., Neiman, P. E., Lerner, K. G., Glucksberg, H. & Buckner, C. D. (1975). Bone marrow transplantation. *New England Journal of Medicine*, 292, 832–43 and 895–902.

Touraine, J.-L. (1981). The bare lymphocyte syndrome: report on the registry. *Lancet*, i, 319–21.

Touraine, J.-L. (1983). Bone marrow and fetal liver transplantation in immuno-deficiencies and inborn errors of metabolism: lack of significant restriction of T-cell function in long term chimeras despite HLA-mismatch. *Immunology Review*, 1, 103–21.

Touraine, J.-L.(1985). *Hors de la Bulle*, vol. 1. Paris: Flammarion.

Touraine, J.-L. (1989). New strategies in the treatment of immunological and other inherited diseases: allogeneic stem cells transplantation. *Bone Marrow Transplantation*, 4 (suppl. 4), 139–41.

Touraine, J.-L. (1991). The place of fetal liver transplantation in the treatment of inborn errors of metabolism. *Journal of Inherited Metabolic Diseases*, 14, 619–26.

Touraine, J.-L. (1992). Transplantation of fetal haemopoietic and lymphopoietic cells in humans, with special reference to *in utero* transplantation. In *Fetal Tissue Transplants in Medicine*, ed. R. G. Edwards, pp. 155–76. Cambridge: Cambridge University Press.

Touraine, J.-L. (1993). *In utero* transplantation of haemopoietic stem cells into human fetuses. In

Frontiers in Gynaecologic and Obstetric Investigation, ed. A. R. Genazzani, F. Petraglia & A. D. Genazzani, pp. 109–22. Carnforth, UK: Parthenon Publishing.

Touraine, J.-L., Bétuel, H., Souillet, G. & Jeune, M. (1978). Combined immunodeficiency disease associated with absence of cell-surface HLA A and B antigens. *Journal of Pediatrics,* 93, 47–51.

Touraine, J.-L., Raudrant, D., Rebaud, A., Roncarolo, M. G., Laplace, S., Gebuhrer, L., Bétuel, H., Frappaz, D., Freycon, F., Zabot, M. T., Touraine, F., Souillet, G., Philippe, N. & Vullo, C. (1992). *In utero* transplantation of stem cells in humans: immunological aspects and clinical follow-up of patients. *Bone Marrow Transplantation,* 9 (suppl. 1), 121–6.

Touraine, J.-L., Raudrant, D., Royo, C., Rebaud, A., Roncarolo, M. G., Souillet, G., Philippe, N., Touraine, F. & Bétuel, H. (1989). *In utero* transplantation of stem cells in the bare lymphocyte syndrome. *Lancet,* i, 1382.

Touraine, J.-L., Raudrant, D., Vullo, C., Frappaz, D., Freycon, F., Rebaud, A., Barbier, F., Roncarolo, M. G., Gebuhrer, L., Bétuel, H. & Zabot, M. T. (1991). New developments in stem cell transplantation with special reference to the first *in utero* transplants in humans. *Bone Marrow Transplant.*ation, 7, 92–7.

Touraine, J.-L., Roncarolo, M. G., Plotnicky, H., Bacchetta, R., Spits, H., Gebuhrer, L. & Bétuel, H. (1994). Tolerance to alloantigens and recognition for 'allo + X' induced in humans by fetal stem cell transplantation. In *Transplantation and Clinical Immunology, Rejection and Tolerance,* XXV, ed. J.-L. Touraine, J. Traeger, H. Bétuel, J. M. Dubernard, J. P. Revillard & C. Dupuy, pp. 265–77. Dordrecht: Kluwer Academic.

Touraine, J.-L., Roncarolo, M. G., Royo, C. & Touraine, F. (1987). Fetal tissue transplantation, bone marrow transplantation and prospective gene therapy in severe immunodeficiencies and enzyme deficiencies. *Thymus,* 10, 75–87.

Touraine, J.-L., Royo, C. & Gitton, X. (1990). Are fetal liver cells able to amount graft-versus-leukaemia effect? *Experimental Hematology,* 18, 657.

Uphoff, D. E. (1958). Preclusion of secondary phase of irradiation syndrome by inoculation of fetal hematopoietic tissue following total-body-X-irradiation. *Journal of the National Cancer Institute,* 20, 625–32.

Veyron, P. & Touraine, J.-L. (1990). Fetal liver cell transplantation: survival of affected grafted Balb/c LSD mice. *Transplantation Proceedings,* 22, 2253–4.

21 Gene therapy

JAMES D. GOLDBERG

Introduction

The human genome comprises over three billion base pairs encoding an estimated 50 000 to 200 000 genes. As the Human Genome Project attempts to map this enormous number of genes, much is already known regarding the structure of many genes and the mutations which cause the disease states. It is a natural progression from this knowledge to the attempt to cure genetic disease by gene therapy.

The demonstration in the 1960s that mammalian cells could integrate and express foreign DNA (Szybalska & Szybalski, 1962) has led to the rapid expansion of investigation into gene therapy in various animal systems. Based on the success of these animal studies, limited human studies involving gene therapy are currently underway. Much work, however, remains in optimizing these experimental protocols.

Gene therapy has not yet been attempted *in utero*. This chapter addresses an overview of the techniques and *ex utero* applications of gene therapy before addressing potential applications *in utero*.

Approaches for gene transfer

Physical methods

Two basic strategies exist for gene therapy, *ex vivo* and *in vivo*. In the *ex vivo* approach, cells are removed from an individual and then genetically modified *in vitro* by one of the techniques described below. The modified cells are then replaced in the donor and expression is determined. With the *in vivo* approach, agents, which are typically viral vectors which incorporate the gene of interest, are directly administered to the individual. Integration or incorporation of the foreign gene then takes place *in vivo* and expression is monitored.

Direct DNA injection
The direct injection of foreign DNA has been reported in both skeletal and cardiac tissue (Lin *et al.*, 1990; Wolff *et al.*, 1990). This has resulted in stable gene expression in these tissues. Unfortunately, the efficiency of incorporation of the DNA is quite low. The injected DNA appears to exist episomally rather than being integrated into the host genome. This approach may prove useful in situations where the local production of a gene product is important.

Liposome fusion
Liposomes are artificially created phospholipid vesicles. DNA which is encapsulated in these large unilamellar vesicles is efficiently transferred into cells in a manner that protects the DNA from intracellular nucleases (Wang & Huang, 1987; Hyde *et al.*, 1993). The liposomes may be conjugated with various antibodies or ligands to increase the specificity of cellular uptake.

Biological vectors

Retroviruses
The use of retroviral vectors has been the most widely used approach for gene therapy (McLachlin *et al.*, 1990; Salmons & Gunzburg, 1993). These viruses are small RNA viruses with a single-stranded RNA genome that is converted to DNA by reverse transcriptase carried in the viral particle. Retroviruses infect a wide range of cell

types and efficiently integrate into the host genome, making them effective transfer agents for gene transfer into foreign cells. One limiting factor is that retroviral integration only occurs in dividing cells, thus limiting the use of this vector to certain cell types.

Retroviruses have been extensively studied and much is known regarding their structure and life cycle. After infecting a cell, the retrovirus begins replication in the cytoplasm of the host cell. Viral-derived reverse transcriptase synthesizes a DNA copy of the single-stranded RNA genome. This viral DNA is then transferred to the nucleus of the cell where it becomes randomly integrated into the host genome as a provirus. The integrated provirus utilizes long terminal repeat sequences (LTRs), which are located at the 5' and 3' ends of the viral genome, to direct host enzymes to produce new retroviral particles. In addition, a packaging sequence and three translational units consisting of the three viral genes (*gag*, *pol* and *env*) are necessary to produce new virion particles. The *gag* sequence codes for specific internal structural proteins of the virus. The *pol* sequence codes for reverse transcriptase and a viral

integrase which helps proviral integration into the host genome. The *env* gene codes for the envelope glycoproteins needed for binding of the virus to the cell surface and the entry of particles into cells. The viral particle is assembled in the cytoplasm of the host cell and is released by budding without killing the host. This information has been helpful in adapting these agents into useful gene transfer vector (Fig. 21.1).

Modification of retroviruses for use as vectors has generally involved deletion of coding sequences of the virus (primarily the *gag*, *pol* and *env* packaging genes) and replacement with the genes of interest, including a selectable marker gene (Fig. 21.2). The genomes of naturally occurring retroviruses generally do not exceed 9 to 10 kb in size. Because of this, the upper limit of genome size that can be inserted into a retroviral capsid is approximately 13 kb. Because of the deletion of the coding sequences for the viral structural genes, helper cell lines are necessary to allow viral replication in the host cell. These packaging cell lines do not produce their own viral progeny because they lack key sequences, usually the site necessary for viral packaging.

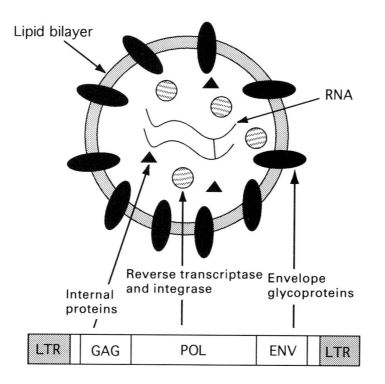

Fig. 21.1 *Retroviral structure. The RNA sequence at the bottom consists of the* gag, pol *and* env *genes flanked by long terminal repeat (LTR) sequences. The viral strand of RNA is shown alongside with its transcribed cDNA.*

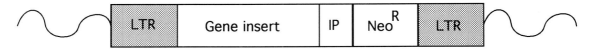

Fig. 21.2 *Typical retroviral vector. The retroviral genes have been replaced by a foreign gene insert, an internal promoter (IP) and a selectable marker for neomycin resistance (NeoR).*

The helper cell line is infected with the replication-deficient viral vector carrying the foreign gene of interest. The DNA produced by reverse transcriptase is integrated into the helper cell genome. An infectious viral particle is then formed utilizing the structural genes of the helper cell line. These infectious particles are then able to infect a normal cell and integrate the foreign gene of interest into the genome. New transmissible particles, however, will not be produced because of the lack of the structural sequences in the infecting virus or in the normal cell which is being infected.

Attempts have been made to target specific cells for retroviral integration. This would provide for enhanced tissue-specific production of the transduced gene. Neda *et al.* (1991), for example, have reported the modification of the surface of a retroviral vector to bind to the asialoglycoprotein receptor which is found in liver cells. Other investigators are using this method to direct cells to the liver for gene therapy of a wide range of liver disorders.

Adenoviruses

Adenoviruses are double-stranded DNA viruses with a 36 kb genome (Berkner, 1991). Unlike retroviruses, adenoviruses can infect non-dividing cells and have an increased affinity for cells of the airway. In addition, adenoviruses have been used for many years in live virus vaccines and have an excellent safety record.

The adenovirus genome includes a subset of genes (*E1A*) which are expressed early and serve as regulators of other genes required for adenovirus replication. In most gene therapy constructs, the *E1A* region is replaced with the foreign DNA of choice. Infective particles are then produced by infecting a helper cell line containing the missing *E1A* region.

As mentioned above, one of the major advantages of adenovirus-mediated gene transfer is the ability to infect both non-dividing and dividing cells. Unfortunately, the adenoviral vectors remain episomal and do not integrate efficiently into nuclear DNA. This can result in transient expression of the gene product. There are also possible toxic effects to the cell which have not been well studied.

Adeno-associated viruses

Adeno-associated viruses (AAV) are small double-stranded DNA viruses of the parvovirus family (Muzyczka, 1991). Unlike parvovirus B19, which is known to cause disease in humans, especially in fetuses, AAV are not known to cause human disease. Approximately 85% of adults are seropositive for AAV capsid proteins.

AAV have the unique property of site-specific integration on chromosome 19 in host cells (Samulski *et al.*, 1991). This site specificity may be lost in some recombinant AAV vectors. AAV are also defective viruses which require coinfection with another virus to complete their life cycle. Because of their small size, AAV can only accommodate inserts of approximately 4.7 kb.

Herpes simplex virus

Herpes virus type 1 (HSV-1) has been studied as a potential vector. Following infection with HSV-1, the virus enters a latent stage in sensory nerve ganglia. Thus, it may be an effective means of introducing DNA into neural cells. HSV-1 is a large, double-stranded DNA virus with a genome of 150 kb.

HSV-1 vectors share similarities with adenoviral vectors. Both can infect non-dividing cells and both remain episomal in location instead of integrating into the host DNA. HSV-1 vectors have the advantage of being able to incorporate much larger pieces of DNA. Problems with duration of expression and possible cytotoxic effects remain under investigation (Breakefield & DeLuca, 1991; Breakefield, 1993).

Selected disease models

Defects in haematopoietic cell function

Much of the work in the area of gene therapy has been related to defects in haematopoietic cell function. This is because haematopoietic stem cells (HSCs) are able to renew themselves and differentiate into progeny after transplantation. This has been well demonstrated in traditional bone marrow transplantation (Chang & Johnson, 1989; Williams, 1990). By transducing HSCs, it should be possible to achieve long-term therapy for a wide range of disorders currently treatable by bone marrow transplantation. These include β-thalassaemia (Lucarelli *et al.*, 1987), and adenosine deaminase (ADA) and purine nucleoside phosphorylase (PNP) deficiencies (Markert *et al.*, 1987), chronic granulomatous disease (Foroozanfar *et al.*, 1977), leukocyte adhesion deficiency (Fischer *et al.*, 1983), and a number of lysosomal storage disorders (Hobbs, 1988; Ringdén *et al.*, 1988; 1990; Kirkpatrick *et al.*, 1990; Krivit *et al.*, 1990).

Efficient gene transfer into HSCs require a high titre of the viral vector and HSCs which are actively dividing. A high titre is necessary because HSCs are relatively rare in bone marrow, 1 in 1×10^5 to 1 in 2×10^5 cells (Harrison, Astle & Lerner, 1988). The maximal titre is determined by several factors including size of the retroviral vector, length of the *gag* region and stability of the vector after gene insertion (Armentano *et al.*, 1987; Bender *et al.*, 1987). Unfortunately, HSCs are usually in the G_0 or non-dividing phase of the cell cycle and are, therefore, not ideal candidates for viral transduction (Ogawa, 1989; Miller, Adam & Miller, 1990). The use of various growth factors to induce HSC division has significantly increased their transduction efficiency (Nolta & Kohn, 1990). Bienzle *et al.* (1994) have shown that HSCs in long-term bone marrow culture may be simultaneously transduced and stimulated into active cell cycling *in vitro*. When these cells were transfused back into dogs without prior marrow ablation, expression was noted for up to 24 months. Thus it may be possible to achieve engraftment of genetically altered HSCs without prior marrow ablation and the risks associated with bone marrow suppression.

Severe combined immunodeficiency caused by ADA deficiency has served a model for a variety of therapeutic trials. Bone marrow transplantation is currently the preferred treatment method and can result in a complete cure, albeit with a significant risk of complications. Fewer than 30% of patients, however, have an HLA-matched donor source.

Enzyme therapy is another therapeutic option. A form of adenosine deaminase linked to polyethylene glycol has been developed. This has provided clinical improvement for many patients. In some cases, however, antibodies are formed which render the therapy ineffective. Because of these problems, gene therapy has been attempted in this disorder.

Two patients have undergone *in vitro* transduction of their peripheral T lymphocytes (Anderson, 1992; Blaese, 1993). Because transduction was in a differentiated cell type with a limited lifespan, infusions were performed every few weeks. Both patients have shown clinical and immune function improvement (Anderson, 1992). Currents efforts are being directed at transduction of HSCs for therapy in this disorder. Bodine *et al.* (1993) have demonstrated long-term *in vivo* expression in multiple cell lineages of transduced surface antigen CD34[+] bone marrow stem cells.

Haemophilia

Haemophilia A and haemophilia B result from deficiencies in coagulation factor VIII and IX, respectively. Both of these genes have been cloned and localized to the long arm of the X chromosome. Unfortunately, no single gene defect or group of gene defects have been found to account for the disease state. A variety of mutations, including partial or complete gene deletions, point mutations, insertions and an inversion mutation in the factor VIII gene, have been found. Haemophilia is considered to be a prime candidate for gene therapy in that there appears to be no significant regulation of the factor proteins and there is no requirement for tissue-specific expression (Thompson, 1991; Brinkhous, 1992). Individuals with severe haemophilia A or B have less than 1% of normal activity. Levels of greater than 5% seem to protect against spontaneous bleeding. Therefore, in attempting gene therapy in these individuals, it would be necessary to provide only greater than 5% activity.

Both *ex vivo* and *in vivo* approaches have been attempted in animal models for gene therapy in haemophilia A and B. Most investigators have used an *ex vivo* approach, which has the advantage of performing gene transduction or transfection under more controlled conditions. Using an *ex vivo* approach, factor IX expression has been demonstrated by a transduced cell line in a hollow fibre tissue culture apparatus. Factor IX was present in the recirculating fluid for several weeks (Lozier *et al.*, 1991). Human factor IX has also been demonstrated following the subcutaneous implantation of transduced cells in rodents (StLouis & Verma, 1988; Palmer, Thompson & Miller, 1989). Unfortunately, in most of these experiments, expression of factor IX has only been demonstrated for a few weeks (St Louis & Verma, 1988; Palmer *et al.*, 1989; Carr-Brendel *et al.*, 1993).

An exception to this short-term expression has been reported by Dai *et al.* (1992). A retroviral vector was constructed with the cytomegalovirus promoter, two copies of the muscle-specific creatine kinase enhancer of gene expression and the cDNA for factor IX. Levels of expression were less than 1%; however, the expression lasted for greater than six months.

A successful *in vivo* approach for gene therapy of factor IX has been reported by Kay *et al.* (1993). A retroviral vector containing canine factor IX was delivered directly to the liver after partial hepatectomy to stimulate hepatocyte regeneration. A less severe form of haemophilia B was noted in the animals. This has persisted for over 13 months (Lozier & Brinkhous, 1994).

Efforts at achieving expression of factor VIII have been somewhat more disappointing. Functional factor VIII has been produced in a number of cell lines following transduction with retroviral vectors (Wood *et al.*, 1984; Kaufman *et al.*, 1989; Hoeben *et al.*, 1990; 1993; Israel & Kaufman, 1990; Sandberg, Lind & Spira, 1991). Unfortunately, following implantation of modified skin fibroblasts into athymic rats there has been no evidence of expression of the factor VIII gene (Hoeben *et al.*, 1993).

Familial hypercholesterolaemia

Familial hypercholesterolaemia results from a deficiency of the receptor for low density lipoprotein (LDL), which carries cholesterol from the intestine to the liver. Indi-viduals homozygous for the LDL receptor deficiency have extremely high levels of cholesterol and manifest accelerated atherosclerosis. Since the LDL receptor is found on the surface of the liver, this disorder has become a model for hepatocyte-directed gene therapy.

Much work has been done utilizing the LDL receptor-deficient Watanabe rabbit model (Chowdhury *et al.*, 1991). In this model, rabbits undergo partial hepatectomy and the removed hepatocytes are transduced *in vitro* with a retroviral vector containing the LDL receptor. These cells are then directly injected into the portal vein of the animal. Stable reductions of 35% to 50% have been reported in these treated animals. A report from the first human patient treated in this manner indicated a 17% reduction in LDL levels (Grossman *et al.*, 1994). This had remained stable for 18 months post-procedure at the time of the report.

Growth deficiency

Another candidate for gene therapy is the administration of growth hormone. Extremely low levels of hormone activity are adequate to produce clinical results. Current therapy involves daily injection of expensive recombinant human growth hormone. Initial studies have shown that the growth hormone gene can be inserted into muscle cells and primary myoblasts and then be transplanted *in vivo* (Barr & Leiden, 1991; Dhawan *et al.*, 1991). Levels of human growth hormone were detected in serum for up to 80 days.

Cancer

There has been much interest in the area of gene therapy for cancer. The earliest gene therapy attempts involved following genetically altered cells *in vivo* in cancer patients to assess various treatment modalities. Rosenberg *et al.* (1990) injected genetically modified tumour-infiltrating lymphocytes, TIL, which had a *neo* gene inserted to determine whether the TIL cells actually were targeted back to the tumour. These studies demonstrated that a small percentage of TIL cells were found in the tumour. This gene-marking approach had also been used for follow-up in cases of autologous bone marrow transplantation (Brenner *et al.*, 1993).

In addition to the gene marker studies described

above, several therapeutic gene therapy trials are under-way. One approach has been to try to augment the host antitumour immune response by inserting foreign genes in the tumour cells themselves or in cells placed in close proximity to the tumour cells (Pardoll, 1992). These studies have shown promise in preliminary animal work (Gansbacher et al., 1990; Golumbek et al., 1991). A related approach is to insert genes into tumour cells that render the cells sensitive to other agents. Studies have been performed that have inserted the herpes simplex virus thymidine kinase gene, which when expressed makes the cell sensitive to the drug ganciclovir. This gene has been inserted into rat brain tumour cells. These animals exhibited a dramatic response to ganciclovir (Culver et al., 1992).

Other, more direct, approaches for cancer therapy are also being investigated. Attempts are being made to downregulate the expression of an oncogene by anti-sense technology (Trojan et al., 1992). In addition, investigators are attempting to insert tumour suppressor genes, which are missing or mutated in many types of cancer. This has been attempted with the p53 sup-pressor gene (Cheng et al., 1992). The difficulty with these types of approach is in transducing the foreign gene into a sufficient number of tumour cells to effect a response.

Cystic fibrosis

Cystic fibrosis is one of the most common genetic diseases in the northern European-derived Caucasian population. The gene for this disorder, cystic fibrosis transmembrane regulator (CFTR), has been cloned and has been shown to code for a transmembrane protein that functions as a chloride transporter. Both adenoviral (Rosenfeld et al., 1991) vectors and cationic liposomes (Hyde et al., 1993) have been used in attempts to transfer the CFTR gene in vivo to airway epithelial cells. Flotte et al. (1993) have recently demonstrated the stable in vivo integration of the CFTR gene with an adeno-associated virus vector in rabbit lungs. The vector was delivered through a fibreoptic bronchoscope into a single lobe of the rabbit lung. It still remains to be shown which cells are necessary to be transduced to provide clinical im-provement in this disorder. This will have to be demon-strated in well-designed human experimentation trials.

A significant advance in this area was reported by Zabner et al. (1993). An adenovirus containing the CFTR gene was applied to the nasal mucosa of three individuals with cystic fibrosis. This therapy was shown to correct the chloride transport defect present in these individuals. These changes were noted for at least three weeks. There were no adverse effects noted. This report is the first to demonstrate in vivo gene therapy to correct the defect in cystic fibrosis.

Muscle gene therapy

Most of the interest in gene therapy for muscle disease has focused on Duchenne muscular dystrophy (DMD). This is the most severe and common form of genetic muscle disease in children. DMD is caused by a defi-ciency of the protein dystrophin (Hoffman, Brown & Kunkel, 1987). This protein is coded for by an extremely large gene of 2.4 megabases on the X chromosome (Koenig et al., 1987; Koenig, Monaco & Kunkel, 1988). The lack of dystrophin causes necrosis of muscle fibre segments (Carpenter & Karpati, 1979).

Much experimental work has been performed on the inbred mdx strain of mice. This strain lacks skeletal muscle dystrophin as a result of a spontaneous mutation of the dystrophin gene (Sicinski et al., 1989). Several investigators have demonstrated low level expression of reporter genes (Wolff et al., 1990; Quantin et al., 1992) or dystrophin gene constructs (Acsadi et al., 1991; Dun-ckley et al., 1992) from DNA directly injected into the muscle of the mdx mouse.

Efforts are being directed towards increasing the level and duration of expression in these cells. With improve-ments in these areas, human therapy trials are likely to follow.

Perinatal considerations

Advances in the in utero evaluation and therapy of the fetus have provided new possibilities for prenatal therapy of abnormal fetuses. Several important areas must be evaluated before considering in utero therapy. The most important issue is whether in utero therapy provides any benefit over postnatal therapy. Traditionally, this type of analysis has focused on whether there is ongoing damage *in utero* that could best be treated by *in utero* therapy. In considering *in utero* gene therapy, other considerations become important. For example, is prenatal therapy more effective or does it have fewer complications than postnatal therapy?

Several approaches have been utilized in experimental animal models for *in utero* gene therapy. The efficiency of transduction of haematopoietic stem cells extracted from fetal liver rather than adult cells has been shown to be higher in dogs, sheep and humans (Eglitis *et al.*, 1987; Kohn *et al.*, 1987; al-Lebban *et al.*, 1990; Ekhterae *et al.*, 1990). In addition, because of the ontogeny of bone marrow development in the fetus, seeding of the marrow with transfused genetically altered stem cells may be possible without the marrow ablation needed after birth (Metcalf & Moore, 1971; Clapp *et al.*, 1991). Direct injection of retroviral vectors in the liver of fetal rats has also been reported (Clapp *et al.*, 1991). Recombinant cells were present in the animals up to 26 weeks after delivery.

As mentioned above, several studies have been performed by *ex vivo* hepatic gene therapy. Investigators have shown that it is possible to do a partial liver resection *in utero* (Harrison, Langer & Adzick, 1990). Other investigators have demonstrated the cultivation and transduction *in vitro* of these cells in a variety of different species including humans (Soriano *et al.*, 1993; Ledley *et al.*, 1987; Koch *et al.*, 1991; Ledley, 1993). The transduced cells could then be infused back into the fetus through the umbilical vein. In fetal lambs, it has been shown that it is possible to constitute up to 3 to 5% of the hepatocyte population with this approach (Soriano *et al.*, 1993). Unfortunately, the presence of isolated hepatocytes was also seen in other non-hepatic tissues. Other investigators have demonstrated the expression of recombinant genes in fetal rat brain after *in utero* injection (Jiao *et al.*, 1992). If these transplants could be performed early *in utero* before the fetus is immunocompetent, it would allow the use of heterologous genetically modified cells without the need for immunosuppression.

Ethical issues

The ethical issues surrounding gene therapy in general are complex. When gene therapy is proposed for the

fetus, the additional consideration of maternal rights needs to be addressed.

A distinction must be made between somatic and germ cell therapy when discussing the ethics of gene therapy. All attempts to date in humans have involved somatic cell therapy. This type of modification does not affect germ cells and, therefore, cannot be passed on from generation to generation. Advances in micromanipulation of the early embryo have made it technically possible to consider germ line therapy. Wivel and Walters (1993) have summarized many of the arguments for and against germ line therapy. Their arguments in support of germ line therapy are as follows: (i) the moral obligation of the health profession to use the best available treatment methods, (ii) parental autonomy and access to available technologies for the purposes of having a health child, (iii) germ line gene modification is more efficient and cost effective than somatic cell gene therapy, and (iv) the freedom of scientific inquiry and intrinsic value of knowledge. Their arguments against germ line therapy include: (i) expensive intervention with limited applicability, (ii) availability of alternative strategies for preventing genetic disease, (iii) unavoidable risks, irreversible mistakes, and (iv) inevitable pressures to use germ line gene modification for enhancement. These issues outline a forum for continued discussion in this area. At present, it is unlikely that germ line therapy in humans will be attempted in the near future.

Conclusion

The goal of gene therapy is treatment of disease. Work to date has demonstrated the feasibility of this approach for the potential therapy of a large number of disorders, such as cystic fibrosis and cancer. Major issues which are still unresolved include the length of time for which interventions will provide the desired therapeutic effect and whether expression of the transferred gene will truly provide clinical benefit. Gene therapy is likely to have applications *in utero* not only for genetic diseases, but also for conditions that cause morbidity and in which transfection of the fetus is likely to be more efficient than that performed postnatally.

References

Acsadi, G., Dickson, G., Love, D. R., Jani, A., Walsh, F. S., Gurusinghe, A., Wolff, J. A. & Davies, K. E. (1991). Human dystrophin expression in mdx mice after injection of DNA constructs. *Nature*, 352, 815–8.

al-Lebban, Z. S., Henry, J. M., Jones, J. B., Eglitis, M. A., Anderson, W. F. & Lothrop, C. D., Jr (1990). Increased efficiency of gene transfer with retroviral vectors in neonatal hematopoietic progenitor cells. *Experimental Hematology*, 18, 180–4.

Anderson, W. F. (1992). Human gene therapy. *Science*, 256, 808–13.

Armentano, D., Yu, S.-F., Kantoff, P. W., von Ruden, T., Anderson, W. F. & Gilboa, E. (1987). Effect of internal viral sequences on the utility of retroviral vectors. *Journal of Virology*, 61, 1647–50.

Barr, E. & Leiden, J. M. (1991). Systemic delivery of recombinant proteins by genetically modified myoblasts. *Science*, 254, 1507–9.

Bender, M. A., Palmer, T. D., Gelinas, R. E. & Miller, A. D. (1987). Evidence that the packaging signal of Moloney murine leukemia virus extends into the *gag* region. *Journal of Virology*, 61, 1639–46.

Berkner, K. L. (1991). Expression of heterologous sequences in adenoviral vectors. *Current Topics in Microbiology and Immunology*, 158, 39–66.

Bienzle, D., Abrams-Ogg, A. C. G., Kruth, S. A., Ackland-Snow, J., Carter, R. F., Dick, J. E., Jacobs, R. M., Kamel-Reid, S. & Dube, I. D. (1994). Gene transfer into hematopoietic stem cells: long-term maintenance of in-vitro activated progenitors without marrow ablation. *Proceedings of the National Academy of Sciences of the USA*, 91, 350–4.

Blaese, R. M. (1993). Development of gene therapy for immunodeficiency: adenosine deaminase deficiency. *Pediatric Research*, 33, 549–55.

Bodine, D. M., Moritz, T., Donahue, R. E., Luskey, B. D., Kessler, S. W., Martin, D. I., Orkin, S. H., Nienhuis, A. W. & Williams, D. A. (1993). Long-term *in vivo* expression of a murine adenosine deaminase gene in Rhesus monkey hematopoietic cells of multiple lineages after retroviral mediated gene transfer into CD34+ bone marrow cells. *Blood*, 82, 1975–80.

Breakefield, X. O. (1993). Gene delivery into the brain using virus vectors. *Nature Genetics*, 3, 187–9.

Breakefield, X. O. & DeLuca, N. A. (1991). Herpes simplex virus for gene delivery to neurons. *New Biologist*, 3, 203–18.

Brenner, M. K., Rill, D. R., Moen, R. C., Krance, R. A., Mirro, J. Jr, Anderson, W. F. & Ihle, J. N. (1993). Gene-marking to trace origin of relapse after autologous bone-marrow transplantation. *Lancet*, 341, 85–6.

Brinkhous, K. M. (1992). Gene transfer in the hemophilias: retrospect and prospect. *Thrombosis Research*, 67, 329–38.

Carpenter, S. & Karpati, G. (1979). Duchenne muscular dystrophy: plasma membrane loss initiates muscle cell necrosis unless it is repaired. *Brain*, 102, 147–61.

Carr-Brendel, V., Lozier, J. N., Thomas, T. J., Young, S. S., Crudele, J., Martinson, L., Roche, B., Boggs, D., Pauley, R., Maryonov, D., Josephs, S., High, K., Johnson, B. & Brauker, J. (1993). An immunoisolation device for implantation of genetically engineered cells: long term expression of factor IX in rats. *Journal of Cellular Biochemistry*, 17E, 224.

Chang, J. M. & Johnson, G. R. (1989). Gene transfer into hemopoietic stem cells using retroviral vectors. *International Journal of Cell Cloning*, 7, 264–80.

Cheng, J., Yee, J.-K., Yeargin, J., Friedmann, T. & Haas, M. (1992). Suppression of acute lymphoblastic leukemia by the human wild-type p53 gene. *Cancer Research*, 52, 222–6.

Chowdhury, J. R., Grossamn, M., Gupta, S., Chowdhury, N. R., Baker, J. R., Jr & Wilson, J. M. (1991). Long-term improvement of hypercholesterolemia after *ex vivo* gene therapy in LDLR-deficient rabbits. *Science*, 254, 1802–5.

Clapp, D. W., Dumenco, L. L., Hatzoglou, M. & Gerson, S. L. (1991). Fetal liver hematopoietic stem cells as a target for *in utero* retroviral gene transfer. *Blood*, 78, 1132–9.

Culver, K. W., Ram, Z., Wallbridge, S., Ishii, H., Oldfield, E. H. & Blaese, R. M. (1992). *In vivo* gene transfer with retroviral vector producer cells for treatment of experimental brain tumors. *Science*, 256, 1550–2.

Dai, Y., Roman, M., Naviaux, R. K. & Verma, I. M. (1992). Gene therapy via primary myoblasts: long-term expression of factor IX protein following transplantation *in vivo*. *Proceedings of the National Academy of Sciences of the USA*, 89, 10892–5.

Dhawan, J., Pan, L. C., Pavlath, G. K., Travis, M. A., Lanctot, A. M. & Blau, H. M. (1991). Systemic delivery of human growth hormone by injection of genetically altered myoblasts. *Science*, 254, 1509–12.

Dunckley, M. G., Love, D. R., Davies, K. E., Walsh, F. S., Morris, G. E. & Dickson, G. (1992). Retroviral-mediated transfer of a dystrophin minigene into mdx mouse myoblasts *in vitro*. *FEBS Letters*, 296, 128–34.

Eglitis, M. A., Kantoff, P. W., McLachlin, J. R., Gillio, A., Flake, A. W., Bordignon, C., Moen, R. C., Karson, E. M., Zwiebel, J. A., Kohn, D. B., Gilboa, E., Blaese, R. M., Harrison, M. R., Zanjani, E. D., O'Reilly, R. O. & Anderson, W. F. (1987). Gene therapy: efforts at developing large animal models for autologous bone marrow transplant and gene transfer with retroviral vectors. *Ciba Foundation Symposium*, 130, 229–46.

Ekhterae, D., Crumbleholme, T., Karson, E., Harrison, M. R., Anderson, W. F. & Zanjani, E. D. (1990). Retroviral vector-mediated transfer of the bacterial neomycin resistance gene into fetal and adult sheep and human hematopoietic progenitors *in vitro*. *Blood*, 75, 365–9.

Fischer, A., Trung, P. H., Descamps-Latscha, B., Lisowska-Grospierre, B., Gerota, I., Perrez, N., Scheinmetzler, C., Durandy, A., Virelizier, J. L. & Griscelli, C. (1983). Bone marrow transplantation for inborn errors of phagocytic cells associated with defective adherence, chemotaxis, and oxidative response during opsonized particle phagocytosis. *Lancet*, ii, 473–6.

Flotte, T. R., Afione, S. A., Conrad, C., McGrath, S. A., Solow, R., Oka, H., Zeitlin, P. L., Guggino, W. B. & Carter, B. J. (1993). Stable *in vivo* expression fo the cystic fibrosis transmembrane conductance regulator with an adeno-associated vector. *Proceedings of the National Academy of Sciences of the USA*, 90, 10613–17.

Foroozanfar, N., Hobbs, J. R., Hugh-Jones, K., Humble, J. G., James, C. D., Selwyn, S., Watson, J. G. & Yamamura, M. (1977). Bone marrow transplantation from an unrelated donor for chronic granulomatous disease. *Lancet*, i, 210–13.

Gansbacher, B., Zier, K., Daniels, B., Cronin K., Bannerji, R. & Gilboa, E. (1990). Interleukin 2 gene transfer into tumor cells abrogates tumorigenicity and induces protective immunity. *Journal of Experimental Medicine*, 172, 1217–24.

Golumbek, P. T., Lazenby, A. J., Levitsky, H. I., Jaffee, L. M., Karasuyama, H., Baker, M. & Pardoll, D. M. (1991). Treatment of established renal cancer by tumor cell engineered to secrete interleukin-4. *Science*, 254, 713–16.

Grossman, M., Raper, S. E., Kozarsky, K., Stein, E. A., Engelhardt, J. F., Muller, D., Lupien, P. J. & Wilson, J. M. (1994). Successful *ex vivo* gene therapy directed to liver in a patient with familial hypercholesterolemia. *Nature Genetics*, 6, 335–41.

Harrison, D. E., Astle, C. M. & Lerner, C. (1988). Number and continuous proliferative pattern of transplanted primitive immunohematopoietic stem cells. *Proceedings of the National Academy of Sciences of the USA*, 85, 822–6.

Harrison, M. R., Langer, J. C., Adzick, N. S., Golbus, M. S., Filly, R. A., Anderson, R. L., Rosen, M. A., Callen, P. W., Goldstein, R. B. & de Lorimier, A. A. (1990). Correction of congenital diaphragmatic hernia *in utero*. *Journal of Pediatric Surgery*, 25, 47–55.

Hobbs, J. R. (1988). Displacement bone marrow transplantation and immunoprophylaxis for genetic diseases. *Advances in Internal Medicine*, 33, 81–118.

Hoeben, R. C., Fallaux, F. J., Van-Tilburg, N. H., Cramer, S. J., van Ormondt, H., Briet, E. & van-der-Eb, A. J. (1993). Toward gene therapy for hemophilia A: long-term persistence of factor VIII-secreting fibroblasts after transplantation into immunodeficient mice. *Human Gene Therapy*, 4, 179–86.

Hoeben, R. C., van der Jagt, R. C. M., Schoute, F., van Tilburg, N. H., Verbeet, M. P., Briet, E., vanOrmondt, H. & van der Eb, A. J. (1990). Expression of functional factor VIII in primary human skin fibroblasts after retro-virus-mediated gene transfer. *Journal of Biological Chemistry*, 265, 7318–23.

Hoffman, E. P., Brown, R. H. & Kunkel, L. M. (1987). Dystrophin: the protein product on the Duchenne muscular dystrophy locus. *Cell*, 51, 919–28.

Hyde, S. C., Gill, D. R., Higgins, C. F., Trezise, A. E., MacVinish, L. J., Cuthbert, A. W., Ratciff, R., Evans, M. J. & Colledge, W. H. (1993). Correction of the ion transport defect in cystic fibrosis transgenic mice by gene therapy. *Nature*, 362, 250–5.

Israel, D. I. & Kaufman, R. J. (1990). Retroviral-mediated transfer and amplification of a functional human factor VIII gene. *Blood*, 1990, 1074–80.

Jiao, S., Acsadi, G., Jani, A., Felgner, P. L. & Wolff, J. A. (1992). Persistence of plasmid DNA and expression in rat brain cells *in vivo*. *Experimental Neurology*, 115, 400–13.

Kaufman, R. J., Wasley, L. C., Davies, M. V., Wise, R. J., Israel, D. I. & Dorner, A. J. (1989). Effect of von Willebrand factor coexpression on the synthesis and secretion of factor VIII in Chinese hamster ovary cells. *Molecular and Cell Biology*, 9, 1233–42.

Kay, M. A., Rothenberg, S., Landen, C. N., Bellinger, D. A., Leland, F., Toman, C., Finegold, M., Thompson, A. R., Read, M. S., Brinkhous, K. M. & Woo, S.-L. C. (1993). In vivo therapy of hemophilia B: sustained partial correction in factor IX-deficient dogs. *Science*, 262, 117–19.

Kirkpatrick, D. V., Barrios, N. J., Shapira, E. & Humbert, J. R. (1990). Treatment of enzyme storage diseases with matched and partially matched bone marrow transplantation: the Tulane marrow transplant group experience. *Blood*, 76, 548a.

Koch, K. S., Brownlee, G. G., Goss, S. J., Martinez Conde, A. & Leffert, H. L. (1991). Retroviral vector infection and transplantation in rats of primary fetal rat hepatocytes. *Journal of Cell Science*, 99, 121–30.

Koenig, M., Hoffman, E. P., Bertelson, C. J., Monaco, A. P., Feener, C. & Kunkel, L. M. (1987). Complete cloning of the Duchenne muscular dystrophy (DMD) cDNA and preliminary genomic organisation of the DMD gene in normal and affected individuals. *Cell*, 50, 509–17.

Koenig, M., Monaco, A. P. & Kunkel, L. M. (1988). The complete sequence of dystrophin predicts a rod-shaped cytoskeletal protein. *Cell*, 53, 219–28.

Kohn, D. B., Kantoff, P. W., Eglitis, M. A., McLachlin, J. R., Moen, R. C., Karson, E., Zwiebel, J. A., Nienhuis, A., Karlsson, S., O'Reilly, R., Gillid, A., Bordignon, C., Gilboa, E., Zanjani, R., Blaese, R. M. & Anderson, W. F. (1987). Retroviral-mediated gene transfer into mamalian cells. *Blood Cells*, 13, 285–98.

Krivit, W., Shapiro, E., Kennedy, W., Lipton, M. Lockman, L., Smith, S., Summers, C. G. Wenger, D.A., Tsai, M.Y. & Ramsay, N.K. (1990). Treatment of late infantile metachromatic leukodystrophy by bone marrow transplantation. *New England Journal of Medicine*, 322, 28–32.

Ledley, F. D. (1993). Prenatal application of somatic gene therapy. *Obstetrics and Gynecology Clinics of North America*, 20, 611–20.

Ledley, F. D., Darlington, G. J., Hahn, T. & Woo, S. C. (1987). Retroviral gene transfer into primary hepatocytes: implications for genetic therapy of liver specific functions. *Proceedings of the National Academy of Sciences of the USA*, 84, 5335–9.

Lin, H., Parmacek, M. S., Morle, G., Bolling, S. & Leiden, J. M. (1990). Expression of recombinant genes in myocardium *in vivo* after direct injection of DNA. *Circulation*, 82, 2217–21.

Lozier, J. N. & Brinkhous, K. M. (1994). Gene therapy and the hemophilias. *Journal of American Medical Association*, 271, 47–51.

Lozier, J. N., Palmer, T. D., Thompson, A. R., Miller, A. D., Brinkous, K. M. & High, K. A.

(1991). Production of recombinant factor IX by hollow fiber tissue culture. *Thrombosis and Haemostasis*, 65, 1158.

Lucarelli, G., Galimberti, M., Polchi, P., Giardini, C., Politi, P., Baronciani, D., Angelucci, E., Manenti, F., Delfini, C., Auereli, G. & Muretto, P. (1987). Marrow transplantation in patients with advanced thalassemia. *New England Journal of Medicine*, 316, 1050–5.

Markert, M. L., Hershfield, M. S., Schiff, R. I. & Buckley, R. H. (1987). Adenosine deaminase and purine nucleoside phosphorylase deficiency: evaluation of therapeutic interventions in eight patients. *Journal of Clinical Immunology*, 7, 389–99.

McLachlin, J. R., Cornetta, K., Eglitis, M. A. & Anderson, W. F. (1990). Retroviral-mediated gene transfer. *Progress in Nucleic Acid Research and Molecular Biology*, 38, 91–135.

Metcalf, D. & Moore, M. S. (1971). *Haemopoietic cells*. Amsterdam: North-Holland.

Miller, D. G., Adam, M. A. & Miller, A. D. (1990). Gene transfer by retrovirus vectors occurs only in cells that are actively replicating at the time of infection. *Molecular and Cellular Biology*, 10, 4239–42.

Muzyczka, N. (1991). Use of adeno-associated virus as a general transduction vector for mammalian cells. *Current Topics in Microbiology and Immunology*, 158, 97–129.

Neda, H., Wu, C. H. & Wu, G. Y. (1991). Chemical modification of an ecotropic murine leukemic virus results in redirection of its target cell specificity. *Journal of Biological Chemistry*, 266, 14143–6.

Nolta, J. A. & Kohn, D. B. (1990). Comparison of the effects of growth factors on retroviral vector-mediated gene transfer and the proliferative status of human hematopoietic progenitor cells. *Human Gene Therapy*, 1, 257–68.

Ogawa, M. (1989). Effects of hemopoietic growth factors on stem cells *in vitro*. *Hematology/Oncology Clinics of North America*, 3, 453–64.

Palmer, T. D., Thompson, A. R. & Miller, A. D. (1989). Production of human factor IX in animals by genetically modified skin fibroblasts: potential therapy for hemophilia B. *Blood*, 73, 438–45.

Pardoll, D. (1992). Immunotherapy with cytokine gene-transduced tumor cells: the next wave in gene therapy for cancer. *Current Opinion in Oncology*, 4, 1124–9.

Quantin, B., Perricaudet, L. D., Tajbakhsh, S. & Mandel, J. L. (1992). Adenovirus as an expression vector in muscle cells *in vivo*. *Proceedings of the National Academy of Sciences of the USA*, 89, 2581–4.

Ringdén, O., Groth, C.-G., Aschan, J., Bolme, P., Ljungman, P., Lönnqvist, B., Malm, G., Mansson, J. E., Shanwell, A., Svennerholm, L., Tollemar, J. & Winiarski, J. (1990). Bone marrow transplantation for metabolic disorders at Huddinge Hospital. *Transplantation Proceedings*, 22, 198–202.

Ringdén, O., Groth, C.-G., Erikson, A., Backman, L., Granqvist, S., Mansson, J. E. & Svennerholm, L. (1988). Long-term follow-up of the first successful bone marrow transplantation in Gaucher disease. *Transplantation*, 46, 66–70.

Rosenberg, S. A., Aebersold, P., Cornetta, K., Kasid, A., Morgan, R. A., Moen, R., Karson, E. M., Lotze, M. T., Yang, J. C., Topalian, S. L. (1990). Gene transfer into humans: immunotherapy of patients with advanced melanoma, using tumor-infiltrating lymphocytes modified by retroviral gene transduction. *New England Journal of Medicine*, 323, 570–8.

Rosenfeld, M. A., Siegfried, W., Yoshimura, K., Yoneyama, K., Fukayama, J., Stier, L. E., Paako, P. K., Gilardi, P., Stratford-Perricaudet, L. D., Perricaudet, M., Jallat, S., Pavirani, A., Lecoco, J.-P. & Crystal, R. G. (1991). Adenovirus-mediated transfer of a recombinant 1-antitrypsin gene to the lung epithelium *in vivo*. *Science*, 252, 431–4.

Salmons, B. & Gunzburg, W. H. (1993). Targeting of retroviral vectors for gene therapy. *Human Gene Therapy*, 4, 129–41.

Samulski, R. J., Zhu, X., Xiao, X., Brook, J. D., Housman, D. E., Epstein, N. & Hunter, L. A. (1991). Targeted integration of adeno-associated virus (AAV) into human chromosome 19. *EMBO Journal*, 10, 3941–50.

Sandberg, H., Lind, P. & Spira, J. (1991). Characteristics of a new recombinant factor VIII deriviative. *Thrombosis and Haemostasis*, 65, 942.

Sicinski, P., Geng, Y., Ryder-Cook, A. S., Barnard, E. A., Darlison, M. G. & Barnard, P. J. (1989). The molecular basis of muscular dystrophy in the mdx mouse: a point mutation. *Science*, 244, 1578–80.

Soriano, H. E., Gest, A. L., Bair, D. K., Vander-Straten, M., Lewis, D. E., Darlington, G. J., Finegold, M. J. & Ledley, F. D. (1993). Feasibility of hepatcellular transplantation via the umbilical vein in prenatal and perinatal lambs. *Fetal Diagnosis and Therapy*, 8, 293–304.

St Louis, D. & Verma, I. M. (1988). An alternative approach to somatic gene cell therapy. *Proceedings of the National Academy of Sciences of the USA*, 85, 3150–4.

Szybalska, E. H. & Szybalski, W. (1962). Genetics of human cell lines, IV: DNA-mediated heritable transformation of a biochemical trait. *Proceedings of the National Academy of Sciences of the USA*, 48, 2026–34.

Thompson, A. R. (1991). Status of gene transfer for hemophilia A and B. *Thrombosis and Haemostasis*, 66, 119–22.

Trojan, J., Blossey, B. K., Johnson, T. R., Rudin, S. D., Tykocinski, M., Ilan, J. & Ilan, J. (1992). Loss of tumorigenicity of rat glioblastoma directed by episome-based antisense cDNA transcription of insulin-like growth factor I. *Proceedings of the National Academy of Sciences of the USA*, 89, 4874–8.

Wang, C.-Y. & Huang, L. (1987). pH-sensitive immunoliposomes mediate target-cell-specific delivery and controlled expression of a foreign gene in mouse. *Proceedings of the National Academy of Sciences of the USA*, 84,7 851–5.

Williams, D. A. (1990). Expression of introduced gentic sequences in hematopoietic cells following retroviral-mediated gene transfer. *Human Gene Therapy*, 1, 229–39.

Wivel, N. A. & Walters, L. (1993). Germ-line gene modification and disease prevention: some medical and ethical perspectives. *Science*, 262, 533–8.

Wolff, J. A., Malone, R., Malone, R. W., Williams, P., Chong, W., Acsadi, G., Jani, A. & Felgner, P. L. (1990). Direct gene transfer into mouse muscle *in vivo*. *Science*, 247, 1465–8.

Wood, W. I., Capon, D. J., Simonsen, C. C., Eaton, D. L., Gitschier, J., Keyt, B., Seeburg, P. H., Smith, D. H., Hollingshead, P., Wion, K. L., Delwart, E., Tuddenham, E. D., Vehar, G. A. & Lawn, R. M. (1984). Expression of active human factor VIII from recombinant DNA clones. *Nature*, 312, 330–7.

Zabner, J., Couture, L. A., Gregory, R. J., Graham, S. M., Smith, A. E. & Welsh, M. J. (1993). Adenovirus-mediated gene transfer transiently corrects the chloride transport defect in the nasal epithelia of patients with cystic fibrosis. *Cell*, 75, 207–16.

Part five

Ethics

22 Ethics of fetal therapy

FRANK A. CHERVENAK AND
LAURENCE B. MCCULLOUGH

Introduction

Invasive and transplacental fetal therapy is increasingly able to undertake a wide array of diagnostic and therapeutic interventions and to conduct research on new interventions. As a consequence, the fetus seems just as much a patient as any other patient, save for its locale (Liley, 1972; American College of Obstetricians and Gynecologists, 1987; 1989; American Academy of Pediatrics, 1988; Harrison, Golbus & Filly, 1988). References to the fetus as a patient have become increasingly commonplace in the literature and practice of maternal fetal medicine (Mahoney, 1978; 1989; Newton, 1980; Fletcher, 1981; Pritchard, MacDonald & Gant, 1985; Walters, 1986; Murray, 1987).

The concept and language of the fetus as a patient have developed primarily as an effect of the technological advances and not as a result of careful ethical investigation of the concept of the fetus as a patient and its clinical implications. The purpose of this chapter is to set out the ethical dimensions of the concept of the fetus as patient and to identify its clinical implications for recommending and offering invasive and transplacental fetal therapy.

A précis of medical ethics

The concept of the fetus as a patient involves the language and concepts of medical ethics, because concern for protecting and promoting the interests of the patient has constituted the foundation for medical ethics since the days of the Hippocratic oath. In the oath the physician swore to do what would benefit the sick, while preventing harm to them (Edelstein, 1967). In more precise ethical terms, the Hippocratic oath should be understood as asserting beneficence-based ethical obligations to patients. Beneficence requires the physician to act in such a way as to produce a greater balance of goods over harms, as those goods and harms are understood from a clinical perspective (Beauchamp & McCullough, 1984; Beauchamp & Childress, 1989). The definition of these goods and harms has been clarified over time on the basis of what medicine as a profession can reasonably claim as its competencies. The goods that medicine is competent to achieve are the prevention of premature death, and the prevention, cure or, at least, management of disease, injury, handicap and unnecessary pain and suffering (Beauchamp & McCullough, 1984; McCullough & Chervenak, 1994). Acting on these goods provides concrete, clinically applicable meaning to the fundamental ethical obligation of protecting and promoting the interests of patients.

Beneficence-based clinical judgment and ethical obligations constituted the whole of medical ethics until the twentieth century. Under the influences of United States common law and philosophical ethics, medical ethics in the United States has increasingly come to acknowledge and emphasize the importance of the patients' perspective on their interests and what should count as protecting and promoting their interests (Faden & Beauchamp, 1986). This emphasis is not uniform around the world. Indeed, there is lively debate about the 'American' approach to medical ethics, i.e. an approach that places strong emphasis on respect for the patient's autonomy. European medical ethics, as well as medical ethics in Japan and other Pacific Rim countries, has tended to place greater emphasis on beneficence. In the

Table 22.1 *A framework for obstetric ethics*

Pregnant woman		Fetal patient	
Beneficence-based obligations of the physician	Autonomy-based obligations of the physician	Beneficence-based obligations of the physician	Beneficence-based obligations of the pregnant woman

United States, autonomy has been developed as a bulwark against physician paternalism, i.e. acting on beneficence-based obligations to the patient in violation of the patient's autonomy (Beauchamp & McCullough, 1984; Beauchamp & Childress, 1989). By contrast, European and Asian medical ethics have been more willing to allow an important clinical role for medical paternalism.

According to the principle of respect for autonomy, the pregnant patient should be presumed to be able to form her judgments about her interests on the basis of her own values and express those judgments in value-based preferences. The ethical principle of respect for autonomy translates this fact into autonomy-based ethical obligations of the physician in clinical practice. Respect for autonomy requires the physician to acknowledge the integrity of the patient's values in her life, to ascertain the patient's value-based preferences and to assist the patient to put her preference into effect. Respect for autonomy is thus put into clinical practice by the informed consent process. This process is usually understood to have three elements: (i) disclosure by the physician to the patient of adequate information about the patient's condition and its management; (ii) understanding of that information by the patient; and (iii) a voluntary decision by the patient to authorize or refuse clinical management (Faden & Beauchamp, 1986).

The concepts of autonomy-based clinical judgment and ethical obligations and of beneficence-based clinical judgment and ethical obligations provide a framework for obstetric ethics in terms of which the concept of the fetus as a patient can be articulated and its clinical implications identified (Chervenak & McCullough, 1985) (Table 22.1).

The fetus as a patient

A prominent approach in the medical ethics' literature to understanding the concept of the fetus as a patient has involved attempts to establish whether or not the fetus has independent moral status (Hellegers, 1970; Noonan, 1970; Ruddick & Wilcox, 1982; Dunstan, 1984; Engelhardt, 1986; Curran, 1987; Elias & Annas, 1987; Fleming, 1987; Strong, 1987; Anderson & Strong, 1988; Evans *et al.*, 1988; Ford, 1988; Strong & Anderson, 1989). Independent moral status for the fetus means that one or more characteristics that the fetus possesses in and of itself, and, therefore, independently of the pregnant woman or any other factor, generate and, therefore, ground obligations to the fetus on the part of the pregnant woman and her physician.

There are three main views about when the fetus does or does not acquire independent moral status. One view is that the fetus possesses independent moral status from the moment of conception or implantation (Noonan, 1979; Bopp, 1984; 1985). Another view is that the fetus acquires independent moral status in degrees, thus resulting in 'graded' moral status (Dunstan, 1984; Evans *et al.*, 1988). A third view, usually held implicitly, is that the fetus never has independent moral status so long as it is *in utero* (Elias & Annas, 1987).

Despite an enormous philosophical and theological literature on this subject, there has been no agreement on a single authoritative account of the independent moral status of the fetus (*Roe* v. *Wade*, 1973; Callahan & Callahan, 1984). This function is an outcome of the intellectual fact there is no single methodology that is authoritative for all of the markedly diverse theological and philosophical schools of thought involved in this centuries-old debate. Without such an authoritative methodology, agreement on the independent moral status of the fetus is impossible. For agreement ever to be possible, deep disagreements about such a final authority within and between theological and philosophical traditions would have to be resolved in a way satisfactory to all. This is an inconceivable event. It is best, therefore, to set aside futile attempts to understand the fetus as a patient in terms of whether or not the fetus possesses independent moral status and whether or not there are autonomy-based obligations to the fetus and turn to an alternative approach. This alternative approach makes it possible to identify ethically distinct senses of the fetus as a patient and their clinical implications. Thus, the framework to obstetric ethics in this chapter makes reference to autonomy-based obligations to the fetus (Table 22.1).

This alternative approach starts with the claim that being a patient does not require that one possesses independent moral status (Ruddick & Wilcox, 1982). Instead, being a patient means that one can benefit from the application of the clinical skills of the physician. Put more precisely, a human being without independent moral status is properly regarded as a patient when two conditions are met: (i) that a human being is presented to the physician, and (ii) the presentation is for the purpose of applying clinical interventions that are reliably expected to be efficacious, in that they are reliably expected to result in a greater balance of goods over harms in the future of the human being in question. In other words, someone is a patient when a physician has beneficence-based ethical obligations to that individual (Chervenak & McCullough, 1985; 1990b; McCullough & Chervenak, 1994). To clarify the concept of the fetus as patient, it is, therefore, appropriate to turn to an account of when there are beneficence-based obligations to the fetus.

This clarification builds on the argument that beneficence-based obligations to the fetus exist when the fetus can become a child with independent moral status (Chervenak & McCullough, 1985; 1990b; McCullough & Chervenak, 1994). That is, the fetus is a patient when medical interventions reasonably can be expected to result in a greater balance of goods over harms for the child the fetus can become. When the fetus is a patient, both the physician and the pregnant woman have beneficence-based obligations to it (Table 22.1). They are the moral fiduciaries of the patient, i.e. they are expected to act primarily to protect and promote the

Table 22.2 *The fetus as a patient*

Viable fetus	Previable fetus
Patienthood status is a function of the biological and technological capacity to become a child with independent moral status	Patienthood status is a function of the pregnant woman's autonomy to take the pregnancy to viability

interests of the fetal patient (McCullough & Chervenak, 1994). Those interests are defined by beneficence-based clinical judgment and the woman's judgment about the fetus' interests. This beneficence-based approach to the concept of the fetus as a patient is not distinctively 'American,' because beneficence is an internationally accepted medical ethical principle.

The viable fetus as a patient

The ethical significance of the concept of the fetus as patient, therefore, depends on links that can be established between the fetus and the child it can become and not on the alleged, and always disputable, independent moral status of the fetus (Table 22.2). One such link is viability. Viability establishes a basis for the first ethical sense of the fetus as a patient. Viability must be understood in terms of both biological and technological factors (*Roe* v. *Wade*, 1973; Fast, Chudwin & Wikler, 1980; Mahowald, 1989). Both factors are required for a viable fetus to exist *ex utero* and become a child with independent moral status (McCullough & Chervenak, 1994). These two factors do not exist as a function of the autonomy of the pregnant woman. When a fetus is viable, i.e. when it is of sufficient maturity so that it can survive into the neonatal period and become a child with independent moral status, even if it requires technological support, the fetus is a patient (McCullough & Chervenak, 1994). Beneficence-based obligations to the viable fetus must, of course, be considered together with beneficence-based and autonomy-based obligations to the pregnant woman (Chervenak & McCullough, 1985; McCullough & Chervenak, 1994).

The previable fetus as a patient

The only possible link between the previable fetus and the child it can become is the pregnant woman's autonomy. This provides the sole basis for the second ethical sense of the fetus as a patient. Technological factors cannot result in the previable fetus becoming a child, because this is what previable means. A link, therefore, between a previable fetus and the child it can become can be established only by the pregnant woman's decision to confer the status of being a patient on her previable fetus. The previable fetus, because it cannot reliably be thought to possess independent moral status, has no claim to the status of being a patient independently of the pregnant woman's autonomy. It follows that the previable fetus is a patient solely as a function of the pregnant woman's autonomy to take the pregnancy to viability, at which time the fetus becomes a patient independently of the pregnant woman's autonomy (McCullough & Chervenak, 1994).

It is important to appreciate that the second sense of the fetus as patient includes *in vitro* embryos. It might seem that the *in vitro* embryo is a patient because such an embryo is presented to the physician. However, simply being presented to a physician does not make the *in vitro* embryo a patient. This is because, in terms of beneficence, whether the fetus is a patient depends as well on links that can be established between the fetus and its future, i.e. the child with independent moral status it can become. Therefore, the reasonableness of medical interventions on the *in vitro* embryo turns on whether that embryo later becomes viable. Otherwise, no benefit of such intervention can meaningfully be said to result. An *in vitro* embryo, therefore, becomes viable only when it survives *in vitro* cell division, transfer, implantation and subsequent gestation to such a time as it becomes viable.

This process of achieving viability occurs *in vivo* and is, therefore, entirely dependent on the woman's decision regarding the status of the fetus(es) as a patient, should assisted conception successfully result in the gestation of the previable fetus(es). Whether an *in vitro* embryo will become a viable fetus and whether medical intervention on such an embryo will benefit the fetus are both functions of the pregnant woman's autonomy. It, therefore, is appropriate to regard the *in vitro* embryo as a previable fetus rather than as a viable fetus. As a consequence, any *in vitro* embryo(s) should be regarded as a patient only when the woman into whose reproductive tract the embryo(s) will be transferred confers that status (McCullough & Chervenak, 1994). Whether the *in vitro* embryo is a patient is, therefore, not a function of the sperm donor's autonomy. The woman is free to confer with the sperm donor as she chooses.

In summary, the viable fetus is a patient. The previable fetus, including the *in vitro* embryo, is a patient solely as a function of the exercise of the woman's autonomy.

An ethical standard of care for invasive and transplacental therapy

Whether fetal therapy can be judged to be standard of care on ethical grounds depends on the clinical implications of the concept of the fetus as a patient. Such fetal therapy must reliably be thought, on the basis of documented clinical experience, to benefit the child that the fetus can become. Recall that the ethical content of this concept is to be understood not simply in terms of physical accessibility but also in terms of whether clinical interventions on the fetus are reliably thought to be efficacious, in that they are reliably expected to result in a greater balance of goods over harms for the child the fetus can reliably be expected to become.

Satisfying this condition establishes standard of care in its initial, beneficence-based sense. This ethical concept of standard of care, however, cannot be completely understood until its autonomy-based dimensions are considered.

The pregnant woman is under no ethical obligation to confer the status of being a patient on her previable fetus simply because there exists a fetal therapy that meets the preceding beneficence-based condition. Whether such therapy is, on ethical grounds, to be judged standard of care for her fetus is entirely a function of the pregnant woman's autonomy. That is, satisfying both beneficence-based and autonomy-based conditions are necessary for fetal therapy to be reliably judged to be the ethical standard of care for previable fetuses on ethical grounds.

The same is true for fetal therapy on the viable fetus. Such a fetus is properly judged to be a patient. However, as noted above, beneficence-based obligations to the fetus must be negotiated with beneficence-based and autonomy-based obligations to the pregnant woman. This is because of a factual consideration; fetal therapy necessarily involves physical, and perhaps mental, health risks to the pregnant woman, and an ethical consideration is that she is ethically obligated only to accept reasonable risks to herself in order to attempt to benefit her fetus (Chervenak & McCullough, 1985; McCullough & Chervenak, 1994).

The above helps to distinguish an ethical from a legal standard of care for fetal therapy. An ethical standard must take account not only of beneficence-based considerations applied to the fetus but also of both beneficence-based and autonomy-based considerations applied to the pregnant woman. A legal standard of care tends to focus on efficacy and safety, which are beneficence-based considerations applied to both the fetus and, perhaps, the pregnant woman. A legal standard of care tends to ignore autonomy-based considerations applied to the pregnant woman. This constitutes the fundamental difference between a legal and an ethical standard of care for fetal therapy.

Given what is at stake in fetal therapy, physicians understandably may have concerns about risks of litigation. The law in each country differs in its state of development and clinical sophistication in the area of fetal therapy. Developing law is usefully informed by ethical analysis and argument of the sort advanced in this chapter. The physician concerned about litigation should obtain appropriate legal consultation and inquire as to whether the ethical framework of this chapter is applicable in the relevant jurisdiction. In any case, practising medicine on the basis of rigorous clinical ethical judgment should be the physician's primary goal, not the avoidance of litigation. Failure to maintain this priority risks the integrity of the medical profession.

Recommending and offering therapy for the viable fetus

Fetal therapy should be recommended when the intervention will benefit the fetus and the risks of the intervention are those the pregnant woman ought to accept. The authors caution that there is no simple algorithm by which a pregnant woman or her physician can conclude that she is obligated to accept risk to herself on behalf of her viable fetus. In the authors' view, such an ethical obligation, which should *not* be automatically equated with a legal obligation, exists when three criteria are satisfied: (i) when invasive therapy of the viable fetus is reliably judged to have a very high probability of being life saving or of preventing serious and irreversible disease, injury, or handicap for the fetus and for the child the fetus can become; (ii) when such therapy is reliably judged to involve low mortality risk and low or manageable risk of serious disease, injury or handicap to the viable fetus and the child it can become; and (iii) when the mortality risk to the pregnant woman is reliably judged to be very low, and when the risk of disease, injury or handicap to the pregnant woman is reliably judged to be low or manageable (Chervenak & McCullough, 1991b; McCullough & Chervenak, 1994).

The justifications for these criteria are both beneficence based and autonomy based. When the first two criteria are satisfied, there is expected to be a clear and substantial net benefit to the viable fetus and the child it can become. When the third criterion is satisfied there is expected to be no clear and substantial net harm to the pregnant woman. Given the expected net benefit to the viable fetus and the low risk of harm to the pregnant woman, the latter are risks she should reasonably be expected to accept (McCullough & Chervenak, 1994), for example, as in intravascular transfusion for severe alloimmunization. This moral fact shapes how she should exercise her autonomy in response to her beneficence-based fiduciary ethical obligations to her fetus (Chervenak & McCullough, 1990b; McCullough & Chervenak, 1994).

Under beneficence-based and autonomy-based clinical judgment, therefore, recommending treatment of the viable fetus is ethically justified when these three criteria are satisfied. The burden of ethical proof rests with those who would propose recommending intervention when one or more of these three criteria cannot be satisfied. This should be a matter of further careful investigation and debate in the ethics of fetal therapy.

Forms of fetal therapy for which an ethical obligation, as defined above, on the part of the pregnant woman to accept them cannot be established should be regarded as experimental. For example, because open abdominal fetal surgery involves risks that no pregnant woman can be understood, at this time, to be *obligated* to accept in an attempt to benefit her viable fetus, all such surgery must, on ethical grounds, be regarded as experimental. There is no ethical justification for recommending this experimental fetal therapy because none of the three conditions above is satisfied.

How should the physician respond if the pregnant woman rejects a recommendation of fetal therapy for a viable fetus that satisfies an ethically justified standard of care? Certainly, informed consent as an ongoing dialogue with the pregnant woman should be the first response. In undertaking a further response, negotiation, the physician should acknowledge and take into account the pregnant woman's assessment of the risks and benefits of invasive fetal therapy to herself and her fetus. It is justified to go beyond negotiation to respectful persuasion, and perhaps even to an ethics committee, as part of a preventive ethics clinical strategy (Chervenak & McCullough, 1990a; McCullough & Chervenak, 1994).

Investigational invasive fetal therapy should be scientifically sound and meet ethical and legal requirements for research with human subjects. These legal requirements vary internationally, but the clear trend is to require review and approval by an institutional review board. To proceed in the absence of such review not only risks disrespect for the pregnant woman and grave risk to the fetus, but loss of scientific rigour as well. Therefore, to proceed with experimental therapy without appropriate institutional review is not ethically justified. So called 'innovative' therapy is subject to the same stringent ethical requirement. Notwithstanding this, institutional review boards are not common outside the United States where ethics committees confine their activity to investigational research protocols.

Experimental therapy, that is, situations in which one or more of the above mentioned criteria are not satisfied, of the viable fetus can justifiably be *offered* to the pregnant woman, only with the approval of an institutional review board. The ethical justification for doing so rests on the three criteria for ethical standard of care defined above. By definition, if the first two criteria are not satisfied, there is no net fetal benefit and, therefore, there is no beneficence-based obligation to the fetus to offer experimental therapy. If the third criterion is not met, even if the first two are, there is only net harm to the pregnant patient and no beneficence-based obligation to her to offer experimental fetal therapy.

The principal justification for offering fetal therapy that does not meet the three criteria is twofold: (i) to benefit future patients, and (ii) to enhance the pregnant woman's autonomy by expanding the range of her options. The first part of this justification appeals to a beneficence-based obligation to provide quality medical care to future fetal patients. This two-part justification must be made clear to the pregnant woman as part of the informed consent process, so she does not subscribe to the mistaken belief that experimental fetal interventions will benefit her fetus or herself. When there are well-developed clinical trials that are requesting referrals from one's geographical area, the authors believe that there is an obligation to offer the opportunity for enrollment as a research subject, again only on the justification that research benefits future patients, that the woman's autonomy will be enhanced and that approval is granted by the appropriate institutional review board.

In cases in which the first two criteria are satisfied but the third is not, intervention should be regarded as experimental and only offered, not recommended, to the pregnant woman. This is because respect for her autonomy requires that she be accorded the opportunity to decide for herself whether the unavoidable risk of serious harm to her is warranted for the sake of possibly benefitting the fetus and the child it can become. Medicine has no competence to make this judgement. Therefore, a pregnant woman's refusal to enroll as a subject in experimental fetal therapy should always be respected and she should be assured her subsequent care will not be affected by her refusal.

Recommending and offering therapy for the previable fetus

There are two subgroups of previable fetuses. The first comprises those upon whom the pregnant woman has conferred the status of being a patient. When she has done so and the above mentioned ethical criteria are also satisfied, it is ethically justified to recommend fetal therapy. This situation is directly analogous to informed consent to therapy for the viable fetus and the strategies discussed above apply.

When the pregnant woman withholds or withdraws the status of being a patient from her previable fetus, the situation is directly analogous to experimental fetal therapy. This is so because there is no ethical obligation on the part of the pregnant woman or the physician to regard the previable fetus as a patient. It follows that any discussion of experimental fetal intervention must be strictly non-directive, which is consistent with offering but not with recommending enrollment as a research subject in a clinical investigation trial (Chervenak & McCullough, 1991a; McCullough & Chervenak, 1994).

Multifetal pregnancy reduction

Multifetal pregnancy reduction (MPR) has recently emerged as an effective and commonly employed management option for multiple gestations (Dumez & Oury, 1986; Berkowitz et al., 1988; Evans et al., 1988; 1990; 1991; Golbus et al., 1988; Hobbins, 1988; Overall, 1990; Zaner, Boetin & Hill, 1990; American College of Obstetricians and Gynecologists, 1991; Wapner et al., 1991; Chervenak, McCullough & Wapner, 1992). The framework for obstetrical ethics developed in this chapter can be effectively applied to this topic. We do so to illustrate the clinical utility of this framework. The approach illustrated here can be adapted readily, the authors believe, to the other controversial clinical topics addressed in this book.

Evans et al. (1988), in a landmark article, first addressed the ethical implications of MPR. There is widespread agreement to support their general view that MPR of high order, four or more, to twins or selective termination of an anomalous fetus should be an option for the pregnant woman (Dumez & Oury, 1986; Berkowitz et al., 1988; Evans et al., 1988; 1990; 1991; Golbus, et al., 1988; Hobbins, 1988; Overall, 1990; Zaner, Boetin & Hill, 1990; American College of Obstetricians and Gynecologists, 1991; Wapner et al., 1991, Chervenak et al., 1992). Ethical debate centres on the justification of MPR to a singleton either from a multiple gestation of high order or from a triplet or even twin pregnancy when a woman requests this procedure.

Recently reported data suggest that MPR of high-order pregnancies is regarded as ethically acceptable, but that this is not the case for twin and triplet pregnancies (Evans et al., 1991). By themselves, such data are not decisive ethically, because they *describe* moral views about MPR to a singleton, they do not *justify* such views.

That is, descriptive ethics cannot perform the task of normative ethics. That task involves arguments.

Arguments have been made in the literature to oppose MPR to a singleton (Evans et al., 1988; 1991; Zaner et al., 1990). The purpose of this section of the chapter is to show how these arguments fail and that MPR to a singleton is ethically justifiable when a woman requests this procedure and, therefore, it should be an option for pregnant women with multiple gestations, whether they are of high order or triplets or twins (Chervenak et al., 1992).

Evans et al. (1988) have made an important argument against MPR to a singleton. They base their argument on the principle of proportionality. As they put it, 'Proportionality is the source of the duty, when taking actions involving risks of harm, to balance risks and benefits so that actions have the greatest chance to cause the least harm and the most benefit to persons directly involved' (Evans et al., 1988). They clearly intend to include the human fetus, or, at least the fetus without anomalies, in the category of persons. This is because they take the view that the fetus possesses what they call, 'graded moral status' (Evans et al., 1988).

This argument is based on questionable assumptions. One is that they assume but do not argue that the fetus is a person. This assumption is hotly contested in the literature on abortion and, therefore, should be defended. Evans et al. (1988) nowhere argue against views, such as Engelhardt's (1986), that it is incoherent to treat the fetus as a person.

In their defence, one might say that the fetus is only to some degree a person in virtue of its graded, not full, moral status. This claim, however, is based on a further questionable assumption, namely that the fetus possesses independent moral status to at least some degree. Claims about the independent moral status of the fetus necessarily involve the further claim that some characteristic of the fetus that it possesses in and of itself, and independent of the pregnant woman or any other factor, grounds obligations to the fetus on the part of the pregnant woman and her physician. Among these obligations, on the principle of proportionality, would be the prevention of unnecessary death. In particular, independent moral status means that reducing a multiple pregnancy to a singleton is not justified unless there is some overwhelming reason. Since mortality risks for a twin pregnancy do not greatly exceed those for a singleton pregnancy, Evans *et al.* (1988) conclude that no such reason exists. Hence, MPR to a singleton, they conclude, is ethically unjustifiable. Recently, they have modified their opposition to MPR to a singleton (Fletcher & Evans, 1987; Evans *et al.*, 1993).

The problem with this argument is that any claim that the fetus possesses independent moral status, whether graded or not, is made against a background of the striking inability to reach closure on a single authoritative account of the independent moral status of the fetus in the history of either philosophical or theological ethics, which we described earlier in this chapter. For closure on such an account ever to be possible, a single, universally accepted methodological authority for philosophical and/or theological traditions would have to be irrefutably established. Evans *et al.* (1988) offer an argument that in effect presumes that this inconceivable event has occurred and, so, their argument does not succeed.

Zaner *et al.* (1990) basically support the position of Evans *et al.* (1988) and they add the argument that a woman who undergoes ovulation induction 'is desirous of becoming pregnant and would incur an increased risk of aborting both fetuses of a twin gestation by selective termination'. Any objection to taking such a risk assumes some degree of independent moral status of the fetus, an assumption that, as we have shown above, cannot be sustained. Alternatively, the argument of Zaner *et al.* (1990) implicitly assumes that beneficence-based ethical judgment is the sole basis for analysing the ethical issues involved. That is, they assume that availing herself of assisted reproduction techniques means that the pregnant woman has irrevocably conferred the status of being a patient on at least two of the fetuses in a multiple gestation.

The fundamental problem with this assumption is that its adherents misunderstand the concept of the fetus as a patient and the relationship between that concept and the autonomy of the pregnant woman. We pointed out above that any attempt to understand the moral status as a fetus in terms of its independent moral status of the fetus is bound to fail. We, therefore, take the only alternative approach, one that is based on the recognition that being a patient does not require that one possess independent moral status (Ruddick & Wilcox, 1982).

MPR involves previable fetuses and the only link between the previable fetus and the child it can become is the pregnant woman's autonomy. This is because, unlike the case of viable fetuses, there are no factors, e.g. technological factors, that can result in the previable fetus becoming a child. The link between a previable fetus and the child it can become, therefore, can be established *only* by the decision of the pregnant woman to confer the status of being a patient on her previable fetus. Because independent moral status of the fetus cannot be reliably established, the previable fetus has no independent claim to the status of being a patient and, therefore, to being a factor in beneficence-based clinical judgment independently of the pregnant woman's autonomy. That is, a pregnant woman is free to withhold, confer or, having once conferred, withdraw the status of being a patient on or from the previable fetus according to her own values and beliefs. Overall has recently provided a useful account of the sort of considerations that women might find relevant in making such a decision (Overall, 1990). The previable fetus is presented to the physician as a potential beneficiary of obstetric management solely as a function of the pregnant woman's autonomy. Beneficence-based clinical judgments about what is in the fetus's interest, therefore, come into play only *after* the woman confers the status of being a patient on the fetus(es) that she intends to take to term.

In contrast, Evans *et al.* (1988) assume that the previable fetus can have moral status independently of the pregnant woman's autonomy. Zaner *et al.* (1990) assume that once the moral status of being a patient is conferred by the pregnant woman on a previable fetus she is not free to withdraw such status. Both assumptions, we have now shown, are unfounded. The general lesson is that the ethics of invasive and transplacental fetal therapy should never be based on the assumption that the fetus at any stage of its development possesses independent moral status. Rather, ethical issues should be framed in terms of whether there are beneficence-based obligations to a fetal patient.

The pregnant woman does confer the status of being a patient on the fetus that survives MPR to the singleton that she intends to take to term. As a consequence, there are beneficence-based obligations on her part and her physician's part to the singleton fetus to avoid significant harm that might result from the MPR. The medical facts never supported the clinical judgment that harm would occur with high probability. In the case of MPR of twins to a singleton, a randomized clinical trial would be necessary to assess clearly whether the survivor would fare slightly better or slightly worse than twins without intervention. Given that the alternative to MPR of twin gestation is often complete termination, any minor risk of harm of the procedure becomes moot under beneficence-based judgment when balanced against 100% mortality. Hence, there are no beneficence-based obligations to the surviving singleton fetus not to reduce the pregnancy to a singleton.

Evans *et al.* (1988) also consider the benefits and burdens of MPR to parents, including the benefits of having one child versus having two. Medicine possesses no competence to reach a beneficence-based judgment about whether it is better for prospective parents to have two children rather than just one child resulting from a pregnancy. There are, therefore, no grounds for including such a benefit in a beneficence-based calculus. Such matters are solely a function of the autonomy of the prospective parents and, therefore, in this area autonomy-based obligations of the physician are decisive.

Nothing in what we have argued obliges the physician in all cases to carry out the request of a pregnant woman for MPR of her pregnancy to a singleton. No patient has a positive right to oblige a physician to act in a way that violates his or her individual private conscience, i.e.,those moral convictions and beliefs that he or she possesses independently of being a physician (Chervenak & McCullough, 1985; 1990a). At the same time, it is not justified to impose one's individual private conscience on the pregnant woman or to base claims of professional ethics on private conscience.

The implications of our argument for clinical practice are the following. Since MPR of a multifetal pregnancy of any order to a singleton is ethically justifiable, a pregnant woman's request for MPR to a singleton either from twins or a higher order multiple gestation should be respected and implemented. Physicians who object to MPR to a singleton in private conscience should not feel compelled to perform the procedure but are obligated to make an appropriate referral (Chervenak *et al.*, 1992).

Conclusion

Clinical ethical judgment and decision making about invasive and transplacental fetal therapy are complex matters. Despite their complexity, these matters are conceptually and clinically manageable with the contribution of the concepts and language of medical ethics. These clarify obligations owed to the pregnant woman and to the fetal patient and when the fetus is a patient. They also provide the basis for identification when it is appropriate to recommend and offer fetal therapy for the viable and previable fetus. Finally, they can be applied clinically to such matters as multifetal pregnancy reduction. As experience with the topics addressed in this book grows, the concepts and language of medical ethics will be an essential dimension of the developing field of invasive and transplacental fetal therapy.

References

American Academy of Pediatrics, Committee on Bioethics (1988). Fetal therapy: ethical considerations. *Pediatrics*, 81, 898–9.

American College of Obstetricians and Gynecologists. Committee on Ethics (1987). *Patient Choice: Maternal–fetal Conflict.* Washington DC: American College of Obstetricians and Gynecologists.

American College of Obstetricians and Gynecologists. Technical Bulletin (1989). *Ethical Decision-Making in Obstetrics and Gynecology.* Washington DC: American College of Obstetricians and Gynecologists.

American College of Obstetricians and Gynecologists (1991). *Multifetal Pregnancy Reduction and Selective Fetal Termination.* Washington, DC: American College of Obstetricians and Gynecologists.

Anderson, G. & Strong, C. (1988). The premature breech: Caesarean section or trial of labour? *Journal of Medical Ethics*, 14, 18–24.

Beauchamp, T. L., & Childress, J. F. (1989). *Principles of Biomedical Ethics*, 3rd edn. New York: Oxford University Press.

Beauchamp, T. L. & McCullough, L. B. (1984). *Medical Ethics: The Moral Responsibilities of Physicians*. Norwalk, NJ: Englewood Cliffs.

Berkowitz, R. L., Lynch L., Chitkara U., Wilkins, I. A., Mehalek, K. E. & Alvarez, E. (1988). Selective reduction of multifetal pregnancies in the first trimester. *New England Journal of Medicine*, 318, 1043–7.

Bopp, J. R. (ed.) (1984). *Restoring the Right to Life: The Human Life Amendment*. Provo: Brigham Young University Press.

Bopp, J. R. (ed.) (1985). *Human Life and Health Care Ethics*. Frederick: University Publications of America.

Callahan, S. & Callahan, D. (eds.). (1984). *Abortion: Understanding Differences*. New York: Plenum Press.

Chervenak, F. A. & McCullough, L. B. (1985). Perinatal ethics: a practical method of analysis of obligations to mother and fetus. *Obstetrics and Gynecology*, 66, 442–6.

Chervenak, F. A. & McCullough, L. B. (1990a). Does obstetric ethics have any role in the obstetrician's response to the abortion controversy? *American Journal of Obstetrics and Gynecology*, 163, 1425.

Chervenak, F. A. & McCullough, L. B. (1990b). Clinical guides to preventing ethical conflicts between pregnant women and their physicians. *American Journal of Obstetrics and Gynecology*, 162, 303–7.

Chervenak, F. A. & McCullough, L. B. (1991a). The fetus as patient: implications for directive versus nondirective counseling for fetal benefit. *Fetal Diagnosis and Therapy*, 6, 93–100.

Chervenak, F.A. & McCullough, L.B. (1991b). An ethically based standard of care for fetal therapy. *Journal of Maternal–Fetal Investigation*, 1, 185–90.

Chervenak, F. A., McCullough L. B. & Wapner, R. J. (1992). Selective termination to a singleton pregnancy is ethically justified. *Ultrasound in Obstetrics and Gynecology*, 2, 84–7.

Curran, C.E. (1978). Abortion: contemporary debate in philosophical and religious ethics. In *Encyclopedia of Bioethics*, 1st edn, ed. W. T. Reich, pp. 1–32. New York: Macmillan.

Dumez, Y. & Oury, J. F. (1986). Method for first trimester selective abortion in multiple pregnancy. *Contributions to Gynecology and Obstetrics*, 15, 50–3.

Dunstan, G .R. (1984). The moral status of the human embryo: a tradition recalled. *Journal of Medical Ethics*, 10, 38–44.

Edelstein, L. (1967). The Hippocratic oath: text, translation, and interpretation. In *Ancient Medicine: Selected Papers of Ludwig Edelstein*, ed. O. Temkin & C. L. Temkin, pp. 6–63. Baltimore, MD: The Johns Hopkins Press.

Elias, S. & Annas, G. J. (1987). *Reproductive Genetics and the Law*. Chicago, II: Year Book Medical Publishers.

Engelhardt, H. T., Jr (1986). *The Foundations of Bioethics*. New York: Oxford University Press.

Evans, M. I., Dommergues, M., Wapner, R. J. *et al.* (1993). Efficacy of multifetal pregnancy reduction: collaborative experience of the world's largest centres. *Obstetrics and Gynecology*, 82, 61–6.

Evans, M. I., Drugan, A., Bottoms, S. F. *et al.* (1991). Attitudes on the ethics of abortion, sex selection, and selective pregnancy termination among health care professionals, ethicists, and clergy likely to encounter such situation. *American Journal of Obstetrics and Gynecology*, 164, 1092–9.

Evans, M. I., Fletcher, J. C., Zador, I. E., Newton, B. W., Quigg, M. H. & Struyk, C. D. (1988). Selective first-trimester termination in octuplet and quadruplet pregnancies: clinical and ethical issues. *Obstetrics and Gynecology*, 71, 289–96.

Faden, R. R. & Beauchamp, T. L. (1986). *A History and Theory of Informed Consent*. New York: Oxford University Press.

Fleming, L. (1987). The moral status of the foetus: a reappraisal. *Bioethics*, 1, 15–34.

Fletcher, J. C. (1981). The fetus as patient: ethical issues (editorial). *Journal of the American Medical Association*, 246, 772–3.

Fletcher, J. C. & Evans, M. I. (1992). Ethics in reproductive genetics. *Clinical Obstetrics and Gynecology*, 35, 763–82.

Ford, N. M. (1988). When Did I Begin? *Conception of the Human Individual in History, Philosophy and Science*. Cambridge: Cambridge University Press.

Fost, N., Chudwin, D. & Wikler, D. (1980). The limited moral significance of fetal viability. *Hastings Centre Report*, 10, 10–13.

Golbus, M. S., Cunningham, N., Goldberg, J. D., Anderson, R., Filly, R. & Callen, P. (1988). Selective termination of multiple gestations. *American Journal of Medical Genetics*, 31, 339–48.

Harrison, M. R., Golbus, M. S. & Filly, R. A. (eds.) (1990). *The Unborn Patient: Prenatal Diagnosis and Treatment*, 2nd edn. New York: Grune & Stratton.

Hellegers, A. E. (1970). Fetal Development. *Theological Studies*, 31, 3–9.

Hobbins, J. C. (1988). Selective reduction – a perinatal necessity? *New England Journal of Medicine*, 318, 1062–3.

Liley, A. W. (1972). The foetus as a personality. *Australian and New Zealand Journal of Psychiatry*, 6, 99–105.

Mahoney, M. J. (1978). Fetal–maternal relationship. In *Encyclopedia of Bioethics*, ed. W. T. Reich. New York: Macmillan.

Mahoney, M. J. (1989). The fetus as patient. *Western Journal of Medicine*, 150, 459–60.

Mahowald, M. (1989). Beyond abortion: refusal of caesarean section. *Bioethics*, 3, 106–21.

McCullough, L. B. & Chervenak, F. A. (1994). *Ethics in Obstetrics and Gynecology*. New York: Oxford University Press.

Murray, T.H. (1987). Moral obligations to the not-yet born: the fetus as patient. *Clinics in Perinatology*, 14, 313–28.

Newton, E. R. (1989). The fetus as patient. *Medical Clinics of North America*, 73, 517–40.

Noonan, J. T. (ed.) (1970). *The Morality of Abortion: Legal and Historial Perspectives*. Cambridge, MA: Harvard University Press.

Noonan, J. T. (1979). *A Private Choice: Abortion in America in the Seventies*. New York: The Free Press.

Overall, C. (1990). Selective termination of pregnancy and women's reproductive autonomy. *Hastings Centre Report*, 20, 6–11.

Pritchard, J. A., MacDonald, P. C. & Gant, N. F. (1985). *Williams' Obstetrics*, 17th edn. Norwalk, NJ: Appleton-Century-Crofts.

Roe v. *Wade*, 410 US 113 (1973).

Ruddick, W. & Wilcox, W. (1982). Operating on the fetus. *Hastings Centre Report*, 12, 10–14.

Strong, C. (1987). Ethical conflicts between mother and fetus in obstetrics. *Clinics in Perinatology*, 14, 313–28.

Strong, C. & Anderson, G. (1989). The moral status of the near-term fetus. *Journal of Medical Ethics*, 15, 25–7.

Walters, L. (1986). Ethical issues in intrauterine diagnosis and therapy. *Fetal Therapy*, 1, 32–7.

Wapner, R.J., Davis, G.H., Johnson, A. *et al.* (1990). Selective reduction of multifetal pregnancies. *Lancet*, 335, 90–3.

Zaner, R. M., Boehm, F. H. & Hill, G. A. (1990). Selective termination in multiple pregnancies: ethical considerations. *Fertility and Sterility*, 54, 203–5.

Index